PLAUT

ADVANCES IN THE BIOSCIENCES

Volume 51

FRONTIERS IN HISTAMINE RESEARCH

ADVANCES IN THE BIOSCIENCES

Latest volumes in the series:

Volume 39: PSYCHOBIOLOGY OF SCHIZOPHRENIA
Editors: M. Namba and H. Kaiya

Volume 40: NEW VISTAS IN DEPRESSION
Editors: S. Z. Langer, R. Takahashi, T. Segawa and M. Briley

Volume 41: TOWARD CHRONOPHARMACOLOGY
Editors: R. Takahashi, F. Halberg and C. A. Walker

Volume 42: BIOLOGICAL AND PSYCHOLOGICAL BASIS OF PSYCHOSOMATIC DISEASE
Editors: H. Ursin and R. Murison

Volume 43: STROKE: ANIMAL MODELS
Editor: V. Stefanovich

Volume 44: RECEPTORS AS SUPRAMOLECULAR ENTITIES
Editors: G. Biggio, E. Costa, G. L. Gessa and P. F. Spano

Volume 45: MICROWAVE FIXATION OF LABILE METABOLITES
Editors: C. L. Blank, W. B. Stavinoha and Y. Maruyama

Volume 46: NEUROBEHAVIORAL METHODS IN OCCUPATIONAL HEALTH
Editors: R. Gilioli, M. G. Cassitto and V. Foà

Volume 47: ADVANCED CONCEPTS IN ALCOHOLISM
Editor: H.-G. Tittmar

Volume 48: NEUROMODULATION AND BRAIN FUNCTION
Editors: G. Biggio, P. F. Spano, G. Toffano and G. L. Gessa

Volume 49: PSYCHOLOGICAL ASPECTS OF CANCER
Editors: M. Watson and T. Morris

Volume 50: PATHOPHYSIOLOGICAL ASPECTS OF CANCER EPIDEMIOLOGY
Editors: G. Mathé and P. Reizenstein

Volume 51: FRONTIERS IN HISTAMINE RESEARCH
Editors: C. R. Ganellin and J. C. Schwartz

Volume 52: ORO-FACIAL PAIN AND NEUROMUSCULAR DYSFUNCTION
Editors: I. Klineberg and B. Sessle

Volume 53: THE PINEAL GLAND AND ITS ENDOCRINE
Editors: M. Brown and S. D. Wainwright

NOTICE TO READERS

Dear Reader

An Invitation to Publish in and Recommend the Placing of a Standing Order to Volumes Published in this Valuable Series

If your library is not already a standing/continuation order customer to this series, may we recommend that you place a standing/continuation order to receive immediately upon publication all new volumes. Should you find that these volumes no longer serve your needs, your order can be cancelled at any time without notice.

The Editors and the Publisher will be glad to receive suggestions or outlines of suitable titles, reviews or symposia for editorial consideration: if found acceptable, rapid publication is guaranteed.

ROBERT MAXWELL
Publisher at Pergamon Press

FRONTIERS IN HISTAMINE RESEARCH

A TRIBUTE TO HEINZ SCHILD

Based on an International Symposium
held at Jouy-en-Josas (near Paris), France,
25–27 July 1984

Editors

C. ROBIN GANELLIN
Vice President of Chemical Research,
Smith Kline & French Research Limited, The Frythe, Welwyn,
Hertfordshire, England
Honorary Professor of Medicinal Chemistry, University of Kent at Canterbury

JEAN-CHARLES SCHWARTZ
Professor, Université René Descartes
Head, Unité 109 de Neurobiologie, Centre Paul Broca de l'INSERM,
2 ter rue d'Alésia, 75014 Paris, France

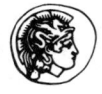

PERGAMON PRESS
OXFORD · NEW YORK · TORONTO · SYDNEY · PARIS · FRANKFURT

U.K.	Pergamon Press Ltd., Headington Hill Hall, Oxford OX3 0BW, England
U.S.A.	Pergamon Press Inc., Maxwell House, Fairview Park, Elmsford, New York 10523, U.S.A.
CANADA	Pergamon Press Canada Ltd., Suite 104, 150 Consumers Road, Willowdale, Ontario M2J 1P9, Canada
AUSTRALIA	Pergamon Press (Aust.) Pty. Ltd., P.O. Box 544, Potts Point, N.S.W. 2011, Australia
FRANCE	Pergamon Press SARL, 24 rue des Ecoles, 75240 Paris, Cedex 05, France
FEDERAL REPUBLIC OF GERMANY	Pergamon Press GmbH, Hammerweg 6, D-6242 Kronberg-Taunus, Federal Republic of Germany

Copyright © 1985 Pergamon Press Ltd.

All Rights Reserved. *No part of this publication may be reproduced, stored in a retrieval system or transmitted in any form or by any means: electronic, electrostatic, magnetic tape, mechanical, photocopying, recording or otherwise, without permission in writing from the publishers.*

First edition 1985

Library of Congress Cataloging in Publication Data
Frontiers in histamine research.
(Advances in the biosciences; v. 51)
Includes index.
1. Histamine—Physiological effect—Congresses.
2. Brain chemistry—Congresses. I. Schild, Heinz O.
(Heinz Otto), 1906-   . II. Ganellin, C. R.
(C. Robin). III. Schwartz, Jean-Charles. IV. Series.
QP801.H5F76   1986   615'.7   84-26368

British Library Cataloguing in Publication Data
Frontiers in histamine research: a tribute to
Heinz Schild: based on an international symposium
held at Jouy-en-Josas (near Paris) France 25–27
July 1984.—(Advances in the biosciences; v.51)
1. Histamine
I. Ganellin, C. R.   II. Schwartz, Jean-Charles
III. Schild, H. O.   IV. Series
612'0157   QP801.H5
ISBN 0-08-031989-0

Printed in Great Britain by A. Wheaton & Co. Ltd., Exeter

SCIENTIFIC ADVISORS

MICHAEL A. BEAVEN, Ph.D.
Deputy Chief, Laboratory of Chemical Pharmacology,
National Heart, Lung and Blood Institute,
National Institutes of Health, Bethesda, USA

ROBERTO LEVI, M.D.
Professor of Pharmacology,
Department of Pharmacology,
Cornell University Medical College, New York, USA

ROSS E. ROCKLIN, M.D.
Allergy Division, Department of Medicine,
Tufts University School of Medicine, Boston, USA

KARL-FRIEDRICH SEWING, Dr. Med.
Professor of Pharmacology,
Zentrum Pharmakologie und Toxikologie,
Medizinische Hochschule Hannover, West Germany

BORJE UVNÄS, M.D.
Emeritus Professor of Pharmacology,
Department of Pharmacology,
Karolinska Institute, Stockholm, Sweden

CONTENTS

Preface   xi
    C.R.GANELLIN & J.-C.SCHWARTZ

Heinz Schild and the Histamine Affair   xiii
    SIR JAMES BLACK

RECEPTOR BIOCHEMISTRY AND PHARMACOCHEMISTRY

Some newer H_1-receptor histamine antagonists   3
    G.J. DURANT, C.R.GANELLIN, R. GRIFFITHS, C.A. HARVEY,
    D.A.A. OWEN & G.S. SACH

Interaction of 4(5)-[2-(4-azido-2-nitroanilino)ethyl]imidazole,
a histamine receptor photoaffinity label, with H_1-histamine
receptors in intact smooth muscle and in cerebral cortical
membranes   13
    G.K.HOGABOOM, K.S.ICE, D.L.HORSTEMEYER, J.P.O'DONNEL &
    J.S.FEDAN

Biochemical studies of cerebral H_1-receptors   19
    M. GARBARG, E. YERAMIAN, M. KORNER & J-C. SCHWARTZ

Histamine H_1-agonist stimulated breakdown of inositol
phospholipids   27
    H.CARSWELL, P.R.DAUM & J.M.YOUNG

Chiral agonists of histamine   39
    W.SCHUNACK, S.SCHWARZ, G.GERHARD, S.BUYUKTIMKIN & S.ELZ

A survey of recently described H_2-receptor histamine
antagonists   47
    C.R.GANELLIN

Histamine H_2-receptor radioligand binding studies   61
    T.J.RISING & D.B.NORRIS

Cognitive properties of H_2 receptors revealed by
[^{3}H]histamine   69
    J.W.WELLS, D.L. CYBULSKY, M.KANDEL, S.I.KANDEL & G.H.STEINBERG

Desensitization of histamine H_2 receptors in human leukemia
cells 79
C.L.JOHNSON & D.G.SAWUTZ

HISTAMINE IN THE BRAIN : LOCALISATION

Purification of and antibodies against L-histidine decarboxylase 91
T.WATANABE, Y.TAGUCHI, N.TAKEDA, S.SHIOSAKA, M.TOHYAMA &
H.WADA

Development of a monoclonal antibody against
L-histidine-decarboxylase as a selective tool for the
localisation of histamine-synthesising cells 103
H POLLARD, I. PACHOT, P. LEGRAIN, G. BUTTIN & J-C. SCHWARTZ

Localization and projections of histamine-immunoreactive
neurons in the central nervous system of the rat 119
H.W.M. STEINBUSCH & A.H. MULDER

Mast cells in rat brain: characterization, localization, and
histamine content 131
L.B.HOUGH, R.C.GOLDSCHMIDT, S.D.GLICK & J.PADAWER

HISTAMINE IN THE BRAIN : RELEASE AND METABOLISM

Histamine synthesis and release in CNS : control by
autoreceptors (H_3) 143
J-M. ARRANG, M. GARBARG & J-C. SCHWARTZ

Neuronal uptake and release of histamine in the central nervous
system 155
A.H.MULDER, R.P.J.M.SMITS & H.W.M.STEINBUSCH

S-Adenosylmethionine-dependent transmethylations of histamine:
purification and partial characterization of guinea pig brain
and kidney histamine N-methyltransferase 163
R.T.BORCHARDT & B.MATUSZEWSKA

Simultaneous determination of histamine and tele-methylhistamine
in the mammalian central nervous system and histamine turnover
measurements 173
K.SAEKI, R.OISHI & M.NISHIBORI

Histamine turnover in regions of rat brain 185
J.P.GREEN & J.K.KHANDELWAL

Histamine metabolites in cerebrospinal fluid, the rationale for
studying them and analytical aspects 197
C-G.SWAHN & G.SEDVALL

HISTAMINE IN THE BRAIN : ACTIONS AND ROLE

Neurobiology of a histaminergic neuron in the CNS of the mollusk
Aplysia californica 205
D.WEINREICH

Contents

Histamine actions in the mammalian central nervous system 215
H.L.HAAS

Physiological functions of histamine in the brain 225
H.WADA, T.WATANABE, A.YAMATODANI, K.MAEYAMA, N.ITOI,
R.CACABELOS, M.SEO, S.KIYONO, K. NAGAI & H.NAKAGAWA

Histamine receptors, cyclic nucleotides and psychotropic drugs 237
E.RICHELSON

ACTIONS AND ROLE OF HISTAMINE IN THE GASTROINTESTINAL TRACT

Actions and the role of histamine in the gastrointestinal tract 251
B.I.HIRSCHOWITZ

Receptors regulating acid secretory function in canine fundic
mucosa: a reductionist approach 253
A.H.SOLL

Histamine H_2 receptors and gastric cells 265
C. GESPACH & S. EMAMI

Stimulus-secretion coupling in the parietal cell 275
K.-FR.SEWING & W.BEIL

Histamine action in isolated gastric glands and its interaction
with metabolically active substances 281
O.NYLANDER & K.J.OBRINK

Properties and function of mucosal mast cells 289
L.ENERBACK

ACTIONS AND ROLE OF HISTAMINE IN THE CARDIOVASCULAR SYSTEM

Physiology and pharmacology of cardiac histamine, revisited 301
P.F.MANNAIONI

IgE-Mediated hypersensitivity and ischemia as causes of
endogenous cardiac histamine release 305
R.LEVI, A.A.WOLFF, D.A.ROBERTSON & L.M.GRAVER

Histamine and myocardial dysfunction 309
R.W.GRISTWOOD, D.A.A.OWEN, P.ROMANEC & K.A.SAMPFORD

Histamine modulation of cardiac sympathetic responses 317
S.S.GROSS & R.LEVI

A new therapeutic approach in congestive heart failure:
combined phosphodiesterase-inhibition with simultaneous
H_2-receptor stimulation 325
G.BAUMANN, D.MERCADER, B.PERMANETTER, U.BUSCH, K.NINGEL,
A.WIRTZFELD & H.BLOMER

Possible involvement of brain histamine in the regulation of
blood pressure 335
A.PHILIPPU

Multiple actions of histamine on cerebral blood vessels 341
P.M.GROSS

ROLE OF HISTAMINE IN IMMUNE RESPONSES

Lymphocytes and histamine, a new entry to immunoregulation 353
J-F. BACH, L. CHATENOUD & M. DY

Histamine-induced suppressor cell responses in normal and atopic subjects 357
R.E.ROCKLIN

Histamine induced inhibition of interleukin-2 synthesis and activity in man 365
R.HUCHET

Histamine-induced human lymphokines affecting T-lymphocyte motility 371
D.J.BEER, W.W.CRUIKSHANK, J.S.BERMAN, & D.M.CENTER

Modulation of cytotoxic T lympocyte responses by histamine 379
M.PLAUT, A.KAGEY-SOBOTKA & A.R.JACQUES

Alterations in immunoregulatory T-lymphocyte phenotype and function: action of H_1 and H_2 histamine agonists 389
R.E.BIRCH & S.H.POLMAR

MECHANISMS OF HISTAMINE RELEASE

Molecular and biochemical mechanisms of IgE-mediated histamine release from mast cells 401
T.ISHIZAKA

Mast cell heterogeneity, differential responsivity to histamine liberators and anti-allergic drugs 411
F.L.PEARCE, H.ALI, K.E.BARRETT, A.D.BEFUS, J.BIENENSTOCK,
J.BROSTOFF, M.ENNIS, K.C.FLINT, N.MCI.JOHNSON, K.B.P.LEUNG &
P.T.PEACHELL

Studies of the calcium signal (quin 2 fluorescence), phospholipid turnover and histamine release in rat basophil leukemic (2H3) cells 423
M.A.BEAVEN & E.WOLDEMUSSIE

Author Index 433

Subject Index 437

PREFACE

C. R. Ganellin* and J. C. Schwartz**

*Smith Kline and French Research Limited, The Frythe,
Welwyn, Hertfordshire, UK
**Unité 109 de Neurobiologie, Centre Paul Broca de
l'INSERM, 2ter rue d'Alesia, 75014 Paris, France

Histamine is an important extracellular messenger, participating in the control of a variety of biological responses in, for example, the gastrointestinal, cardiovascular, central nervous, and immune systems. Yet histamine has been relatively neglected by scientists in recent times in comparison with the effort expended on messengers such as the catecholamines, indolylalkylamines, and peptides.

The reason for the neglect lies partly with the paucity of suitable research tools for histamine; for a long time the histochemical methods lacked the necessary power for an adequate study of histamine localisation, or to even identify the cells which store and release it, and to differentiate the cells upon which it acts. Similarly, powerful agents to block specifically the synthesis, release, or metabolism of histamine have been lacking. The impact that chemical tools may have on biological research is well illustrated by the rapid research progress made immediately after the respective introductions of the specific H_1 and H_2 receptor histamine antagonists.

Recently, however, we have seen several new immunohistochemical approaches to the visualisation of histamine-synthesising and storing cells, which suggests that we may be about to witness another major breakthrough in the various fields of histamine research. We also see the emergence of several non-isotopic methods for studying histamine catabolism which will extend the well known and highly reliable isotopic procedures, and these developments complement the recent identification of potent selective inhibitors of histamine biosynthesis and metabolism. These improvements in the techniques available should lead directly to more effective investigation of histamine's function.

Recent studies of receptor-ligand interaction have been especially interesting in the histamine field and we continue to see the development of new ligands. Much new information on histamine receptor taxonomy has come to light; there have been exciting discoveries regarding the secondary events following receptor stimulation, and there is the prospect of developing agents to modify histamine release from a new class (H_3) of histamine receptors.

In drug therapy, there is a renewal of interest in the 'antihistamines,' now renamed as H_1-receptor histamine antagonists, since compounds have been identified which either do not penetrate the brain or, at least, apparently have a much lower propensity to cause sedation as a 'side-effect.' There has also been an explosive increase in the interest of pharmaceutical companies wishing to exploit the discoveries made with H_2-receptor histamine antagonists in controlling gastric acid secretion.

Potential therapeutic applications of our knowledge about histamine have clearly served to heighten our interest in its role in both physiology and pathology. This has been very obvious in such clinical areas as allergy, inflammation, and gastroenterology. So it is with great expectation that we continue to see other areas emerge to direct our attention, as in neurobiology and immunology where histamine appears to exert complex and finely adjusted controls. We anticipate further exciting opportunities for improvements in therapy in the coming years.

The above represents some of the changing frontiers in histamine research and it seems to be at a point at which important advances can be anticipated. Therefore we felt it to be an opportune time to convene a conference where those responsible for expanding our frontiers could come together to present their results, exchange information, and learn what is new in histamine research outside of their own immediate area of investigation.

This book is based upon the contributions of some fifty invited speakers and chairmen to an International Symposium held on a picturesque campus location at Jouy-en-Josas, some twenty kilometres south west of Paris, France. The chairmen and speakers, all leaders in the field of histamine resarch, were selected with the assistance of a committee of scientific advisors, which included M.A. Beaven, R. Levi, R.E. Rocklin, K.-F. Sewing, and B. Uvnäs, and we are grateful to them for their sound advice and help. The result was spectacularly successful, and this volume reflects their perspicacity. We thank the chairmen of the various sessions for their active participation: J.F. Bach, J.P. Green, B.I. Hirschowitz, W. Lorenz, P.F. Mannaioni, M.E. Parsons, B. Uvnäs and G.B. West, and we thank our colleagues who presented papers for their excellent contributions and for so promptly writing articles for inclusion in this volume.

We owe much to SK&F France for giving help with the organisation and for the financial support needed to keep the registration costs for attendees within reasonable bounds. But it was not a 'company' meeting; the meeting was open to all, it was international, and provided a good mix of academic and industrial researchers. This assistance was generously given as a contribution to research to assist the free exchange of ideas and dissemination of scientific information.

We gratefully acknowledge the help of the local organising committee, J.M. Arrang, M. Garbarg, and H. Pollard (from INSERM), and Mlle C. Finet of Medicongres for attending to the myriad of details that ensured that things went smoothly and we thank Mlle Dominique Saveaux and Mrs Lilian Peduto for their considerable secretarial skills and effort.

Sadly, the meeting was held too late to permit the attendance of Professor Heinz Schild, one of the revered architects of histamine pharmacology, and we have dedicated this volume to his memory. The contents of this book certainly illustrate that the field he helped to nurture is alive and growing well. We are grateful to another great contributor to histamine research and his close colleague, Sir James Black, for writing an appreciation to be included in this book. We hope that this volume will prove informative and stimulating to all 'histaminologists.' In the progress of their research they will be honouring Heinz Schild in the manner which he would surely have liked best.

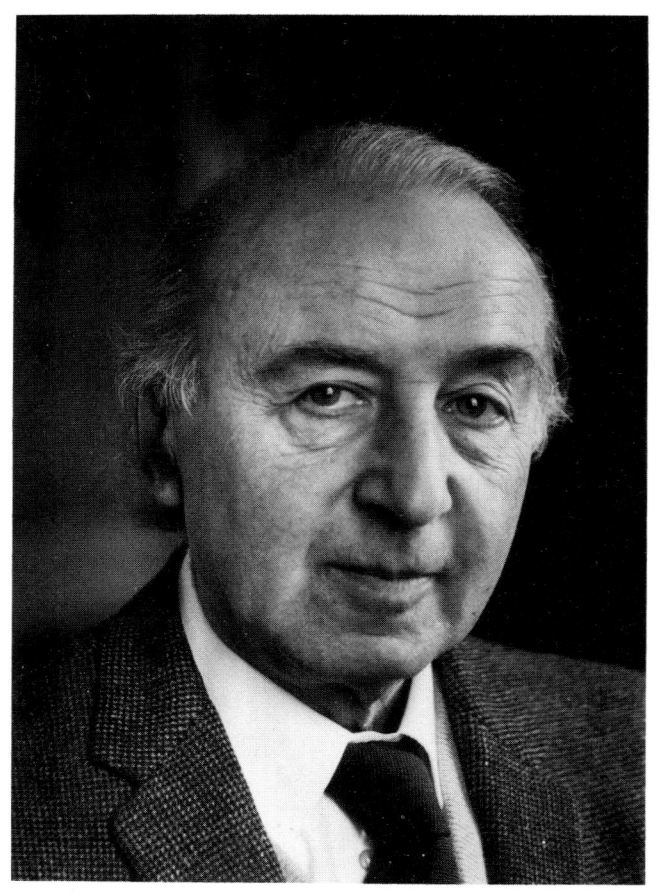

HEINZ OTTO SCHILD, M.D., PhD, DSc, FRS,
Professor of Pharmacology and Emeritus
Professor, University College, London 1961 - 1984

HEINZ SCHILD AND THE HISTAMINE AFFAIR

Sir James Black

Analytical Pharmacology Unit, King's College School of
Medicine and Dentistry, Rayne Institute,
123 Coldharbour Lane, London SE5 9NU, UK

I. de Burgh Daly introduced Heinz Schild to the problem of histamine and anaphylaxis when he joined Daly in Edinburgh in 1933, but before that his contacts and collaboration had prepared him for the challenge. He had had two years in Straub's laboratory in Munich where he met Georg Kahlson and he had had a year in Dale's laboratory at Hampstead where he had worked with Gaddum and Feldberg. His work with Gaddum had a particular impact on him. Heinz Schild had always had a passion for physics and mathematics and was clearly influenced by Gaddum's analytical approach. The foundations of his lifelong interest in bioassay started then.

He put his skill in bioassay to work straightaway at Edinburgh. Feldberg's work on the release of histamine from the perfused guinea-pig lung during anaphylaxis was confirmed by them (de Burgh Daly, Peat and Schild, 1935) and then they showed that the anaphylactic "shock substance" was destroyed by histaminase (de Burgh Daly and Schild, 1934), providing strong evidence that it was indeed histamine. However, he also found that when guinea-pig uterus is immersed in a high concentration of histamine it becomes, after wash out, insensitive to histamine but still responds to antigen (Schild, 1936a), thus anticipating the discovery of SRSA by Brocklehurst. At this time, he tried to persuade his chemical colleagues to make a specific histamine antagonist - an "atropine" for histamine - but he failed to raise any enthusiasm. Meanwhile Bovet, in Fourneau's laboratory in Paris was doing just that.

Nevertheless, Schild continued to attack the problem of histamine and anaphylaxis. He first of all showed that it really was "release" and not due to decarboxylation of the antigen's histidine (Schild, 1936b) or a consequence of smooth muscle contractions (Schild, 1936c). He showed that histamine release in guinea-pigs varied with the tissues (aorta most, gut least), developing a new technique en route (Schild, 1939).

Gaddum returned from Cairo in 1937 to the Chair at University College London and invited Schild to join them. The team was expanded to include Georg Kahlson from Sweden, and Smith and Gregory from the College. The problem chosen by Gaddum was to see if elevated blood histamine during exercise was the cause of reactive hyperaemia. The results were negative but two tremendous developments came out of it.

One was the discovery of histamine-releasing agents. Kahlson found that in eliminating the muscle contractions with tubocurarine, the blood histamine rose dramatically. Schild then showed that while strychnine methiodide, a powerful curarising agent, did the same, strychnine, which had practically no curarising action, also had powerful histamine-releasing activity (Schild and Gregory, 1947). So opened up a life-long interest and research into mechanisms of histamine release.

The other development was in the improvement of the design and technique of bioassay. In the course of the work on histamine release he became progressively disillusioned about the "matching assay" which was generally used at that time. Although the matching assay had the merit of directness it was soon obvious to Schild that it suffered badly from lack of precision. The inability of the method reliably to measure small changes in histamine concentrations was particularly frustrating. He tackled the problem in two ways. He developed an automatic assay apparatus to reduce experimental error (Schild, 1946) and he developed a statistically-controlled assay design so that the error-variance could be estimated on a single preparation. Fisher had developed the experimental design using randomised blocks in space to meet the need of agricultural research. Schild applied Fisher's methods to a randomised sequence in time to meet the needs of pharmacological assay; a remarkable achievement for someone untrained in statistics to have gotten there unaided (Schild, 1942).

Schild's research during the second World war led him into his famous studies on drug receptors and their antagonists. This work began, like many other of his fruitful ventures, in his enthusiasm for dealing with practical problems. He has testified that applied problems are not only stimulating but they also provide a unique entree into fundamental studies - in this case, into the quantification of drug antagonism. The kind of question he tried to tackle was, for example, "What do we mean when we say that mepyramine is 10,000 times as active against histamine as against acetylcholine?" His answer was the development first of the pA notation as a measure of drug antagonism and then the use of drug antagonists for the development of pharmacological classification (Schild, 1947a, 1947b). This work reached its peak in 1959 with his paper with Mme Arunlakshana. That paper defined the necessary conditions for the operational classification of competitive antagonism and then showed how antagonists can be used to identify agonists acting on the same receptors and then to establish if the same receptors occur in different tissues (Arunlakshana and Schild, 1959). All these developments eventually came together in 1966 in his work with Ash when he classified the H_1-set of histamine receptors. He was appointed a consultant to SK&F Laboratories in 1969 and I think he was delighted to see the way his development of pharmacological theory was being put to practical use in the selection of H_2-receptor histamine antagonists (Ash and Schild, 1966).

After the second World war Heinz Schild had a long and fruitful collaboration with Jack Mongar on anaphylaxis and histamine secretion (Mongar and Schild, 1957). They showed the fundamentally different nature of histamine release by organic bases, and histamine secretion induced by anaphylaxis. They studied some of the main factors which influence histamine secretion and some of the ways, generally non-specific, for its inhibition. With Herxheimer and Hawkins, they were the first to show histamine secretion by human lung tissue in vitro - the tissue from a sensitised individual responding to the specific antigen (Hawkins and co-workers, 1951). They also showed the "antihistamine paradox" in this tissue whereby mepyramine could block the contractile effects in the bronchial muscle of added histamine but not, apparently, the effects of histamine released by the antigen.

In over 30 years Heinz Schild was involved in tackling one aspect or another of the histamine affair. His work has had profound effects, both theoretical and practical, on our appreciation of the biology of histamine. I doubt if any one could study any aspect of histamine's role today without being influenced by Schild's ideas - a fitting commentary for someone who was a founder member of the famous Histamine Club. As Sir William Paton pointed out in his citation at the presentation of the Wellcome Gold Medal to Professor H.O. Schild "... it's fascinating ..... to see how often he was at the start of things".

REFERENCES

Arunlakshana, O. and H.O. Schild (1959). Some quantitative uses of drug antagonists. Brit. J. Pharmacol., 14, 43-58.

Ash, A.S.F. and H.O. Schild (1966). Receptors mediating some actions of histamine. Brit. J. Pharmac. Chemother., 27, 427-439.

de Burgh Daly, I., S. Peat and H.O. Schild (1935). The release of a histamine-like substance from the lungs of guinea-pigs during anaphylactic shock. Quart J. exp. Physiol., XXV, 33-59.

de Burgh Daly, I., and H.O Schild (1934). Inactivation by histaminase preparations of the histamine-like substance recovered from lungs during anaphylactic schock. J. Physiol., 83, 3P.

Hawkins, D.F., H. Herxheimer, J.L. Mongar and H.O Schild (1951). Reactions of isolated human asthmatic lung and bronchial tissue to a specific antigen. Lancet, 2, 376-382.

Mongar, J.L. and H.O. Schild (1957). Inhibition of the anaphylactic reaction. J. Physiol., 135, 301-319.

Schild, H.O. (1936a). The reaction of the guinea-pig uterus immersed in a histamine solution to histamine and anaphylaxis. J. Physiol., 86, 51P.

Schild, H.O. (1936b). The origin of the histamine-like substance released in anaphylactic shock. J. Physiol., 86, 50P.

Schild, H.O. (1936c). Histamine release and anaphylactic shock in isolated lungs of guinea-pigs. Quart J. exp. Physiol., XXVI, 166-179.

Schild, H.O. (1939). Histamine release in anaphylactic shock from various tissues of the guinea-pig. J. Physiol., 95, 393-403.

Schild, H.O. (1942). A method of conducting a biological assay on a preparation giving repeated graded responses illustrated by the estimation of histamine. J. Physiol., 101, 115-130.

Schild, H.O. (1946). Automatic apparatus for pharmacological assays on isolated preparations. Brit. J. Pharmacol., 1, 135-138.

Schild, H.O. (1947a). pA, a new scale for the measurement of drug antagonism. Brit. J. Pharmacol., 2, 189-206.

Schild, H.O. (1947b). The use of drug antagonists for the identification and classification of drugs. Brit. J. Pharmacol., 2, 251-258.

Schild, H.O. and R.A. Gregory (1947). Liberation of histamine from striated muscle by curarine, strychnine and related substances. Int. Physiol. Congr., Abstr. XVII, p. 288.

Receptor Biochemistry and Pharmacochemistry

SOME NEWER H_1-RECEPTOR HISTAMINE ANTAGONISTS

G. J. Durant, C. R. Ganellin, R. Griffiths,
C. A. Harvey, D. A. A. Owen and G. S. Sach

Smith Kline & French Research Ltd., The Frythe, Welwyn,
Hertfordshire, UK

ABSTRACT

H_1-Receptor histamine antagonists are in widespread use for the treatment of allergic rhinitis and related disorders. Certain of the newer antagonists, e.g. ketotifen, oxatomide and azelastine, also exhibit pronounced anti-anaphylactic effects and inhibit the release of histamine and other allergic mediators from mast cells; there is evidence for the clinical utility of ketotifen in the prophylaxis of bronchial asthma. Additionally, attempts have been made to develop H_1-receptor antagonists (e.g. terfenadine and astemizole) with increased selectivity and reduced centrally-mediated side-effects. SK&F 93944, which is chemically unrelated to previously described H_1-receptor antagonists, is potent and selective and penetrates the central nervous system to an insignificant extent in animal models.

KEYWORDS

Antihistamines; H_1-receptor antagonist; histamine; ketotifen; oxatomide; azelastine; terfenadine; astemizole, SK&F 93944.

INTRODUCTION

The first antihistaminic substances were discovered in France by Bovet and collaborators who reported in 1937 that 2-(N-piperidinomethyl)-1,4-benzodioxan (piperoxan, Fig. 1) and related aryl ethers such as 929F, protected guinea-pigs against lethal doses of histamine. Further work at the Pasteur Institute (Staub, 1939) demonstrated that -NH- was an effective isosteric replacement for -O- in these antihistaminic aryl ethers (e.g. 1571F, Fig. 1) and the results on these early compounds prompted intensive research activity in Europe and the United States to discover clinically effective antihistaminics. Some notable compounds discovered during the 1940's and 1950's which were introduced into therapy include mepyramine, diphenhydramine, chlorpheniramine, tripolidine and promethazine (Fig. 1). A fuller discussion of these classical studies and a critique of structure-activity relationships is contained in recent reviews (Ganellin, 1982; Witiak and Cavestri, 1981). A general structure which compromises most conventional antihistaminic drugs is included in Fig. 1 which indicates the requirement for two aromatic ring systems Ar_1 and Ar_2 linked by a short side-chain to a tertiary amino group. A degree of conformational rigidity can be introduced into the ring systems (as in tricyclic phenothiazines e.g. promethazine) and into the side-chain (triprolidine as _trans_ isomer).

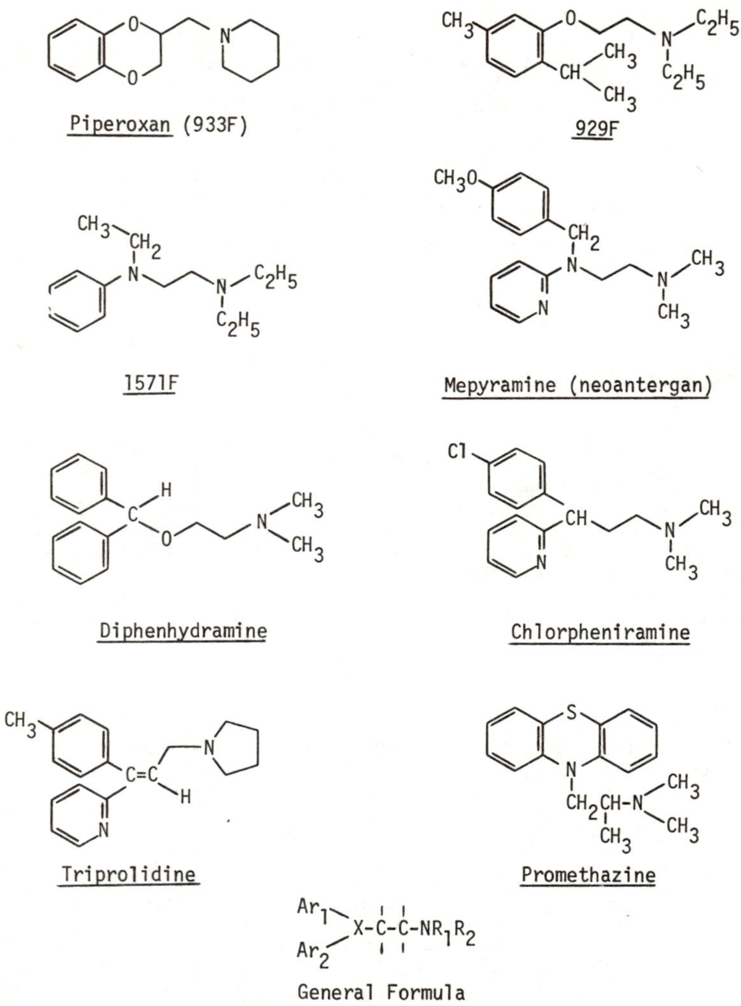

Piperoxan (933F)

929F

1571F

Mepyramine (neoantergan)

Diphenhydramine

Chlorpheniramine

Triprolidine

Promethazine

General Formula

Fig. 1. Some early antihistamines

Pharmacological studies showed that in addition to protecting guinea-pigs against histamine-induced bronchospasm, these compounds also antagonised histamine-induced contraction of various smooth muscles and lessened the symptoms of anaphylactic shock. Quantitative pharmacological studies showed that the mode of action was competitive and Schild (1947) introduced pA_x values to characterise this antagonism. Two typical compounds, mepyramine and diphenhydramine, were shown to be specific in antagonising histamine-induced contractions of guinea-pig ileum and bronchi. The pharmacological receptors involved in these mepyramine- and diphenhydramine-sensitive responses were subsequently defined as histamine H_1 receptors by Ash and Schild (1966).

Antihistamines Combining H_1-Receptor Antagonism and Anti-Anaphylactic Activity

In recent years two general approaches have been adopted in attempts to identify H_1-receptor histamine antagonists with potentially greater clinical efficacy than existing agents. The first approach attempts to identify pharmacologically useful properties in addition to H_1-receptor antagonism that could broaden the clinical application of drug candidates into more severe allergic conditions, such as bronchial asthma in which conventional antihistamines are ineffective. This approach includes attempts to combine H_1-receptor antagonism, either with antagonism of other mediators of the allergic response including 5-hydroxy-tryptamine, bradykinin and leukotrienes, or alternatively (or additionally) to inhibit anaphylactic release of histamine and other chemical mediators. Some examples are included in Fig. 2.

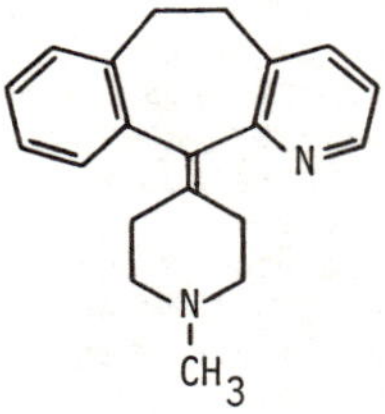

Azatadine

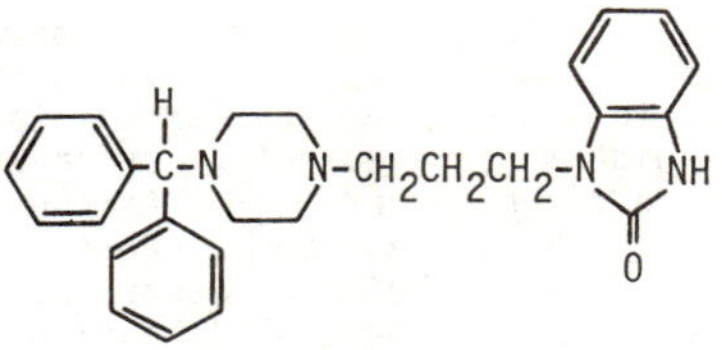

Oxatomide

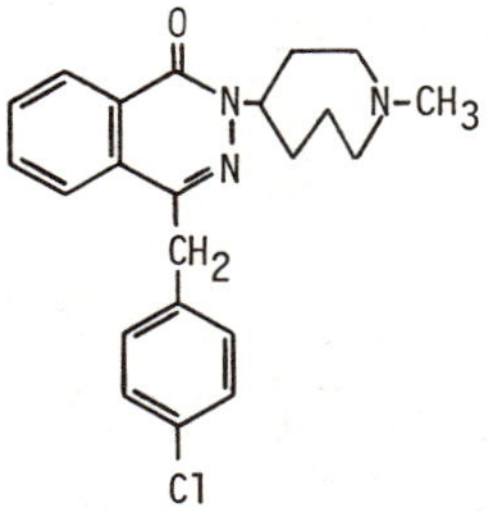

Azelastine

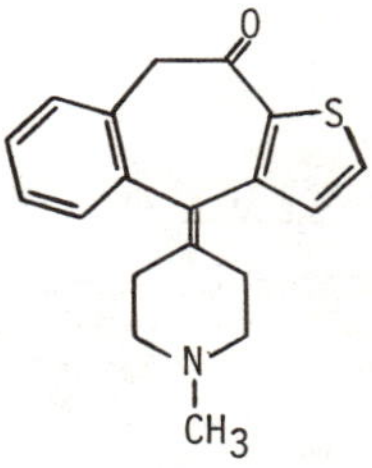

Ketotifen

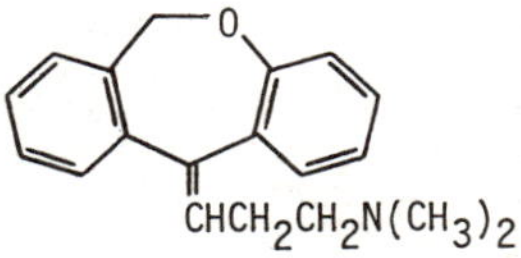

Doxepine

Fig. 2. Some newer H_1-receptor histamine antagonists with additional pharmacological actions.

Azatadine, an analogue of cyproheptadine, is reported (Tozzi, Roth and Tabachnick, 1974) to combine antagonism of histamine H_1-receptors with anti-5HT and anticholinergic activity. Oxatomide (Emanuel and Towse, 1980) reportedly combines antagonism of histamine H_1-, 5-HT and leucotriene receptors. Oxatomide also inhibits the release of histamine and other mediators from human lung tissue and sensitised mast cells. This inhibition occurs with other H_1-receptor histamine antagonists including chlorpheniramine (Church and Gradidge, 1980) but the relationship between antihistaminic activity and mast cell stabilising activity is unclear. Many H_1-receptor histamine antagonists (and other lipophilic cationic structures) exert a biphasic effect on anti-IgE-induced histamine release from human lung fragments in vitro, eliciting a dose-related inhibition of histamine release at low concentrations and a liberation of histamine at higher concentrations. Azelastine (Zechel and others, 1981) and ketotifen (Fig. 2) are further examples of histamine H_1-receptor antagonists which exert a pronounced mast-cell stabilising effect. Ketotifen has been extensively studied (Martin and Romer, 1978; Martin and others, 1981) and unlike many other tricyclic structures, it appears to exhibit relatively weak anti-5HT or anticholinergic activity. Ketotifen is reported to be a potent anti-anaphylactic agent in animal tests (e.g. rat PCA test) and to be considerably more potent than the 'selective' H_1-receptor histamine antagonist clemastine in these tests. Ketotifen is also reported to inhibit cAMP phosphodiesterase from different organs and 48/80 induced histamine release from isolated rat peritoneal mast cells in a manner similar to disodium chromoglycate whereas clemastine increases the 48/80 effect. It appears that the actions of ketotifen as an H_1-receptor histamine antagonist and as an anti-anaphylactic agent are distinct and separable. Clinical studies in bronchial asthma have given equivocal results but long-term administration of ketotifen is reported to be effective. A recently published post-marketing surveillance study (Maclay and others, 1984) has reported that ketotifen was efficacious in the prophylaxis of bronchial asthma in subjects studied for 1 year. The tricyclic structure of ketotifen bears some structural resemblance to antidepressants such as doxepine (Fig. 2) which have recently been shown to have extremely high affinity for histamine H_1 receptors (Richelson, 1978). The main side-effect of ketotifen is sedation which is a common problem and can be a limiting side-effect in the clinical use of many H_1-receptor histamine antagonists.

'Non-Sedative' H_1-Receptor Histamine Antagonists

The second approach adopted in attempts to develop improved H_1-receptor antagonists has been to identify molecules with greater selectivity particularly with regard to sedative side-effects. Most antihistamines readily penetrate the blood-brain barrier but it has not been established whether sedation is directly related to the occupation of central histamine H_1 receptors. A reduced incidence of sedative side-effects reported for the phenothiazine derivative mequitazine (Fig. 3) has been attributed to a greater affinity for peripheral than central H_1 receptors (Le Fur, Malgouris and Uzan, 1981). However, Quach and co-workers (1979) attribute the low in vivo occupation of cerebral histamine H_1 receptors by mequitazine to poor penetration of the blood-brain barrier. Terfenadine (Fig. 2), which has also been described as an antihistaminic agent with a low incidence of sedative side-effects, appears to interact with both cerebral and peripheral H_1 receptors with a similar affinity but appears to occupy cerebral H_1 receptors to a small extent when administered to mice at normal clinical doses (Rose and co-workers, 1982). The relatively low incidence of sedation with terfenadine may therefore also be due to difficulty in penetrating the blood-brain barrier.

Astemizole (Fig. 3) which has a slow onset and an exceptionally long duration of action is another recently introduced H_1-receptor antagonist with a reportedly low incidence of sedative side-effects which has been attributed to difficulty of access to the central nervous system (Laduron and co-workers, 1981). Further recently reported "non-sedative" H_1-receptor histamine antagonists (Fig. 3) include acrivastine (BW 825C; Leighton, Butz and Findlay, 1983) which is an acrylic acid derivative of tripolidine and SCH 29851, an analogue of azatidine (Barrett and co-workers, 1984).

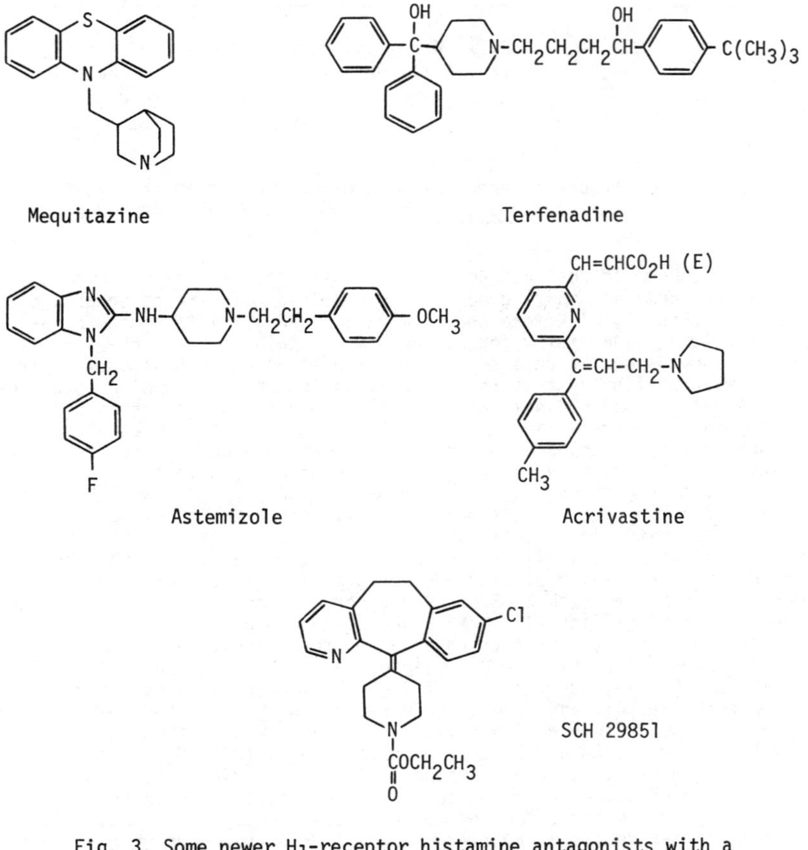

Fig. 3. Some newer H_1-receptor histamine antagonists with a reportedly low incidence of sedative side-effects.

SK&F 93944

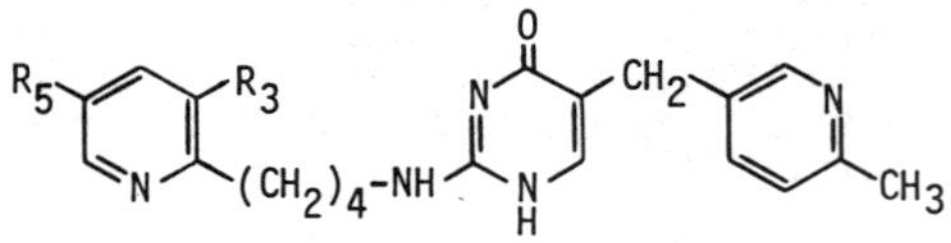

Fig. 4. Structures and histamine H_1- and H_2-receptor antagonist activity *in vitro* of SK&F 93319 and 93944

SK&F	R_3	R_5	(H$_1$, Ileum) pA$_2$	(H$_2$, Atrium)
93319	OCH$_3$	H	7.77 (6.85 - 8.39) (slope = 1.05 ± 0.33)	7.49 (7.00 - 8.50) (slope = 0.95 ±0.17)
93944	CH$_3$	Br	9.55 (9.38 - 9.82) (slope = 0.89 ± 0.26)	ca 5.9 (slope = 0.3)

In our own studies to design a non-sedative H_1-receptor histamine antagonist we chose as our chemical starting point, the combined H_1/H_2-receptor antagonist SK&F 93319, (Fig. 4, Blakemore and co-workers, 1983). This compound has approximately equal affinity for H_1 and H_2 receptors, but its chemical structure, based on isocytosine, is unusual for an H_1-receptor antagonist and of particular interest was the finding that the molecule did not cross the blood-brain barrier. SK&F 93319 also possessed only weak anticholinergic activity and provided a lead for designing a selective and non-CNS penetrating H_1-receptor antagonist. Structure-activity studies demonstrated that both H_1- and H_2-receptor antagonist activity are separately sensitive to substituent effects in the pyridine ring and particularly to substituent size in the 3-position (R_3). By suitable choice of substituents R_3 and R_5, H_1 antagonist activity could be increased and H_2-antagonist activity reduced. This work led to SK&F 93944 (R_3 = CH$_3$, R_5 = Br; Durant and co-workers, 1984), which contains a combination of substituents (R_3 = CH$_3$, R_5 = Br) which elevates H_1-receptor antagonist activity by two orders of magnitude compared with SK&F 93319 and concomitantly reduces H_2-receptor antagonist activity (Fig. 4). SK&F 93944 is also highly active as an H_1-receptor antagonist *in vivo*, e.g. in causing dose-dependant inhibition of histamine-induced bronchoconstriction in guinea-pigs over the dose-range 1.25×10^{-9} - 7.5×10^{-8} mol/kg, iv. Regressions of log [DR-1] upon log [dose] for SK&F 93944 and mepyramine in this assay were non-parallel, but, using the dose to produce [DR-1]=10 as the criterion of activity, SK&F 93944 was equi-potent with mepyramine ([DR-1]=10 of 30nmol/kg and 28nmol/kg respectively) (Fig. 5). SK&F 93944 is also a highly effective H_1-receptor antagonist in anaesthetised cats, determined by its inhibition of depressor responses to 2-(2-aminoethyl)pyridine, when a potency approximately twenty times that of mepyramine was determined. SK&F 93944 is also an effective H_1-receptor antagonist in conscious guinea-pigs when administered orally and in conscious rats, administered either intravenously or orally, when measured by its inhibition of cutaneous vascular permeability.

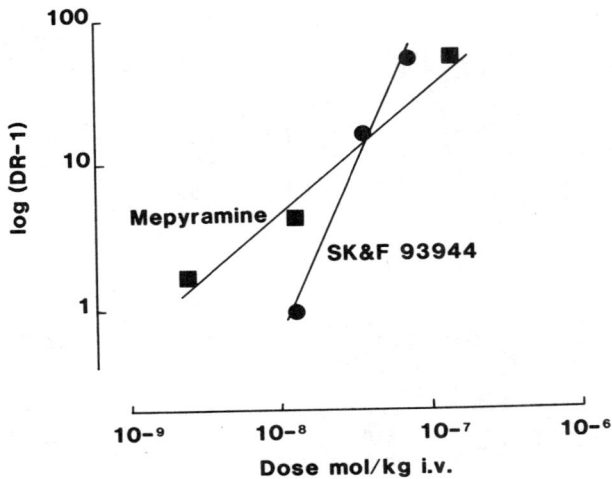

Fig. 5. Inhibition of histamine-induced bronchoconstriction by SK&F 93944 and mepyramine in anaesthetised guinea-pigs.

SK&F 93944 is a weak non-competitive antagonist of carbachol on guinea-pig ileum (a dose-ratio of 2 requiring a concentration of 1.07×10^{-4}M). In guinea-pigs, a dose of 7.5×10^{-8}mol/kg of SK&F 93944 which shifted the dose-response curve to histamine with a dose-ratio in excess of 50 had no effect on carbachol-induced bronchoconstriction. The lack of anticholinergic activity was also determined in cats by its effect on bradycardia during vagus nerve stimulation, no significant activity being exhibited by SK&F 93944 at doses up to 10mg/kg.

Penetration into the central nervous system was measured in anaesthetised male rats during intravenous administration of ^{14}C-SK&F 93944 or ^{3}H-mepyramine. At steady-state blood concentrations of about 3×10^{-9}mol/ml the whole brain concentration of mepyramine was approximately 7×10^{-9}mol/g wet weight, whereas that for SK&F 93944 was less than 1.5×10^{-11}mol/g wet weight, which is the limit of detection. In this rat model, there is therefore insignificant brain penetration by SK&F 93944.

SK&F 93944 differs chemically from previously described H_1-receptor antagonists in that the molecule does not possess a tertiary amino group. The most basic centre in SK&F 93944 has a pK_a of 5.9 compared with pK_a's of around 9 for most conventional H_1-receptor antagonists (Fig. 6). Thus, whereas the protonated form of most conventional H_1-receptor antagonists will predominate at physiological pH, SK&F 93944 will exist largely as the neutral form under these conditions.

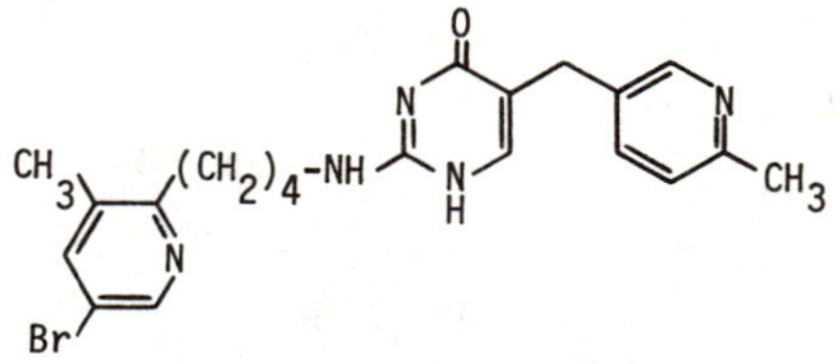

SK&F 93944

pK_a's (37°, U.V. method)	3.7	2.6	5.9

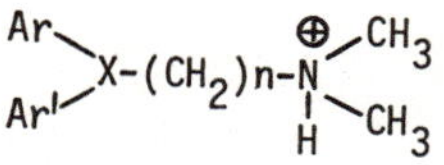

($pK_a \approx 9$)

Conventional H_1-Antagonists

Fig. 6. pK_a's of SK&F 93944 and comparison with conventional H_1-receptor antagonists.

SK&F 93944 offers the prospect of a novel non-sedating and effective H_1-receptor histamine antagonist and is being actively studied clinically. The effects of single oral doses of SK&F 93944 on cardiovascular responses to the H_1-receptor agonist betahistine in healthy human subjects have been reported (Boyce, 1984).

REFERENCES

Ash, A.S.F., and H.O. Schild (1966). Br. J. Pharmacol., 27, 427-439.

Barnett, A., L.C. Iorio, W. Kreutner, S. Tozzi, H.S. Ahn, and A. Gulbenkian (1984). Agents and Actions, 14, 590-597.

Blakemore, R.C., T.H. Brown, D.G. Cooper, G.J. Durant, C.R. Ganellin, R.J. Ife, A.C. Rasmussen, M.E. Parsons, and G.S. Sach (1983). Br. J. Pharmacol., 80, 437P.

Bovet, D., and A.M. Staub (1937). C.R. Soc. Biol. (Paris), 124, 547-549.

Boyce, M. (1984). Br. J. Clin. Pharmacol., 18, 277-278P.

Church, M.K., and C.F. Gradidge (1980). Br. J. Pharmacol., 69, 663-667.

Durant, G.J., C.R. Ganellin, R. Griffiths, C.A. Harvey, R.J. Ife, D.A.A. Owen, M.E. Parsons, and G.S. Sach (1984). Br. J. Pharmacol., 82, 232P.

Emanuel, M.B., and G.D.W. Towse (1980). Drugs of Today, 16, 219-229.

Ganellin, C.R. (1982). In C.R. Ganellin and M.E. Parsons (Ed.) Pharmacology of Histamine Receptors, Wright, London, Chapter 2, pp 10-102.

Laduron, P.M., P.F.M. Janssen, W. Gommeron and J.E. Leysen (1982). Mol. Pharmacol., 21, 294-300.

Leighton, H.J., R.F. Butz, and J.W.A. Findlay (1983). Pharmacologist, 25, 163, abstract 328.

Le Fur, G., C. Malgouris and A. Uzan (1981). Life Sciences, 29, 547-552.

Maclay, W.P., D. Crowder, S. Spiro, and P. Turner (1984). Br. M. J., (288), 911-914.

Martin, U., C. Greenwood, L.P. Craps and M. Bagglioni (1981). In M.E. Goldberg (Ed.) Pharmacological and Biochemical Properties of Drug Substances, Vol. 3, Am. Pharm. Assoc., Washington D.C., pp 424-460.

Martin, U., and D. Romer (1978). *Arz. Forsch.* 28, 770-782.
Quach, T.T., A.M. Duchemin, C. Rose, and J.C. Schwartz (1979). *Eur. J. Pharmacol.*, 60, 391-392.
Richelson, E. (1978). *Nature,* 274, 176-177.
Rose, C., T.T. Quach, C. Llorens and J.C. Schwartz (1982). *Arz. Forsch.*, 32, 1171-1173.
Schild, H.O. (1947). *Br. J. Pharmacol.*, 2, 189-206.
Staub, A.M. (1939). *Ann. Inst. Pasteur (Paris)*, 63, 400-524.
Tozzi, S., F.E. Roth, and I.L.A. Tabachnick (1974). *Agents and Actions*, 4/4, 264-270.
Trureh, A., J.R. White and F.L. Pearce (1982). *Agents and Actions,* 12, 206-209.
Ungar, G.; J. -L. Parrot and D. Bovet (1937). *C. R. Soc. Biol., (Paris)*, 124, 445-446.
Witiak, D.T., and R.C. Cavestri (1981). In M.E. Wolff (Ed.) Burger's Medicinal Chemistry, 4th Ed., Part III, Wiley-Interscience, New York, Chapter 49, pp 553-622.
Zechel, H. -J., N. Brock, D. Lenke, and U. Achterrath-Tuckermann (1981). *Arz. Forsch.*, 31, 1184-1193.

INTERACTION OF 4(5)-[2-(4-AZIDO-2-NITROANILINO)ETHYL]IMIDAZOLE, A HISTAMINE RECEPTOR PHOTOAFFINITY LABEL, WITH H_1-HISTAMINE RECEPTORS IN INTACT SMOOTH MUSCLE AND IN CEREBRAL CORTICAL MEMBRANES

G. K. Hogaboom*, K. S. Ice**, D. L. Horstemeyer***,
J. P. O'Donnell**** and J. S. Fedan**,*****

*Department of Molecular Pharmacology, Smith Kline and French Laboratories, P.O. Box 7929 (L-108), Philadelphia, PA 19101, USA
**Department of Pharmacological Toxicology, West Virginia University Medical Centre, Morgantown, WV 26JO6, USA
***Department of Biology, West Virginia University Medical Centre, Morgantown, WV 26JO6, USA
****School of Pharmacy, West Virginia University Medical Centre, Morgantown, WV 26JO6, USA
*****Physiology Section, Lab. Invest. Br., DRDS, NIOSH, 944 Chestnut Ridge Rd, Morgantown, WV 26505, USA

ABSTRACT

A photoaffinity analog of histamine, 4(5)-[2-(4-azido-2-nitroanilo)ethyl imidazole or arylazide histamine (AAH), was synthesized and its ability to interact with H_1-histamine receptors in intact smooth muscles and in cerebral cortical membranes was determined. Photolysis of AAH in organ chambers containing intact guinea-pig vas deferens and aortic strips produced, after washout, a specific and irreversible antagonism of histamine-induced contractions. Nonirradiated AAH produced a reversible antagonism of histamine-induced contractions in the vas deferens and aorta. In contrast, photolyzed AAH had no effect on histamine-induced contractions of the canine trachealis but nonirradiated AAH was a competitive antagonist to histamine in the same preparation. Additional studies determined the effect of AAH on the binding of [^{3}H]-histamine ([^{3}H]-HA), [^{3}H]-mepyramine ([^{3}H]-MEP) and [^{3}H]-tiotidine ([^{3}H]-TIOT) to rat cerebral cortical membranes. Competition binding assays determined rank order K_i's for [^{3}H]-HA binding as HA > AAH >> MEP = TIOT, [^{3}H]-MEP binding as MEP >> AAH > HA > TIOT and [^{3}H]-TIOT binding as TIOT >> MEP > HA = AAH. These studies suggest that AAH may be a useful probe in determining molecular and biochemical characteristics of the H_1-histamine receptor in intact tissues or membrane preparations.

KEYWORDS

Histamine; H_1-histamine receptor; Histamine antagonist; Photoaffinity label; Rat cerebral cortex; Guinea-pig vas deferens; Guinea-pig aorta; Dog trachealis; Arylazide histamine

INTRODUCTION

Photoaffinity labels are ligands that contain a photosensitive functional group which, when photoactivated with light, are able to form a covalent bond at or near a binding site. These agents have an inherent affinity for the binding site and can possess biological activity. Our interests originated in utilizing photoaffinity labels as pharmacological probes in functional studies with intact smooth muscle preparations. As there are many pharmacological agonists which presumably induce responses via receptor-mediated events but for which no specific receptor antagonist exists, it is conceivable that any agonist agent could be made into a specific pharmacological antagonist by the addition of a photosensitive moiety. With this idea in mind, the role of adenosine 5'-triphosphate (ATP) was evaluated in autonomic neurotransmission utilizing an ATP photoaffinity analog synthesized originally by Jeng and Guillory (1975). The ATP photoaffinity label, referred to as ANAPP$_3$, antagonized specifically ATP-induced responses in the guinea-pig vas deferens and allowed the pharmacological determination of P$_2$-purinergic receptors as well as defining a role for ATP as a co-transmitter in this tissue (Hogaboom, O'Donnell, Fedan, 1980; Fedan and coworkers, 1981). Additional applications of photoaffinity labels as pharmacological tools in intact tissues, whole cells or membrane fractions have been recently reviewed (Fedan, Hogaboom, O'Donnell, 1984).

This communication describes the pharmacological characteristics of arylazide histamine (AAH), a photoaffinity analog of histamine. In studies with intact smooth muscles, AAH, after photolysis, is a specific, irreversible H$_1$-histamine receptor antagonist. In radioligand binding studies with histamine agonists and antagonists, AAH interacts with H$_1$-histamine receptors in cerebral cortical membranes.

MATERIALS AND METHODS

4(5)-[2(4-Azido-2-nitroanilo)ethyl]imidazole hydrochloride (AAH) was synthesized in our laboratory as described by Fedan, Hogaboom, O'Donnell (1981). The structure of AAH is shown in Fig. 1. The tissues were prepared for pharmacological experiments as described by O'Donnell, Hogaboom, Fedan (1981) for guinea-pig vas deferens and as described by Fedan, Hogaboom, O'Donnell (1982) for guinea-pig aorta and dog trachealis. The effects of AAH on the responses of the smooth muscle of the vas deferens, aorta and trachealis to the various agonists were determined using protocols and guidelines described by Fedan and coworkers (1983). For radioligand binding studies, the cerebral cortex was removed from male guinea pigs and polytron-homogenized in 50 mM phosphate buffer (pH 7.5). The homogenate was centrifuged 50,000 X g for 10 min and the pellet resuspended in 50 vol of 50 mM phosphate buffer and centrifuged as described above. The pellet was resuspended in 50 vol of 50 mM phosphate buffer to give the membrane fraction used in the radioligand binding experiments. Binding assays were conducted at 30° C in a final volume of 1 ml and nonspecific binding was determined by the addition of 10 μM excess unlabeled ligands.

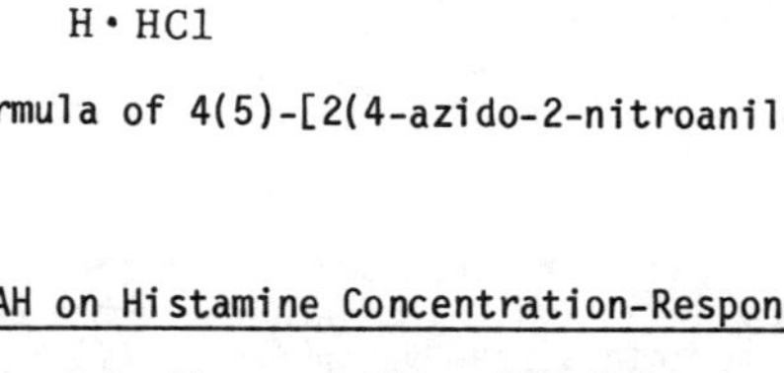

Fig. 1. Structural formula of 4(5)-[2(4-azido-2-nitroanilo)ethyl]imidazole HCl.

RESULTS

Effect of Photolyzed AAH on Histamine Concentration-Response Relationships

In the concentrations used in these studies, AAH did not cause contraction of the guinea-pig vas deferens, guinea-pig aorta or dog trachealis upon its addition to the organ bath. The ability of AAH, after photolysis and in the absence of photolysis, to antagonize histamine-induced contractions was tested in several intact smooth muscle preparations. The guinea-pig vas deferens was chosen initially as this tissue preparation had been used in our laboratory to characterize the actions of the ATP photoaffinity label, $ANAPP_3$ (Hogaboom, O'Donnell, Fedan, 1980). After its photolysis and washout, 30 μM AAH abolished the response of the tissues to histamine (O'Donnell, Hogaboom, Fedan, 1981). There was no effect of photolysis per se on the contraction of the vas deferens and the antagonism by photolyzed AAH was not reversed by repeated washing of the tissues. When compared to control tissues, the transient exposure of the tissue to AAH without photolysis had no effect on subsequent histamine concentration-response curves. The antagonism by photolyzed AAH was specific for histamine receptors as responses to KCl, norepinephrine and MgATP were unaffected whilst responses to acetylcholine were only slightly affected. To determine on a more molecular basis the site to which AAH was bound, protection studies were conducted with a histamine receptor agonist and histamine receptor antagonists. The presence of diphenhydramine during photolysis reversed the antagonistic actions of photolyzed AAH. In contrast, the presence of histamine provided no protection whilst cimetidine provided only slight protection.

Photolyzed AAH (30 μM) produced an 11.5-fold shift of the histamine concentration response curve to the right of control and reduced the maximum response by 38 percent in the isolated guinea-pig aortic strip (Fig. 2). When normalized with regard to the tissue's maximum response (Fig. 1, right-hand panel), photolyzed AAH produced a parallel shift to the right of the histamine concentration

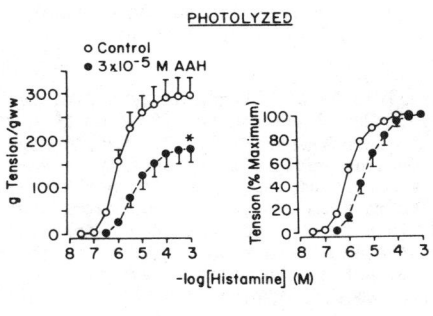

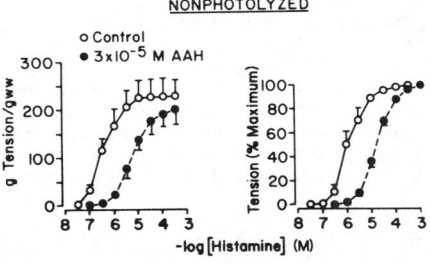

Fig. 2. Effect of 30 μM AAH on histamine concentration-response curves of guinea-pig aorta. Upper panels: AAH was photolyzed and washed out before the addition of histamine. Lower panels: Concentration-response curves were obtained in the presence of non-photolyzed AAH. *Significantly less than irradiated control. Reproduced with permission from European Journal of Pharmacology (Copyright 1982 Elsevier/North-Holland Biomedical Press).

TABLE 1 Radioligand Agonist and Antagonist Binding Characteristics of Rat Cortical Membranes

[^{3}H]-LIGAND	K_D (nM)	LIGAND	K_I	
[^{3}H]-HA[a]	5.0	HA	15.7	nM
		AAH	157	nM
(Two-Site Model; High Affinity Site)		MEP	14.3	μM
		TIOT	49.4	μM
[^{3}H]-MEP	0.61	MEP	1.53	nM
		AAH	3.14	μM
(Two-Site Model; High Affinity Site)		HA	10.1	μM
		TIOT	170	μM
[^{3}H]-TIOT	18.1	TIOT	10.6	nM
		MEP	8.51	μM
(One-Site Model)		HA	45.9	μM
		AAH	42.5	μM

[a] Competition binding assays used [^{3}H]-ligand concentrations of 6, 1 and 2 nM for [^{3}H]-HA, [^{3}H]-MEP and [^{3}H]-TIOT, respectively.

response curve. The specificity of antagonism by photolyzed AAH also was determined. Photolysis of 30 μM AAH had no effect on EC_{50} values or maximum responses of the aorta to norepinephrine or KCl (Fedan, Hogaboom, O'Donnell, 1982). The histamine-specific antagonism by photolyzed AAH was photolysis dependent as transient exposure of the tissues to non-irradiated AAH had no effect on EC_{50} values and maximum responses. Concentration response curves to histamine were also obtained in the presence of non-irradiated AAH (Fig. 2). Histamine concentration-response curves were shifted to the right of control in a parallel manner with no effect on the maximum response. Non-irradiated AAH, thus, produces an equilibrium competitive antagonism in this tissue.

In contrast to the antagonism produced by photolyzed AAH in the guinea-pig vas deferens and aorta, photolyzed AAH had no effect on the EC_{50} or maximum response to histamine in dog trachealis (Fedan, Hogaboom, O'Donnell, 1982). This lack of antagonism was not explained by a lack of affinity of the H_1-histamine receptors in the trachealis for AAH as the K_B values for AAH in the aorta and trachealis were not significantly different. pA_2 values for diphenhydramine indicated a slightly greater potency in the aorta versus the trachealis. However, the difference in diphenhydramine potencies does not explain the complete lack of effect of photolyzed AAH in the dog trachealis.

Interactions of AAH with Histamine Receptors in Cerebral Cortical Membranes

To characterize further the interaction of AAH with histamine receptors, the effect of AAH on the binding of [^{3}H]-HA, [^{3}H]-MEP and [^{3}H]-TIOT was studied. The K_D values obtained (Horstemeyer and coworkers, 1984) for [^{3}H]-HA, [^{3}H]-MEP and [^{3}H]-TIOT were similar to previous reports (Barbin and coworkers, 1980; Table 1). Competition binding studies with [^{3}H]-HA indicated an order of potency of HA > AAH >> MEP = TIOT. Because of the greater potency of AAH than MEP, AAH may interact with the high affinity state of the H_1-histamine receptor. In addition, as guanine nucleotides were not present in these assays, AAH may possess partial agonist activity. The potency series for displacement of [^{3}H]-MEP and [^{3}H]-TIOT binding (Table 1) indicate that AAH had a greater affinity for H_1 versus H_2-histamine receptors in the cortical membranes. These data support the results of previous studies and further suggest that AAH preferentially interacts with H_1-histamine receptor sites.

SUMMARY

The results of these studies indicate that photoactivated AAH is a specific and irreversible H_1-histamine receptor antagonist in intact smooth muscles. These studies are supported by the findings that AAH interacts preferentially with H_1-histamine binding sites in cerebral cortical membranes. The data indicate that photolyzed AAH inserts covalently in or near the H_1-histamine receptor in the guinea-pig aorta and vas deferens. In addition, a variety of biochemical and pharmacological criteria, which apply to the use of photoaffinity labels, have been satisfied (see Fedan and coworkers, 1983). 1) The histamine receptors in the intact tissues are not altered by photolysis. 2) Non-photolyzed AAH interacts reversibly with histamine receptors in intact tissues and interacts preferentially with the H_1-histamine receptor in ligand binding studies using brain membranes. 3) The exposure of the tissues to non-irradiated AAH does not result in a non-specific toxicity. 4) AAH does not interact to any great degree with the agonist-induced action of chemically unrelated agents. 5) Prior occupancy of the binding site with diphenhydramine prevents the covalent insertion of AAH into the histamine receptor site. In conclusion, these studies provide evidence that arylazide histamine may be useful in determining molecular and biochemical properties of the H_1-histamine receptor either in intact tissues or membrane preparations.

ACKNOWLEDGEMENTS

The authors thank Judy Seaman for expert assistance in the preparation of this manuscript. This work was supported, in part, by NIGMS 5 T32 GM07039.

REFERENCES

Barbin, G., J.M. Palacios, E. Rodergas, J.C. Schwartz, and G. Garbag (1980) Mol. Pharmacol., 33, 1167-1180.
Fedan, J.S., G.K. Hogaboom, J.P. O'Donnell, J. Colby, and D.P. Westfall (1981) Eur. J. Pharmacol., 69, 41-53.
Fedan, J.S., G.K. Hogaboom, and J.P. O'Donnell (1982) Eur. J. Pharmacol., 81, 393-402.
Fedan, J.S., G.K. Hogaboom, D.P. Westfall, and J.P. O'Donnell (1983) Fed. Proc., 42, 2846-2850.
Fedan, J.S., G.K. Hogaboom, and J.P. O'Donnell (1984) Biochem. Pharmacol., 33, 1167-1180.
Hogaboom, G.K., J.P. O'Donnell, and J.S. Fedan (1980) Science, 208, 1273-1276.
Horstemeyer, D.L., K.S. Ice, G.K. Hogaboom, J.P. O'Donnell, and J.S. Fedan (1984) Fed. Proc., 43, 689.
Jeng, S.J., and R.J. Guillory (1975) J. Supramolec. Struct., 3, 448-458.
O'Donnell, J.P., G.K. Hogaboom, J.S. Fedan. (1981) Eur. J. Pharmacol., 73, 261-271.

BIOCHEMICAL STUDIES OF CEREBRAL H_1-RECEPTORS

M. Garbarg, E. Yeramian, M. Korner and
J-C. Schwartz

Unité 109 de Neurobiologie, Centre Paul Broca de l'INSERM,
2ter rue d'Alésia, 75014 Paris, France

ABSTRACT

The presence of an essential thiol group at H_1-receptors has been investigated by treating guinea-pig cerebellar membranes with N-ethylmaleimide (NEM). The binding of ^{3}H-mepyramine or other H_1-antihistamines (Kd or Bmax values) was not modified. In marked contrast, binding of agonists was modified : NEM caused a shift to the left of the competition binding curve for histamine and decreased the pseudo-Hill slope coefficient of competition curve from unit to 0.69. These findings suggest that NEM induced a heterogeneity in the ^{3}H-mepyramine binding sites with a fraction of H_1-receptors being converted to a form of high affinity for the agonist. The shift of the IC_{50} and the decrease of the pseudo-Hill coefficient were also observed with the full H_1-receptor agonist 2-thiazolylethylamine, whereas binding of partial agonists was less affected. These changes could not be prevented by a preincubation with H_1-receptor agonists or antagonists but were still present in a solubilised preparation suggesting that the NEM-sensitive residues are located within the receptor complex but distant from the ligand-binding domain. Partial purification of the digitonin-solubilised ^{3}H-mepyramine binding sites was undertaken using affinity chromatography. The H_1-receptors were retained on wheat germ lectin columns and eluted with N-acetyl-D-glucosamine with a 4-fold enrichment. This suggests the glycoprotein nature of H_1-receptors.

KEYWORDS

Histamine ; H_1-receptors ; Thiols ; Glycoprotein

INTRODUCTION

Studies of receptors at the molecular level have started with the advent of selective radioligands which allows not only to undertake purification of these macromolecules but even biochemical studies when they are still in their membrane-bound state. For instance covalent chemical modifications of receptor proteins have been proved to be useful to get information about functional groups. The most widely used are reagents modifying sulfhydryl groups and disulfide bonds. Agonist and antagonist binding to receptors are often differentially affected, suggesting a role of thiol groups or disulfide bonds in the changes of conformation of the receptor protein elicited only by agonists (see review by Strauss, 1984). The reactive groups may play a critical role for ligand binding as well as for events involved in the transduction system. For instance, there are now strong evidences that critical thiol

groups are located on the stimulatory guanine nucleotide regulatory protein from β- noradrenergic receptors (Andre and co-workers, 1982 ; Korner, Gilon and Schramm, 1982) and on the inhibitory guanine nucleotide regulatory protein from muscarinic and opiate receptors (Smith and Harden, 1984). In the case of histamine (HA) receptor alkylation of sulfhydryl groups by N-ethylmaleimide (NEM) inhibits the H_1-receptor mediated contractions of rabbit aorta, whereas reduction of disulfide bonds by dithiothreitol potentiates both this response (Fleisch, Krzan and Titus, 1973, 1974), and the guinea-pig ileum contraction (Glover, 1979). However the specificity of the dithiothreitol effects was recently questioned (Fontaine, Famaey and Reuse 1984) and the effects of these reagents on intact cell preparations cannot be easily interpreted.
The development of ^{3}H-mepyramine as a suitable radioligand for H_1-receptors and the realisation that the guinea-pig cerebellum is a reasonably enriched tissue (Hill, Emson and Young, 1978) now allows direct biochemical studies of this receptor.

ANTAGONIST BINDING AT H_1-RECEPTOR IN NEM-TREATED MEMBRANES

Pretreatment of membranes from guinea-pig cerebellum with the thiol-alkylating agent did not apparently modify the binding of antagonists at H_1-receptors. Thus the apparent dissociation constant and the maximal number of specific ^{3}H-mepyramine binding remained unchanged after 2 mM NEM (Fig. 1). Increasing the concentration of NEM up to 5 mM led to similar results. Moreover inhibition studies performed with d-chlorpheniramine and mianserin showed that the IC_{50} values of these H_1-receptor antagonists were not altered under these conditions (data not shown).

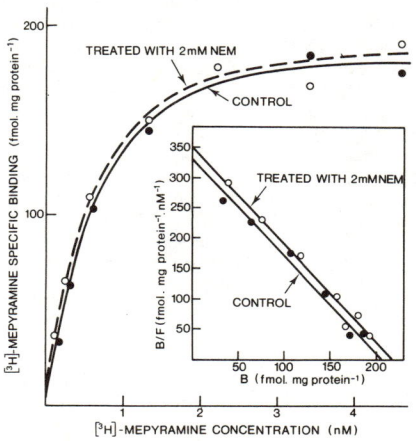

Fig. 1. Saturation curve of ^{3}H-mepyramine binding on guinea-pig cerebellar membranes untreated or treated with 2 mM NEM.
Membranes from guinea-pig cerebellum were first preincubated with 2 mM NEM. After addition of 2-mercaptoethanol and centrifugation, they were resuspended in phosphate buffer and incubated with increasing concentrations of ^{3}H-mepyramine alone (total binding) or together with 0.2 µM mianserin (non specific binding). Bound ligand was isolated from free ligand by a filter separation technique.
The inset represents the Scatchard plot of the data from the saturation curve.

This suggests the absence of any critical thiol group in the binding of the tested antagonists to the H_1-receptors. This seems as well the case for β-adrenergic (Stadel and Lefkowitz, 1979) and muscarinic receptors (Aronstam, Abood and Hoss, 1978 ; Nukada and co-workers, 1983) whereas the alkylating agent impairs antagonist binding to opiate (Simon and Groth, 1975) and dopamine receptors (Freedman, Poat and Woodruff, 1982).
However structure-activity studies among H_1-antihistamines belonging to various classes have strongly suggested that the binding domain of these compounds overlaps only partially that of HA itself or of agonists (Ariens, 1979). In addition it is generally admitted that bindings of agonists and antagonists differ in the sense that only the former is accompanied by a conformational change. All these considerations prompted us to study agonist binding following the NEM pretreatment.

MODIFICATION OF AGONIST BINDING AT H_1-RECEPTOR IN NEM-TREATED MEMBRANES

In membranes pretreated with NEM the inhibition curve of HA was modified in a complex manner (Fig. 2). First it was clearly shifted to the left, and this effect was even more marked after 5 mM than after 2 mM NEM-treatment. Hence, the shift factor of IC_{50} value was 2.8 after 2 mM NEM-treatment and 3.7 after 5 mM NEM-treatment.

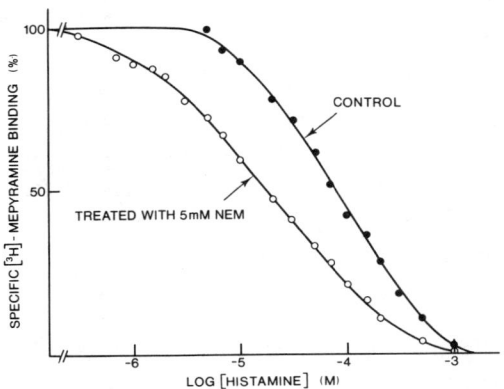

Fig. 2 Histamine inhibition curve of specific ^{3}H-mepyramine binding after treatment of guinea-pig cerebellar membranes with 5 mM NEM.
The specific binding at 0.6 nM ^{3}H-mepyramine was (in fmoles.mg protein^{-1}) 108 $\pm$ 2 for control membranes (o) and 98 $\pm$ 9 for NEM-treated membranes (x). The mean IC_{50} values for HA were 78 µM for control membranes and 21 µM for NEM-treated membranes.

In addition there was a shallowing of the inhibition curve indicated by a decrease in the pseudo-Hill coefficients which were 1.00 ± 0.03 for control membranes, 0.77 ± 0.06 after 2 mM NEM and 0.69 ± 0.03 after 5 mM NEM. The value equal to unit indicates that HA binds to a single population of sites in control membranes, whereas NEM seems to induce an heterogeneity in these binding sites. This is also illustrated by the Scatchard plot of these data linear for control membranes and curvilinear for NEM-treated membranes (not shown).

Hence the HA inhibition curve in NEM-treated membranes, when analysed either by the Scatchard plot or a computerised program could be resolved into two populations of sites, the first one with an affinity similar to the single component in control membranes and the second one with an affinity increased by about 30-fold . The size of the latter component was progressively increased with the NEM-concentration. This suggests that the effect of the thiol-alkylating agent was to shift a fraction of the H_1-receptors from a state of low affinity for the agonist into a state of higher affinity. The fact that, even at the highest NEM-concentration tested (5 mM) only 50 % of the receptors were shifted might indicate an heterogeneity of the binding sites, with only a fraction of them sensitive to NEM. A similar observation was reported for β-adrenoreceptors and related to the existence of a NEM-resistant subpopulation of sites not functionally coupled to the adenylate cyclase (Vauquelin and Maguire, 1980). In the case of H_1-receptors the effector system is not a cyclase but, presumably a calcium translocation system (Schwartz, 1979) and, therefore, it is difficult to draw any parallel.

TABLE 1 Effect of 5 mM NEM-treatment on the inhibition of ^{3}H-mepyramine binding to membranes of guinea-pig cerebellum by various H_1-receptor agonists

AGONIST	IC_{50} VALUE (μM)	
	CONTROL	NEM-TREATED
Histamine	78 ± 3	21 ± 2*
2-Thiazolylethylamine	112 ± 6	49 ± 7*
Betahistine	101 ± 5	63 ± 4*
2-methylhistamine	226 ± 2	198 ± 21
2-phenylhistamine (SKF 71491)	11 ± 1	7 ± 1
2-(2-aminoethyl)imidazo [1,2-a] pyridine (SKF 71473)	16 ± 1	15 ± 1

Inhibition curves were performed in the presence of 0.6 nM ^{3}H-mepyramine. The overall IC_{50} value was determined from 10-14 different concentrations for each agonist.

From the EC_{50} values of HA in several H_1-receptor mediated systems (Palacios and co-workers, 1978 ; Daum, Hill and Young, 1982 ; Daum, Downes and Young, 1984) similar to its IC_{50} value in ^{3}H-mepyramine binding inhibition, it can be concluded that the low affinity component presumably corresponds to the receptor in a functional state. The lower EC_{50} values of HA regarding responses like guinea-pig ileum contraction or glycogen hydrolysis in brain slices seem related to a "receptor reserve" in these responses (Quach and co-workers, 1980). Therefore it is likely that NEM stabilises the H_1-receptors in a conformation distinct from that of the active state as previously proposed for other receptor types (see, for instance, Andre and co-workers, 1982 ; Blume, Mullikin-Kilpatrick and Larsen, 1983), an effect possibly related with the role of a critical thiol in agonist-mediated conformational transitions (Raftery and Moore, 1979). In agreement with this view, the NEM effects were well marked on the inhibition curve of HA or a full agonist like 2-thiazolylethylamine but less apparent on that of partial agonist like betahistine and inapparent on that of SKF 71473 a very partial agonist (Table 1).

Because neither agonists nor antagonists added even in high concentration with NEM were able to protect the receptor from the alkylating agent, the critical thiol group is presumably distant from the ligand binding domain. However the persistence of NEM effects on a digitonin solubilised preparation suggests that it is located on the receptor molecule itself or, at least, on a tightly bound protein. In contrast, for several receptors regulated by a guanylnucleotide binding protein, the effect of NEM, lost upon solubilisation, is attributed to the presence of a critical thiol on this protein (reviewed by Strauss, 1984). Our finding is, therefore, consistent with the hardly detectable effect of GTP on ^{3}H-mepyramine binding (Chang and Snyder, 1980).

GLYCOPROTEIN NATURE OF THE H_1-RECEPTOR DEMONSTRATED BY AFFINITY CHROMATOGRAPHY

The first step in the purification of membrane-bound receptors consists in obtaining them in soluble form. After several trials with various detergents (CHAPS, sodium cholate, octylglucoside lysolecithine, tween 80, digitonin) we have confirmed that the best agent was digitonin (Toll and Snyder, 1982), allowing a 50 % solubilisation of ^{3}H-mepyramine sites from guinea-pig cerebellar membranes.

The adsorption of these sites to lectin affinity columns was tested.
When the solubilised preparation was applied to Concanavalin A column, a large part of the ^{3}H-mepyramine binding sites were not bound to the lectin and only 2% were eluted with the specific sugar (Table II).
In contrast, most of the applied ^{3}H-mepyramine binding sites were retained onto a column of Wheat Germ Agglutinin, a lectin known to bind macromolecules containing N-acetyl-D-glucosamine. The specificity of the elution by N-acetyl-D-glucosamine was checked by the absence of retention of H_1-receptors on a column previously equilibrated with this sugar.
The poor recovery of ^{3}H-mepyramine binding sites for both lectins could not be attributed to a limited capacity of the column but rather suggested an unspecific tight adsorption to the lectin or a partial denaturation of the receptors. Nevertheless the specific sugar elution of the H_1-receptors clearly shows that the solubilised HA H_1-receptors are glycoproteins with a N-acetyl-D-glucosamine like glucosidic part.

TABLE 2 Affinity chromatography of solubilised ^{3}H-mepyramine binding sites from guinea-pig cerebellum on lectin column

FRACTION	^{3}H-MEPYRAMINE BINDING SITES (fmoles)	PROTEINS (mg)	PURIFICATION FACTOR
I - CONCANAVALIN A COLUMN			
Crude Solubilisate	1,695 (100 %)	11.3 (100 %)	1
Unbound	645 (38 %)	9.5 (84 %)	
α-methyl-D-mannoside eluted	35 (2 %)	1.0 (9 %)	
II - WHEAT GERM AGGLUTININ COLUMN			
Crude solubilisate	1,400 (100 %)	9.4 (100 %)	1
Unbound	107 (8 %)	7.9 (84 %)	
N-acetyl-D-glucosamine eluted	522 (37 %)	1.0 (10 %)	3.7

After solubilisation with 0.5 % digitonin, membranes were applied on the lectin column equilibrated with phosphate buffer containing 0.1% digitonin. After a washing step, specific elution was performed with the appropriate sugar (0.1 M). Binding assays were performed using 3 nM ^{3}H-mepyramine and the separation of bound from free ligand was achieved by using activated charcoal.

REFERENCES

Andre, C., Vauquelin, G., Severne, Y., De Backer, J.P., and Strosberg, A.D. (1982). Dual effect of N-ethylmaleimide on agonist-mediated conformational changes of β-adrenergic receptors. Biochem. Pharmacol., 31, 3657-3662.

Ariens, E.J., Beld, A.J., Rodrigues, D.E., Miranda, J.F., and Simonis, A.M. (1979). The pharmacon-effector concept. A basis for understanding the transmission of information in biological systems. In R.D. O'Brien (Ed.), The receptors, a comprehensive treatise, vol. 1. Plenum Press, New York and London. pp. 33-92.

Aronstam, R.S., Abood, L.G., and Hoss, W. (1978). Influence of sulfhydryl reagents and heavy metals on the functional state of the muscarinic acetylcholine receptor in rat brain. Mol. Pharmacol., 14, 575-588.

Blume, A.J., Mullikin-Kilpatrick, D., and Larsen, N.E. (1983). Involvement of sulfhydryl groups in the functional integrity of the opiate receptors of neuroblastoma x glioma hybrid. In Segawa et al. (Eds.), Molecular Pharmacology of neurotransmitter receptors. Raven Press, New York. pp. 259-268.

Chang, R.S.L., and Snyder, S.H. (1980). Histamine H_1-receptor binding sites in guinea-pig brain membranes : regulation of agonist interactions by guanine nucleotides and cations. J. Neurochem., 34, 916-922.

Daum, P.R., Hill, S.J., and Young, J.M. (1982). Histamine H_1-agonist potentiation of adenosine-stimulated cyclic AMP accumulation in slices of guinea-pig cerebral cortex : comparison of response and binding parameters. Brit. J. Pharmacol., 77, 347-357.

Daum, P.R., Downes, C.P., and Young, J.M. (1984). Histamine stimulation of inositol-1-phosphate accumulation in lithium-treated slices from regions of guinea-pig brain. J. Neurochem., 43, 25-31.

Fleisch, J.H., Krzan, M.C., and Titus, E. (1973). Pharmacologic receptor activity of rabbit aorta : effect of dithiothreitol and N-ethylmaleimide. Circulation Res., 33, 284-290.

Fleisch, J.H., Krzan, M.C., and Titus, E. (1974). Alterations in pharmacologic receptor activity by dithiothreitol. Am. J. Physiol., 227, 1243-1248.

Fontaine, J., Famaey, J.P., and Reuse, J. (1984). Potentiation by sulphydryl agents of the responses of guinea-pig isolated ileum to various agonists. J. Pharm. Pharmacol., 36, 450-453.

Freedman, S.B., Poat, J.A., and Woodruff, G.N. (1982). Influence of sodium and sulphydryl group on ^{3}H-sulpiride binding sites in rat striatal membranes. J. Neurochem., 38, 1459-1464.

Glover, W.E. (1979). Effect of dithiothreitol on histamine receptors in rabbit colon and guinea-pig ileum. Clin. and Exp. Pharmacol. and Physiol., 6, 151-157.

Hill, S.J., Emson, P.C., and Young, J.M. (1978). The binding of ^{3}H -mepyramine to histamine H_1-receptors in guinea-pig brain. J. Neurochem., 31, 997-1004.

Korner, M., Gilon, C., and Schramm, M. (1982). Locking of hormone in the β - adrenergic receptor by attack on a sulfhydryl in an associated component. J. Biol. Chem., 259, 3389-3396.

Nukada, T., Haga, T., and Ichiyama, A. (1983). Muscarinic receptors in porcine caudate nucleus II different effects of N-ethylmaleimide on ^{3}H-Cis-methyldioxolane binding to heat-labile (guanylnucleotie sensitive) sites and heat-stable (guanyl nucleotide-insensitive) sites. Mol. Pharmacol., 24, 374-379.

Palacios, J.M., Garbarg, M., Barbin, G., and Schwartz, J.C. (1978). Pharmacological characterization of histamine receptors mediating the stimulation of cyclic AMP accumulation in slices from guinea-pig hippocampus. Mol. Pharmacol., 14, 971-982.

Quach, T.T., Duchemin, A.M., Rose, C., and Schwartz, J.C. (1980). ^{3}H-glycogen hydrolysis elicited by histamine in mouse brain slices : selective involvement of H_1-receptors. Mol. Pharmacol., 17, 301-308.

Raftery, M.A., and Moore, H.G.H. (1979). Ligand-induced interconversion of affinity states in membrane-bound acetylcholine receptor from Torpedo californica. Effects of sulfhydryl and disulfide reagents. Biochemistry, 18, 1907-1911.

Schwartz, J.C. (1979). Histamine receptors in brain. Life Sci., 25, 895-912.

Simon, E.J., and Groth, J. (1975). Kinetics of opiate receptor inactivation by sulfhydryl reagents : evidence for conformational change in the presence of sodium ions. Proc. Nat. Acad. Sci., USA, 72, 2404-2407.

Smith, M., and Harden, T.K. (1984). Modification of receptor-mediated inhibition of adenylate cyclase in NG 108-15 neuroblastoma x glioma cells by N-ethylmaleimide. J. Pharmacol. Exp. Ther., 228, 425-433.

Stadel, J.M., and Lefkowitz, R.J. (1979). Multiple reactive sulfhydryl groups modulate the function of adenylate cyclase coupled to beta-adrenergic receptors. Mol. Pharmacol., 16, 709-718.

Strauss, W.L. (1984). Sulfhydryl groups and disulfide bonds : modification of amino acid residues in studies of receptor structure and function. In J.C. Venter and L.C. Harrison (Eds.), Membranes detergents and receptor solubilization. Alan P. Liss, Inc., New York. pp. 85-97.

Toll, L., and Snyder, S.H. (1982). Solubilization and characterization of histamine H_1-receptors in brain. J. Biol. Chem., 257, 13593-13629.

Vauquelin, G., and Maguire, M.E. (1980). Inactivation of β-adrenergic receptors by N-ethylmaleimide in S49 lymphoma cells. Agonist induction of functional receptor heterogeneity. Mol. Pharmacol., 18, 362-369.

HISTAMINE H_1-AGONIST STIMULATED BREAKDOWN OF INOSITOL PHOSPHOLIPIDS

H. Carswell, P. R. Daum and J. M. Young

Department of Pharmacology, University of Cambridge,
Hills Road, Cambridge, UK

ABSTRACT

The histamine-induced breakdown of inositol phospholipids in slices of guinea-pig brain has been investigated by measurement of the accumulation of inositol 1-phosphate which occurs in the presence of 10 mM Li^+ ion. The response has the properties expected for an H_1-receptor mediated process and is greatest in those brain regions with the highest H_1-receptor density. However, the characteristics of the response to histamine seem to differ in cerebellum and cerebral cortex. Marked differences are also observed between the two regions in the extent of the response to the partial agonists 2-methylhistamine and N,N-dimethylhistamine. These observations suggest that the mechanism of the histamine-induced formation of inositol 1-phosphate in guinea-pig brain regions might be more complex than purely activation of the inositol cycle.

KEYWORDS

Histamine; H_1-receptors; inositol phospholipids; lithium; inositol phosphates; 2-methylhistamine; N,N-dimethylhistamine;

INTRODUCTION

Activation of histamine H_1-receptors can lead to a wide variety of cellular responses, including such diverse effects as contraction of smooth muscle cells, stimulation of glycogen breakdown, induction of the release of derivatives of arachidonic acid, stimulation of cyclic GMP formation and potentiation of the actions of directly acting activators of adenylate cyclase. However, there is evidence to suggest that the primary action of H_1-agonists on all cell types is to increase the intracellular concentration of free Ca^{2+} ions and that most, if not all, of the cellular responses are secondary to this change in the Ca^{2+} concentration. What has remained more controversial is the biochemical mechanism by which H_1-receptor activation is coupled to calcium mobilisation. For nearly a decade Michell has argued vigorously and cogently that the essential step in this process, and one common to all receptors which act via changes in the intracellular Ca^{2+} concentration, is the agonist-stimulated breakdown of inositol phospholipids (Michell, 1975). In the last year or so there has been a quite dramatic accumulation of evidence to support this proposition.

The original observations of agonist-induced changes in inositol phospholipid metabolism were made by the Hokins some thirty years ago (Hokin and Hokin,

1953, 1955) who found that muscarinic agonists caused an enhanced incorporation of ^{32}Pi into phosphatidylinositol. The current view of the cycle of reactions involved in this response is shown in Fig. 1.

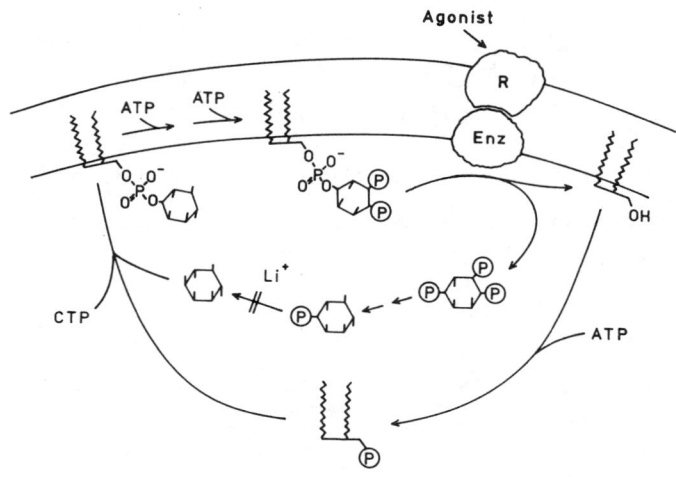

Fig. 1. Agonist-stimulated inositol phospholipid metabolism. Combination of agonist with its receptor activates a phosphodiesterase which catalyses the breakdown of phosphatidylinositol 4,5-bisphosphate to give myo-inositol 1,4,5-trisphosphate and 1,2-diacylglycerol. The 1,4,5-trisphosphate is broken down stepwise by phosphatases to yield inositol 1-phosphate and free myo-inositol. Phosphatidic acid, formed by the action of a kinase on 1,2-diacylglycerol, is activated by reaction with CTP to form CDP-diacylglycerol (not shown), which combines with inositol to form phosphatidylinositol. This in turn is phosphorylated by kinases in the plasma membrane to complete the cycle by forming phosphatidylinositol 4,5-bisphosphate. The action of Li^+ is to inhibit inositol 1-phosphatase and thus cause accumulation of inositol 1-phosphate.

The evidence for this scheme has been admirably reviewed recently by Berridge (1984) and will not be repeated here. The only essential difference from the original scheme proposed by Michell (1975) is that the step catalysed by the agonist is considered to be the breakdown of phosphatidylinositol 4,5-bisphosphate rather than that of phosphatidylinositol itself. The rapid equilibration between the phosphoinositides had been observed by early workers (see Michell, 1975) as had the agonist-stimulated breakdown of the 4,5-bisphosphate (see Berridge, 1984), but the significance of these observations only became clear when it was demonstrated that the agonist-induced breakdown of phosphatidylinositol 4,5-bisphosphate occurs much more rapidly than that of phosphatidylinositol (Michell and others, 1981). A considerable impulse to the acceptance of the central role of agonist-stimulated phosphoinositide breakdown in cellular response has been given by the discovery that both of the products of the cleavage, inositol 1,4,5-trisphosphate and 1,2-diacylglycerol, appear to have a role as second messengers. Inositol 1,4,5-trisphosphate has been shown to induce the release of Ca^{2+} from non-mitochondrial intracellular membranes (Berridge, 1984), while diacylglycerol activates protein kinase C (reviewed by Nishizuka, 1984), which is also the target for tumour promoting phorbol esters. A further way in which inositol phospholipid breakdown may be linked to cellular response depends on the fact that the fatty acid at carbon 2 in the phosphoinositides is usually arachidonate. Cleavage at this position through the action of a diacylglycerol lipase or a phospholipase acting on phosphatidic acid may be important pathways for the agonist-induced release of arachidonic acid (Berridge, 1984).

Despite the volume of the literature on the agonist-stimulated breakdown of inositol phospholipids, the response to histamine has been relatively little explored, probably because of the lack of any pronounced action on the secretory tissues on which many of the early experiments concentrated. Some ten years ago Friedel and Schanberg (1975) observed that histamine injected intracisternally in rats stimulated the incorporation of ^{33}Pi into phosphatidic acid and phosphatidylinositol, although some stimulation of the labelling of phosphatidylcholine was also noted. The enhanced phospholipid labelling was blocked by prior administration of the H_1-antagonist tripelennamine. These observations have been confirmed and extended by Subramanian and others (1980), who also used the receptor selective agonists, 2-pyridylethylamine (H_1) and dimaprit (H_2), and antagonists, mepyramine (H_1) and cimetidine (H_2) to provide further evidence of the H_1-receptor selectivity of the response. The development of the histamine-stimulated incorporation of ^{33}Pi into brain phospholipids in newborn rats paralleled the increase in [^3H]mepyraminebinding sites (Subramanian and others, 1981). Peripherally histamine has been shown to produce a mepyramine-sensitive increase in ^{32}Pi incorporation into phosphatidylinositol in guinea-pig intestinal smooth muscle in vitro (Jafferji and Michell, 1976) and, more recently, in rabbit aortic rings (Villalobos-Molina and Garcia-Sainz, 1983).

While there can be little doubt that these studies do provide good evidence for an H_1-receptor-mediated response, determination of the incorporation of ^{32}Pi or [^3H]inositol into phosphatidylinositol is only an indirect measure of the actual step catalysed by the agonist, namely the hydrolysis of phosphatidylinositol 4,5-bisphosphate (Fig. 1). Further, in brain tissues accurate measurement of the relatively small agonist-stimulated increase in inositol phospholipid labelling has often proved difficult. A distinct methodological breakthrough has come with the development of a more direct and sensitive method of monitoring the agonist-stimulated step (Berridge, Downes and Hanley, 1982). The crux of this method is the presence in the incubation medium of 5-10 mM Li^+ ion, which earlier workers have shown to cause the accumulation of inositol 1-phosphate in cells (Allison and others, 1976) as a result of the selective inhibition of inositol 1-phosphatase (Naccarato, Ray and Wells, 1974; Hallcher and Sherman, 1980; Sherman and others, 1981). The tissue is preincubated with [^3H]inositol and the course of the agonist-stimulated breakdown of [^3H]phosphatidylinositol 4,5-bisphosphate monitored by measuring the accumulated [^3H]inositol 1-phosphate, which is separated from other water soluble phosphates by anion-exchange chromatography (Berridge and others, 1982). Using this assay histamine has been shown to stimulate [^3H]inositol 1-phosphate accumulation in slices of rat cerebral cortex (Berridge and others, 1982; Brown, Kendall and Nahorski, 1984). The assay has also formed the basis for our own studies in guinea-pig brain (Daum, Downes and Young, 1983, 1984).

Our interest in histamine-induced inositol phospholipid breakdown was originally stimulated by the proposition that this reaction is an invariable consequence of H_1-receptor activation. If this is true then histamine-induced inositol phospholipid breakdown should be a test of H_1-receptor functionality analagous to that provided by the stimulation of adenylate cyclase by H_2-receptor activation. This has the potential to be of particular utility in studies of H_1-receptors in the CNS, where the relationship between [^3H]mepyramine binding sites and functional receptors has been uncertain and where other biochemical responses to H_1-receptor activation are limited in number and tissue or species dependent.

METHODS

All measurements have been carried out at 37° on cross-chopped slices (300 x 300 μm or, more recently, 350 x 350 μm) prepared on a McIlwain tissue chopper. Measurement of [^{3}H]inositol 1-phosphate accumulation in the presence of 10 mM LiCl following preincubation of the slices with 0.33 μM myo-[2-^{3}H]inositol was made using the method of Berridge and others (1982). The incubation conditions are decribed in detail elsewhere (Daum and others, 1984). Incubation with histamine was routinely for 60 min. In the first series of experiments [^{3}H]inositol 1-phosphate was separated from other water-soluble reaction products on Dowex-1 anion exchange resin (formate form) using the simplified batch elution procedure, but more recently the 1-phosphate has been separated on columns essentially as decribed by Berridge and others (1982).

RESULTS AND DISCUSSION

Quantitation of the Response to Histamine

Within a series of experiments carried out under similar experimental conditions the response of brain slices to histamine is usually fairly constant. However, occasionally the magnitude of the response may vary quite markedly. This raises the fundamental question of how the extent of the response to histamine should be expressed. In an early series of experiments using cerebral cortical slices it was apparent that although the absolute magnitude of the response to histamine (stimulated-basal) differed between experiments the response to histamine expressed as percentage of basal was much less variable. The success of this measure is presumably that it allows for differing viabilities of slice preparations. Thus if 50% of the cells are non-functional in a preparation the absolute magnitude of the response to histamine is clearly less than in a fully viable slice preparation, but the percentage stimulation over basal may be the same. It must be borne in mind, however, that the relationship of the agonist-induced increase in the level of [^{3}H]inositol 1-phosphate to the accumulation in the absence of agonist (basal) is unknown. The basal level may reflect accumulation in a much wider population of cells than those stimulated by histamine and may not occur by the same biochemical pathways. If experimental conditions vary between two experiments then comparison of the agonist induced responses as percentage of basal may give a misleading impression. This point is discussed below with respect to the action of lithium in cerebellar slices. A more trivial way in which stimulation of basal can be misleading is that batches of [^{3}H]inositol from different suppliers can give widely differing levels of basal accumulation even though the absolute magnitude of the histamine-stimulated accumulation may be the same. Even if charged impurities are removed from the [^{3}H]inositol by passage through ion-exchange columns the stabilities of the purified material can vary markedly.

Characterisation and Time Course of the Response to Histamine

The accumulation of [^{3}H]inositol 1-phosphate induced by 100 μM histamine is blocked by 1 μM mepyramine, but not by 100 μM cimetidine. Similarly the H_2-selective agonist dimaprit (1 mM) produced no significant accumulation whereas 2-thiazolylethylamine (400 μM) gave a response in cerebellar slices of the same order as that given by histamine. These data are all consistent with an H_1-receptor mediated response, as earlier workers have demonstrated for enhanced incorporation of ^{32}Pi or ^{33}Pi into phosphatidylinositol (Friedel and Schanberg, 1975; Jafferji and Michell, 1976; Subramanian and others, 1980). The best evidence, discussed later, is the agreement of the affinity constant derived for mepyramine with that determined for other H_1-responses (Daum and others, 1984). The same was true for methapyrilene, although the agreement was not quite so good.

The effect of increasing the incubation time with histamine on the accumulation of the three inositol phosphates, separated by stepwise elution from Dowex-1 (formate form) ion exchange resin, is shown in Fig. 2. The four peaks correspond to glycerophosphoinositol, inositol 1-phosphate, inositol 1,4-

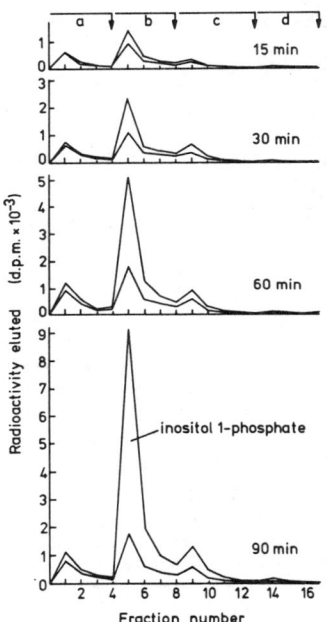

Fig. 2. Separation of [^{3}H]inositol phosphates on Dowex-1 formate anion exchange columns. The upper trace on each panel is from incubations containing 100 μM histamine. The lower trace is the basal level in the absence of agonist. Stepwise elution with: a, 5 mM sodium tetraborate/60 mM ammonium formate: b, 5 mM sodium tetraborate/200 mM ammonium formate; c, 100 mM formic acid/300 mM ammonium formate and d, 100 mM formic acid/1 M ammonium formate. (Reproduced with permission from the Journal of Neurochemistry).

bisphosphate and (barely visible except at 90 min), inositol 1,4,5-trisphosphate. At all times measured the greatest stimulation is in the inositol 1-phosphate peak, consistent with the action of Li$^+$ as an inhibitor of inositol 1-phosphatase. A more detailed time-course from a similar experiment with cerebral cortical slices is shown in Fig. 3 (note the differing scales on the ordinates of the three graphs). The most striking feature is the apparent

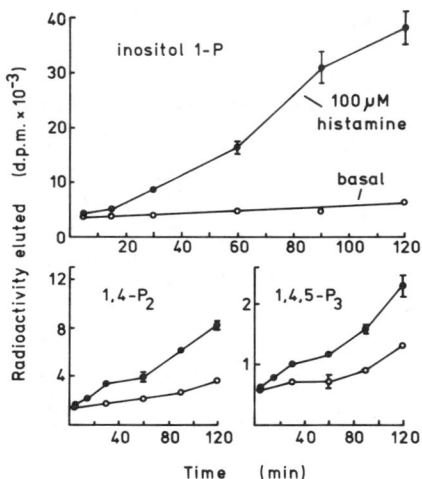

Fig. 3. Time course of the response to 100 μM histamine in cerebral cortical slices. Error bars represent ± S.E. Where no bar is drawn the error was within the size of the symbol. The lower graphs show the levels of inositol 1,4-bisphosphate (1,4-P_2) and inositol 1,4,5-trisphosphate (1,4,5-P_3).

lack of any desensitisation in the stimulation produced by 100 μM histamine even after 120 min incubation. If desensitisation occurs, as might be expected, then it cannot be at the receptor level. A similar time course of agonist-stimulated inositol 1-phosphate accumulation has been observed for other neurotransmitters (e.g. carbachol, Berridge and others, 1982). The lack of any desensitation also implies that curves of agonist binding, usually determined from inhibition of [^{3}H]mepyramine binding, should represent binding to the active conformation of the receptor and gives grounds for hope that it may ultimately be possible to correlate parameters of binding and response.

Histamine does cause some accumulation of inositol 1,4-bisphosphate and inositol 1,4,5-trisphosphate, but the effect is small.

Calcium Dependence of the Response to Histamine

In rat cerebral cortical slices the response to histamine is completely abolished simply by omission of calcium from the medium (Kendall and Nahorski, 1984). This is not what would be expected if [^{3}H]inositol 1-phosphate is generated solely by the pathway indicated in Fig. 1. The results of a similar experiment carried out on slices from ginea-pig cerebral cortex in which incubation was initially in calcium-free Krebs-Henseleit medium, followed by incubation with 200 μM histamine in the presence or absence of 2.5 mM Ca^{2+} or in the presence of 0.5 mM EGTA are set out in Table 1.

Table 1. Calcium-dependence of the response to histamine in cerebral cortical slices

	[^{3}H]Inositol 1-phosphate accumulated (d.p.m)		
	2.5mM Ca^{2+}	No Ca^{2+}	0.5mM EGTA
Basal	988 ± 29	881 ± 33	763 ± 21
200 μM histamine	1933 ± 161	1407 ± 43	809 ± 47
Histamine-basal	945 ± 164	526 ± 54	46 ± 51

Cerebral cortical slices were preincubated in calcium-free Krebs-Henseleit medium before incubation for 60 min with or without 200 μM histamine with or without 2.5 mM Ca^{2+} or with 0.5 mM EGTA (no Ca^{2+}).

Omitting Ca^{2+} from the medium reduces the response to histamine, but does not abolish it. As in the rat (Kendall and Nahorski, 1984) the response to histamine disappears in the presence of 0.5 mM EGTA, as did the response to 200 μM carbachol measured in a parallel experiment. The response to histamine in the guinea-pig may thus differ from that in the rat, but there are several fators which complicate the interpretation of this type of experiment. The most important one is that an appreciable Ca^{2+} concentration in the medium occurs even in the absence of added Ca^{2+} as a result of release from the slices (26 μM in the experiment in Table 2). A proper evaluation of the role of added Ca^{2+} in the response to histamine in guinea-pig slices will require close control of the concentration of free Ca^{2+}.

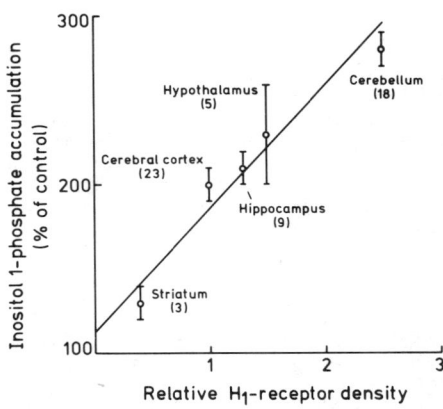

Fig. 4. Correlation between stimulation of [^{3}H]inositol 1-phosphate accumulation by histamine and H$_1$-receptor density.

Relationship of the Magnitude of the Response to H_1-Receptor Density

The relationship between [^{3}H]inositol 1-phosphate accumulation stimulated by 100 M histamine in slices from various regions of guinea-pig brain and the relative density of histamine H_1-receptors (cerebral cortex = 1), taken from Hill, Emson and Young (1978), is shown in Fig. 4. The measurements on [^{3}H]inositol, 1-phosphate accumulation encompass all the experiments which used the simplified batch procedure for isolation of the 1-phosphate (see Methods). The good correlation is encouraging and suggests that H_1-receptor sites labelled by [^{3}H]mepyramine do represent functional receptors. Conversely it is consistent with the proposition that inositol phospholipid breakdown is always associated with H_1-receptor activation. However, caution needs to be exercised in quantitative interpretation of the data. Reservations have already been expressed over the use of percentage stimulation over basal, particularly here in comparing different brain regions, even though in any one region the response expressed in this way is much less variable. The other difficulty which has emerged more recently, and which is discussed below, is that the characteristics of the response to histamine may differ between brain areas.

Li^+ Amplification of the Response to Histamine

The response to histamine in slices of guinea-pig cerebellum is much less dependent of the presence of Li^+ ions than the response in cerebral cortical slices (Table 2). In contrast the accumulation of [^{3}H]inositol 1-phosphate

Table 2. Li^+-Dependence of the Response to Histamine.

Region	Ratio of accumulated levels of [^{3}H]-inositol 1-P (+Li/-Li).	
	Basal	Histamine-Basal
Cerebellum (5)	1.6 ± 0.2	1.8 ± 0.2
Cerebral cortex (3)	1.1 ± 0.1	5.3 ± 0.7

Each value is the mean $\pm$ S.E. (number of determinations) of the ratio of the amount of [^{3}H]inositol 1-phosphate accumulated in the presence of 10 mM LiCl to the amount accumulated in the absence of lithium measured on the same slice preparation. Incubation with or without (basal) 100 μM histamine was for 60 min. Histamine-basal is the difference in the amount accumulated in the presence and absence of histamine.

in the absence of histamine (basal) is increased in cerebellar slices in the presence of lithium, but not significantly in cerebral cortical slices. As a result of this, if the accumulation in the presence of histamine is expressed as a percentage of basal, then in cerebellum the value is practically the same in the presence or absence of Li^+. The effect of Li^+ on the response in hippocampal slices was intermediate between those of cerebellum and cerebral cortex (Daum and others, 1984). Interestingly Brown and others (1984) have reported that the response to histamine in slices of rat cerebral cortex is little altered by the presence of Li^+.

The ability to obtain an appreciable response to histamine in cerebellar slices in the absence of lithium has provided an opportunity to test whether 10 mM Li^+ has any direct effect on H_1-receptor function. A dose-response curve to histamine measured in the absence of lithium was practically superimposable on a curve obtained from the combined data from 3 independent experiments in the presence of Li$^+$ (Fig. 5).

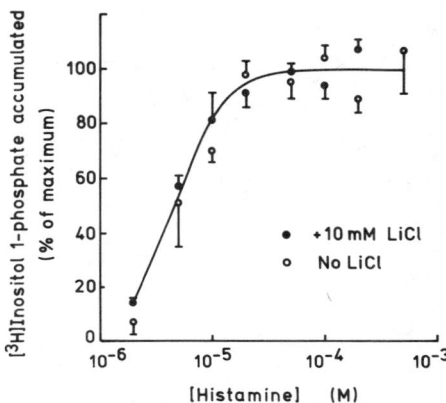

Fig. 5. Effect of Li$^+$ on the dose-response curve to histamine in cerebellar slices. Incubation with histamine was for 60 min. (●), Combined data from 3 independent determinations in the presence of 10 mM LiCl. (o), Values obtained from a single experiment with no Li$^+$ present.

Differences in the Response of H$_1$ Agonists in Cerebellum and Cerebral Cortex

In early experiments it was not apparent that there was any significant difference in the characteristics of the dose-response curve to histamine in cerebellum, cerebral cortex, hippocampus or hypothalamus. However, a more detailed re-evaluation of the response to histamine has shown that dose-response curves for histamine in cerebellar and cerebral cortical slices differ both in position and shape (Fig. 6). Best-fit values of the EC_{50} are 20 ± 3 μM in cerebral cortex and 5 ±1 μM in cerebellum. The EC_{50} for histamine is similar to the value 16 μM, derived from histamine inhibition of the binding of [^{3}H]mepyramine to a cerebral cortical homogenate (Daum, Hill and Young, 1982). This suggests that while the accumulation of [^{3}H]inositol 1-phosphate in cerebral cortex may occur via the inositol cycle depicted in Fig. 1, the process in cerebellum, where the EC_{50} is lower, may be more complex. Consistent with this, whereas the Hill coefficient for the histamine dose-response curve in cerebral cortex was 1.1 ± 0.1, that in cerebellum, 2.1 ± 0.1, was significantly greater than unity.

Further evidence for a difference in the nature of the response in cerebellum and cerebral cortex has come from an investigation of the action of 2-methylhistamine and N^α,N^α-dimethylhistamine, both of which were partial agonists on the H$_1$-agonist potentiation of adenosine-stimulated accumulation of cyclic AMP in guinea-pig cerebral cortical slices, where the EC_{50} for histamine was 5 ± 1 μM (Hill coefficient 0.97 ± 0.12) (Daum and others, 1982). On both cerebellar and cerebral cortical slices 2-methylhistamine and N^α,N^α-dimethylhistamine were partial agonists (Table 3), but reached a greater percentage of the maximum response to histamine than in cerebral cortex. In analogy to histamine the EC_{50} for 2-methylhistamine and N,N-dimethylhistamine was greater in cerebral cortex,

75 ± 15 and 90 ± 40 μM, respectively, than in cerebellum, 13 ± 2 and 22 ± 14 μM. The potency ratios with respect to histamine did not differ significantly between the two tissues (26 ± 6 and 36 ± 7 for 2-methylhistamine and 22 ± 10 and 21 ± 14 for N,N-dimethylhistamine).

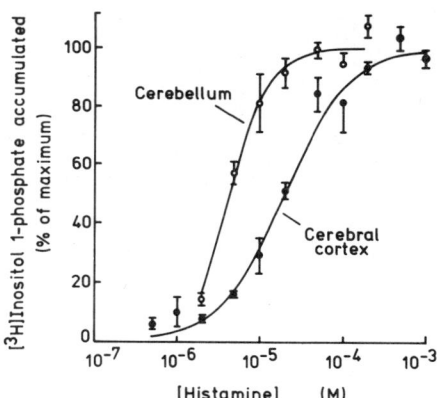

Fig. 6 Comparison of dose-response curves to histamine in cerebellum and cerebral cortex. Each curve is a weighted best-fit line to the combined data from 3 experiments.

Table 3. Responses to H_1-agonists in cerebellum and cerebral cortex

	Maximum Response (%)	
	Cerebellum	Cerebral cortex
Histamine	100	100
2-Methylhistamine	84 ± 6	32 ± 2
N^α,N^α-Dimethylhistamine	70 ± 13	23 ± 3

The quantitative evaluation of the dose-response curves for the partial agonists is complicated by the apparent presence of a non-H_1-receptor mediated component at the high concentrations needed to define the top of the curve. The same is true for high concentrations of histamine. The response to histamine in cerebellum up to concentrations of approximately 100 μM appears to be almost entirely H_1-receptor mediated. The best evidence for this is that the approximately 10 fold shift of the dose-response curve to histamine in the presence of 5 nM mepyramine yields an affinity constant, $2.3 \times 10^9 M^{-1}$, of the same order as that, $1.4 \times 10^9 M^{-1}$ determined from mepyramine inhibition of [^{3}H] mepyramine binding in cerebellar homogenates and the value, $1.6 \times 10^9 M^{-1}$, from mepyramine antagonism of the histamine-induced contraction of intestinal smooth muscle (Daum and others, 1984). However, if a dose-response curve for histamine stimulated accumulation of [^{3}H]inositol 1-phosphate is measured in the presence of 1 μM mepyramine the apparent affinity constant for mepyramine falls to $5.3 \times 10^8 M^{-1}$. A similar experiment with 2-methylhistamine as agonist yielded an even lower constant of $2.3 \times 10^8 M^{-1}$.

Although the likely presence of a non-H_1 component complicates the interpretation of the dose-response curves for the partial agonists it seems probable that the difference in response between the two brain regions is real. Certainly the histamine dose-response curves do not extend to concentrations at which there is any evidence for any marked non-H_1-receptor mechanism.

CONCLUSION AND PROSPECTS

It will be evident from the modest amount of information on H_1-agonist stimulated inositol phospholipid hydrolysis, summarised in this chapter, and from the small number of references that can be cited, that the study of histamine interaction with inositol phospholipid metabolism is still very much in its infancy. It seems a safe prophesy that a review on this topic written in five years time will look very different. However, even at this stage there are signs in the differing effects of lithium in different regions and in the apparent differences in the response to histamine, 2-methylhistamine and N,N-dimethylhistamine in cerebellum and cerebral cortex that the response may prove to be more complex than the scheme in Fig. 1 suggests. The relationship of calcium gating to inositol phospholipid metabolism remains obscure, but calcium gating and large amounts of calcium entering the cell from the external medium during prolonged stimulation could well be central to understanding complexities of the histamine response still only dimly perceived.

ACKNOWLEDGEMENTS

Our thanks are due to the Medical Research Council for the financial support of this project.

REFERENCES

Allison, J.H., M.E. Blisner, W.H. Holland, P.P. Hipps and W.R. Sherman (1976). Increased brain myo-inositol 1-phosphate in lithium-treated rats. Biochem.Biophys.Res.Commun., 71, 664-676.
Berridge, M.J. (1984). Inositol trisphosphate and diacylglycerol as second messengers. Biochem.J., 220, 345-360.
Berridge, M.J., C.P. Downes and M.R. Hanley (1982). Lithium amplified agonist-dependent phosphatidylinositol responses in brain and salivary glands. Biochem.J., 206, 587-595.
Brown, E., D.A. Kendall and S.R. Nahorski (1984). Inositol phospholipid hydrolysis in rat cerebral cortical slices: I. Receptor characterisation. J.Neurochem., 42, 1379-1387.
Daum, P.R., C.P. Downes and J.M. Young (1983). Histamine induced inositol phospholipid breakdown mirrors H_1-receptor density in brain. Eur.J.Pharmacol., 87, 497-498.
Daum, P.R., C.P. Downes and J.M. Young (1984). Histamine stimulation of inositol 1-phosphate accumulation in lithium-treated slices from regions of guinea-pig brain. J.Neurochem., 25, 25-32.
Daum, P.R., S.J. Hill and J.M. Young (1982). Histamine H_1-agonist potentiation of adenosine-stimulated cyclic AMP accumulation in slices of guinea-pig cerebral cortex: comparison of response and binding parameters. Br.J.Pharmacol., 77, 347-357.
Friedel, R.O. and S.M. Schanberg (1975). Effects of histamine on phospholipid metabolism in rat brain in vivo. J.Neurochem., 24, 819-820.

Hallcher, L.M. and W.R. Sherman (1980). The effects of lithium and other agents on the activity of myo-inositol-1-phosphatase from bovine brain. J.Biol.Chem., 255, 10896-10901.

Hill, S.J, P.C. Emson and J.M. Young (1978). The binding of [^{3}H]mepyramine to histamine H_1-receptors in guinea-pig brain. J.Neurochem., 31, 997-1004.

Hokin, M.R. and L.E. Hokin (1953). Enzyme secretion and the incorporation of P^{32} into phospholipides of pancreas slices. J.Biol.Chem., 203, 967-977.

Hokin, L.E. and M.R. Hokin (1955). Effects of acetylcholine on the turnover of phosphoryl units in individual phospholipids of pancreas slices and brain cortex slices. Biochim.Biophys.Acta, 18, 102-110.

Jafferji, S.S. and R.H. Michell (1976). Stimulation of phospatidylinositol turnover by histamine, 5-hydroxytryptamine and adrenaline in the longitudinal smooth muscle of the guinea-pig ileum. Biochem.Pharmacol., 25, 1429-1430.

Kendall, D.A. and S.R. Nahorski (1984). Inositol phospholipid hydrolysis in rat cerebral cortical slices: II. Calcium requirement. J.Neurochem., 42, 1388-1394.

Michell, R.H. (1975). Inositol phospholipids and cell surface receptor function. Biochim.Biophys.Acta, 415, 81-147.

Michell, R.H., C.J. Kirk, L.M. Jones, C.P. Downes and J.A. Creba (1981). The stimulation of inositol phospholipid metabolism that accompanies calcium mobilization in stimulated cells: defined characteristics and unanswered questions. Philos.Trans.R.Soc.Lond.(Biol.), 296, 123-137.

Naccarato, W.F., R.E. Ray and W.W. Wells (1974). Biosynthesis of myo-inositol in rat mammary gland. Isolation and properties of the enzymes. Arch.Biochem.Biophys., 164, 194-201.

Nishizuka, Y. (1984). The role of protein kinase C in cell surface signal transduction and tumour promotion. Nature, 308, 693-698.

Sherman, W.R., A.L. Leavitt, M.P. Honchar, L.M. Hallcher and B.E. Phillips (1981). Evidence that lithium alters phosphoinositide metabolism; chronic administration elevates primarily D-myo-inositol 1-phosphate in cerebral cortex of the rat. J.Neurochem., 36, 1947-1951.

Subramanian, N., W.L. Whitmore, F.J. Seidler and T.A. Slotkin (1980). Histamine stimulates brain phospholipid turnover through a direct H-1 receptor mechanism. Life Sci., 27, 1315-1319.

Subramanian, N., W.L. Whitmore, F.J. Seidler and T.A. Slotkin (1981). Ontogeny of histaminergic neurotransmission in the rat brain: concomitant development of neuronal histamine, H_1-receptors, and H_1-receptor mediated stimulation of phospholipid turnover. J.Neurochem., 36, 1137-1141.

Villalobos-Molina, R. and J.A. Garcia-Sainz (1983). H_1-Histaminergic activation stimulates phosphatidylinositol labeling in rabbit aorta. Eur.J.Pharmacol., 90, 457-459.

CHIRAL AGONISTS OF HISTAMINE

W. Schunack*, S. Schwarz**, G. Gerhard**,
S. Büyüktimkin** and S. Elz**

*Institute of Pharmacy, Free University of Berlin, D-1000
Berlin 33, Federal Republic of Germany
**Institute of Pharmacy, Johannes Gutenberg-Universität,
Mainz, Federal Republic of Germany

ABSTRACT

The synthesis of chiral histamine analogues is described. The optically pure enantiomers were prepared outgoing from L- and D-histidine, or by resolution using either dibenzoyl- respectively di-O-(p-toluoyl)tartaric acid or p-chlorotartranilic acid. The absolute configuration was determined through ORD-measurements as well as by X-ray structure analysis. The enantiomers were tested on the isolated guinea-pig ileum for H_1- and on the isolated spontaneously beating guinea-pig atrium for H_2-agonistic activity. At the H_1-receptor all enantiomeric pairs show an activity ratio of S/R=1. At the H_2-receptor those chiral derivatives of histamine having an absolute configuration corresponding to R-configurated D-histidine, possess greater activity. From the chiral isomers of Impromidine, the R-configurated Sopromidine (which corresponds to S-configurated L-histidine) has 7.4 times the activity of histamine on the atrium whereas the S-enantiomer shows H_2-antagonistic action. The results illustrate, a high degree of stereoselectivity is characteristic of the H_2-receptor.

KEYWORDS

Chiral histamine agonists; enantiomeric histamine agonists; Sopromidine; Impromidine isomers; chiral guanidines; chiral α-substituted histamines.

INTRODUCTION

Histamine is an achiral substance. The purpose of this investigation was the preparation of chiral agonists of histamine and the research of their activity concerning histamine H_1- and H_2-receptors. Important questions to be answered were:
Which degree of stereoselectivity do the two receptor types show? Do the enantiomers possess the same H_2:H_1 activity ratio?

When we started our experiments only one pair of enantiomers had been investigated. Chapman and Williams (1953) have described the synthesis of 2-(2-aminopropyl)pyridine and its resolution into (+)- and (-)-isomers. Graham and Tonks (1956) found that the (+)-isomer is some three times as active as the (-)-isomer (cat gastric acid secretion; guinea-pig ileum) but the agonist activity is less than 1 % that of histamine.

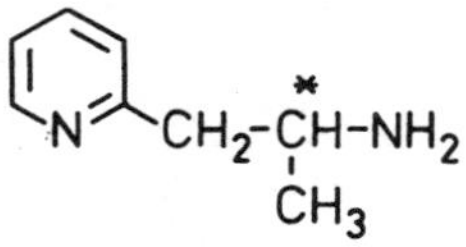

2-(2-aminopropyl)pyridine

CHEMISTRY AND PHARMACOLOGY

In the series of histamine analogues with α-branched side chain the optically pure enantiomers were obtained by resolution or by synthesis outgoing from L- and D-histidine.

Resolution of 5-amino-4,5,6,7-tetrahydrobenzimidazole with (-)-dibenzoyltartaric acid yields the (+)-enantiomer, with (+)-dibenzoyltartaric acid the (-)-enantiomer (Schwarz and Schunack, 1979). 4-(2-Aminopropyl)-5-methylimidazole (5,α-dimethylhistamine) was resolved with p-chlorotartranilic acid. The (+)-enantiomer was obtained with (-)-p-chlorotartranilic acid, the (-)-enantiomer by means of the (+)-acid (Schwarz and Schunack, 1982). The absolute configuration was determined by ORD- and CD-measurements of the phthalimide derivatives.

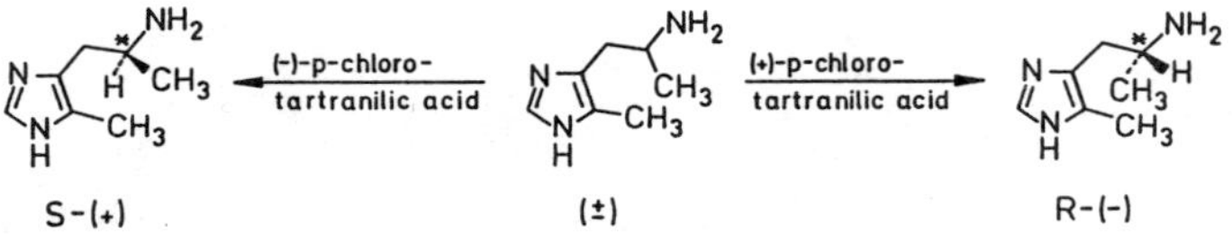

Fig. 1. Resolution of (±)-4-(2-aminopropyl)-5-methylimidazole with (+)- and (-)-p-chlorotartranilic acid

The enantiomeric α-methylhistamines can be synthesized starting from L- and D-histidine. Esterification and reduction with lithium aluminum hydride give the optically active histidinols. Reaction with thionylchloride yield the α-chloromethylhistamines, hydrogenation of which produce the optically pure enantiomers of α-methylhistamine (Gerhard and Schunack, 1980a, 1981). The enantiomeric α,N^α-dimethylhistamines can be prepared without racemisation from the α-methylhistamines by cyclisation with N,N'-carbonyldiimidazole followed by the reduction with lithium aluminum hydride (Gerhard and Schunack, 1980b). The absolute configuration was deduced and confirmed by means of ORD-measurements.

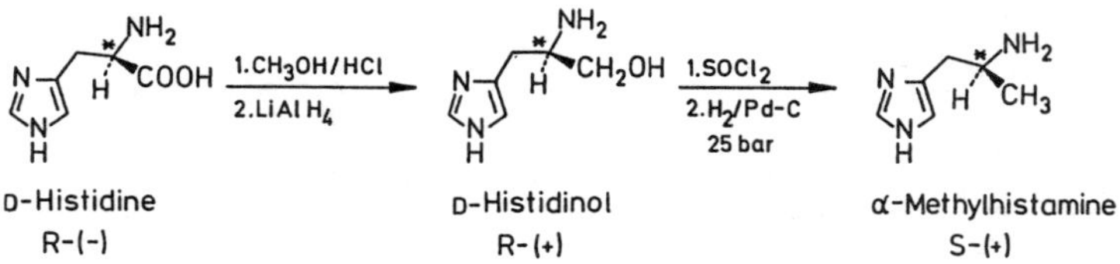

Fig. 2. Synthesis of S-(+)-α-methylhistamine from D-histidine.

The enantiomers were tested on the isolated guinea-pig ileum for H_1- and on the isolated spontaneously beating guinea-pig atrium for H_2-agonistic activity. The results are summarized in Table 1.

TABLE 1 Agonistic Activity at Guinea-pig Ileum (H_1) and Atrium (H_2)

Enantiomer	Configuration	Agonist activity (histamine=100)		$H_2:H_1$
		H_1	H_2	
imidazole-CH(NHCH$_3$)-CH$_3$	S	0.71 (0.51-1.07)	0.98 (0.74-1.26)	1.4:1
	R	0.69 (0.65-0.78)	0.42 (0.25-0.66)	0.6:1
imidazole-CH(NH$_2$)-CH$_3$	S	0.49 (0.21-0.81)	1.74 (1.00-3.47)	3.6:1
	R	0.49 (0.18-0.91)	1.02 (0.68-1.26)	2.1:1
imidazole-cyclic-NH$_2$	S	0.29 (0.25-0.33)	2.09 (1.58-2.75)	7.2:1
	R	0.29 (0.25-0.34)	0.30 (0.14-0.64)	1:1
imidazole-C(NH$_2$)(CH$_3$)-CH$_3$	S	0.26 (0.21-0.31)	8.71 (6.46-11.75)	33:1
	R	0.33 (0.26-0.46)	4.78 (3.98-5.75)	15:1
imidazole-CH(NH$_2$)-CH$_2$Cl	R	0.32 (0.17-0.60)	42.7 (30.2-63.1)	133:1
	S	0.30 (0.23-0.37)	17.4 (7.1-33.1)	58:1
imidazole-CH(NHCH$_3$)-CH$_2$Cl	R	0.30 (0.20-0.35)	51.3 (32.7-89.1)	171:1
	S	0.29 (0.12-1.02)	7.1 (4.0-13.2)	24:1

The first 3 histamine analogues in Table 1 are weak agonists. The 3 compounds listed last are selective agonists for H_2-receptors. In an enantiomeric pair the more effective enantiomer also shows the more marked activity ratio H_2/H_1. All compounds have only weak H_1-agonistic activity. The efficacy of the enantiomeric pairs in regard to H_1- and H_2-receptors as well as the structure and configuration of the more potent enantiomer are represented in Table 2.

As one can see, all enantiomeric pairs show an activity ratio S/R=1 at the H_1-receptor. At the H_2-receptor however, those enantiomers having an absolute configuration corresponding to R-configurated D-histidine, possess greater activity. The results illustrate the pronounced stereoselectivity of the H_2-receptor. If the H_1-receptor does or does not show any stereoselectivity can only be decided by means of highly effective chiral H_1-agonists. Up to now we have not succeeded in preparing substances having such an effect. α- or β-methylated 2-(2-aminoethyl)thiazoles possess weak, corresponding substituted isohistamines no H_1-agonistic potency (Steffens and Schunack, 1984).

TABLE 2 The Activity Ratio of the Enantiomers at H_1- and H_2-Receptors

Configuration	Enantiomer	H_1-receptor	H_2-receptor
S	imidazole-CH₂-C*H(NH₂)(CH₃)	$\frac{S}{R} = 1$	$\frac{S}{R} = 1.7$
S	imidazole-CH₂-C*(NH₂)(CH₃)₂	$\frac{S}{R} = 1$	$\frac{S}{R} = 1.8$
S	imidazole-CH₂-C*H(NHCH₃)(CH₃)	$\frac{S}{R} = 1$	$\frac{S}{R} = 2.3$
S	imidazole-cyclohexyl-NH₂	$\frac{S}{R} = 1$	$\frac{S}{R} = 7$
R	imidazole-CH₂-C*H(NH₂)(CH₂Cl)	$\frac{R}{S} = 1$	$\frac{R}{S} = 2.5$
R	imidazole-CH₂-C*H(NHCH₃)(CH₂Cl)	$\frac{R}{S} = 1$	$\frac{R}{S} = 7.2$
R	imidazole-CH₂-C*H(NH₂)(COOH)	D-Histidine	

In the series of histamine analogues with β-branched side chain the preparation of optically pure enantiomers is very difficult. β-methylhistamine was resolved with di-O-(p-toluoyl)tartaric acid.

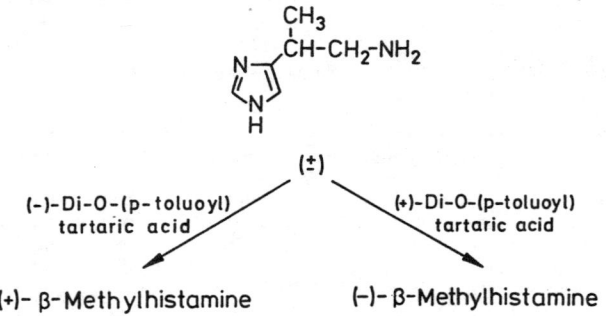

Fig. 3. Resolution of (±)-β-methylhistamine with (+)- and (-)-di-O-(p-toluoyl)tartaric acid

Chiral agonists of histamine

β-Methylhistamine is a weakly active agonist. The enantiomers show equal activity at the H_1-receptor; at the H_2-receptor there is an activity ratio of $(-)/(+) = 7.3:1$ (Büyüktimkin, Schoger, and Schunack, in preparation).

According to our previous results the preparation of extremely effective, chiral agonists of histamine seemed to be desirable. By far the most potent and specific agonist for histamine H_2-receptors is the achiral Impromidine (Durant, Duncan, Ganellin, Parsons, Blakemore and Rasmussen, 1978).

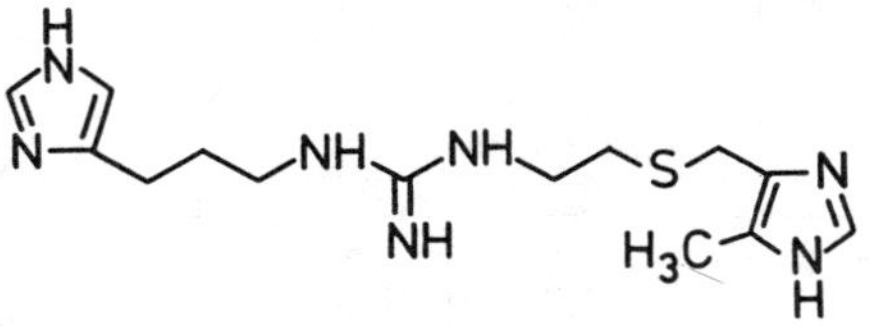

Impromidine

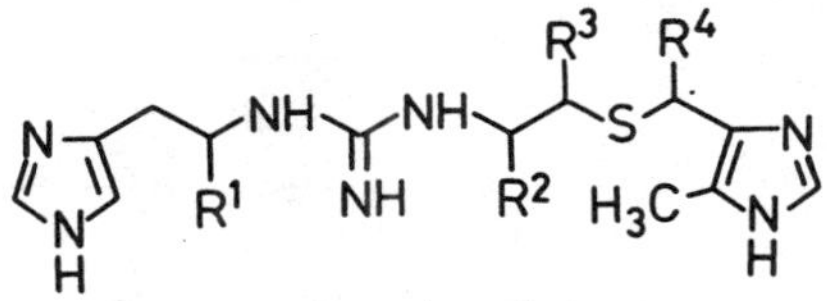

Chiral analogues

Chiral isomers of Impromidine are obtained by chain branching. Replacing the homohistamine element of Impromidine with R-(-)- and S-(+)-α-methylhistamine, as shown in Fig. 4, yields especially interesting compounds.

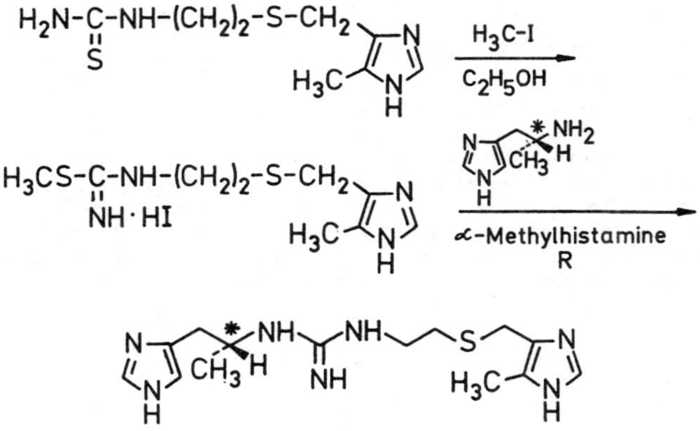

Sopromidine
R

Fig. 4. Synthesis of Sopromidine

Application of R-(-)-α-methylhistamine yields Sopromidine (Schunack and Gerhard, 1982), an R-configurated isomer of Impromidine. S-(+)-α-methylhistamine gives the optically opposite form (S-(+)-enantiomer). The pharmacological results are summarized in Table 3.

Sopromidine has 7.4 times the activity of histamine on the atrium, while the S-enantiomer shows no intrinsic activity but surprisingly, H_2-antagonistic action (24% of Metiamide). The racemate is consequently a partial agonist (intr. act. 0.8) with activity approximately triple to that of histamine. Sopromidine stimulates the acid secretion (mouse) to the same extent as histamine, while the S-enantiomer is inactive. Sopromidine shows weak H_1-agonistic activity, hence follows an activity ratio of $H_2/H_1 = 436:1$. Thus, Sopromidine is a highly stereoselective H_2-agonist. The absolute configuration of Sopromidine, however, corresponds to the S-configurated L-histidine, in contrast to the series of α-branched histamines. The results illustrate, a high degree of stereoselectivity is characteristic of the H_2-receptor.

TABLE 3 Pharmacological Results of Sopromidine and its Enantiomer

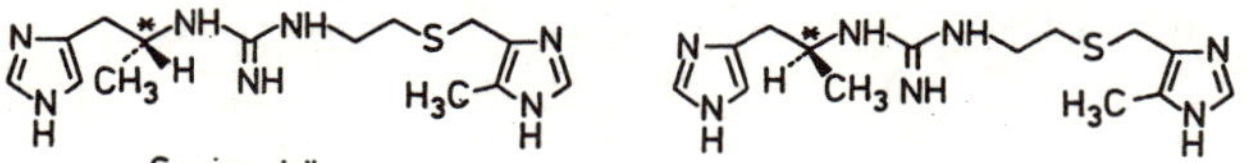

Sopromidine
R-(-)-Enantiomer

S-(+)-Enantiomer

| | H_2-Receptor | | | | | | H_1-Receptor | |
| | Guinea-pig atrium | | | | Acid secretion (mouse) | | Guinea-pig ileum | |
	intrinsic activity	pD_2	rel. act. [%]	H_2-antagon. act. Metiamide=100 [%]	intrinsic activity	pD_2	intrinsic activity	rel. act. [%]
Histamine	1	5.95	100	-	1	5.2	1	100
Sopromidine	1	6.82	741	-	1	4.9	0.2	1.7
S-enantiomer	0	0	0	24	0	0	0	0
racemat	0.8	6.41	288	-	-	-	-	-

The branching of the side chain between sulfur and the imidazole ring leads to a marked decrease of the H_2-agonistic activity. The resolution was realized at the stage of 4-[1-(2-aminoethylmercapto)ethyl]-5-methylimidazole with di-O-(p-toluoyl) tartaric acid. The absolute configuration was determined by X-ray structure determination. Both enantiomers have no H_2-agonistic activity at the guinea-pig atrium. However, the S-(-)-enantiomer has 1.3% of the activity of histamine at the guinea-pig ileum (intr. act. 0.9) while the R-(+)-enantiomer is also inactive at the H_1-receptor (Elz, Schoger, Dräger, and Schunack, 1983). The enantiomeric guanidines were obtained by the following method.

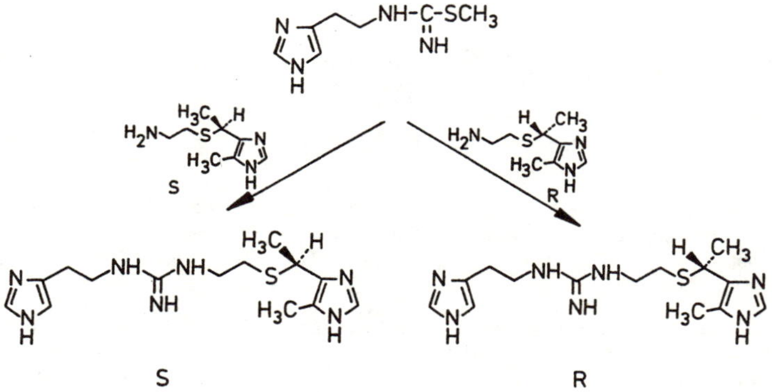

Fig. 5. Preparation of isomers of Sopromidine where the branching of the side chain is between sulfur and imidazole ring.

The introduction of a branching in the group which contributes affinity in antagonist structures decreases the activity of the enantiomers evidently. The S-(-)-enantiomer has 3.2%, the R-(+)-enantiomer 2% of the activity of histamine at the guinea-pig atrium. The activity of both enantiomers at the H_1-receptor lies by 1% of the histamine activity (Büyüktimkin and Schunack, 1983).

In the recent past the chiral α- and β-branched aminoethylthiomethylimidazoles have been obtained and the absolute configurations determined by X-ray structure analysis (Elz, Dräger, Schunack, in preparation). The integration into chiral Sopromidine analogues is in operation.

BIOCHEMISTRY

The inhibitor/activator and substrate properties of the chiral α-methylhistamines and α,$N^α$-dimethylhistamines were investigated using a highly purified histamine methyltransferase preparation. In 1-100 µM concentrations, S- and R-α-methylhistamine were acceptor substrates as good as histamine itself. If substrate concentrations were increased to 1 mM these substances were methylated to an even greater extent than histamine, since they did not exert substrate inhibition on histamine methyltransferase. Introduction of a further methyl-group into the $N^α$-position reduced acceptor substrate properties drastically. A difference in methylation was then seen, since R-α,$N^α$-dimethylhistamine was a better substrate than the S-enantiomer. Whereas α-methylhistamines could not activate histamine methyltransferase, the α,$N^α$-dimethylhistamines did. The poorer the substrate affinity of the investigated substances was, the better they were able to activate histamine methyltransferase (Barth, Schunack, Crombach and Lorenz, 1984).

Latest findings concerning chiral agonists of histamine are also contained in the publications of J. M. Arrang and J. W. Wells.

ACKNOWLEDGEMENT

The authors would like to thank the Verband der Chemischen Industrie, Fonds der Chemischen Industrie, and the Deutsche Forschungsgemeinschaft (Schu 228/6) who supported this work by grants.

REFERENCES

Barth, H., W. Schunack, M. Crombach, and W. Lorenz (1984). Gastric histamine methyltransferase: Different methylation rates for enantiomers of side chain methylated histamine analogues using a highly purified enzyme preparation. <u>Agents and</u>

Actions, 346-350.
Büyüktimkin, S., and W. Schunack (1983). Chirale Guanidine mit histaminartiger Wirkung. Pharm. Ztg. Sci. Ed., 128, 1239-1241.
Chapman, N. B., and J. F. A. Williams (1953). Optically active forms of 1-methyl-2,2'-pyridylethylamine. J. Chem. Soc., 2797-2799.
Durant, G. J., W. A. M. Duncan, C. R. Ganellin, M. E. Parsons, R. C. Blakemore, and A. C. Rasmussen (1978). Impromidine (SK&F 926 76) is a very potent and specific agonist of histamine H_2 receptors. Nature, 276, 403-405.
Elz, S., K. Schoger, M. Dräger, and W. Schunack (1983). Racemattrennung, Kristallstruktur und histaminartige Wirkung von 4-[1-(Aminoethylthio)ethyl]-5-methylimidazol. Justus Liebigs Ann. Chem., 678-683.
Gerhard, G., and W. Schunack (1980a). Absolute Konfiguration und histaminartige Wirkung der enantiomeren α-Methylhistamine. Arch. Pharm. (Weinheim), 313, 709-714.
Gerhard, G., and W. Schunack (1980b). Absolute Konfiguration und histaminartige Wirkung der enantiomeren α,$N^α$-Dimethylhistamine. Arch. Pharm. (Weinheim), 313, 780-784.
Gerhard, G., and W. Schunack (1981). Absolute Konfiguration und histaminartige Wirkung der enantiomeren α-Chlormethylhistamine und $N^α$-Methyl-α-chlormethylhistamine. Arch. Pharm. (Weinheim), 314, 1040-1045.
Graham, J. D. P., and R. S. Tonks (1956). Stereoisomerism and activity in a congener of histamine. Arch. Int. Pharmacodyn. Ther., 106, 457-469.
Schunack, W., and G. Gerhard (1982). Chiral agonists with stereoselective activity at histamine H_2-receptors. Naunyn-Schmiedeberg's Arch. Pharmacol. 319, R 56.
Schwarz, S., and W. Schunack (1979). Absolute Konfiguration und histaminartige Wirkung der Enantiomere von 5-Amino-4,5,6,7-tetrahydro-benzimidazol. Arch. Pharm. (Weinheim), 312, 933-939.
Schwarz, S., and W. Schunack (1982). Absolute Konfiguration und histaminartige Wirkung der Enantiomere von 4-(2-Aminopropyl)-5-methylimidazol. Arch. Pharm. (Weinheim), 315, 674-680.
Steffens, R., and W. Schunack (1984). Racemische Histamin-H_1-Agonisten. Arch. Pharm. (Weinheim), in press.

A SURVEY OF RECENTLY DESCRIBED H_2-RECEPTOR HISTAMINE ANTAGONISTS

C. R. Ganellin

Smith Kline & French Research Ltd., The Frythe, Welwyn, Hertfordshire, UK

ABSTRACT

Recent developments have given rise to a considerable diversity in the chemical structures of active H_2-receptor histamine antagonists. Most of the compounds, however, still comprise an aromatic ring with a flexible four-atom chain joined to a polar group which, characteristically, displays pronounced H-bonding properties. Within this broad structural class, the published compounds can be grouped into four main series according to the aromatic ring, and in each series there are several examples of drugs (or potential drugs) which have been studied in human subjects or are undergoing pharmaceutical development. Reported structure-activity studies suggest that it is unlikely that all these compounds interact in a chemically similar manner, but it is not yet clear whether there really are four distinct series. An interesting further development is the discovery that the four-atom chain can be replaced by a more rigid benzenoid structure to afford active compounds. Here, too, there appears to be more than one chemical series.

KEYWORDS

Structure-activity; H_2 antagonists; K_B atrium; drug development; imidazoles; dimethylaminomethylfurans; guanidinothiazoles; piperidinomethylphenoxy; meta-phenylene.

INTRODUCTION

The highly successful development of cimetidine as an H_2 receptor histamine antagonist, useful as a drug for the treatment of conditions involving gastric hypersecretion of acid, (Brimblecombe et al, 1975) has stimulated a search for other more potent examples from this pharmacological class of agent. Many other potent compounds have now been described although, to date, only one, viz. ranitidine, has made the transition to become a drug introduced into therapy (Bradshaw et al, 1979). However, there is little doubt that other drugs will follow and it may be of interest at this Symposium to have some preview of what chemical structures are under active consideration at this time.

Early structure-activity studies of cimetidine and analogues at SK&F had drawn attention to the apparent special significance of the following structural

features of which cimetidine was a representative example (e.g. see Ganellin, 1981):
(i) An imidazole ring (or similar nitrogen heterocycle)
(ii) A flexible chain, especially -CH$_2$SCH$_2$CH$_2$-
(iii) A planar π-electron group which is very polar and has potential for strong H-bonding (both as acceptor and donor), and contains a 1,3 NH system e.g. -NH-C-NH-
                                                                                              ‖

Subsequent investigations in many other laboratories (and especially those of pharmaceutical companies) have provided examples of other structural features and expanded considerably the scope for active structures. Indeed, there is now a considerable diversity in the chemistry of active H$_2$-receptor histamine antagonists. For ease of presentation in this paper, compounds are divided into two main structural classes, viz:
1. Compounds containing a flexible connecting chain.
2. Conformationally restricted analogues.

STRUCTURES WITH A FLEXIBLE CONNECTING CHAIN

Compounds with structures containing a flexible connecting chain are represented by the general formula in Fig. 1, i.e. comprising an 'aromatic ring', a 'flexible chain', and a 'polar group'. The compounds are grouped conveniently into four main series according to the aromatic ring of the archetypal member of the series, viz: imidazoles, dimethylaminomethylfurans, guanidinothiazoles and piperidinomethylphenoxy derivatives. These are shown with respective examples in Tables 1-4, together with the reference and published K$_B$ values for in vitro antagonism of histamine stimulated increase in the rate of beating of the isolated right atrium from the guinea-pig.

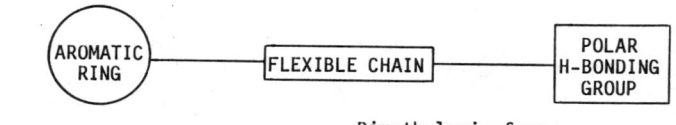

Fig. 1. General formula of H$_2$-receptor histamine antagonists containing a flexible connecting chain; there are four main series, according to the aromatic ring.

All the compounds of Table 1 have been administered to man (volunteer studies or in patients). The archetypal structure is cimetidine having a 4(5)-methyl-substituted imidazole ring, methylthioethyl connecting chain, and methylcyano-guanidine polar group. Bristol Laboratories introduced the propargyl group to give etintidine.

Shortly after cimetidine was discovered, we investigated the diamino-nitroethene analogue SK&F 92456 but saw insufficient advantage in it. However, the nitroethene group was taken up by Glaxo chemists and is incorporated in the structure of ranitidine (see Table 2).

We extended the range of structures for the 'polar' group to ring systems which had the advantage of permitting the introduction of additional substituents, e.g. the methylenedioxybenzyl group in the 5 position of isocytosine afforded oxmetidine. This compound was taken through an active programme of drug development which, unfortunately, had to be curtailed last year (1983) when, after it had been administered to some 2000 patients, several cases of liver sensitivity were reported.

In the above structures, the imidazole ring can be replaced by other heterocycles to give active compounds, e.g. thiazole and pyridine, preferably with a substituent in the position ortho to the side chain. A special example is the 3-methoxypyridine SK&F 93319, which has a picolylmethyl substituent in the isocytosine ring and combines into one molecule the ability to block both H_1 and H_2 receptor-mediated actions of histamine.

TABLE 1   Imidazole Series of H_2 Antagonists

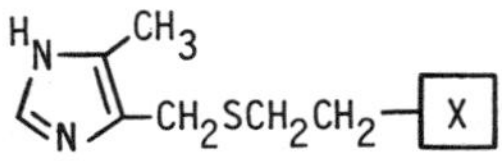

Name	X	*Guinea-pig atrium in vitro K_B	Reference
Cimetidine SK&F 92334	NCN ‖ -NHCNHCH$_3$	0.8 μM	Brimblecombe et al (1975)
Etintidine BL 5641 A	NCN ‖ -NHCNHCH$_2$C≡CH	0.2	Cavanagh et al (1980, 1983)
SK&F 92456	CHNO$_2$ ‖ -NHCNHCH$_3$	1.4	Durant et al (1976, 1982)
Oxmetidine SK&F 92994	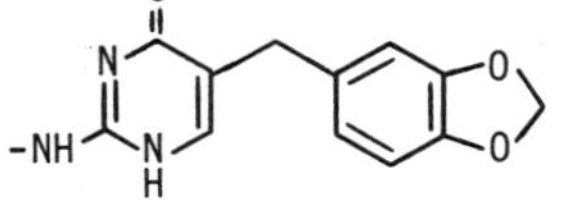 (methylenedioxybenzyl-isocytosine structure)	16 x cimetidine	Blakemore et al (1980)
			Pyridine analogue
SK&F 93319	(3-methoxypyridine structure with picolylmethyl isocytosine)	0.032	Blakemore et al (1983) Harvey and Owen (1983)

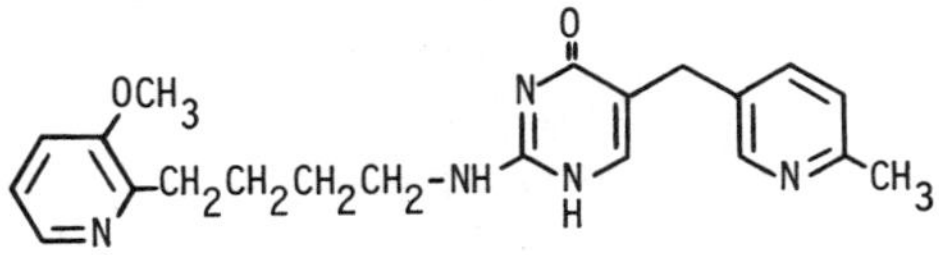

*In Tables 1 - 9, unless otherwise indicated, the K_B value is that published in the given reference, for antagonism of histamine or dimaprit stimulated increase in rate for the spontaneously beating guinea-pig right atrium in vitro.

Glaxo chemists investigated the possibility that the basic imidazole ring in cimetidine might not be essential for H_2-receptor blockade and they replaced it with alternative ring systems to which a basic function was attached as a substituent, i.e. moving the nitrogen from within the ring to an exocyclic position (Bradshaw et al, 1982). They found that replacement of the imidazole ring by furan substituted by a dimethylaminomethyl group, afforded compounds of potency comparable with those of the imidazoles, e.g. in cyanoguanidine and thioureas. Replacement of the 'polar' group by diamino-nitroethene, however afforded a substantial increase in activity compared with the imidazole derivative. This compound was selected for drug development and is ranitidine (Table 2). Although ranitidine is somewhat more active than cimetidine as an inhibitor of stimulated gastric acid secretion, its time course for inhibition is very similar.

A further development at SK&F combined the dimethylaminomethylfuran ring with the picolylmethylisocytosine group that had been developed in the imidazole series (e.g. SK&F 93319) to obtain a potent antagonist, SK&F 93479, which also showed evidence of prolonged duration of action relative to cimetidine in vivo as an inhibitor of stimulated gastric acid secretion. A sustained inhibition by SK&F 93479 was also obtained in human subjects, but further trials were suspended (1983) after the observation of mucosal changes in the forestomachs of rats which had been given very high doses of drug for at least six months (Betton and Salmon, 1984).

TABLE 2 Furan Series of H_2 Antagonists

Me_2NCH_2—[furan]—$CH_2SCH_2CH_2$—X

Name	X	Guinea-pig atrium in vitro K_B	Reference
Ranitidine AH 19065	$-NHCNHCH_3$ with $=CHNO_2$	0.063 μM	Bradshaw et al (1979)
Lupitidine SK&F 93479	[isocytosine-picolyl group]	0.016	Blakemore et al (1981)
BMY 25271	[thiadiazole-NH₂ group]	0.026 0.006	Algieri et al (1982) Lumma et al (1982)
		Rat uterus K_B	Thiazole analogue
Nizatidine LY 139037		0.08	Lin et al (1983)

Me_2NCH_2—[thiazole]—$CH_2SCH_2CH_2$—$NHCNHCH_3$ with $=CHNO_2$

Chemists at Bristol Laboratories and almost simultaneously at Merck Sharpe and Dohme identified 1,2 diamino-thiadiazole sulphoxide as an alternative 'polar' group, and the dimethylaminomethylfuran derivative (BMY 25271) appears to be under further study at Bristol.

Nizatidine, being developed by Eli Lilly, is structurally a close analogue of ranitidine in which dimethylaminomethylfuran has been replaced by dimethylaminomethylthiazole. It probably should not be regarded as being closely related to the guanidinothiazoles of Table 3.

The discovery of guanidinothiazole as an imidazole-replacement (Table 3) was made at ICI as a result of a screening programme in which compounds were selected from the chemist's collection of samples on file. Activity was found for 2-guanidino-4-methylthiazole and investigation of derivatives revealed that the cimetidine analogue (i.e. with the methylthioethyl-cyanoguanidine side chain) tiotidine, was very potent, with an apparent dissociation constant (K_B) of approximately 10^{-8} M.

TABLE 3   Guanidinothiazole Series of H_2 Antagonists

Name	X	Guinea-pig atrium in vitro K_B	Reference
Tiotidine ICI 125211	NCN ‖ -NHCNHCH$_3$	0.015 µM	Yellin et al (1979)
BL 6341 A	(thiadiazole sulphoxide: -NH...NH$_2$)	0.027 0.007	Cavanagh et al (1981) Lumma et al (1982)
Famotidine YM 11170	NSO$_2$NH$_2$ ‖ -CNH$_2$	0.017*	Takeda et al, (1981, 1982)
	Guinea-pig brain cortex in vitro K_i		
E 821308 Hoechst	(thiadiazole dioxide: -NH...N(CH$_3$)...NHCH$_2$CH$_2$Ph)	ca 0.03	Norris et al (1984)
E 82980 Hoechst	(imidazolone: -NH...=CHCHCH$_2$CH$_3$, CH$_3$)	ca 0.008	Norris et al (1984)

*SK&F Result

Unfortunately, clinical studies with this compound had to be discontinued when lesions were discovered in the gastric mucosa of rats after chronic administration at high doses (Streett et al, 1984).

The guanidinothiazole group appears to confer high affinity at the H_2 receptor and many active derivatives are now known. The 'polar' group encompasses a wider diversity of chemical structures than obtains for the imidazole series, and examples of compounds under active pharmaceutical development are BL 6341A (Bristol Laboratories) and famotidine (Yamanouchi). Recently described compounds from Hoechst Laboratories, E821308 and E82980, illustrate that there is also considerable scope for modifying these structures. BL 6341A also shows extended duration of action in vivo (relative to cimetidine) as an inhibitor of stimulated gastric acid secretion, and is not easily washed out from the guinea-pig atrium (Buyniski et al 1984).

A further development from the Glaxo chemists was the replacement of the furan ring by phenoxy; in effect, moving the oxygen atom from within the ring to outside of the ring. Activity is also dependant upon the amine substituent and a meta piperidinomethyl group was found to be particularly favourable. Use of m-piperidinomethylphenoxypropyl attached to the 'polar' group considerably expanded the scope for active structures (Table 4) e.g. lamtidine, and loxtidine, and this finding has been applied by chemists in many other pharmaceutical companies e.g.TZU 0460 (Teikoku), TAS (Wakamoto), BMY 25260 (Bristol Laboratories) = L 643441 (Merck Sharpe and Dohme), BMY 25368, Wy 45086 (Wyeth).

It appears that m-piperidinomethylphenoxypropyl confers high affinity at the H_2 receptor and many active derivatives have been made. Particularly noteworthy was the finding by Teikoku researchers that the 'polar' group need only contain one N atom and they reported that a simple derivative such as -NHCOCH$_3$ has a K_B value of 0.22 µM determined in vitro on the guinea-pig atrium.

Depending upon the 'polar' group there is also considerable change in the kinetics of interaction and it appears that compounds such as lamtidine, loxtidine, BMY 25260 = L 643441, and BMY 25368 are long lasting in vivo as inhibitors of stimulated acid secretion. They are also very difficult to displace by washing in vitro from guinea-pig atria and appear to induce a nearly irreversible blockade of receptor function, (see Stables et al 1983, Torchiana et al 1983, Buyniski et al 1984).

The question arises as to whether one is justified in categorising these compounds into four chemical classes. It is convenient to see them this way but is there any real basis for it? Indeed, the division may be arbitrary since a pyridine derivative (SK&F 93319) is included along with imidazoles in Table 1, and a thiazole derivative (nizatidine) is included with furans in Table 2, rather than with the thiazoles of Table 3. Furthermore thiazole could be considered an isostere of imidazole.

There are examples in each chemical class which appear to act specifically and competitively in vitro as antagonists of histamine-induced responses on the guinea-pig atrium and rat uterus, so that there is no biological basis for such subdivision.

It is clear, however, that the contribution of the 'polar' group to affinity differs between the series and that affinity is much more sensitive to structural change of the polar group in the imidazole series than in the guanidinothiazoles or m-piperidinomethylphenoxypropyl derivatives. In the last two series, the aromatic ring systems appear to make a greater contribution to affinity than does the imidazole ring so that comparisons between series of the effects of molecular change are made from different base lines, and may

TABLE 4 m-Piperidinomethylphenoxy Series of H_2 Antagonists

Name	X	Guinea-pig atrium in vitro K_B	Reference
Lamtidine AH 22216	-NH-C(=N-N(CH₃))-N=C-NH₂ (3-amino-5-methylamino-1-methyl-1,2,4-triazole)	0.07 μM (DR=2)	Brittain et al (1982) Stables et al (1983)
Loxtidine AH 23844	1-methyl-3-(hydroxymethyl)-5-amino-1,2,4-triazole -NH linkage, CH₂OH substituent	non-competitive	Stables & Humphray (1983)
TAS (Wakamoto)	-NH-(1,3,4-thiadiazol-2-yl)-NH₂	0.054	Tsuritani et al (1984)
TZU 0460 (Teikoku)	-NHCCH₂OCCH₃ (with two C=O)	0.11	Shibata (1984)
BMY 25260 L 643441	-NH-(1,2,5-thiadiazole-1-oxide)-NH₂	0.04 0.02	Algieri et al (1982) Lumma et al (1982) Torchiana et al (1983)
BMY 25368	-NH-(squaramide)-NH₂	0.013	Buyniski et al (1984)*
Wy 45086	-NH-(benzisothiazole-1,1-dioxide)	0.008	Nielsen et al (1984)

*The squaramide group was first introduced into antagonist structures in the imidazole series (Ganellin and Young, 1980)

therefore be misleading. Even so, the structure-activity patterns suggest that not all the aromatic ring systems interact at the receptor in the same manner chemically. This is particularly apparent after examining certain detailed stereochemical differences.

In the imidazoles related to cimetidine, methyl substitution in the ring at the 4(5)-position (adjacent to the flexible chain) gave compounds having enhanced activity (Durant et al 1977). In ranitidine, however, analogous substitution (3 position in the furan) is reported to give a much less active compound whereas the isomeric 4-methyl derivative was active (Table 5). Furthermore, the 4-isopropyl compound was also active, in contrast to the imidazole thiourea

TABLE 5 Effect of Substituents in the Furan Ring of Ranitidine*

Parent structure: Me$_2$NCH$_2$-[furan(4,3)]-O-CH$_2$SCH$_2$CH$_2$NHC(=CHNO$_2$)NHCH$_3$

Furan substitution	ID$_{50}$[†]
(unsubstituted)	0.18 mg/kg
3-CH$_3$	>10 [§]
4-CH$_3$	0.25
4-CH(CH$_3$)$_2$	0.33

*Bradshaw et al, 1982; †Compounds tested intravenously against histamine stimulated gastric acid secretion in the anaesthetised rat, perfused stomach preparation; §Also reported by Leonardi et al (1982) to have ca 10% of the potency of ranitidine in vitro on the guinea-pig atrium.

series where a 4(5)-isopropyl group considerably reduces activity (Impicciatore et al 1979). Thus the furan and imidazole rings are apparently not simply analogues in which -O- replaces -N=.

DIARYL STRUCTURES

An interesting further development is the discovery that the flexible connecting four-atom chain can be replaced by a more rigid benzenoid structure to afford active diaryl compounds. Structure-activity studies reported by Gilman et al (1982) suggest that for analogues of tiotidine the -CH$_2$SCH$_2$CH$_2$- chain can be replaced by meta-phenylene with retention or even enhancement of antagonist potency, as in the cyanoguanidine ICI 127032 (Table 6). There is, however, some discrepancy in the activities reported for this compound; see footnotes to Table 6.

Similarly, meta-phenylene analogues of methylthiourea and diamino-nitroethene are active. There also appears to be a considerable degree of stereochemical specificity since ortho- and para- phenylene isomers of the methylthiourea were not active. Interestingly, the cis-1,3-cyclohexane and cyclopentane analogues of ICI 127032 were also found to be active; these results emphasise the importance of stereochemical factors rather than the electronic effects which arise from the π-electron system of the benzene ring.

In contrast, imidazolylphenylene and dimethylaminomethyl-furanylphenylene derivatives (Table 7) were only weakly active (Gilman et al 1982, Hoffman et al

TABLE 6 meta-Phenylene Analogues of Tiotidine*

Name	Structure	Guinea-pig atrium in vitro K_B
Tiotidine		0.018 μM
ICI 127032		0.002 0.014† 0.32 §
	cis	0.009
	meta X=CHNO$_2$ meta X=S ortho X=S para X=S	0.001 0.2 § 0.008 weak weak

*Gilman et al, 1982; †SK&F result; §Hoffman et al (1983) report K_I

1983), suggesting that in receptor interaction the relationship between the thiazole ring and 'polar' group is different from that between the imidazole or furan and 'polar' group; i.e. despite the formal similarity in structure between cimetidine and tiotidine the heteroaromatic rings undergo chemically different interactions at the receptor and perhaps they 'see' a somewhat different view of the receptor site. However, caution is needed in these interpretations, particularly since there is some indication that, as with the tiotidine analogues, activity is associated only with imidazolylphenylene meta-isomers for cyanoguanidine, guanidine, or amidine derivatives i.e. similar stereochemical discrimination may operate (Table 7).

Another type of diaryl structure exists for mifentidine (DA 4577, Table 8). Here the imidazole ring is retained, the flexible chain is replaced by phenylene, but the 'polar' group is a formamidine and activity is reported to reside with the para isomer, rather than the meta (Donetti et al 1984). Formamidine is a basic group which is mainly in the cationic form at physiological pH and it is probable that this is the active form at the receptor. It is surprising therefore that reported activity of guanidine and benzamidine analogues, which are also cationic at physiological pH, resides in the meta isomers but not in the para (Table 7). Activity of these formamidines

TABLE 7 meta-Phenylene Analogues of Cimetidine

Structure	R	Guinea-pig atrium in vitro K_B	Reference
4-methylimidazole-5-yl linked to phenyl-R (meta)	$-NHC(=NCN)NHCH_3$ ortho and para isomers	40*μM 80*	Hoffman et al (1983) ibid
	$-NHC(=CHNO_2)NHCH_3$	16*	ibid
	$-NH-$(4-amino-1,2,5-thiadiazole 1-oxide)	0.79*	ibid
imidazol-4-yl—phenyl(meta)—NHC(=S)NHCH$_3$		weak	Gilman et al (1982)
imidazol-4-yl—phenyl(meta)—NHC(=NHR)NHCNH$_2$ (guanidine)	H CH$_3$ para isomers	5.5† 4.4 >30	Donetti et al (1984) ibid ibid
imidazol-4-yl—phenyl(meta)—C(=NH)NHR (benzamidine)	H CH$_3$ para isomers	7.2 8.7 >30	Donetti et al (1984) ibid ibid
imidazol-4-yl—phenyl(meta)—N=CH—NHR (formamidine)	H CH$_3$ CH(CH$_3$)$_2$ CN	>30 >30 >100 >30	Donetti et al (1984) ibid Cereda et al (1983) Donetti et al (1984)
	para isomers active, see Table 8		

* K_I (cf. cimetidine 0.5 μM); †cf. cimetidine 0.47 μM.

also appears to be extraordinarily sensitive to N-alkyl substituents, and within the series R=H<Me<Et the reported antagonist potency in vitro on the guinea-pig atrium increases respectively by factors of approximately 25 and 60, i.e. an overall range of three orders of magnitude. In this respect, the formamidines also appear to differ from the analogous guanidines and benzamidines. Hence, it is likely that the specific chemical interactions contributing to receptor binding are somewhat different for the phenylformamidines in comparison with the guanidines and bezamidines.

A third type of diaryl structure has been described by Lipinski (1983), viz amino-triazolyl-pyridines (Table 9). Here it is extremely difficult to decide on which ring mimics the aromatic ring of the flexible antagonists and whether the other ring is simulating the 'polar' group or binding in some other way. Lipinski modelled the molecule in comparison with cimetidine but was unable to distinguish between these possibilities.

TABLE 8   Imidazolyl-phenylformamidines as H_2 Antagonists*

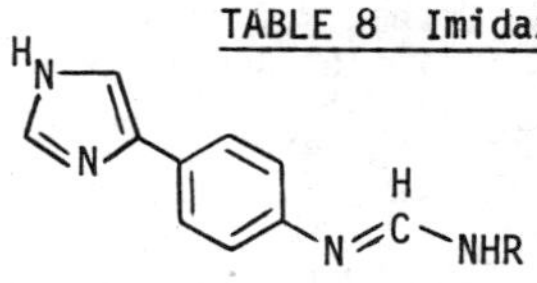

	R	K_B
		Guinea-pig atrium, in vitro
1. Activity is sensitive to R	H	30 µM
	Me	1.2
	Et	0.019
	n-Pr	0.032
Mifentidine, DA 4577 =	i-Pr	0.024
	t-Bu	0.017
2. Activity requires a basic amidine	CN >	30
3. Activity resides with para isomer	meta >	30 R=H, Me
4. Activity requires a tautomeric amidine†		
N-methyl analogues of DA 4577	>	100

*Donetti et al (1984); †Cereda et al (1983)

TABLE 9   Aminotriazolyl-pyridines as H_2 Antagonists*

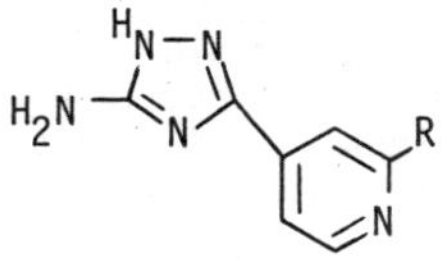

R	K_B
	Guinea-pig atrium in vitro
H	42 µM
NH_2	2.2
$NHCH_2CH_3$	0.24

*Lipinski, (1983)

Hopefully, in the near future, we may see a more concerted effort to analyse the structure-activity relationships between these series so that we may form a clearer view of how the compounds interact at the receptor level.

REFERENCES

Algieri, A.A., Luke, G.M., Standridge, R.T., Brown, M., Partyka, R.A. and Crenshaw, R.R. (1982). J. Med. Chem., 25, 210-212.
Betton, G.R. and Salmon, G.K. (1984). Scand. J. Gastroenterol., 19, Suppl. 101 103-108.
Blakemore R.C., Brown, T.H., Durant, G.J., Emmett, J.C., Ganellin, C.R., Parsons, M.E. and Rasmussen, A.C. (1980). Brit. J. Pharmacol, 70, 105P.
Blakemore R.C., Brown, T.H., Durant, G.J., Emmett, J.C., Ganellin, C.R., Parsons, M.E., Rasmussen, A.C. and Rawlings, D.A. (1981). Brit. J. Pharmacol, 74, 200P.
Blakemore R.C., Brown, T.H., Cooper, D.G., Durant, G.J., Ganellin, C.R., Ife, R.J., Parsons, M.E., Rasmussen, A.C. and Sach, G.S. (1983). Brit. J. Pharmacol, 80, 437P.
Bradshaw, J., Brittain, R.T., Clitherow, J.W., Daly, M.J., Jack, D., Price, B.J. and Stables, R. (1979). Brit J. Pharmacol 66, 464P.

Bradshaw, J., Butcher, M.E., Clitherow, J.W., Dowle, M.D., Hayes, R., Judd, D.B., McKinnon, J.M. and Price, B.J. (1982). In: A.M. Creighton and S. Turner (Eds.), The Chemical Regulation of Biological Systems. Special Publication No. 42 The Royal Society of Chemistry, London. pp. 45-57.
Brimblecombe, R.W., Duncan, W.A.M., Durant, G.J., Ganellin, C.R., Parsons, M.E. and Black, J.W. (1975a). Brit. J. Pharmacol. 53, 435P.
Brimblecombe, R.W., Duncan, W.A.M., Durant, G.J., Emmett, J.C., Ganellin, C.R. and Parsons, M.E. (1975b). J. Int. Med. Res. 3, 86-92.
Brittain, R.T., Daly, M.J., Humphray, J.M. and Stables, R. (1982). Brit. J. Pharmacol. 76, 195P.
Buyniski, J.P., Cavanagh, R.L., Pircio, A.W., Algieri, A.A. and Crenshaw, R.R. (1984). Structure-activity relationships among newer histamine H_2-receptor antagonists. In: C. Melchiorre and M. Giannella (Eds.), Elsevier, Amsterdam, New York, Oxford. Highlights in Receptor Chemistry. pp. 195-215
Cavanagh, R.L., Usakewicz, J.J. and Buyniski, J.P. (1980). Fed. Proc., 39, 768, Abstr. 2638.
Cavanagh, R.L., Usakewicz, J.J. and Buyniski, J.P. (1981). Fed. Proc., 40, 693, Abstr. 2652.
Cavanagh, R.L., Usakewicz, J.J. and Buyniski, J.P. (1983). J. Pharmacol. Exp. Therap., 224, 171-179.
Cereda, E., Donetti, A. Bellora, E., Giachetti, A., Micheletti, R. and Pagani, F. (1983). Poster Communication (P18) at "Highlights in Receptor Chemistry" Camerino.
Donnetti, A., Cereda, E. Bellora, E., Gallazzi, A. Bazzano, C., Vanoni, P., Del Soldato, P., Micheletti, R., Pagani, F. and Giachetti, A. (1984) J. Med. Chem., 27, 380-386.
Durant, G.J., Emmett, J.C., Ganellin, C.R., and Prain, H.D. (1976). Brit. Pat., 1421792
Durant, G.J., Emmett, J.C., Ganellin, C.R., Miles, P.D., Prain, H.D., Parsons, M.E. and White, G.R. (1977). J. Medicin. Chem., 20, 901-906.
Durant, G.J., Brown, T.H., Emmett, J.C., Ganellin, C.R., Prain, H.D., and Young, R.C. (1982). Some Structure-Activity Considerations in H_2-Receptor Antagonists. In: A.M. Creighton and S. Turner (Eds.), The Chemical Regulation of Biological Systems. Special Publication No. 42. The Royal Society of Chemistry, London. pp. 27-44.
Ganellin, C.R. (1981). J. Med. Chem., 24, 913-920.
Ganellin, C.R. and Young, R.C. (Smith Kline & French Laboratories Ltd.) (1980). Brit. Pat., 15363090.
Gilman, D.J., Jones, D.F., Oldham, K., Wardleworth, J.M. and Yellin, T.O. (1982). 2-Guanidinothiazoles at H_2-receptor antagonists. In: A.M. Creighton and S. Turner (Eds.) The Chemical Regulation of Biological Systems. Special Publication No. 42. The Royal Society of Chemistry, London. pp. 58-76.
Harvey, C.A. and Owen, D.A.A. (1983). Brit. J. Pharmacol., 80, 438P.
Hoffman, J.M., Pietruszkiewicz, A.M., Habecker, C.N., Phillips, B.T., Bolhofer, W.A., Cragoe, E.J., Torchiana, M.L., Lumma, W.C. and Baldwin, J.J. (1983). J. Med. Chem., 26, 140-144.
Impicciatore, M., Chiavarini, M., Razzetti, R. and Vitali, T. (1979). Eur. J. Pharmacol., 57, 79-82.
Leonardi, A., Cazzulani, P. and Nardi, D. (1982). Boll. Chim. Farm., 121, 1-9.
Lin, T.M., Evans, D.C., Warrick, M.W., Pioch, R.P. and Ruffalo, R.R. (1983). Gastroenterol., 84, 1231.
Lipinski, C.A. (1982). J.Med. Chem., 26, 1-6.
Lumma, W.C., Anderson, P.S., Baldwin, J.J., Bolhofer, W.A., Habecker, C.N., Hirshfield, J.M., Pietruszkiewicz, A.M., Randall, W.C., Torchiana, M.W., Britcher, S.F., Clineschmidt, B.V., Denny, G.H., Hirschmann, R., Hoffman, J.M., Phillips, B.T. and Streeter, K.B. (1982). J. Med. Chem., 25, 207-210.
Nielson, S.T., Dove, P., Palumbo, G., Sandor, A., Buonato, C., Schiehser, G., Santilli, A. and Strike, D. (1984). Fed. Proc., 43, 1074, Abstr. 4617.
Norris, D.B., Gajtkowski, Wood, T.P. and Rising, T.J. (1984). Poster communication (P17) 13th meeting of European Histamine Research Society, Florence.

Shibata, T. et al. (1984). Abstract 29N1-2S, Communication to 104th Ann. Meeting Japan Pharmaceutical Soc. Sendai.
Stables, R., Daly, M.J. and Humphray, J.M. (1983). Agents and Actions, 13, 166-169.
Stables, R. and Humphray, J.M. (1983). Abstr. 012, 12th Meeting European Histamine Research Society, Brighton.
Streett, C.S., Cimprich, R.E. and Robertson, J.L. (1984). Scand. J. Gastroenterol., 19, Suppl. 101, 109-117.
Takagi, T., Takeda, M. and Maeno, H. (1982). Arch. Int. Pharmacodyn., 256, 49-58.
Takeda, M., Takagi, T. and Maeno, H. (1981). Jap. J. Pharmacol., 31, 222P.
Takeda, M., Takagi, T. Yashima, Y. and Maeno, H. (1982). Arzneim. Forsch., 32(ii), 734-737.
Torchiana, M.L., Pendleton, R.G., Cook, P.G., Hanson, C.A. and Clineschmidt, B.V. (1983). J. Pharmacol. Exp. Therap., 224, 514-519.
Tsuritani, M. (1984). Abstract 0-92, 57th Ann. Meeting of Japan Pharmacological Society, Kyoto.
Yellin, T.O., Buck, S.H., Gilman, D.J., Jones, D.F. and Wardleworth, J.M. (1979a). Pharmacologist, 21, 266, Abstr. 635.
Yellin, T.O., Buck, S.H., Gilman, D.J., Jones, D.F. and Wardleworth, J.M. (1979b). Life Sciences, 25, 2001-2009.

HISTAMINE H$_2$-RECEPTOR RADIOLIGAND BINDING STUDIES

T. J. Rising and D. B. Norris

Hoechst Pharmaceutical Research Laboratories, Walton Manor, Walton, Milton Keynes MK7 7AJ, UK

ABSTRACT

The availability of a valid radioligand binding assay for the histamine H$_2$-receptor, using ^{3}H-tiotidine, has led to further studies on the role of this receptor in the central nervous system. However extending the investigations to peripheral tissues, employing similar experimental procedures, has, with the exception of guinea-pig lung parenchymal preparations, led to problems. The recent data derived from central and peripheral tissues are presented.

KEYWORDS

Histamine H$_2$-receptor; ^{3}H-tiotidine; ^{3}H-cimetidine; binding assay; central nervous system; guinea-pig; kidney; lung; anti-depressants.

INTRODUCTION

Over the last few years a number of different radioligands have been employed in binding studies for the identification of the histamine H$_2$-receptor (Burkard, 1978; Kendall, Ferkany and Enna, 1980; Osband and McCaffrey, 1979; Rosenfeld, Thompson and Jacobson, 1976). Although today ^{3}H-tiotidine meets the criteria for labelling the H$_2$-receptor (Gajtkowski and colleagues, 1983), claims had previously been made for the validity of using other tritiated H$_2$-compounds, particularly ^{3}H-histamine and ^{3}H-cimetidine. The two major disadvantages with employing ^{3}H-histamine are the high dissociation constant and the problems associated with other histamine receptors. Tritiated histamine is however not without its uses as will be discussed by others at this symposium.

In our hands ^{3}H-cimetidine gave binding which was saturable, reversible and showed protein linearity. Thus some of the criteria that must be satisfied for valid radioligand binding studies were achieved. However, other data found by us (Norris and colleagues, 1980; Rising and colleagues, 1980) and others (Smith and colleagues, 1980), questioned whether in fact ^{3}H-cimetidine was labelling the H$_2$-receptor. High affinity was observed, but the values determined in different tissues were not only different, but lower than those found using other <u>in vitro</u> biochemical and pharmacological measurements.

Regarding H_2-antagonists with different chemical structures, when ranitidine and tiotidine became available, possessing furan and guanidinothiazole moeities, no true displacement of ^3H-cimetidine was seen. Finally, when histamine stimulated adenylate cyclase and ^3H-cimetidine binding activity were compared in sub-cellular fractions of the gastric mucosa, the enzyme activity was found predominantly in the 1000g membrane fraction, but the highest ^3H-cimetidine binding was observed in the 100,000g pellet. All these studies confirmed that the observed binding of ^3H-cimetidine was not to the H_2-receptor, but to an imidazole recognition site (Warrander and colleagues, 1983).

^3H-TIOTIDINE BINDING - EARLY STUDIES

When the tritiated form of the more potent H_2-antagonist tiotidine became available, hopes of authentic radioligand binding studies were raised. However, early attempts, as tried by several workers in the field, failed. This was predominantly due to the labelled tiotidine available at the time. However, with the chemically stable form of the radioligand and slight modifications to the method, we were able to demonstrate the validity of using ^3H-tiotidine for labelling the H_2-receptor in guinea-pig cerebral cortex membranes (Gajtkowski and colleagues, 1983).

Perhaps the most convincing evidence was the excellent correlation found between binding constants and those derived using other procedures (Table 1).

TABLE 1 Comparison of the Activity of H_2-Compounds

Compound	Tiotidine binding # K_i (μM)	Adenylate cyclase * K_B (μM)	G.P. right atrium K_B (μM)
TIOTIDINE	0.034	0.02	0.037
RANITIDINE	0.39	0.20	0.12
CIMETIDINE	0.47	0.79	0.48
BURIMAMIDE	3.0	3.2	7.4
SKF 91581	160	72	210
HISTAMINE	43		
DIMAPRIT	44		
4-METHYLHISTAMINE	270		
2-METHYLHISTAMINE	>1000		

\# Guinea-pig cerebral cortex
* Guinea-pig gastric mucosa (histamine stimulated)

For H_2-antagonists of different structures and possessing a wide range of activities, the agreement between binding, cyclase activity and chronotropic effects was very good. The H_2-agonists also showed inhibition of binding, with specificity observed between 4- and 2-methylhistamine.

THE H_2-RECEPTOR IN THE CNS

How has the method been used in further investigation of the histamine H_2-receptor?

About a year ago we reported on the distribution of H_1 and H_2-receptors in five different areas of guinea-pig brain (Norris, Gajtkowski and Rising, 1984).

This study basically revealed that whereas the concentration of the
H_1-receptor was fairly similar in all the areas examined, that was not the
case for the H_2-receptor. No binding was seen in the cerebellum or pons plus
medulla areas, with the highest level observed in the corpus striatum.

When we screened compounds that have been reported to be associated on occasions
with the H_2-receptor, we found that prostaglandins, muscarinic and adrenergic
compounds and benzodiazepines, had no activity at the H_2-receptor. The two
exceptions were atropine, where the calculated K_i value was a thousand fold
greater than at the muscarinic receptor, and clonidine, where the affinity was
similar to that reported for H_2-agonist activity (Audigier, Virion and Schwartz,
1976).

For H_1-antagonists, including the more recent compounds ketotifen and
astemizole, some displacement of binding was seen. However the K_i values were
well above those for the H_1-receptor.

TABLE 2 Binding Affinities of Anti-depressants

Compound	K_i (µM)	Hill coefficient	Adenylate# cyclase
DESIPRAMINE	8.5	0.85*	12
IPRINDOLE	3.9	0.60	8.1
DOXEPIN	1.8	0.81	1.4
IMIPRAMINE	1.7	0.77	3.3
AMITRIPTYLINE	0.83	0.74	1.9
MIANSERIN	0.29	0.60	2.8

\# Dissociated tissue (Kanba and Richelson, 1983)
* Significantly different ($P < 0.01$) from 1.0

Table 2 lists some anti-depressants which we have screened for H_2-activity.

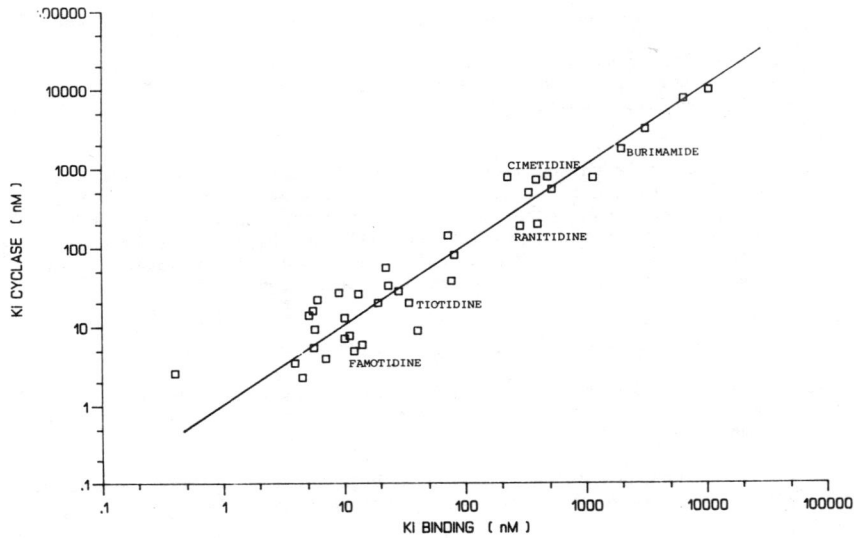

Fig. 1.   A comparison of ^3H-tiotidine binding and adenylate cyclase
activities for compounds of diverse chemical structure.

The K_i values for binding have been compared with those from adenylate cyclase as measured in dissociated tissue. With the exception of mianserin, the correlation is very good. Although it is unlikely that the H_2-receptor is primarily responsible for the therapeutic actions of these compounds, these micromolar levels are reached in patients undergoing chronic therapy (Schwartz, Quach and Garbarg, 1982).

Finally we have looked at a series of our own H_2-antagonists (Fig. 1). A comparison of adenylate cyclase activity as measured in the gastric mucosa with ^{3}H-tiotidine binding in the cerebral cortex gave a correlation of r = 0.99 and a slope of 1.03. The compounds included the known H_2-antagonists as indicated, but also different structural types - phenoxypropyl derivatives, guanidinothiazoles and hydantoins.

More recently we have investigated the role of mono- and di-valent cations on the ^{3}H-tiotidine binding (Fig. 2). The various ions were added at concentrations similar to those found in normal serum.

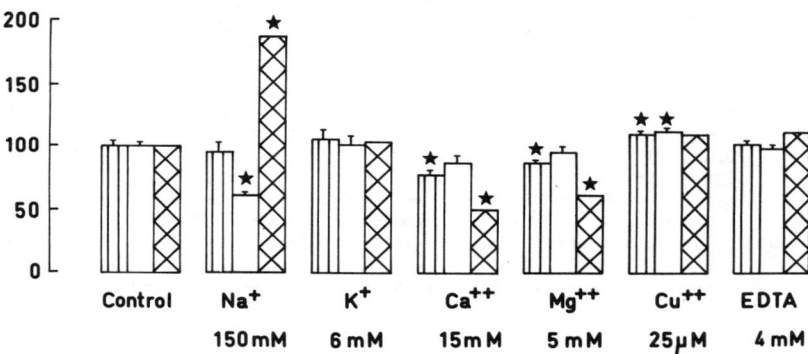

Fig. 2. The effect of mono- and di-valent cations on total and specific ^{3}H-tiotidine binding. ■, total binding; □, non specific binding; ▨, specific binding. ★ $P < 0.01$.

The divalent cations calcium and magnesium depressed both the total and non specific binding, resulting in a large reduction in specific binding. Copper had a marked effect on both the total and NSB, with the resultant specific binding being unchanged. Most significant of all was the result with sodium ions, where specific binding was dramatically increased. A similar event was not observed with the other mono-valent cation, potassium.

H_2-RECEPTOR BINDING IN PERIPHERAL TISSUES

Described so far, relating to ^{3}H-tiotidine binding, has been work in the cerebral cortex. Attempts have also been made to establish the ^{3}H-tiotidine assay in a number of peripheral tissues.

Little success to date has been achieved when using either the gastric mucosa or right atrium and limited attempts with platelets have failed.

The early results with the kidney were encouraging, where saturable binding was obtained which also showed protein linearity. Looking at the inhibition of binding of known H_2-antagonists (Fig. 3) the displacements for some of the compounds, namely tiotidine, burimamide and cimetidine appeared acceptable.

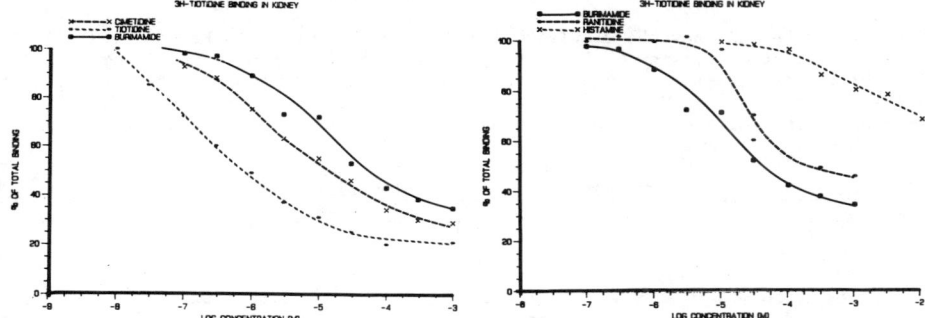

Fig. 3. The inhibition of ^{3}H-tiotidine binding in the kidney by (left hand graph) cimetidine, tiotidine and burimamide and (right hand graph) histamine, ranitidine and burimamide.

However, when we assayed ranitidine and histamine, the results did not appear to be so encouraging, with ranitidine and histamine being much weaker than expected.

These apparent differences between kidney and cerebral cortex could not be due to an imidazole or guanidinothiazole recognition site and the ratio of IC_{50} values in kidney and cerebral cortex, with a few exceptions, was about 10. After a number of unsuccessful modifications to the procedure we were fortunate enough to screen one of our own compounds E1346. Both in <u>in vitro</u> and <u>in vivo</u> estimates of H_2-activity, E1346 was about 20 times less active than cimetidine.

TABLE 3 H_2-Activity of 1346

Assay	Activity	
	E1346	Cimetidine
^{3}H-tiotidine binding, brain K_i (µM)	15	0.47
Adenylate cyclase, mucosa IC_{50} (µM)	700	29
Rat perfused stomach, ID_{50} (µmol/kg)	>25	10
^{3}H-tiotidine binding, kidney K_i (µM)	0.1	3.0

However, in the kidney binding system it was 30 times more active, and hence this clearly indicated it was not in fact the H_2-receptor being labelled by ^{3}H-tiotidine. We can make no definitive conclusions to explain the data.

Turning to the last peripheral tissue lung, our colleages, John Foreman and Steve Webber at University College, London, have obtained some encouraging initial findings (Webber and colleagues, 1984). In Table 4 are listed the K_i values of the standard H_2-agonists and H_2-antagonists. It can be seen that the compounds displace with the right potency and specificity is found between 2- and 4-methylhistamine.

TABLE 4   Inhibition Constants for ^{3}H-tiotidine Binding in Guinea-Pig Lung

Compound	K_i(M)	Hill Slope
YM 11170	$4.1 \pm 1.1 \times 10^{-8}$	1.08 ± 0.14
Tiotidine	$6.4 \pm 0.5 \times 10^{-9}$	1.05 ± 0.16
Ranitidine	$8.1 \pm 2.8 \times 10^{-7}$	1.21 ± 0.10
Metiamide	$7.6 \pm 3.4 \times 10^{-7}$	1.03 ± 0.04
Cimetidine	$8.2 \pm 1.5 \times 10^{-7}$	1.03 ± 0.10
Burimamide	$4.2 \pm 0.8 \times 10^{-6}$	0.94 ± 0.05
4-Methylhistamine	$1.2 \pm 0.5 \times 10^{-5}$	1.05 ± 0.13
Histamine	$3.4 \pm 1.5 \times 10^{-5}$	1.06 ± 0.16
Dimaprit	$1.9 \pm 0.3 \times 10^{-5}$	0.95 ± 0.19
Mepyramine	$> 10^{-4}$ M	
2-Methylhistamine	$> 10^{-4}$ M	

Results are mean values $\pm$ SE from 3 determinations

Why then does ^{3}H-tiotidine label the H_2-receptor in lung and cerebral cortex but not other peripheral tissues? It is not merely a case of transferring the method in toto from one tissue to another. This point is illustrated in Table 5 which shows that the experimental conditions have to be changed for the lung in order to obtain H_2-binding.

TABLE 5   Modifications to Lung Experimental Conditions

Buffer : 50 mM Na/K phosphate → 150 mM Na phosphate
Tissue preparation : lung parenchyma
Protein concentration : 2 → 1 mg/ml
Temperature : R.T. → 4°C

The reduction in temperature as well as the choice of buffer appear to be important.

Perhaps the buffer and the associated ion content might be the change necessary in other tissues to achieve valid H_2-binding using ^{3}H-tiotidine. An alternative strategy is to label another H_2-antagonist of higher affinity. An authentic binding assay for the histamine H_2-receptor in other tissues would allow us to explore the role of this receptor in the many systems in which it is now found.

REFERENCES

Audigier, Y., A. Virion, and J.C. Schwartz (1976). Stimulation of cerebral histamine H_2-receptors by clonidine. Nature, 262, 307-308.

Burkard, W.P. (1978). Histamine H_2-receptor binding with ^{3}H-cimetidine in brain. Eur. J. Pharmac., 50, 449-450.

Gajtkowski, G.A., D.B. Norris, T.J. Rising and T.P. Wood (1983). Specific binding of (^{3}H-tiotidine to histamine H_2-receptors in guinea pig cerebral cortex. Nature, 304, 65-67.

Kanba, S., and E. Richelson (1983). Antidepressants are weak competitive antagonists of histamine H_2-receptors in dissociated brain tissue. Eur. J. Pharmac., 94, 313-318.

Kendall, D.A., J.W. Ferkany and S.J. Enna (1980). Properties of ^{3}H-cimetidine binding in rat brain membrane fractions. Life Sci., 26, 1293-1302.

Norris, D.B., T.J. Rising, S.W. Warrander, and T.P. Wood (1980). ^{3}H-cimetidine binding in guinea pig gastric mucosa. Br. J. Pharmac. 72, 548P.

Norris, D.B., G.A. Gajtkowski, and T.J. Rising (1984). Histamine H_2-binding studies in the guinea pig brain. Agents and Actions, 14, 543-545.

Osband, M., and R. McCaffrey (1979). Solubilization, separation and partial characterization of histamine H_1 and H_2 receptors from calf thymocyte membranes. J. biol. Chem., 254, 9970-9972.

Rising, T.J., D.B. Norris, S.E. Warrander, and T.P. Wood (1980). High affinity ^{3}H-cimetidine binding in guinea pig tissues. Life. Sci., 27, 199-206.

Rosenfeld, G.C., E.D. Jacobson, and W.J. Thompson (1976). Gastric mucosal binding of ^{3}H-metiamide to putative histamine H_2-receptors. Gastroenterology, 70, 832-835.

Schwartz, J.C. T.T. Quach, and M. Garbarg (1982). Histamine receptors and actions in mammalian brain. In G. Biggio, E. Costa, G.L. Gessa, and P.F. Spano (Eds.), Advances in the biosciences, Vol. 44 Pergamon Press, 359-420.

Smith, I.R., M. Cleverley, C.R. Ganellin, and K. Metlers (1980). Binding of ^{3}H-cimetidine to rat brain tissue. Agents and Actions, 10, 422-426.

Warrander, S.E., D.B. Norris, T.J. Rising, and T.P. Wood (1983). ^{3}H-cimetidine and the H_2-receptor. Life Sci., 33, 1119-1126.

Webber, S.E., D.B. Norris, T.J. Rising, and J.C. Foreman (1984). Submitted to J. biol. Chem.

COGNITIVE PROPERTIES OF H_2 RECEPTORS REVEALED BY [^{3}H]HISTAMINE

J. W. Wells, D. L. Cybulsky, M. Kandel,
S. I. Kandel and G. H. Steinberg

Faculty of Pharmacy, University of Toronto, Toronto,
Ontario M5S 1A1, Canada

ABSTRACT

Homogenates of washed tissue from rat cerebral cortex bind low concentrations of [^{3}H]histamine at an apparently uniform population of sites with an affinity of 3.9 ± 0.5 nM and a capacity of 80-100 pmol/g protein. H_2 antagonists inhibit the interaction with Hill coefficients from 0.57 to 1.0; inhibitory potency (IC_{50}) correlates well with H_2 pharmacological potency in guinea-pig right atrium ($r = 0.992$, $n = 13$, $P < 0.00001$). All H_2 agonists other than histamine inhibit in a characteristic and distinctly biphasic manner that is not observed with compounds devoid of H_2 activity. The sites therefore can be identified as H_2 histaminic receptors. Upon solubilisation in 1% digitonin, the receptors behave in every respect as a single and uniform population of sites. Moreover, a new pharmacological specificity of binding emerges for H_2 antagonists but not for H_2 agonists. This divergence and other properties of the binding patterns suggest that H_2 agonists and antagonists bind at different sites in the membrane.

KEYWORDS

[^{3}H]Histamine binding; H_2 histaminic receptors; H_2 agonists; H_2 antagonists

INTRODUCTION

Sites with nanomolar affinity for [^{3}H]histamine first were reported by Palacios, Schwartz and Garbarg (1978) in homogenates of mammalian brain, and were found to bind H_2 agonists more tightly than H_1 agonists or catabolites of histamine. Barbin and co-workers (1980) subsequently demonstrated that the sites possess several properties indicative of histaminic receptors, but concluded that the pharmacological specificity was neither H_1 nor H_2. Studies in our own laboratory revealed good agreement between binding affinity and H_2 pharmacological potency for several H_2 agonists, excluding histamine, but not for the H_2 antagonists cimetidine and metiamide (Kandel and co-workers, 1980). The inconclusive nature of our preliminary work arose in part from the narrow selection of histaminic drugs, particularly antagonists, and in part from the technical problems associated with high levels of non-specific binding. In recent years, however, the selection of H_2-specific drugs has broadened considerably with respect both to structural diversity and to the range of pharmacological potency. Moreover, the sites have been solubilised (Cybulsky and co-workers, 1981), and levels of non-specific binding in suspension have been reduced. These developments have permitted us not only to identify the sites as H_2 receptors, but also to investigate some novel aspects of their interaction with histaminic drugs.

MATERIALS AND METHODS

Binding Assays

[^{3}H]Histamine was obtained from either Amersham Corporation (40-54 Ci/mmol) or New England Nuclear (32.2 Ci/mmol), and unlabelled histamine from Sigma. Ranitidine was kindly donated by Glaxo Canada Limited, Toronto; tiotidine by ICI Americas Inc., Wilmington, Delaware; and etintidine by Ortho Pharmaceutical Corporation, Raritan, New Jersey. All other histaminic drugs were the generous gift of Smith Kline and French Research Limited, Welwyn Garden City, U.K. P_2 pellets were prepared from the cerebral cortex of male Wistar rats, washed extensively, and either resuspended (100 mM Tris, 10 mM $MgCl_2$, 1 mM EDTA, pH 7.48, 0.4-2.0 mg protein per ml) or solubilised (1% digitonin, 50 mM Tris, 1 mM $MgCl_2$, pH 7.4, 0.9-1.6 mg protein per ml; Cybulsky and co-workers, 1981) for the binding assays. Binding was measured at 30° essentially according to reported procedures (Hulme and co-workers, 1978; Cybulsky and co-workers, 1981). Reaction mixtures were equilibrated for 45 min in suspension and 30 min in solution; bound radioligand was separated by microcentrifugation and gel filtration, respectively. Standard errors typically were less than 1% on quintuplicate determinations in suspension, and less than 2% on triplicate determinations in solution. Saturating concentrations of all drugs tested reduced the binding of [^{3}H]histamine to the same level, as expected if all drugs preclude access of the radioligand to the same population of sites. Non-specific binding generally constituted about 40% of the total signal at 1.4 nM [^{3}H]histamine in suspension, and 5-10% at 10 nM [^{3}H]histamine in solution; total binding usually did not represent more than 3% and 1%, respectively, of the radioligand added. Protein was measured according to the method of Lowry. Further details will be described elsewhere.[1,2]

Analysis of the Data

All data were analysed in non-linear form according to the Hill equation or to the expressions shown below. For histamine in suspension and for all compounds in solution, the radioligand (P) and the unlabelled drug (A) appear to compete for a uniform population of sites (R). Total binding of the radioligand at equilibrium ($[P]_{b,obs}$) is described by Eq. 1, in which K_P and K_A are the dissociation constants for P and A, respectively, and C is the fraction of free radioligand that appears as non-specific binding. P and A represent the quantities ($[P]_t-[P]_{b,s}$) and ($[A]_t-[A]_{b,s}$), respectively; $[P]_{b,s}$ and $[A]_{b,s}$ represent the specific binding of each ligand and were negligible relative to $[P]_t$ and $[A]_t$ in most experiments. Total concentrations are indicated by the subscript t. K_P was substituted for K_A in studies on the inhibition of [^{3}H]histamine by unlabelled histamine at low concentrations of the radioligand.

$$[P]_{b,obs} = \{[R]_t PK_A/(PK_A+AK_P+K_AK_P)\} + CP \quad (1)$$

For inhibition in suspension by ligands other than histamine, the data were analysed assuming one or two classes of non-interconverting sites as appropriate. Total binding of [^{3}H]histamine was described according to Eq. 2, in which $[P]_{b,max}$ and $[P]_{b,min}$ represent the asymptotic levels of binding at limiting concentrations of unlabelled drug; F_H and F_L sum to one and represent the fraction of sites exhibiting affinity K_H and K_L, respectively. F_H or F_L was set to zero when only one class of sites was justified by the data. The expression mirrors the binding of A only when $[A]_t$ approximates the free concentration and when the radioligand is essentially without effect on the shape or position of the curve.

$$[P]_{b,obs} = ([P]_{b,max}-[P]_{b,min})\{F_H K_H/(K_H+[A]_t) + F_L K_L(K_L+[A]_t)\} + [P]_{b,min} \quad (2)$$

All functions were fitted to experimental data according to the non-linear, least-squares algorithm of Marquardt (1963); Eq. 1 was solved numerically. Standard errors on replicate

---

[1]Steinberg, G.H., M. Kandel, S.I. Kandel and J.W. Wells, manuscript in preparation.
[2]Cybulsky, D.L., S.I. Kandel and J.W. Wells, manuscript in preparation.

determinations of total binding proved to be a constant percentage of the mean and the data were weighted accordingly. Statistical variation is indicated throughout by the standard error.

RESULTS

Binding of Histamine

Suspension. Histamine-specific sites in homogenates of washed tissue from rat cortex resemble those found in unwashed preparations studied previously (Barbin and co-workers, 1980; Kandel and co-workers, 1980). Maximal binding of [^{3}H]histamine is attained within 45 min at the concentrations used, and remains unchanged thereafter for up to 6 hr. Total binding at equilibrium includes a specific component that is precluded in the presence of 1 mM unlabelled histamine, and a non-specific component that increases linearly with the concentration of radioligand (Fig. 1A). As illustrated in Fig. 1C, the specific component can be described adequately assuming a single population of sites (Eq. 1); the mean dissociation constant (K_D) from three experiments is 3.9 ± 0.4 nM (log K_D = -8.41 ± 0.04), with capacities of 80-100 pmol/g protein.

The relative values of $[R]_t/K_D$ and C preclude the acquisition of data at concentrations of [^{3}H]histamine much above 10 nM. There accordingly is considerable uncertainty over the true shape of the binding profile, and hence over the appropriateness of the assumption that one class of non-interacting sites is involved. The data can be shown to be internally consistent at low concentrations of [^{3}H]histamine (< 1.5 nM) through competitive experiments with the unlabelled analogue. Seven experiments similar to that illustrated in Fig. 2A yield a mean Hill coefficient of 0.96 ± 0.03; the mean value of K_D for a single class of sites (Eq. 1) is 3.9 ± 0.7 nM (log K_D = -8.41 ± 0.08), which is identical to that obtained by varying the concentration of radioligand. At higher concentrations of [^{3}H]histamine, however, the competitive binding patterns become more complex and indicate that this model is overly simplistic.[1]

Solution. It has been noted previously that a single class of sites is inadequate to describe the saturable binding of histamine to the solubilised preparation (Cybulsky and co-workers, 1981). More recent work has indicated, however, that appreciable binding of the radioligand occurs in solutions of 1% digitonin lacking the membrane, and that the interaction is blocked by 0.1 mM unlabelled histamine. This non-specific but ostensibly saturable effect is concentration-dependent and can be described empirically assuming a single class of sites with an apparent affinity of 69 μM and a capacity of 5.3 nM. Total binding of [^{3}H]histamine to the solubilised preparation from rat cortex is illustrated in Fig. 1B, where 0.024% of the total radioligand is seen to bind in the presence of excess, unlabelled drug. A further 0.0076% binds in a saturable manner to the detergent, resulting in the total, non-specific contribution illustrated by the dashed line. Although negligible at concentrations of [^{3}H]histamine below 10-15 nM, binding to the detergent becomes appreciable at higher concentrations and gives rise to the heterogeneity reported previously.

Saturable binding attributable to the solubilised membrane attains equilibrium within 30 min and shows the concentration-dependence illustrated in Fig. 1D. The mean Hill coefficient from five experiments is 0.94 ± 0.05 and the data are well described assuming a single population of sites. The mean value for K_D is 4.8 ± 0.4 nM (log K_D = -8.31 ± 0.03) and capacities vary from 30 to 80 pmol/g protein. These results agree well with those obtained from studies on the inhibition of [^{3}H]histamine by its unlabelled analogue. Data from several experiments reveal a mean Hill coefficient of 1.03 ± 0.03 (n = 16) and good descriptions are obtained assuming a single class of sites (Fig. 2B). The mean value of K_D is 5.3 ± 0.9 nM (log K_D = -8.30 ± 0.04) from five experiments in which the concentration of [^{3}H]histamine was below 9 nM. Estimates of the Hill coefficient, K_D and capacity compare favourably in suspension and solution, suggesting that [^{3}H]histamine labels the same sites in both preparations.

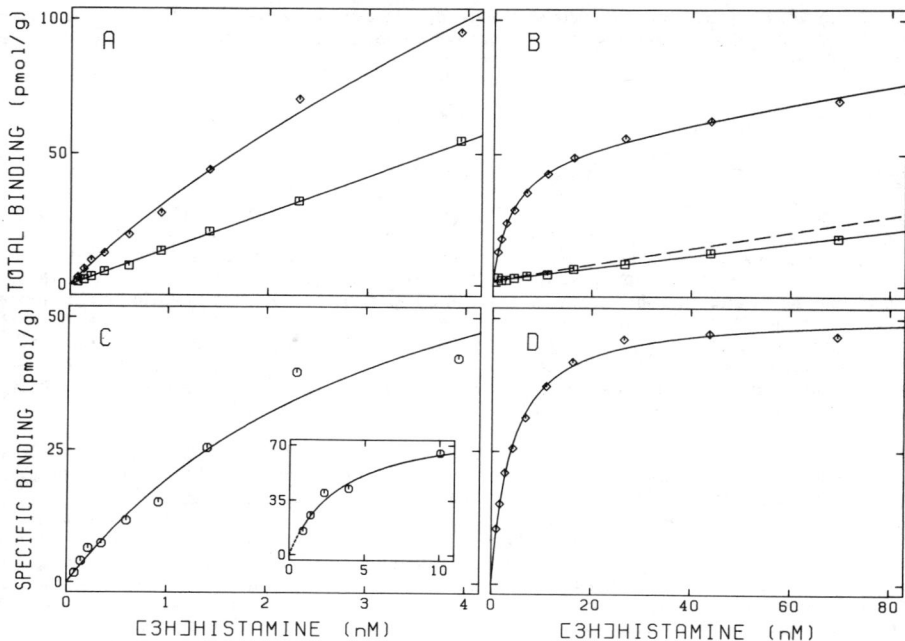

Fig. 1. Binding of [^{3}H]histamine in suspension (A and C) and solution (B and D). Total binding (A and B) was measured in the absence (◇) and presence (□) of 1 mM (A) or 0.1 mM (B) unlabelled histamine. The lines in A represent the best fit of Eq. 1 to the experimental data and the corresponding, parametric values are as follows: $K_P = 3.2 \pm 0.4$ nM, $[R]_t = 85 \pm 7$ pmol/g protein (2.0 mg protein per ml), $C = 13.8 \pm 0.2$ pmol·g^{-1}·nM^{-1}. The lines in B represent the best fit of an expression related to Eq. 1, but with two additional contributions to total binding. Firstly, a non-specific but apparently saturable component reflects the binding of [^{3}H]histamine to digitonin; values of K_P and $[R]_t$ for this component were determined independently and included as constants during successive iterations of the fitting procedure. Secondly, a y-intercept reflects the presence of a small background signal that is observed in some experiments. Parametric values obtained by regression for saturable binding attributable to the solubilised membrane are $K_P = 4.0 \pm 0.2$ nM and $[R]_t = 51 \pm 1$ pmol/g protein (1.0 mg protein per ml). The value of C is 0.24 ± 0.01 pmol·g^{-1}·nM^{-1} and the y-intercept is 2.0 ± 0.1 pmol/g protein. Total non-specific binding including that to digitonin is indicated by the dashed line. Specific binding is illustrated in C and D for suspension and for solution, respectively; values plotted on the ordinate represent total binding less the fitted estimate of non-specific binding. A point at 10 nM [^{3}H]histamine omitted from A and C is shown in the inset.

Binding of H$_2$ Agonists

<u>Suspension.</u> In competition with 1.4 nM [^{3}H]histamine, all H$_2$ agonists tested to date reveal the distinctly biphasic pattern illustrated for impromidine and 4-methylhistamine in Fig. 2A. The data are well described assuming two classes of sites differing in affinity for the drug (Eq. 2). The differences between K_H and K_L are substantial, and vary from nine hundredfold with N^α,N^α-dimethylhistamine (log $K_L/K_H = 2.95$) to over three millionfold with thiazolylethylamine (log $K_L/K_H = 6.49$). This behaviour evidently is peculiar to H$_2$ agonists, since N-methyldimaprit and telemethylhistamine both yield Hill coefficients indistinguishable from one (Fig. 2A); both compounds are structurally related to H$_2$ agonists but lack H$_2$ activity. Monophasic patterns also are obtained with unrelated, neurohumoral agents such as serotonin, dopamine and epinephrine.

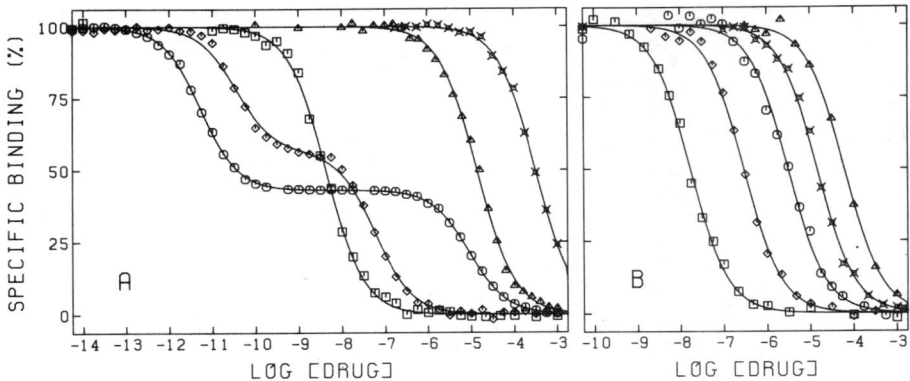

Fig. 2. Inhibition of [^{3}H]histamine by H$_2$ agonists and structurally related compounds in suspension (A) and solution (B). The lines represent best fits of Eq. 1 or Eq. 2 to experimental data obtained at different concentrations of the unlabelled drug. Values plotted on the ordinate are normalised at 100% and 0% to the asymptotes obtained from the fitting procedure. Points at the lower limit on the abscissa were determined in the absence of unlabelled drug. The total concentration of [^{3}H]histamine was 1.4 nM in suspension and 2-12 nM in solution. Parametric values obtained by regression are as follows: 4-methylhistamine (○) in (A), log K_H = -11.28 ± 0.01, log K_L = -5.04 ± 0.01, F_L = 0.43 ± 0.002; in (B), log K_A = -5.70 ± 0.03; impromidine (◇) in (A), log K_H = -10.45 ± 0.04, log K_L = -7.23 ± 0.03, F_L = 0.57 ± 0.01; in (B), log K_A = -7.01 ± 0.03; histamine (□) in (A), log K_P = -8.50 ± 0.02; in (B), log K_P = -8.30 ± 0.08; N-methyldimaprit (×) in (A), log K_L = -3.50 ± 0.01 (F_H = 0); in (B), log K_A = -5.33 ± 0.02; telemethylhistamine (△) in (A), log K_L = -4.86 ± 0.01 (F_H = 0); in (B), log K_A = -4.45 ± 0.03.

The data presented in Fig. 2A illustrate that the fraction of sites ostensibly of higher or lower affinity (F_H or F_L, respectively) varies significantly from agonist to agonist, in spite of the fact that the concentration of [^{3}H]histamine was 1.4 nM in all experiments. It therefore seems inappropriate to attribute the biphasic nature of the binding to two classes of non-interconverting sites; rather, the agonist itself appears to determine the distribution of sites between two states of different affinity. Since the multi-site model is based on the simple notion of heterogeneity and includes no provision for an agonist-driven interconversion, the parameters that define this expression must be regarded as empirical and parametric values interpreted with caution.

The determination of affinity is complicated further by the observation with dimaprit that K_H increases but K_L remains unchanged as the concentration of [^{3}H]histamine is raised from 1.4 to 10 nM. Since K_P for [^{3}H]histamine is ostensibly 3.9 nM at all sites, the inhibition by H$_2$ agonists is not attributable exclusively to competitive or to non-competitive effects. Moreover, K_H is markedly less than $[R_H]_t/2$ for three agonists, including 4-methylhistamine, when the capacity corresponding to F_H is calculated from the concentration and affinity of the radioligand. Since the apparent binding constants are in units of total agonist, this discrepancy implies that one equivalent of unlabelled drug precludes the interaction of [^{3}H]histamine with more than one equivalent of binding sites if the system is at thermodynamic equilibrium. While these considerations serve further to illustrate the uncertainty over the significance of K_H and K_L, it may be noteworthy that K_L and H$_2$ pharmacological potency in the guinea-pig right atrium differ by less than threefold for six out of ten agonists (Fig 3A). There is no correlation between K_H and K_L, suggesting that the structural requirements for binding differ at the sites reflected in each parameter.

Solution. H$_2$ agonists inhibit the specific binding of [^{3}H]histamine to the solubilised preparation with Hill coefficients indistinguishable from one. The binding patterns thus are well described assuming a single class of sites (Fig. 2B), in contrast to the two classes

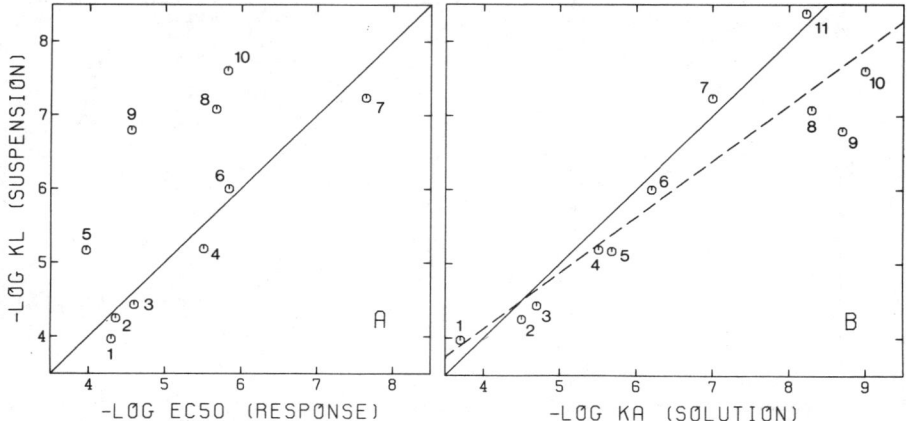

Fig. 3. Comparisons of apparent affinity and potency among H_2 agonists. The apparent affinity for binding in suspension (K_P for histamine, Eq. 1; K_L for other agonists, Eq. 2) is compared in A with the H_2 pharmacological potency in guinea-pig right atrium (EC_{50}), and in B with the apparent affinity for binding in solution (K_P for histamine and K_A for other agonists, Eq. 1). Equivalence and correlation are illustrated by the solid and dashed lines, respectively (in B: r = 0.931, P = 0.00003). Individual compounds are as follows: 1) thiazolylethylamine, 2) pyridylethylamine, 3) 2-methylhistamine, 4) 4-methylhistamine, 5) nordimaprit, 6) dimaprit, 7) impromidine, 8) imidazolylpropylguanidine, 9) N^α,N^α-dimethylhistamine, 10) N^α-methylhistamine, 11) histamine. Estimates of H_2 pharmacological potency were taken from the following sources: Black and co-workers, 1972 (burimamide); Blakemore and co-workers, 1981 (SK&F 93479); Cavanagh, Usakewicz and Buyniski, 1980 (etintidine); Daly, Humphray and Stables, 1981 (ranitidine); Durant and co-workers, 1978 (cimetidine, impromidine and SK&F 92408); Ganellin, Port and Richards, 1976 (N^α,N^α-dimethylhistamine, N^α-methylhistamine, 2-methylhistamine, telemethylhistamine); Ganellin, 1980 (norburimamide, 2-pyridylethylamine, 2-thiazolylethylamine); C.R. Ganellin, Smith Kline and French Research Limited, personal communication (nordimaprit, SK&F 92374, SK&F 92422, SK&F 92540); Kandel and co-workers, 1980 (histamine); Parsons and co-workers, 1975 (imidazolylpropylguanidine); Parsons and co-workers, 1977 (dimaprit); Smith and co-workers, 1980 (SK&F 92629); Trendelenburg, 1960 (mepyramine); Yellin and co-workers, 1979 (tiotidine).

observed in suspension. Moreover, the potency (IC_{50}) of an agonist in solution varies with the concentration of [^{3}H]histamine in a competitive manner commensurate with the measured value of K_P for the radioligand. The single affinity observed in solution (K_A, Eq. 1) correlates well with the weaker of the two affinities (K_L, Eq. 2) observed in suspension (P = 0.00003, Fig. 3B). This comparison argues further that [^{3}H]histamine labels the same sites in both preparations.

Binding of H_2 Antagonists

Suspension. Hill coefficients for the inhibition of 1.4 nM [^{3}H]histamine by fourteen H_2 antagonists vary from 1.0 to 0.57. The data thus can be described assuming either one or two classes of sites (Eq. 2), depending upon the drug (Fig. 4A). Among those antagonists for which the two-site model is justified by the data, there are significant differences in the values of F_L, as illustrated by the comparison between SK&F 92629 and SK&F 92540 in Fig. 4A. The patterns of inhibition thus resemble those observed for agonists in that the apparent distribution of sites among two states depends, at least in part, upon the drug. In other respects, however, agonists and antagonists show marked differences in their behaviour. For both tiotidine (n_H = 0.97 ± 0.01) and cimetidine (n_H = 0.59 ± 0.002), changes in the concentration of [^{3}H]histamine over the practicable range from 1 to 10 nM

Cognitive properties of H$_2$ receptors

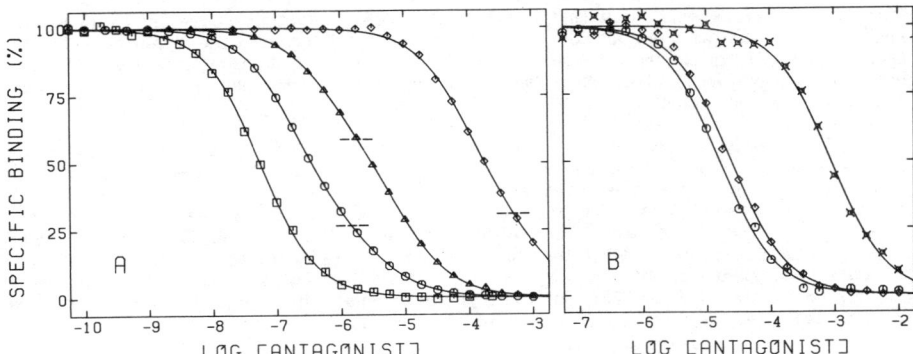

Fig. 4. Inhibition of [^{3}H]histamine by H$_2$ antagonists in suspension (A) and solution (B). The solid lines represent best fits of Eq. 2 (A) or Eq. 1 (B) to the experimental data; the dashed lines in A illustrate the value of F_L for those antagonists that reveal two classes of sites. Further details are given in the legend to Fig. 2. Parametric values obtained by regression are as follows: SK&F 92540 (○) in A, log K_H = -6.71 ± 0.01, log K_L = -5.51 ± 0.03, F_2 = 0.26 ± 0.01; in B, log K_A = -4.95 ± 0.04; SK&F 92374 (◇) in A, log K_H = -3.99 ± 0.05, log K_L = -3.02 ± 0.15, F_2 = 0.28 ± 0.07; in B, log K_A = -5.03 ± 0.02; SK&F 92629 (△) in A, log K_H = -6.19 ± 0.02, log K_L = -5.09 ± 0.02, F_2 = 0.59 ± 0.02; tiotidine (□) in A, log K_L = -7.26 ± 0.01 (F_H = 0); ranitidine (×) in B, log K_A = -3.43 ± 0.02.

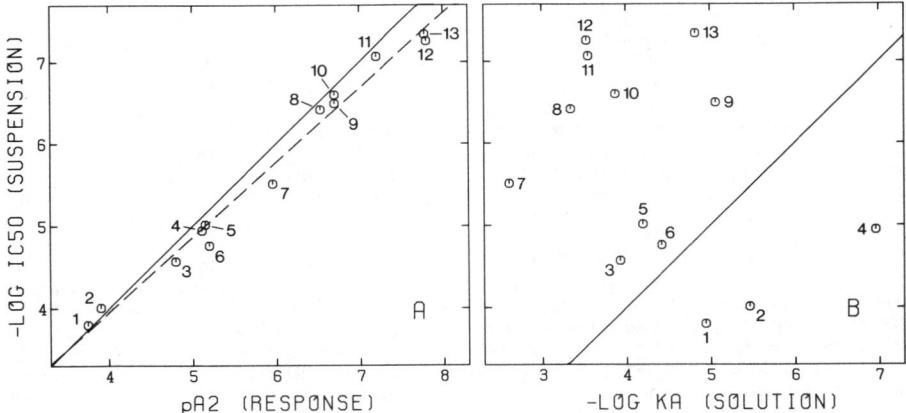

Fig. 5. Comparisons of apparent affinity and potency among H$_2$ antagonists. Inhibitory potency versus the specific binding of [^{3}H]histamine in suspension (-log IC$_{50}$) is compared in A with the H$_2$ pharmacological potency in guinea-pig right atrium (pA$_2$), and in B with the apparent affinity for binding in solution (-log K_A, Eq. 1). Estimates of IC$_{50}$ were calculated from the values of K_H, K_L and F_L that define the best fit of Eq. 2 to the binding curves. Equivalence and correlation are illustrated by the solid and dashed lines, respectively (in A: r = 0.992, P < 0.00001). Individual compounds are as follows: 1) SK&F 92374, 2) norburimamide, 3) SK&F 92408, 4) burimamide, 5) SK&F 92422, 6) mepyramine, 7) SK&F 92629, 8) cimetidine, 9) SK&F 92540, 10) etintidine, 11) ranitidine, 12) SK&F 93479, 13) tiotidine. Estimates of H$_2$ pharmacological potency were taken from the sources listed in the legend to Fig. 3.

are without effect on either the shape of the curve or its position on the abscissa. The data thus are not consistent with the notion of simple competition between an antagonist and a radioligand with an affinity (K_P) of 3.9 nM. Moreover, the shallowest binding profile among all antagonists tested to date is obtained with SK&F 93479; the difference between K_H and K_L is less than 60-fold, in contrast to the much larger differences observed with H_2 agonists.

Figure 5A presents a comparison among H_2 antagonists between inhibitory potency in the binding assay (-log IC_{50}) and reported, pharmacological potency in the guinea-pig right atrium (pA_2). The former was taken as the concentration of antagonist at which specific binding of the radioligand is reduced by 50% according to Eq. 2, assuming one or two classes of sites as appropriate. The excellent correlation (r = 0.992, P < 0.00001) argues strongly that the sites labelled by [^{3}H]histamine are H_2 receptors. The correlation is somewhat less significant if -log IC_{50} is replaced by -log K_H (r = 0.971, P < 0.00001) or -log K_L (R = 0.936, P < 0.00001) for the eight antagonists that reveal two classes of sites; in each case, pA_2 is numerically closer to the former.

Solution. In the solubilised preparation, antagonists are found to inhibit the specific binding of [^{3}H]histamine with Hill coefficients indistinguishable from one whenever the solubility and potency of the drug allow a complete binding curve to be obtained (Fig. 4B). Moreover, the value of IC_{50} increases with the concentration of the radioligand in the manner expected for competitive inhibition. The multiphasic binding patterns and the apparently non-competitive behaviour observed in suspension thus are lost upon solubilisation. Values of K_A obtained for H_2 antagonists in solution are compared in Fig. 5B with the corresponding values of IC_{50} in suspension. The absence of any correlation indicates that solubilisation has altered profoundly the pharmacological specificity for the inhibition of [^{3}H]histamine by H_2 antagonists. Three drugs become more potent and eleven become weaker, with the change in apparent affinity exceeding one thousandfold for some.

DISCUSSION

Two lines of evidence argue that [^{3}H]histamine labels an H_2 receptor in homogenates of rat cerebral cortex. Firstly, there is an excellent correlation (P < 0.00001) among thirteen H_2 antagonists between the concentration that reduces the specific binding of [^{3}H]histamine by 50% (log IC_{50}) and the reported, pharmacological potency (pA_2) in the guinea-pig right atrium;[3] moreover, estimates of -log IC_{50} and pA_2 are numerically similar, suggesting that a linear relationship exists between occlusion of the receptors and inhibition of the response. Secondly, H_2 agonists inhibit the binding of [^{3}H]histamine in a highly characteristic, biphasic manner that has not been observed to date with compounds that lack H_2 activity.

Dissolution of the receptor in 1% digitonin is accompanied by profound changes in the binding properties revealed by histaminic drugs. The radioligand nevertheless appears to label the same sites in both preparations. Binding parameters obtained for histamine itself are similar before and after solubilisation. The apparent affinity in suspension (3.9 nM) agrees well with that in solution (5.1 nM); the capacities compare favourably, with the solubilised preparation showing about 50% fewer sites per unit mass of protein. The sites in both preparations show a common pharmacological specificity for H_2 agonists, as indicated by the good correlation between the single affinity observed in solution (K_A) and the weaker of the two affinities observed in suspension (K_L). For six agonists in addition to histamine, estimates of K_A and K_L agree numerically to within a factor of three.

The two preparations also reveal a number of similarities in the effects of guanylylnucleotides and magnesium on the binding of histamine. Barbin and co-workers

---

[3]Mr. Steven Howorucha in our laboratory recently has extended this comparison to twenty compounds (r = 0.987; P < 0.00001), with the inclusion of S-sopromidine and six other H_2 antagonists kindly provided by Dr. W. Schunack of the Institut für Pharmazie, Freie Universität Berlin.

(1980) have reported that GMP-PNP reduces the capacity for [^{3}H]histamine in crude homogenates by 37% with no significant change in the dissociation constant, which they found to be 5.9 nM; a similar effect has been found in our own laboratory and has been shown to require magnesium.[1] We have reported more recently that the inhibitory effect of GMP-PNP on the specific binding of [^{3}H]histamine is retained in solution and arises from an increase in the rate constant for dissociation of the radioligand (Cybulsky and co-workers, 1981); we subsequently have demonstrated that this action of GMP-PNP also requires magnesium.[2] The removal of magnesium in the absence of nucleotide reduces, but does not eliminate, the specific binding of [^{3}H]histamine in both suspension and solution.[1,2] Magnesium and guanylylnucleotide thus have similar effects in both preparations; their action suggests that [^{3}H]histamine labels the same receptors before and after solubilisation, and also that those receptors interact with a G/F-protein possibly linked to adenylate cyclase.

The changes that accompany solubilisation imply that the inhibition of [^{3}H]histamine by H_2-specific drugs is mechanistically different in the two preparations. With antagonists, a new pharmacological specificity emerges that differs markedly from the H_2 specificity observed in suspension. If the same site mediates the pharmacological action of all H_2-specific drugs in vivo, one might expect a comparable reordering of affinities to occur among H_2 agonists. Histamine itself behaves similarly in both preparations, however, and the pharmacological specificity toward H_2 agonists is retained, at least at the sites of lower affinity. The question of specificity at the sites of higher affinity is moot following solubilisation, as those sites are no longer observed. This differential effect of solubilisation constitutes a paradox that would be resolved were agonists and antagonists to bind at different sites in the membrane. The inhibitory action of the latter on the binding of [^{3}H]histamine in suspension then would reflect an allosteric interaction that becomes uncoupled in solution, with a concomitant change in pharmacological specificity. It has been noted above that the inhibitory potency of antagonists (IC_{50}) is insensitive to the concentration of [^{3}H]histamine in suspension but sensitive in solution; this apparent change from non-competitive to competitive inhibition may reflect binding at the antagonist-specific site in the former, and at the agonist-specific site in the latter. The suggestion of an allosteric mechanism for the antihistaminic action of H_2 antagonists is speculative, but raises the possibility of a yet unrecognised class of H_2 antagonists that inhibit in a competitive manner and may differ therapeutically from existing drugs.

The effects of solubilisation on the binding of H_2 agonists are difficult to rationalise in view of the nature of the binding patterns in suspension. The curves not only are incompatible with a mixture of non-interconverting sites, as pointed out above, but also are difficult to reconcile with co-operative models based on the Adair equation and a ternary complex model suggested for the ß-adrenergic system (De Lean, Stadel and Lefkowitz, 1980). The complex nature of the inhibition is reflected further in the paradoxical sensitivity of the binding profiles to the concentration of [^{3}H]histamine, and also in the observation that the stoichiometry of inhibition at R_H appears to exceed one for some agonists. It seems unlikely that the apparent disappearance of sites of higher affinity reflects simply a failure to solubilise a particular subpopulation of the receptors labelled by [^{3}H]histamine in suspension. Firstly, the biphasic nature of the binding is a property, at least in part, of the agonist and not exclusively of the receptors. Secondly, the selective solubilisation of some receptors is difficult to reconcile with the observed changes in the binding of antagonists. It thus seems reasonable to suggest that the sites of higher affinity are not observed in solution owing to the failure of an unknown component to interact with the receptor. Since the action of GMP-PNP is retained in solution (Cybulsky and co-workers, 1981), the unknown component is presumably not the G/F-protein. If H_2 antagonists indeed bind in suspension at a site distinct from histamine, the same component may be necessary both for the inhibition by antagonists and for the biphasic, inhibitory pattern of agonists.

ACKNOWLEDGEMENTS

The authors are grateful to Dr. C.R. Ganellin and his colleagues at Smith Kline and French Research Limited, Welwyn Garden City, for their interest and for their invaluable contribution of histaminic drugs. Mr. Andras Nagy is thankfully acknowledged for his knowledgeable assistance in various technical matters, and Miss Marybeth Chen for her careful typing of the manuscript. This investigation was supported by the J.P. Bickell Foundation and the Medical Research Council of Canada (Grants MT-3057 and MA-7130). J.W.W. is a Career Scientist of the Ontario Ministry of Health and during the course of this investigation was a Scholar of the Canadian Heart Foundation.

REFERENCES

Barbin, G., J.-M. Palacios, E. Rodergas, J.-C. Schwartz, and M. Garbarg (1980). Characterization of the high-affinity binding sites of [^{3}H]histamine in rat brain. Mol. Pharmacol., 18, 1-10.

Black, J.W., W.A.M. Duncan, G.F. Durant, C.R. Ganellin, and E.M. Parsons (1972). Definition and antagonism of histamine H_2-receptors. Nature, 236, 385-390.

Blakemore, R.C., T.H. Brown, G.J. Durant, C.R. Ganellin, M.E. Parsons, A.C. Rasmussen, and D.A. Rawlings (1981). SK&F 93479, a potent and long acting histamine H_2-receptor antagonist. Br. J. Pharmac., 74, 200P.

Cavanagh, R.L., J.J. Usakewicz, and J.P. Buyniski (1980). Comparative activities of three new histamine H_2-receptor antagonists-BL-5641, ranitidine, and ICI 125,211. Fed. Proc., 39, 768.

Cybulsky, D.L., S.I. Kandel, J.W. Wells, and A.G. Gornall (1981). Guanylylimidodiphosphate modulates [^{3}H]histamine binding in a solubilised preparation from rat brain. Eur. J. Pharmac., 407-409.

Daly, M.J., J.M. Humphray, and R. Stables (1981). Some in vitro and in vivo actions of the new histamine H_2-receptor antagonist, ranitidine. Br. J. Pharmac., 72, 49-54.

De Lean, A., J.M. Stadel, and R.J. Lefkowitz (1980). A ternary complex model explains the agonist-specific binding properties of the adenylate cyclase-coupled ß-adrenergic receptor. J. Biol. Chem., 255, 7108-7117.

Durant, G.J., W.A.M. Duncan, C.R. Ganellin, M.E. Parsons, R.C. Blakemore, and A.C. Rasmussen (1978). Impromidine (SK&F 92676) is a very potent and specific agonist for histamine H_2 receptors. Nature, 276, 403-404.

Ganellin, C.R., G.N.J. Port, and W.G. Richards (1976). Conformation of histamine derivatives. 2. Molecular orbital calculations of preferred conformations in relation to dual receptor activity. J. Med. Chem., 16, 616-620.

Ganellin, C.R. (1980). In A. Torsoli, P.E. Lucchelli, and R.W. Brimblecombe (Eds.), H_2 antagonists, Excerpta Medica, Amsterdam. pp. 231-241.

Hulme, E.C., N.J.M. Birdsall, A.S.V. Burgen, and P. Mehta (1978). The binding of antagonists to brain muscarinic receptors. Mol. Pharmacol., 14, 737-750.

Kandel, S.I., G.H. Steinberg, J.W. Wells, M. Kandel, and A.G. Gornall (1980). Seperate binding sites for histaminic drugs in rat cerebral cortex. Biochem. Pharmacol., 29, 2269-2272.

Marquardt, D.L. (1963). An algorithm for least-squares estimation of nonlinear parameters. J. Soc. Ind. Appl. Math., 11, 431-441.

Palacios, J.-M., J.-C. Schwartz, and M. Garbarg (1978). High affinity binding of [^{3}H]histamine in rat brain. Eur. J. Pharmac., 50, 443-444.

Parsons, M.E., R.C. Blakemore, G.J. Durant, C.R. Ganelin, and A.C. Rasmussen (1975). 3-[4(5)-Imidazolyl]propylguanidine (SK&F 91486) — a partial agonist at histamine H_2-receptors. Agents Actions, 5, 464.

Parsons, M.E., D.A.A. Owen, C.R. Ganellin, and G.J. Durant (1977). Dimaprit — [S-[3-(N,N-dimethylamino)propyl]isothiourea] — a highly specific histamine H_2-receptor agonist. Part 1. Pharmacology. Agents Actions, 7, 31-37.

Smith, I.R., M.T. Cleverley, C.R. Ganellin, and K.M. Metters (1980). Binding of [^{3}H]cimetidine to rat brain tissue. Agents Actions, 10, 422-426.

Trendelenburg, U. (1960). The action of histamine and 5-hydroxytryptamine on isolated mammalian atria. J. Pharmacol., 130, 450-460.

Yellin, T.O., S.H. Buck, D.J. Gilman, D.F. Jones, and J.M. Wardleworth (1979). ICI 125,271: A new gastric antisecretory agent acting on histamine H_2-receptors. Life Sci., 25, 2001-2009.

DESENSITIZATION OF HISTAMINE H_2 RECEPTORS IN HUMAN LEUKEMIA CELLS

C. L. Johnson and D. G. Sawutz

Department of Pharmacology and Cell Biophysics,
University of Cincinnati College of Medicine,
Cincinnati, Ohio 45267, USA

ABSTRACT

The HL-60 cell line was originally derived from a patient with promyelocytic leukemia and consists mainly of promyelocytes with a small proportion of more mature cells formed by a slow rate of spontaneous differentiation under normal culture conditions. The specific H_2 agonist dimaprit, in the concentration range of 10^{-7} to 10^{-4} M, induced partial maturation of HL-60 cells as assessed by morphological appearance and the induction of biochemical markers, including lysozyme, beta-glucuronidase, and NBT reductase. The failure of dimaprit to cause complete differentiation to the terminal neutrophil stage may be due to rapid desensitization of the H_2 receptor response. Exposure of HL-60 cells to 10^{-5} M dimaprit caused an 80-90 % loss of the agonist's ability to stimulate the production of cAMP with a half-time of about 2.5 hours. The desensitization was completely blocked by including 10^{-5} M cimetidine in the initial incubation with dimaprit, and adding cimetidine after desensitization had taken place caused virtually complete recovery within 24 hours. The dimaprit-induced desensitization was largely homologous, but some heterologous desensitization of the PGE_2 stimulated production of cAMP was also seen (usually about 20%). In contrast, 10^{-5} M PGE_2 caused heterologous desensitization to both prostaglandin and dimaprit, and this loss of cAMP response was largely reversed by the phosphodiesterase inhibitor IBMX, suggesting that induction of phophodiesterase may be the mechanism of the PGE_2-induced desensitization. Neither the homologous nor the heterologous component of the dimaprit-induced desensitization was influenced by the phosphodiesterase inhibitor. The microtubule and microfilament inhibitors, colchicine and cytochalasin B (both at 10^{-6} M), did not influence dimaprit-induced desensitization. In addition, binding studies with [^{3}H]-tiotidine failed to show any decrease in number of binding sites after desensitization. Some evidence for the validity of the tiotidine binding assay was provided by the observation that the irreversible H_2 antagonist L-643,441 (10^{-5} M for 1 hour followed by extensive washing of the cells) caused a complete loss of binding sites. These results suggest that receptor internalization was not involved in dimaprit-induced desensitization. The most likely explanation for the desensitization involves a structural change in the receptor such that it is uncoupled from the adenylate cyclase. Both the dimaprit and PGE_2 desensitizations were completely blocked by mepacrine. The possibility that phospholipase-A_2 activation is involved in desensitization is discussed. The physiological relevance of H_2 receptor desensitization is unknown, but evidence exists for its occurance in mouse T lymphocytes after injection of histamine. Since histamine is released during inflammatory reactions, desensitization of H_2

receptors in various tissues could result in a variety of different responses depending on the tissues involved. Correlation of H_2 receptor desensitization with alterations in histamine-mediated function may lead to a clearer understanding of the still poorly defined physiological role of these receptors in various tissues.

KEYWORDS

Desensitization; histamine; H_2 receptor; PGE_1 receptor; cAMP; [^{3}H]-tiotidine binding; cultured cell line; cell differentiation.

INTRODUCTION

Acute myelogenous leukemia (AML) is considered to be a disease primarily involving a block in the differentiation of myeloid cells and it continues to be one of the most difficult leukemias to treat (Collins and co-workers, 1978). The growth advantage of myeloid leukemia cells over normal cells is their failure to differentiate into the normal non-dividing terminal cells, neutrophils and macrophages. Chemical agents which induce differentiation in these blocked cells are of considerable theoretical and practical interest, but research along these lines has been difficult in the past due to the absence of suitable model systems for testing drugs. Animal models of this leukemia do not appear to be very similar to human AML, and fresh human leukemic cells have a limited survival time in vitro. Several human myeloid cell lines have been established, from patients with myelogenous leukemia, which have long term survival in liquid suspension culture. These cells may provide the necessary tools for eventually understanding the regulatory mechanisms involved in growth and differentiation of myeloid cells and how these mechanisms may be modified by pharmacological agents.

The HL-60 cell line was established in 1977 from a patient with AML and has been widely used for cell differentiation studies. The cells grow well in suspension culture, have a mean doubling time of 30-40 hours, and have been reported to maintain distinct myeloid characteristics for at least a year in continuous culture (Collins and co-workers, 1978). The majority of cells in an HL-60 culture are promyelocytes, but a small percentage of more mature cells are present having the morphological and histochemical characteristics of myelocytes, metamyelocytes, and banded and segmented neutrophils (Collins and co-workers, 1977). Recently it was reported that agents which increase cAMP levels in HL-60 cells also cause some degree of cell differentiation (Chaplinski and Niedel, 1982). For example, dibutyryl-cAMP, PGE_2, and theophyllin induced several changes indicative of differentiation: (a) There was an induction of the differentiation-related plasma membrane markers, chemotactic peptide receptor and NBT reductase activity, within a few hours after exposure to the elevated cAMP levels. (b) The increase in these markers appeared before any obvious morphological maturation. (c) Continuous exposure of the cells to elevated cAMP for 1 to 2 days appeared to be required for differentiation to the metamyelocyte stage. (d) PGE_2 and theophyllin induced functional changes similar to db-cAMP but the cells matured only to the myelocyte stage.

A recent study demonstrated that HL-60 cells possess both histamine H_2 and PGE receptors coupled to the production of cAMP (Gespach and co-workers, 1982). More than 20 fold increases in cAMP levels were noted with both agents, even in the absence of a phosphodiesterase inhibitor. The present study was undertaken to determine if H_2 agonists would cause differentiation of the HL-60 cell. Although differentiation to the myelocyte and metamyelocyte stage was observed, terminal maturation to the neutrophil stage was not evident, similar to the results with PGE_2 (Chaplinsky and Niedel, 1982). Our results suggest that one explanation for the failure of both dimaprit and prostaglandin to induce a more extensive maturation is that both the H_2 and PGE receptors are rapidly desensitized after exposure to their respective agonists and that cAMP levels may not remain elevated long enough to insure terminal differentiation. We describe here attempts at defining the molecular mechanism involved in the desensitization process.

METHODS

Cell Culture

HL-60 cells (American Type Culture, Rockville MD) were grown in suspension culture in RPMI-1640 supplemented with 10% heat inactivated fetal calf serum, 2 mM glutamine, 1 mM sodium pyruvate, Minimal Essential Medium vitamins and amino acids, and Tylosine, in 5% CO_2 in air at 37°C. The cells were subcultured every 4-5 days to maintain an approximate density of 0.5 - 3.0 x 10^6 cells/ml. For the desensitization studies, agonists were added directly to the cell culture medium. After various periods of exposure, the cells were collected by centrifugation and resuspended in cold MOPS-Kreb's buffer (pH 7.4) of the following composition (in mM): NaCl (120), KCl (4.7), $CaCL_2$ (1.2), $MgSO_4$ (1.2), MOPS (5), and dextrose (5). The cells were washed three times and resuspended in the same buffer. Trypan blue exclusion was generally greater than 90%.

cAMP Assay

cAMP levels were determined essentially as described by Gespach and co-workers (1982). HL-60 cells (approximately 10^6 cells) were preincubated for 10 min in buffer at 37°C. Following the addition of appropriate agonists, the incubation was continued for an additional 10 min and terminated by the addition of boiling acetate buffer. After centrifugation the supernates were collected and assayed by radioimmune assay using ^{125}I-TME-ScAMP and the standard acetylation procedure (Steiner and co-workers, 1972). The cAMP standard curve was constructed over the range 1 fmole to 2.5 pmoles and fit by the ALLFIT program of DeLean and co-workers (1978) adapted for the Apple computer by one of us (C. L. J).

Protein Kinase

Protein kinase and the protein kinase activity ratio was determined essentially as described by Cherrington and co-workers (1976). After exposure of cells to agonists for various periods of time, the cells were rapidly cooled and centrifuged, the cell pellet was resuspended in MOPS-Kreb's buffer with 10 mM EGTA and 5 mg activated charcoal (to remove free cAMP), the cells were lysed by 2 freeze-thaw cycles, and the supernate obtained after high speed centrifugation was immediately added to the protein kinase assay buffer (50 mM Tris, 10 mM NaF, 3 mM $MgCl_2$, 0.1 mM IBMX, 0.06 mg/ml Kemptide, 0.02 mM [^{32}P]ATP, plus or minus 0.002 mM cAMP). The tubes were incubated at 30°C and aliquots removed at 2 min intervals and applied to 1 cm squares of Whatman P81 phosphocellulose paper (Glass and co-workers, 1978). After extensive washing the paper squares were counted in a liquid scintillation counter.

[^{3}H]-Tiotidine Binding Assay

HL-60 cells in buffer were incubated with 10^{-7} M [^{3}H]-tiotidine (1.8 x 10^6 cpm) for 3 hours at 4°C. The reaction was terminated by addition of 5 ml cold MOPS-Kreb's buffer followed by filtration. The Schleicher and Schuell #25 glass fiber filters were pretreated with a 1% Prosil-28/1% BSA solution for 2 hours as described by Harden and co-workers (1983) which decreased non-specific filter binding by more than a factor of 10. The treated filters were washed with 4 x 5 ml water before applying the sample. After application of the sample, the filters were washed with 3 x 5 ml cold buffer and counted in a scintillation counter. Specific binding was defined as total binding minus the binding observed in the presence of 10^{-4} M cimetidine.

RESULTS

HL-60 Cell Differentiation

Because of the long incubation times involved and the reported presence of histaminase in myeloid cells, we employed the specific H_2 agonist dimaprit in most of the studies described here. Dimaprit in the concentration range 10^{-7} to 10^{-4} M induced the partial maturation of HL-60 cells (Kalinyak and co-workers, 1983). Morphological changes were not evident for the first 2 days after exposure to the agonist. Even after 6 days, most of the cells had matured only to the myelocyte stage, with a small proportion of metamyelocytes but no obvious banded neutrophils. The morphological evidence of maturation was supported by biochemical marker studies: both lysozyme and NBT reductase activities were induced in dimaprit-treated cells.

Effect of Dimaprit on cAMP Levels and Protein Kinase Activity

HL-60 cells were cultured in the presence of 10^{-5} M dimaprit for various periods of time. Aliquots were removed for the determination of cAMP levels and protein kinase activity ratio. For the cAMP determinations, the cells were centrifuged and both the supernatant and cell pellet were analyzed. As shown in Table 1, there was a rapid increase in both the cAMP levels and the protein kinase activity ratio which peaked around a half-hour after addition of the H_2 agonist. This was followed by a drop in the protein kinase activity and cell cAMP levels. It appeared that most of the cellular cAMP was extruded into the external medium within about 2 hours and this cAMP remained detectable by RIA for more than a day.

TABLE 1   Effect of Dimaprit on cAMP and Protein Kinase

Time of Exposure to 10^{-5} M Dimaprit (hours)	cAMP Levels pmoles/10^6 cells		Protein Kinase Activity Ratio -cAMP:+cAMP
	Cells	Medium	
0	0.76	0.66	0.067
1/3	73.1	6.5	0.65
2/3	99.6	16.8	0.41
1	53.0	21.3	0.49
2	4.6	83.6	0.48
3	5.4	63.1	ND
4	3.5	60.7	ND
8	5.5	60.4	0.19
12	3.2	65.1	ND
24	3.3	61.1	0.20

ND = not determined

These results indicate that following exposure to the H_2 agonist there is a rapid loss of the ability of the HL-60 cell to maintain elevated levels of cAMP. There are a number of possible mechanisms for such an effect which will be considered in the following sections.

Specificity of the Loss of cAMP Response

When HL-60 cells were exposed to dimaprit for various periods of time, then extensively washed and assayed for their ability to respond to agonists, it was observed that there was a rapid loss in response to H_2 agonists (either dimaprit or histamine) but very little loss of response to PGE_2 (Table 2). This suggested that an induction of cAMP phosphodiesterase by dimaprit could not be the explanation for the decreased response. In support of this view, we found that inclusion of the phosphodiesterase inhibitor IBMX (0.5 mM) did not reverse the loss of response.

TABLE 2 Time Course of Dimaprit Induced Loss of cAMP Response

Time of Exposure to 10^{-4} M Dimaprit hours	cAMP Response	
	10^{-4} M Dimaprit	10^{-5} M PGE_2
	% of control	
0	100	100
2	62.4	112.5
4	16.7	91.8
6	13.5	78.2
8	16.6	93.5
12	12.0	72.0
24	12.0	69.0
48	15.0	87.0

There was a loss of cAMP from HL-60 cells after exposure to dimaprit (Table 1). Calculations of cell volumes indicated that the movement of cAMP was down a large concentration gradient. Although an increased diffusion of cAMP from the cells could explain the decreased sensitivity to dimaprit, it clearly could not explain the maintainance of PGE_2 sensitivity unless one postulates separate pools of cAMP associated with each receptor. Thus the most likely explanation for the decreased response to H_2 agonists is a specific, homologous receptor desensitization.

Characterization of H_2 Receptor Desensitization

As shown in Table 2, the dimaprit-induced desensitization was rapid, with a half-time of about 2.5 hours using 10^{-5} M dimaprit. In general, 80-90 percent of the response was lost within 4 hours; the remainder appeared to be relatively stable and cAMP levels always remained slightly elevated even days after continuous exposure to dimaprit. Histamine and impromidine induced a desensitization indistinguishable from that of dimaprit, whereas the analog, N-methyl dimaprit (SK&F 92054), which is pharmacologically inactive was incapable of increasing cAMP levels or causing desensitization. The dimaprit-induced desensitization was completely prevented by 10^{-3} M cimetidine but was not affected by 10^{-5} M mepyramine (Table 3). After a 4 hour dimaprit desensitization, addition of cimetidine resulted in virtually complete recovery of sensitivity within 24 hours (data not shown).

TABLE 3 Effect of Cimetidine and Mepyramine on Desensitization

Desensitization Conditions	Stimulation by 10^{-4} M Dimaprit (pmoles cAMP/10^6 cells)
Control	159 +/- 19
10^{-5} M Dimaprit	20 +/- 3
10^{-3} M Cimetidine	173 +/- 5
Dimaprit + Cimetidine	176 +/- 21
Control	242 +/- 26
10^{-5} M Dimaprit	50 +/- 5
10^{-5} M Mepyramine	317 +/- 7
Dimaprit + Mepyramine	62 +/- 3

It has been reported that beta receptor desensitization in ascites cells does not occur at low temperatures, possibly due to a decrease in microtubule function believed to be involved in receptor internalization (Kurokawa and co-workers, 1979). H_2 receptor desensitization in HL-60 cells was also blocked at 4°C (Table 4). However, we did not observe any effect of the microtubule and microfilament inhibitors, colchicine and cytochalasin B, on dimaprit-induced desensitization (Table 4). It is possible that the temperature dependence reflects a metabolic component of the desensitization mechanism, and some support for this view may be provided by the results obtained with dinitrophenol (Table 4). The degree of desensitization appeared to be markedly attenuated by DNP, although the interpretation of these results is complicated by the large DNP-induced decrease in dimaprit sensitivity in the control cells.

TABLE 4   Effect of Various Assay Conditions on Desensitization

Desensitization Conditions	Stimulation by 10^{-4} M Dimaprit (pmoles cAMP/10^6 cells)
37°C	
Control	57.5 +/- 9.0
10^{-5} M Dimaprit	2.9 +/- 0.5
4°C	
Control	67.2 +/- 4.0
10^{-5} M Dimaprit	89.7 +/- 3.0
Control	38.5 +/- 2.5
10^{-5} M Dimaprit	3.2 +/- 0.5
10^{-6} M Colchicine	31.5 +/- 1.0
Dimaprit + Colchicine	7.1 +/- 3.5
Control	136.0 +/- 11.0
10^{-5} M Dimaprit	10.8 +/- 0.5
10^{-6} M Cytochalasin B	87.3 +/- 5.4
Dimaprit + Cytochalasin B	9.6 +/- 2.5
Control	57.5 +/- 9.0
10^{-5} M Dimaprit	2.9 +/- 0.5
10^{-4} M Dinitrophenol	9.7 +/- 0.5
Dimaprit + Dinitrophenol	6.7 +/- 2.7
Control	136.2 +/- 11.0
10^{-5} M Dimaprit	10.8 +/- 1.0
10^{-4} M Mepacrine	146.6 +/- 5.0
Dimaprit + Mepacrine	155.2 +/- 4.0

It has been suggested that beta receptor desensitization in astrocytoma cells is mediated by activation of phospholipase A_2, based on inhibition of desensitization by purported PL-A_2 inhibitors (Mallorga and co-workers, 1980). Mepacrine did completely prevent dimaprit-induced desensitization in HL-60 cells (Table 4). At the concentration of mepacrine used, this compound was also able to partially inhibit (by about 20%) dimaprit stimulated production of cAMP in control cells. This small degree of inhibition did not appear to be sufficient to explain the complete block of desensitization.

[^{3}H]-Tiotidine Binding

By using specially treated glass fiber filters, it was possible to show specific binding of tiotidine to intact HL-60 cells (Table 5). The degree of non-specific binding, determined in the presence of 10^{-4} M cimetidine was still uncomfortably high. Nevertheless, displacement assays using increasing concentrations of cimetidine, impromidine, tiotidine, or histamine all showed the same degree of non-specific binding (approximately 55% using 10^{-7} M [^{3}H]-tiotidine) and the displacement curves were essentially parallel for all the competing ligands (data not shown). HL-60 cells were treated with either 10^{-5} M dimaprit (4 hours) or 10^{-5} M L-643,441 (1 hour), washed extensively and then examined for cAMP sensitivity to dimaprit and for number of tiotidine binding sites. L-643,441 is a long acting antagonist of H_2 receptors (Torchiana and co-workers, 1983). Pretreatment of HL-60 cells with this compound lead to an apparent irreversible blockade of the cAMP response to dimaprit (dimaprit dose response curves, not shown, were depressed in maximum response with no change in EC50). As shown in Table 6, treatment with L-643,441 caused a complete loss of specific tiotidine binding, supporting the view that tiotidine binding was to the H_2 receptor. In contrast, dimaprit treatment did not lead to any change in tiotidine binding despite the obvious loss of cAMP response. These results suggest that desensitization does not involve a loss of H_2 receptors from the HL-60 cell membrane surface.

TABLE 5 [^{3}H]-Tiotidine Binding to Normal HL-60 Cells

	Experiment #				
	1	2	3	4	Mean +/- SEM
CPM Bound					
Total Binding	4132	3728	3542	4117	3880 +/- 146
Non-Specific	2732	2278	2268	2455	2434 +/- 108
Specific Binding	1400	1449	1274	1662	1446 +/- 81
fmoles/mg protein	44.6	63.6	81.6	83.4	68.3 +/- 9.1
fmoles/10^6 cells	5.9	14.3	9.9	8.6	9.7 +/- 1.8

TABLE 6 Effect of Dimaprit and L-643,441 Treatment on Tiotidine Binding

Pretreatment	Stimulation of cAMP by 10^{-4} M Dimaprit (pmoles/10^6 cells)	[^{3}H]-Tiotidine (CPM Bound)	
		Total	Non-Specific
Control	114.0 +/- 1.0	3764 +/- 143	2990 +/- 97
10^{-5} M Dimaprit	4.3 +/- 0.6	3733 +/- 348	2822 +/- 233
Control	248.0 +/- 16.0	3764 +/- 143	2990 +/- 97
10^{-5} M L-643,441	6.1 +/- 2.5	2817 +/- 148	2711 +/- 201

DISCUSSION

Exposure of HL-60 cells to the H_2 agonist dimaprit caused morphological and biochemical changes indicative of partial maturation along the granulocyte pathway. Most of the cells matured to the myelocyte stage, with a smaller proportion maturing to the metamyelocyte stage. Terminal differentiation to the neutrophil-like stage was not observed even with 10^{-4} M dimaprit for as long as 6 days. One possible explanation for this is the rapid desensitization of the H_2 receptor such that cAMP levels remain markedly elevated for only a few hours after addition of dimaprit to the culture medium. Receptor desensitization may also be the cause of the reported failure of prostaglandins to cause terminal maturation (Chaplinski and Niedel, 1982) since we have also observed marked desensitization of the PGE_2 cAMP response in HL-60 cells (unpublished data).

In the case of dimaprit, desensitization was mainly homologous in that the prostaglandin response was largely retained (75 to 80 percent in most experiments) after exposure to the H_2 agonist. However, the degree of retention of the prostaglandin response was quite variable; in some experiments virtually no decrease occurred, whereas in others as much as 50 percent of the response was lost. The explanation for this variability is unknown, but there does appear to be some heterologous desensitization. Neither the homologous nor the heterologous components of desensitization were reversed by including a phosphodiesterase inhibitor in the assay, suggesting that induction of phosphodiesterase could not be the explanation for the desensitization. Our results in the HL-60 cell are distinctly different than those reported in mononuclear leukocytes in which histamine caused a heterologous desensitization of histamine, catecholamine and prostaglandin responses, apparently through activation of a phosphodiesterase (Safko and co-workers, 1981; Chan and co-workers, 1982). However, we did observe that prostaglandin caused heterologous desensitization of both histamine and prostaglandin responses in the HL-60 cell, and this desensitization was largely reversed in the presence of a phosphodiesterase inhibitor (unpublished data).

The dimaprit-induced desensitization was completely blocked by including cimetidine in the incubation medium along with the H_2 agonist and could be reversed within 24 hours by adding cimetidine after desensitization had taken place. Histamine and impromidine caused a desensitization indistinguishable from that of dimaprit, but the chemical control, N-methyl dimaprit (SK&F 92054), was incapable of stimulating cAMP formation, of causing desensitization, and of blocking the dimaprit-induced responses. The H_1 antagonist mepyramine did not influence desensitization.

The mechanism of the dimaprit-induced desensitization remains unclear. We used the radiolabeled antagonist tiotidine to see whether there was a loss of receptor sites as commonly seen with desensitization of other receptor systems. The tiotidine binding assay has apparently been successfully applied to only one tissue that we are aware of, namely guinea pig cerebral cortex membranes (Gajtkowski and co-workers, 1983). Our binding studies with [^{3}H]-tiotidine suggest that there is no loss of binding sites, at least after 4 hours exposure to dimaprit. There are however significant problems with the tiotidine binding assay, including very high non-specific binding and variability in the radiochemical purity of the batches obtained from NEN. In addition, because of the relatively low affinity of tiotidine, high concentrations have to be used to obtain a significant amount of binding and the assay becomes too expensive for large numbers of experiments. Displacement assays indicated that tiotidine, impromidine, cimetidine and histamine blocked ligand binding, the displacement curves were essentially parallel, and the rank order of potencies in displacing the labeled tiotidine were as expected on the basis of pharmacological data and were similar to those reported previously (Gajtkowski and co-workers, 1983). However, the K_D of tiotidine calculated from the displacement curve using unlabeled tiotidine (1.7×10^{-7} M) was considerably greater than would be expected from pharmacological pA_2 data. On the other hand, the K_D of cimetidine (1.0×10^{-6} M) was consistent with pharmacological data. At the present time, the best evidence that we have that tiotidine is labeling the H_2 receptor are the results obtained with the compound L-643,441. The effects of this compound on both cAMP generation and tiotidine binding were consistent with an irreversible binding of this antagonist to the H_2 receptor site. The fact that there was a complete loss of tiotidine binding sites with this compound, but no loss in the dimaprit treated cells provides support for the view that dimaprit-induced desensitization does not involve an (initial) loss of binding sites. The failure of colchicine or cytochalasin B to influence desensitization would be consistent with the absense of receptor internalization. Presumably, the receptors are still present but because of a structural modification, can no longer bind the agonist or are uncoupled from the membrane adenylate cyclase.

One interesting observation of the present study is that mepacrine completely blocked the dimaprit-induced as well as the prostaglandin-induced desensitization. It is claimed that this compound is a phospholipase A_2 inhibitor and that activation of this enzyme is involved in beta receptor desensitization in astrocytoma cells (Mallorga and co-workers, 1980). This compound also interferes with cAMP generation as well, however the concentration used to block desensitization should not have significantly influenced cAMP formation. We were unable to obtain any effect of another reported inhibitor of the phospholipase, tetracaine, on dimaprit-induced desensitization. Although inhibition of phospholipase could be the mechanism for mepacrine's action, it should be noted that undifferentiated HL-60 cells have virtually no measurable $PL-A_2$ activity (Bonser and co-workers, 1981; unpublished data from this laboratory confirmed this report). Thus, the mechanism of action of mepacrine remains unclear at present.

The physiological relevance of H_2 receptor desensitization is unknown, but some evidence for its occurance in vivo can be sited. Cytolytically active T lymphocytes (CTL) will lyse mouse P815 cells and this response is inhibited by histamine via an H_2 receptor mechanism (Plaut and Roszkowski, 1979). However, when mice were treated by I.P. injections of histamine prior to isolating the CTL, there was a marked reduction in histamine's ability to influence the lysis reaction, suggesting that the H_2 receptors may have been desensitized. Since histamine is released during inflammatory responses, desensitization of H_2 receptors in various tissues could result in a variety of different responses depending on the tissues involved. Correlation of H_2 receptor desensitization with alterations in histamine-mediated function may lead to a clearer understanding of the still poorly defined physiological role of histamine H_2 receptors in various tissues.

ACKNOWLEDGEMENTS

The authors wish to thank Mrs. Diane Brockman for technical assistance, Dr. Supriya Ganguli for generous supplies of the cAMP RIA components, and Dr. Robin Ganellin for the H_2 agonists used in this study. This work was supported by grants from the National Institutes of Health, HL-22136 and HL-07382.

REFERENCES

Bonser, R. W., M. I. Siegel, R. T. McConnell, and P. Cuatrecasas (1981) Biochem. Biophys. Res. Comm. 98, 614-620.
Chan, S. C., S. R. Grewe, S. R. Stevens, and H. M. Hanifin (1982). J. Cyc. Nucleotide Res. 8, 211-224.
Cherrington, A. D., F. D. Assimacopoulos, S. C. Harper, J. D. Corbin, C. R. Park, and J. H. Exton (1976). J. Biol. Chem., 251, 5209-5218.
Chaplinski, T. J. and J. E. Niedel (1982). J. Clin. Invest. 70, 953-964.

Collins S. J., R. C. Gallo, and R. E. Gallagher (1977). Nature 270, 347-349.
Collins S. J., F. W. Ruscetti, R. E. Gallagher, and R. C. Gallo (1978). Proc. Natl. Acad. Sci. USA 75, 2458-2462.
DeLean, A., P. J. Munson, and D. Rodbard (1978). Am. J. Physiol. 235, E97-E102.
Gajtkowski, G. A., D. B. Norris, T. J. Risinf, and T. P. Wood (1983). Nature 304, 65-67.
Gespach, C., F. Saal, H. Cost, and J. P. Abita (1982). Mol. Pharmacol. 22, 547-553.
Glass, D. B., R. A. Masaracchia, J. R. Feramisco, and B. E. Kemp (1978). Anal. Biochem. 87, 566-575.
Harden, T. K., R. B. Meeker, and M. N. Martin (1983). J. Pharmacol. Exp. Ther. 227, 570-578.
Kalinyak, K., D. G. Sawutz, C. L. Johnson, B. C. Lampkin, and J. A. Whitsett (1983). J. Cell Bio. 97, 347a.
Kurokawa, T., M. Kurokawa, and S. Ishibashi (1979). Biochim. Biophys. Acta 583, 467-473.
Mallorga, P., J. F. Tallman, R. C. Henneberry, F. Hirata, W. T. Strittmatter, and J. Axelrod (1980). Proc. Natl. Acad. Sci. USA 77, 1341-1345.
Plaut, M. and W. Roszkowski (1979). In: T. O. Yellin (Ed.), Histamine Receptors. Spectrum Publications, New York. pp. 361-376.
Safko, M. J., S. C. Chan, K. D. Cooper, and J. M. Hanifin (1981). J. Allergy Clin. Immunol 68, 218-225.
Steiner, A. H., C. W. Parker, and D. M. Kipnis (1972). J. Biol. Chem. 247, 1106-1113.
Torchiana, M. L., R. G. Pendelton, P. G. Cook, C. A. Hanson, and B. V. Clineschmidt (1983). J. Pharmacol. Exp. Ther. 224, 514-519.

Histamine in the Brain: Localisation

PURIFICATION OF AND ANTIBODIES AGAINST L-HISTIDINE DECARBOXYLASE

T. Watanabe, Y. Taguchi, N. Takeda, S. Shiosaka*, M. Tohyama* and H. Wada

Department of Pharmacology II, and Department of Neuroanatomy, Institute of Higher Nervous Activity, Osaka University School of Medicine, Kita-ku, Osaka 530, Japan

ABSTRACT

L-Histidine decarboxylase was purified from fetal rat liver to apparent homogeneity. The native enzyme had a molecular weight of 110,000 and consisted of a dimer of 54,000 subunits. Antibody was raised against it in rabbits. In an Ouchterlony double diffusion test, its precipitin lines with histidine decarboxylases from fetal rat liver and adult rat stomach and brain fused completely. The antibody inhibited the enzymatic activity of the three sources to similar degrees. On indirect fluorescent immunohistochemical examination, the antibody showed the presence of histidine decarboxylase-like immunoreactive structures in rat brain. The immunoreactive cell bodies were found only in the posterior hypothalamus, i.e., the tuberal, caudal and postmammillary caudal magnocellular nuclei. Immunoreactive nerve fibers were widely but unevenly distributed throughout the brain, being especially dense in the following areas: Rostrally, in the hypothalamus, cerebral cortex, olfactory bulb and amygdaloid complex, and caudally in the central grey matter, auditory system, and nucleus tractus solitarii.

KEYWORDS

Histamine; histidine decarboxylase; immunohistochemistry; rat brain; hypothalamus; magnocellular nuclei.

INTRODUCTION

L-Histidine decarboxylase (HDC, L-histidine carboxylyase, E.C.4.1.1.22) catalyzes decarboxylation of L-histidine to histamine, and thus is important as the only and therefore rate-limiting enzyme in the formation of histamine. Histamine has many actions in physiological, pharmacological and pathological states (Beaven, 1978). Therefore, many studies have been carried out on HDC, especially its activation under various conditions as summarized by Beaven (1982) and Watanabe and Wada (1983). However, there have been few studies on this enzyme at the molecular level, because it is very difficult to purify HDC since it is very unstable and its content in tissues is very low (Aures and Håkanson, 1971; Schayer, 1972). HDC was partially purified from rat fetuses (Burkhalter, 1962; Håkanson, 1963; Tran and Snyder, 1981 Watanabe and coworkers, 1979), hamster placenta (Håkanson, 1967a), mouse mastocytoma (Hammar and Hjertén, 1980), rat gastric mucosa (Savany and Cronenberger, 1982a, 1982b), and gastric carcinoid of Mastomys (Hosoda and others, 1971), all of which contain relatively high HDC activities.

Many neurochemical, neurophysiological and neuropharmacological studies have suggested that histamine is a putative neurotransmitter (Hough and Green, 1984; Roberts and Calcutt, 1983; Schwartz and coworkers, 1980, 1982). However, little is known about the fundamental problem of the morphological location of the histaminergic neuron system in the brain, because histamine, unlike catecholamines and serotonin, does not form a fluorescent conjugate with formaldehyde. However, antibody against HDC can be used as a marker in immunohistochemical studies on the histaminergic neuron system. The first attempt to do this was made by Fukui, Watanabe and Wada (1980), who showed that the antibody raised against HDC purified from whole bodies of fetal rats cross-reacted with HDC from rat brain; namely on Ouchterlony's double diffusion the precipitin lines with HDC's from fetus and brain fused. However, spur formation was observed, suggesting only partial identity of the antigenic determinants of the two HDC's. Moreover, the antibody did inhibit brain HDC but less strongly than fetal HDC. This is the reason why this antibody showed positive immunostaining of mast cells and the stomach, but not of the brain (Watanabe and coworkers, 1982). Subsequently, Tran and Snyder (1981) purified HDC from fetal rat liver, which contains about 75% of the total HDC activity of whole fetuses, and raised antibody against it. This antibody cross-reacted completely with HDC's from the brain and stomach and showed positive immunostaining of both parietal cells of the stomach and the stria terminalis of the brain. However, the specificity of their antibody was questioned by Beaven (1982) and discussed previously by Taguchi and others (1984). The problems involved will not be discussed here but one major point is that it is enterochromaffin-like (ECL) cells and not parietal cells that contain high HDC activity in the stomach.

Recently, we purified HDC from fetal rat and raised antibody to it (Taguchi and others, 1984). This antibody was specific and potent enough to enable us to determine the location of the histaminergic neuron system in rat brain (Watanabe and co-workers, 1983, 1984).

PURIFICATION AND PROPERTIES OF HDC OF FETAL RAT LIVER

Table 1 summarizes the protocol of the purification of HDC from fetal rat liver. The Sephacryl S-300 fraction was not pure and was purified further by

TABLE 1 Purification of HDC from Fetal Rat Liver

Procedure	Total Activity (U)*	Total Protein (mg)	Specific Activity (U/mg)
Crude extract**	2,250	26,200	0.086
Ammonium Sulfate	2,070	8,090	0.26
Phospho-cellulose	1,940	3,760	0.52
DEAE-cellulose	1,060	359	2.95
Bio-Gel A-0.5m	729	57.2	12.7
Carnosine Agarose	414	17.8	23.3
DEAE-cellulose	226	1.94	116
Sephacryl-300	120	0.94	128

* One unit catalyzes formation of one nmole of histamine per min.
** Starting from 400 g of liver.

polyacrylamide gel electrophoresis. The final preparation appeared pure on SDS polyacrylamide gel electrophoresis (Taguchi and others, 1984). Due to extensive inactivation during electrophoresis, the specific activity of the pure preparation could not be determined. The procedure is long and gives low recovery of activity, and thus it obviously requires further improvement, such as by use of affinity

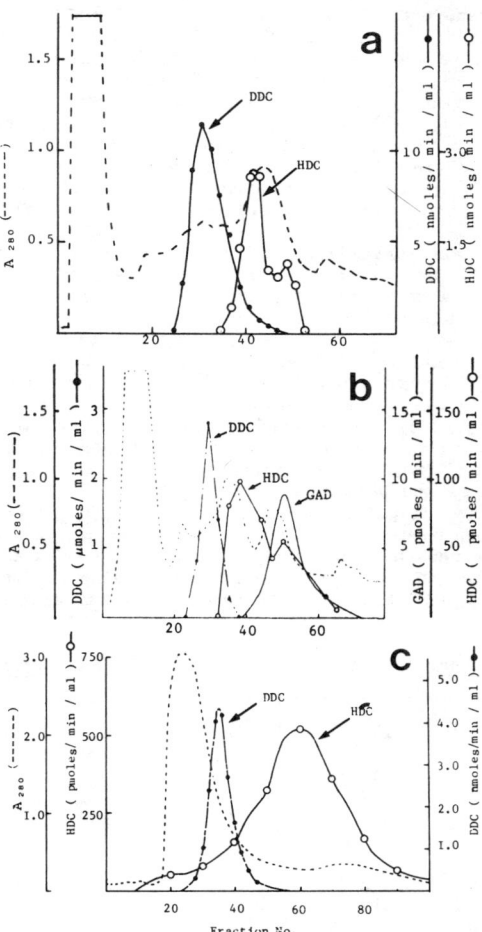

Fig. 1. Comparison of HDC with DOPA and glutamate decarboxylases. A crude extract of fetal rat liver (a) or carcass (b) was applied to a column of DEAE cellulose (1 x 10 cm), which was developed with a linear gradient of 0.02 M to 0.2 M potassium phosphate buffer, pH 6.8, as described previously (Taguchi and others, 1984). (c) The HDC fraction from the Bio-Gel 0.5m step was applied to a carnosine agarose column (2 x 30 cm) equilibrated with 0.4 M sodium citrate buffer, as described previously (Taguchi and others, 1984). DDC, DOPA decarboxylase; GAD, glutamate decarboxylase.

chromatography with anti HDC antibody or histamine or pyridoxal 5'-phosphate as a ligand, or HPLC on an ion exchanger such as DEAE, or a gel permeation column.
Since the identity of HDC with other decarboxylases, especially DOPA decarboxylase and glutamate decarboxylase, has been a matter of controversy, we examined this problem (Nakanishi and others, unpublished). The crude extract of fetal rat liver was applied to a DEAE-cellulose column which was developed as shown in Fig. 1a. As previously reported for stomach and brain (Yamada et al. 1984), DOPA decarboxylase was eluted earlier than HDC on DEAE chromatography. No glutamate decarboxylase activity was detected. However, similar chromatography of a crude extract of the carcass of fetal rats, that is their whole body without the liver, resulted in a similar elution pattern and glutamate decarboxylase was well separated from HDC (Fig. 1b). HDC and DOPA decarboxylase were completely separated from each other at the carnosine affinity step as shown in Fig. 1c. But these two decarboxylases were eluted in almost the same region on chromatographies on Sephacryl S-300 and Phenyl-Sepharose (adsorbed with 30 mM potassium phosphate pH 6.8, and eluted with 1 mM buffer; or retarded with 3 mM buffer).

The properties of HDC are summarized in Table 2. The native enzyme had a molecular weight of 110,000 judging from the results of Sephacryl S-300 gel filtration and polyacrylamide gel electrophoresis with different gel concentrations by the method of Hedrick and Smith (1968), and consisted of a dimer of 54,000 subunits. Its isoelectric point was 5.1, confirming a previous result (Yamada and others, 1984). Pyridoxal 5'-phosphate (PLP) was necessary to activate apo-HDC, which was prepared by treating HDC with penicillamine or alkaline phosphatase (Y. Sakamoto and others, unpublished), and its K_D value was 10^{-7}M. To our knowledge, alkaline phosphatase has not previously been used to resolve PLP from pyridoxal enzymes. The K_D value of 10^{-7}M is one or two orders of magnitude greater than that of the other pyridoxal enzymes. So, in the equilibrium, Holo-HDC $\rightleftharpoons$ Apo-HDC + PLP, alkaline phosphatase cleaves the phosphate ester bond of PLP to pyridoxal and Pi, and the equilibrium may by displaced to the right, because pyridoxal has little affinity to the enzyme, resulting in resolution. The Km for L-histidine was 0.25 mM in 0.1 M potassium phosphate buffer, pH 6.8. HDC seemed to be very specific for L-histidine. It had no activity on 1-methylhistidine and only weakly activity on 3-methylhistidine. HDC had no detectable DOPA or glutamate decarboxylase

TABLE 2. Properties of HDC Purified from Fetal Rat Liver

Molecular Weight	110 K (54 K x2)	
pI	5.1	
K_D for PLP	10^{-7}M	
Km for L-His	0.25 mM (0.1 M KPB , pH 6.8)	
Optimal pH	6.8 (0.25 mM His, 0.1 M KPB)	
Substrate Specificity	DOPA	0 %
	Glu	0 %
	3-Me-His	15 %
	1-Me-His	0 %
Inhibitors	α-Methylhistidine	Ki = 0.1 mM[*]
	α-Fluoromethylhistidine	Ki = 0.084mM
	Methionine	Ki = 3.85 mM
	Homocysteine	0.84
	Cysteine	0.61
	Urocanic acid	1.45
	Serine and Homoserine	No inhibition at 10 mM

[*] Kahlson and others (1963)

activity under our assay conditions. α-Methylhistidine and α-fluoromethylhistidine are strong inhibitors as already reported (Kahlson, Rosengren and Thunberg, 1963; Kollonitsch and coworkers, 1978). Details of the mechanism of inhibition of HDC by α-fluoromethylhistidine was reported by Kubota and others (1984) and Wada and co-workers (1984). Of about 100 compounds tested, sulfur containing amino acids, methionine, cysteine and homocysteine, inhibited HDC rather strongly, but the hydroxyl amino acids corresponding to the latter two, serine and homoserine, were not inhibitory at concentrations of 10 mM (Sakamoto and others, submitted to <u>Agents Actions</u>). Cysteine and homocysteine may inhibit HDC by forming a thiazolidine and 1,3-thiazan ring, respectively, with PLP. As reported by Håkanson (1967b), DOPA inhibited HDC by forming isoquinoline with PLP

CHARACTERIZATION OF ANTI HDC ANTIBODY

Anti-HDC antibody was raised by injecting HDC with Freund's complete adjuvant into rabbits as described previously (Taguchi and others, 1984). On Ouchterlony double diffusion, its precipitin line with the HDC's purified from fetal rat liver and adult rat stomach and brain fused as shown in Fig. 2a. The antibody inhibited the three HDC's to similar degrees (Fig. 2b). These results are in contrast to those on the previous antibody (Fukui, Watanabe and Wada 1980) with which the precipitin lines to fetal HDC and brain HDC showed spur formation and which inhibited brain HDC less than fetal HDC. The antibody (up to 1 mg/ml IgG) did not inhibit DOPA decarboxylase activity of rat brain as reported by Watanabe and others (1983). However, when a greater amount of antibody (~10 mg IgG/ml) was used, it inhibited DOPA decarboxylase, especially that of the liver of quinea-pigs (Taguchi and others, unpublished). Further studies are necessary on this problem, but it is probable that these two decarboxylases share some antigenic structure(s). In this sense, monoclonal antibody may be useful.

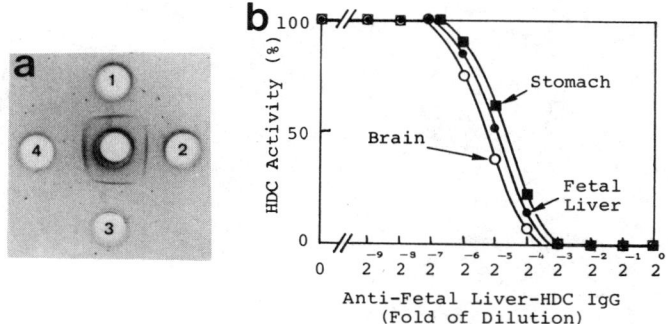

Fig. 2(a) Ouchterlony double diffusion test with anti HDC antibody (center well) and HDC's from various tissues (1,4, fetal liver; 2, adult stomach; 3, adult brain). (b) Inhibition of the HDC activitves by anti HDC. 100% activity = 1 pmole/min. IgG concentration of $2°$ = 0.58 mg/ml.

IMMUNOHISTOCHEMISTRY

Using this antibody as a marker, we examined the HDC-immunoreactive (HDCI) structures in the brain (Watanabe and coworkers 1983, 1984). Fig. 3a and b show

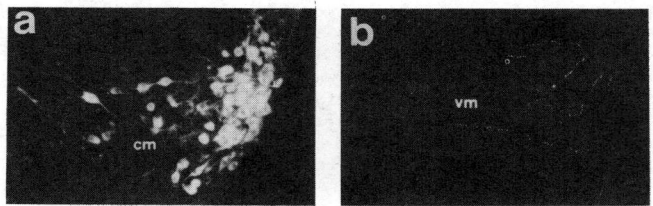

Fig. 3 Indirect immunofluorescent histochemistry of rat brain with anti HDC as a marker. (a) HDCI cell bodies in the caudal magnocellular nucleus of the mammillary body (x 100).
(b) HDCI nerve fibers with varicose appearance in the ventromedial hypothalamic nucleus of the (x 100).

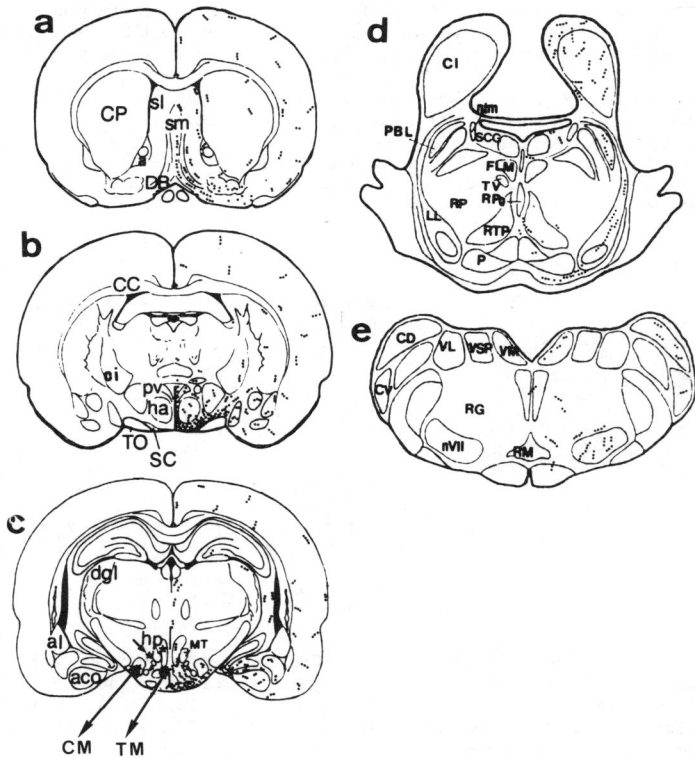

Fig. 4 Diagram of the histaminergic neuron system in rat brain. Frontal sections a, b, c, d, and e are +8.0, +5.5, +3.5, -1.5, and -4.5 mm from ear line (+, rostral; -, caudal). Left half, HDCI cell bodies; right half, HDCI nerve fibers. PCM was found in a region behind c (+3.2 mm).

typical HDCI cell bodies and nerve fibers, respectively, of rat brain. The HDCI cell body in the mammillary body is large and fusiform with two or three well-developed dendrites, and HDCI nerve fibers in the ventromedial hypothalamic nucleus are thin and have clear appearance of varicosity.

Fig. 4a shows a diagram of the distribution of HDCI cell bodies (left half) and nerve fibers (right half) in the frontal sections of rat brain. HDCI cell bodies were concentrated in the posterior hypothalamus in positions corresponding to the tuberal, caudal and postmammillary caudal magnocellular nulcei (TM, CM, and PCM, respectively) named by Bleier, Cohn and Siggelknow (1979). Some scattered cells were found in the posterior and lateral hypothalamic nuclei. HDCI nerve fibers were distributed widely but unevenly throughout the brain. They were most abundant in the hypothalamus, but extended rostrally in the cerebral cortex, olfactory bulb, diagonal band of Broca, amygdaloid complex, bed nucleus of the stria terminalis, with a few in the thalamus and hippocampus. They were also found caudally in the central grey matter of the midbrain and pons, auditory system (colliculus inferior, lateral lemniscus, nucleus corpus trapezoideum, and dorsal cochlear nuclei, with a few in the superior olivary nucleus and medial geniculate body), parabrachial nuclei, medial vestibular nucleus, dorsal raphe nucleus, facial nucleus etc.

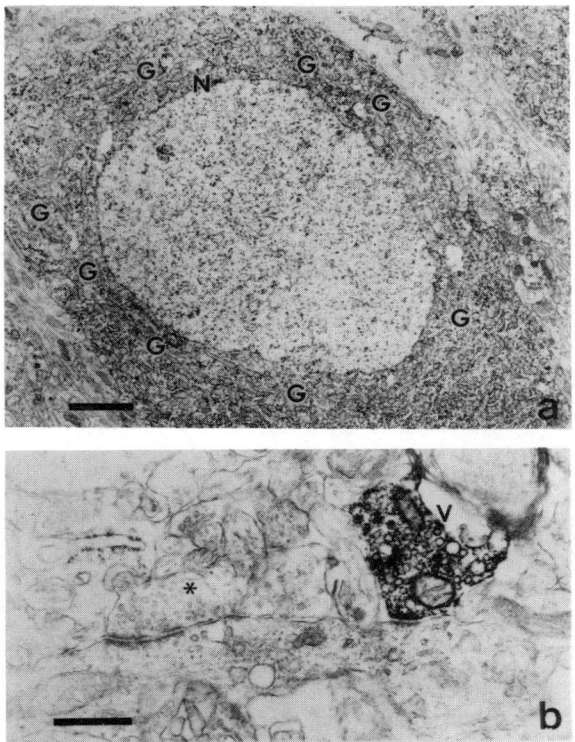

Fig. 5. Electronmicrophotographs of an HDCI cell body (a) and nerve terminal (b) in the caudal magnocellular nucleus. G, golgi apparatus; N, nucleus; V, varicosity. *non-reactive terminal. Scales; (a) 2 µm & (b) 0.5 µm.

Electron Microscopic Observation of HDCI Structures

HDCI structure in the CM were examined by electron microscopy (Fig. 5) (Hayashi and others 1984). The HDCI cell body (a) is large, and has a large oval nucleus, a well-developed Golgi apparatus, many mitochondria and much rough endoplasmic reticulum, suggesting active protein synthesis. The HDCI nerve terminal contained electron-lucent vesicles and made a synaptic contact, but most terminals were free from typical synaptic contact, suggesting the nonsynaptic release of histamine as an autacoid in the periphery.

Fiber Connection of HDCI Neuron System

The fiber connection of the HDCI neuron system was examined by a combination of total or hemitransection and the retrograde tracer technique with horseradish peroxidase (HRP) (Takeda and others, 1984a). Total transection of the brain just rostral to the posterior hypothalamus completely abolished the fluorescence in the

TABLE 3   Comparison of $[^3H]$-Mepyramine Binding Sites and HDC Nerve Fibers

Area	Region	$[^3H]$-Mepyramine binding[a]	HDCI reaction[b]
Cerebrum	Cerebral cortex	++[c]	++[d]
Basal body	Caudate-putamen	±	+
Limbic	Bed nucleus of stria terminalis	+++	++
	Hippocampus	+++	+∧-
	Amygdaloid body	++∧+++	+∧++
	Olfactory bulb	±∧+	++
Thalamus	Paraventricular n.	++	+
	Nn. reuniens & reticularis	+	-
	N. rhomboideum	+	-
Hypothalamus	Supraoptic & suprachiamatic nn.	+++	+
	Ventro-medial nucleus	+++	+++
	Paraventicular n.	++	+
	Lateral & dorsomedial nn.	+	+
Midbrain	N. ruber, Substance nigra	+∧±	-
	N. originis n. oculomotorius	+∧±	-
Pons	Pontine n., N. originis n. facialis	+++	++
	N. vestibularis medialis	+++	++
	N. raphe dorsalis	++	+
	N. raphe magnus	+++	-
	Locus caeruleus, N. olivaris sup.	++	-
	N. vestibularis lateralis	+	-
Medulla	N. tractus solitarii	+++	++
	N. originis n. vagi	+++	±
	N. originis n. hypoglossi	++	-
	N. ambiguus	++	-
	N. olivaris inferior	+	-
Cerebellum		-	-

a) Taken from Palacios, Wamsley and Kuhar (1981)
b) Taken from Watanabe and others (1984)
c) +++, high (40-70 grains per 529 square microns of tissue); ++, moderate (30-39); +, some (20-29); ± little (<20).
d) +++ high, ++ moderate, + some, ± slight, - little.

cerebral cortex, but that transection caudal to the posterior hypothalamus caused no change. Thus, the cell bodies in the posterior hypothalamus are the main site of innervation of histaminergic projections to the cerebral cortex. Hemitransection at the former level reduced the intensity of fluorescence in the cerebral cortex partially but not completely, suggesting bilateral innervation of the histaminergic neurons. By the retrograde tracer technique, HRP injected into the cerebral cortex was demonstrated in the TM, CM, and PCM on both sides, but predominantly in the ipsilateral side. All these results suggest that the histaminergic neuron system is bilateral with ipsilateral predominance. The same experiments showed that the medial vestibular nucleus are also innervated bilaterally with ipsilateral predominance (Takeda and others, 1984b).

COMPARISON OF THE PRESENT DATA WITH THOSE OF OTHERS

The present results on the histaminergic neuron system in rat brain are in good agreement with those obtained by degeneration studies with HDC as a marker by Schwartz and his coworkers (Ben-Ari and others, 1977; Garbarg and others, 1974; Schwartz and coworkers, 1982), except that their cell body in the reticular formation of the midbrain is slightly too caudal and may correspond to our TM. The distribution of H_1-receptors studied with $[^3H]$-mepyramine as a ligand by Palacios, Wamsley and Kuhar (1981) is compared with the distribution of HDCI nerve fibers in Table 3. In general, the distributions of the two are very similar, but there are some differences. Areas with a high density of H_1-receptors but few HDCI nerve fibers were the hippocampus, n. reticularis tegmenti pontis, n. vestibularis lateralis, n. tractus spinalis nervi trigemini, n. reticularis lateralis, inferior olivary complex, n. gracilis, n. cuneatus, n. raphe magnus, n. ambiguus, n. originis nervi vagi, and n. originis nervi hypoglossi. One possible explanation for this is that mepyramine binds to other receptors besides H_1-receptor. Another more likely possibility is that the immunohistochemical technique with antibody against the enzyme is not so sensitive for nerve terminals as for neurons, and thus more sensitive methods like that with anti histamine antibody as a marker may reveal the presence of histamine nerve terminals in these areas. On the contrary, several areas, such as the n. caudatus-putamen, n. accumbens and lateral hypothalamus were found to contain many HDCI nerve fibers, but little mepyramine receptor. These areas are probably rich in H_2-receptor.

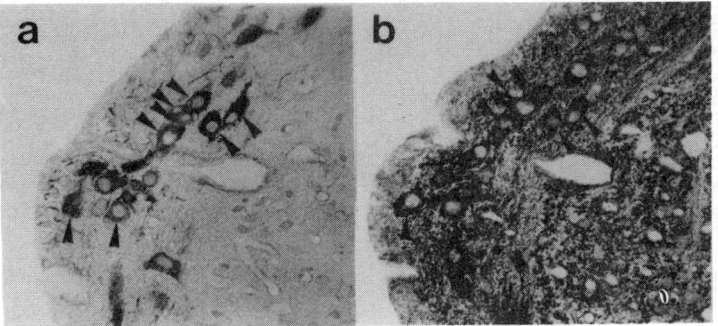

Fig. 6. Coexistence of HDCI and GADI structures in the same neurons in the PCM of rat brain. Two serial frontal sections were stained for HDCI (a) and GADI (b), respectively, as decribed elsewhere (Takeda and others, 1984c). Arrowheads indicate identical neurons. (x225).

Steinbush and Mulder (1984) and subsequently Panula, Yang and Costa (1984) conducted immunohistochemical studies on histamine-containing cells in rat brain with anti-histamine antibody as a marker. Their findings on the histaminergic neuron system are in good agreement with ours. The cell bodies are confined to the posterior hypothalamus and the nerve fibers are widely distributed in the brain.

Recently, Vincent et al. (1983) reported that the TM, CM and PCM also contain glutamate decarboxylase-like immunoreactivity. We found by examination of alternate consecutive sections with anti HDC or anti GAD antibody as a marker (Fig. 6) and the by double labelling technique, that neurons in TM, CM and PCM contained both HDCI and GADI structures suggesting the possible coexistence of histamine and GABA in the same neurons (Takeda and others, 1984c). Furthermore, Nagy et al. (1984) and Shiromizu et al. (1984) demonstrated the presence of adenosine deaminase-like and thyroid stimulating hormone releasing hormone (TRH)-like immunoreactivity, respectively, in these neurons. The coexistence of histamine, GABA, adenosine and TRH in the same neurons and the interactions of these compounds remain to be clarified.

ACKNOWLEDGEMENTS

We thank Drs H. Takagi and H. Hayashi, and Mr. H. Kubota, Y. Sakamoto and A. Nakanishi for their cooperation in this work and Mrs K. Tsuji for typing. We also thank Dr. Oertel for supplying anti GAD. This work was partially supported by a Grant-in-Aid from the Ministry of Education, Science and Culture of Japan.

REFERENCES

Aures, D., and R. Håkanson (1971). Histidine decarboxylase (mammalian). In H. Tabor and C. W. Tabor (Eds), Methods in Enzymology, Vol 17B. Academic Press, New York. pp.667-677.
Beaven, M. A. (1978). Histamine: Its Role in Physiological and Pathological Processes. S. Karger, Basel.
Beaven, M. A. (1982). Factors regulating availability of histamine at tissue receptors. In C. R. Ganellin and M. E. Parsons (Ed.), Pharmacology of Histamine Receptors, Wright PSG, Bristol, London, Boston. pp. 103-145.
Ben-Ari, Y., G. LaSalle Legale, G. Barbin, J. C. Schwartz, and M. Garbarg (1977). Histamine synthesizing afferents within the amygdaloid complex and nucleus of the stria terminalis of the rat. Brain Res., 138, 285-294.
Bleier, R., P. Cohn, and I. R. Siggelkow (1979). A cytoarchitectonic atlas of the hypothalamus and hypothalamic third ventricle of the rat. In P.H. Morgane, and J. Panksepp (Ed.), Handbook of Hypothalamus Vol. 1. Marcel Dekker, New York. pp. 137-220.
Burkhalter, A. (1962). The formation of histamine by fetal rat liver. Biochem. Pharmacol., 11, 315-322.
Fukui, H., T. Watanabe, and H. Wada (1980). Immunochemical crossreaction of the antibody elicited against L-histidine decarboxylase purified from the whole bodies of rats with the enzyme from rat brain. Biochem. Biophys. Res. Commun., 93, 333-339.
Garbarg, M., G. Barbin, J. Feger, and J.C. Schwartz (1974). Histaminergic pathway in rat brain evidenced by lesions of the medial forebrain bundle. Science, 186, 833-835.
Håkanson, R. (1963). Histidine decarboxylase in the fetal rat. Biochem. Pharmacol., 12, 1289-1296.
Håkanson, R. (1967a). Kinetic properties of mammalian histidine decarboxylase. Eur. J. Pharmacol., 1, 42-46.
Håkanson, R. (1967b). Mammalian histidine decarboxylase: Interaction between apoenzyme and pyridoxal-5'phosphate. Eur. J. Pharmacol., 1, 383-390.
Hammar, L., and S. Hjertén (1980). Purification and immunochemical analysis of

histidine decarboxylase from murine mastocytoma. Agents Actions, 10, 92-98.
Hayashi, H., H. Takagi, N. Takeda, Y. Kubota, M. Tohyama, T. Watanabe, and H. Wada (1984). Fine structure of histaminergic neurons in the caudal magnocellular nucleus of the rat as demonstrated by immunocytochemistry using histidine decarboxylase as a marker. J. Comp. Neurol., in press.
Hedrick, J. L., and A.J. Smith (1968). Size and charge isomer separation and estimation of molecular weights of proteins by disc gel electrophoresis. Arch. Biochem. Biophys., 126, 155-164.
Hosoda, S. (1971). Histidine decarboxylase in the transplantable argyrophilic gastric carcinoid of Pramyos (Mastomys) natalensis. Biochem. Pharmacol., 20, 2671-2676.
Hough, L. B., and J. P.Green (1984). Histamine and its receptors in the nervous system. In A. Lajtha (Ed), Handbook of Neurochemistry, Vol. 6, Plenum, New York. pp. 145-211.
Kahlson, G., E. Rosengren, and R. Thunberg (1963). Observations on the inhibition of histamine formation. J. Physiol., 169, 467-486.
Kollonitsch, J., A. A. Patchett, S. Marburg, A. L. Maycock, L. M. Perkins, G. A. Doldouras, D. E. Duggan, and S. A. Aster (1978). Selective inhibitor of biosynthesis of aminergic neurotransmitters. Nature, 274, 906-908.
Kubota, H., H. Hayashi, T. Watanabe, Y. Taguchi, and H. Wada (1984). Mechanism of inactivation of mammalian L-histidine decarboxylase by (S)-α-fluoromethylhistidine. Biochem. Pharmacol., 33, 883-900.
Nagy, J. I., L.A. LaBella, M. Buss, and P. E. Daddona (1984). Immunohistochemistry of adenosine deaminase: implications for adenosine neurotransmission. Science, 224, 166-168.
Palacios, J. M., J. K. Wamsley, M.J. Kuhar (1981). The distribution of histamine H_1-receptors in the rat brain: autoradiographic study. Neuroscience, 6, 15-37.
Panula, P., H-YT. Yang, E. Costa (1984). Histamine-containing neurons in the rat hypothalamus. Proc. Nat. Acad. Sci. USA., 81, 2572-2576.
Roberts, F., and C.R. Calcutt (1983). Histamine and the hypothalamus. Neuroscience, 9, 721-739.
Savany, A., and L. Cronenberger (1982a). Isolation and properties of multiple forms of histidine decarboxylase from rat gastric mucosa. Biochem, J., 52, 405-412.
Savany, A., and L. Cronenberger (1982b). Properties of histidine decarboxylase from rat gastric mucosa. Eur. J. Biochem., 123, 593-599.
Schayer, R. W. (1972) Biogenesis of histamine. In Rocha e Silva (Ed), Handbook of Experimental Pharmacology, Vol. 18/2. Springer-Verlag, Berlin. pp. 109-129.
Schwartz, J.C., H. Pollard, and T. T. Quach (1980). Histamine as a neurotransmitter in mammalian brain: Neurochemical evidence. J. Neurochem., 35, 26-33.
Schwartz, J.C,, G. Barbin, A. M. Duchemin, M. Garbarg, C. Llorens, H. Pollard, T. T. Quach, and C. Rose(1982). Histamine receptors in the brain and their possible functions. In C. R. Ganellin, and M. E. Parsons (Ed.). Pharmacology of Histamine Receptors. Wright . PSG, Bristol, London, Boston. pp. 351-391.
Shiromizu, M., T. Yamamoto, H. Kimura, and J. Ochi (1984). Hypothalamus cortex projection of TRH-containing neuron. Proceeding of the 7th Meeting of the Japanese Neuroscience Society, Chiba (in Japanese), p. 35.
Steinbusch, H. W. M., and A.H. Mulder (1984). Immunohistochemical localization of histamine in neurons and mast cells in the rat brain. In A. Bjorklund, and T. Hokfelt (Ed.). The Handbook of Chemical Neuroanatomy, Vol. 2. Elsevier, Amsterdam. in press.
Taguchi, Y., T. Watanabe, H. Kubota, H. Hayashi, and H. Wada (1984). Purification of histidine decarboxylase from the liver of fetal rats and its immunochemical and immunohistochemical characterization. J. Biol. Chem., 259, 5214-5221.
Takeda, N., S. Inagaki, Y. Taguchi, M. Tohyama, T. Watanabe, and H. Wada H (1984a). Origins of histamine-containing fibers in the cerebral cortex of rats studied by immunohistochemistry with histidine decarboxylase as a marker and transection. Brain Res., in press.
Takeda, N., M. Morita, T. Watanabe, H. Wada, M. Tohyama, T. Kubo, and T. Matsunaga

(1984b). Histaminergic Projection from the posterior hypothalamus to the medial vestibular nucleus of the rat. Neurochem. Res., in press.

Takeda, N., S. Inagaki, S. Shiosaka, Y. Taguchi, W. H. Oertel, M. Tohyama, T. Watanabe, and H. Wada (1984c). Immunochemical evidence for the coexistence of histidine decarboxylase-like and glutamate decarboxylase-like immunoreactivities in nerve cells of the magnocellular nucleus of the posterior hypothalamus of rats. Proc. Nat. Acad. Sci. USA, in press.

Tran, V.T., and S.H. Snyder(1981). Histidine decarboxylase: Purification from fetal rat liver, immunologic porperties, and histochemical localization in brain and stomach. J. Biol. Chem., 256, 680-686.

Vincent, S. R., T. Hokfelt, L.R. Skirboll, and J-Y. Wu (1983). Hypothalamic -aminobutyric acid neurons project to the neocortex. Science, 220, 1309-1311.

Wada, H., T. Watanabe, K. Maeyama, Y. Taguchi and H. Hayashi (1984). Mammalian histidine decarboxylase and its suicide substerate α-fluoromethylhistidine. In A. E. Evangelopoulos (Ed.). Chemical and Biological Aspects of Vitamin B_6 catalysis: Part A. Alan R. Liss, New York. pp. 245-254.

Watanabe, T,, H. Nakamura, L. Y. Liang, A. Yamatodani, and H. Wada (1979). Partial purification and characterization of L-histidine decarboxylase from fetal rats. Biochem. Pharmacol., 28, 1149-1155.

Watanabe, T., M. Yamada, Y. Taguchi, H. Kubota, K. Maeyama, A. Yamatodani, H. Fukui, S. Shiosaka, M.Tohyama and H. Wada (1982). Purification and properties of histidine decarboxylase isozymes and their pharmacological significance. In B. Uvnas, and K. Tasaka (Ed.). Advances in Histamine Research, Pergamon, Oxford, New york. pp.93-106

Watanabe, T., and H. Wada (1983). Histidine decarboxylase and histamine N-methyltransferase. In S. Parvez, T. Nagatsu, I. Nagatsu, and H. Pravez (Ed.), Methods in Biogenic Amine Research, Elsevier, Amsterdam. pp. 689-720.

Watanabe, T., Y. Taguchi, H. Hayashi, J. Tanaka, S. Shiosaka, M. Tohyama, H. Kubota, Y. Terano, and H. Wada (1983). Evidence for the presence of a histaminergic neuron system in the rat brain: An Immunochemical analysis. Neurosci. Lett., 39, 249-254.

Watanabe, T., Y. Taguchi, S. Shiosaka, J. Tanaka, H. Kubota, Y. Terano, M. Tohyama, and H. Wada (1984). Distribution of the histaminergic neuron system in the central nervous system of rats; a fluorescent immunohistochemical analysis with histidine decarboxylase as a marker. Brain Res., 295, 13-25.

Yamada, M., T. Watanabe, H. Fukui, Y. Taguchi, and H. Wada (1984). Comparison of histidine decarboxylase from rat stomach and brain with that from whole bodies of rat fetus. Agents Actions, 14, 143-152.

DEVELOPMENT OF A MONOCLONAL ANTIBODY AGAINST L-HISTIDINE DECARBOXYLASE AS A SELECTIVE TOOL FOR THE LOCALISATION OF HISTAMINE-SYNTHESISING CELLS

H. Pollard*, I. Pachot*, P. Legrain**, G. Buttin**
and J-C. Schwartz*

*Unité 109 de Neurobiologie, Centre Paul Broca de
l'INSERM, 2ter rue d'Alésia, 75014 Paris, France
**Unité de Génétique Somatique, Institut Pasteur,
75015 Paris, France

ABSTRACT

L-histidine decarboxylase (H.D.) from rat stomach was purified by about 1,000-fold in a few steps. A non-precipitant, non-inhibiting monoclonal antibody was developped in mouse against this antigen using the hybridoma technology and immunoprecipitation of H.D. activity as a screening test. It recognised H.D. from various tissues including brain but not a bacterial H.D., glutamate or DOPA decarboxylases. In various preliminary immunohistochemical studies the antibody stained mastocytoma and gastric mast cells as well as neuronal elements in the rat hypothalamus. Particularly magnocellular neuronal perikarya in the posterior hypothalamus were labelled, a localisation in agreement with 1) previous neurochemical and lesion data from this laboratory 2) recent immunohistochemical data from others with polyclonal antibodies against histamine (HA) or H.D. 3) the alleged functions of an ascending histaminergic pathway diffusely projecting to telencephalon, as previously proposed in this laboratory.

KEYWORDS

Histaminergic neurones, L-Histidine decarboxylase, Monoclonal antibody, Immunocytochemistry.

INTRODUCTION

The identification and precise localisation of cellular populations synthesising and releasing chemical messengers constitute important conditions to understand their functions which were, as yet, only partially met in the case of histamine (HA). Whereas its presence in mast-cells from various tissues is well established, namely by histofluorescence techniques (Brody and co-workers, 1972), the existence of non-mast-cell HA stores, not revealed by this relatively insensitive technique is suspected in several tissues. In brain the existence of histaminergic neurones was proposed more than a decade ago since HA apparently fulfilled many criteria used to recognise putative neurotransmitters (reviewed by Schwartz, 1975). Indeed the whole biochemical machinery to synthetise, store, and release the amine was, already shown to be present in isolated nerve-endings. Furthermore the distal changes in H.D. activity occuring after lateral hypothalamic lesions were interpreted as a consequence of an anterograde degeneration process in a system of histaminergic neurones (Garbarg and co-workers, 1974), the gross disposition of which was established in a series of lesion studies (Barbin and co-workers, 1975 and 1976 ; Garbarg and co-workers, 1976 ; Ben Ari and co-workers, 1976 ; Pollard and co-workers, 1976, 1978 ; Schwartz co-workers, 1980,1981 ; Garbarg and co-workers, 1980a). These conclusions were supported by electrophysiological recordings following stimulation of alleged pathways (Sastry and Phillis, 1976 ; Haas and Wolf, 1977) as well as by the recovery pattern of H.D. activity after its irreversible inhibition (Garbarg and co-workers, 1980b). Nevertheless it is clear that the complexity of CNS requires more powerful and precise methods than the neurochemical ones to localise chemically-identified neuronal pathways. In addition histochemical methods are obviously required to visualise other putative HA-storing cells like microvessels (Jarrot and co-workers, 1979 ; Karnyushina co-workers, 1980) in the CNS as in other organs.

In the last few years several experimental approaches to this problem were reported which include immunohistochemical studies with polyclonal antibodies directed against either HA (Wilcox and Seybold, 1982 ; Leslie and co-workers, 1983 ; Panula and co-workers, 1984 ; Steinbusch and Mulder, this symposium) or the enzyme H.D. (Tran and Snyder, 1981 ; Watanabe and co-workers, 1983, 1984) and attempts at localising autoradiographically H.D. with ^{3}H-α-fluoromethyl-histidine (Schwartz and co-workers, 1982b), an irreversible (Kcat) inhibitor (Kollonitsch and co-workers, 1978 ; Garbarg co-workers, 1980b). While the latter approach was unsuccesful, immunohistochemical studies have already provided some consistent informations regarding HA-storing and HA-synthesising cells, particularly in the CNS, but there has already been some discrepancies between data obtained with various antibodies. Thus, for instance, in the rat gastric gland, a tissue with high H.D. activity, parietal cells were stained with one antibody (Tran and Snyder, 1981) whereas enterochromaffin-like cells were stained with another one (Watanabe and co-workers, 1983) and results with antibodies against HA were not reported. Indeed it is difficult to establish that antibodies raised against a small molecule like HA do not cross-react with other cerebral constituents. In the same way the specificity of polyclonal antibodies raised against a purified protein must always be questionned, particularly as long as the latter is not shown to be homogeneous in various sensitive tests, because antisera might contain antibodies directed against impurities in the antigen.

For these various reasons, our own strategy (Pollard and co-workers, 1983) has been to develop monoclonal antibodies against H.D. (EC 4.1.1.22) since 1) the enzyme seems a highly specific marker of HA-synthesising neurones in C.N.S. (Schwartz and co-workers, 1970, 1971 ; Garbarg and co-workers, 1976 ; Martres and co-workers, 1975) 2) due to its instability H.D. is difficult to purify to absolute homogeneity (Aures and co-workers, 1970) 3) with monoclonal antibodies it is possible to avoid the development of antibodies against impurities and, therefore, to start even from a very partially purified antigen, provided that the screening test allows to identify antibodies specifically directed against the enzyme molecule itself.

PARTIAL PURIFICATION OF RAT GASTRIC L-HISTIDINE DECARBOXYLASE

There has been several previous attempts to obtain the mammalian H.D. in pure form, starting from rich sources like the rat gastric mucosa (Savany and Cronenberger, 1978, 1982) rat fetuses (Aures and Håkanson, 1971 ; Watanabe and co-workers, 1979, 1982) mouse mastocytoma (Aures and Håkanson, 1971 ; Hammar and co-workers, 1975, 1980) or rat fetal liver (Tran and Snyder, 1981 ; Taguchi and co-workers, 1984). However these attempts have sometimes met limited success due to great instability of the enzyme. We have deliberately aimed at a partial purification of the enzyme starting from the rat gastric mucosa, a convenient source and selecting for this purpose a few rapid purification steps that will be outlined below :

Development of a monoclonal antibody against L-histidine-decarboxylase   105

a) <u>Extraction</u> : the scrapped mucosa from normally fed rats (which displays a much higher H.D. activity than that of fasting animals) was homogeneised in phosphate buffer containing various stabilising agents either specific (pyridoxal-5'-phosphate, the co-enzyme) or non-specific ones (dithiotreitol, phenylmethyl sulfonyl fluoride, EDTA, polyethylene glycol) that were proposed in previous reports (see ref. above). A clear high-speed (3.10^6 g x min) supernatant of this homogenate contained a large fraction of the starting enzyme, well-known to be in soluble form in most tissues (Aures and Håkanson, 1971) including brain (Schwartz and co-workers, 1970 ; Baudry and co-workers, 1973).

b) <u>Ammonium sulfate fractionation</u> : a double precipitation procedure similar to that initially used by Håkanson (1963) was utilised in which were successively retained the 27 % $SO_4(NH_4)_2$ supernatant and the 43 % $SO_4(NH_4)_2$ pellet. After dialysis the latter retained approximately one third of the original activity and displayed a rather modest enrichment (3-fold over the high-speed supernatant).

c) <u>Chromatofocusing</u> : Starting from the work of Savany and Cronenberger (1982) who concluded to the presence of several H.D. isoenzymes with pI values comprised between 5.3 and 5.9, this mild and efficient technique which associates two important steps of purification (ion exchange chromatography and isofocusing) was used. The purified enzyme preparation was loaded onto a polybuffer exchanger columm (Pharmacia PBE 94) equilibrated at pH 7 and eluted with a polybuffer pH 5.0 containing pyridoxal 5'-phosphate. The major peaks of activity (corresponding to pI values of 5.2-5.6) after being combined led to a preparation with a 25-fold enrichment at this step and an excellent recovery (Table 1).

TABLE 1   Purification of L-histidine decarboxylase from rat gastric mucosa

STEPS	SPECIFIC ACTIVITY (dpm/h/µg protein)	YIELD (%)	PURIFICATION FACTOR
Crude homogenate	188	100	1.0
High Speed Supernatant	434	57	2.3
0-27 % $SO_4(NH_4)_2$ Supernatant	806	48	4.3
27-43 % $SO_4(NH_4)_2$ Pellet	1,766	33	6.5
Chromatofocusing	30,360	32	160
Gel filtration	205,454	30	1,082

All steps were carried out at 4°C in 3 days. Enzyme activity measured by the radiochromatographic assay (Baudry and co-workers, 1973) using 0.1 µM ^{3}H-L-His (50 Ci/mM) as substrate.

d) <u>Gel filtration</u> : this final step was undertaken on an Ultrogel ACA 44 (LKB) column from which the enzyme activity peak eluted at a position corresponding to an apparent M.W. of 90-100 kDa. This value is in rather good agreement with those reported by Hammar and Hjerten (1980) i.e. 110 kDa for H.D. from mouse mastocytoma, by Savany and Cronenberger (1978) i.e. 90-97 kDa for

H.D. from rat stomach and by Yamada et al. (1984) i.e. about 90 kDa for H.D. from rat stomach, brain or fetuses. This suggests that the enzymes from different mammalian sources have similar M.W.. In contrast Tran and Snyder (1981) reported a M.W. of 210 kDa for the enzyme from rat fetal liver, a discrepancy which awaits clarification.

e) <u>Purity</u> : the final preparation was enriched by about 1,000-fold with a final 25-30 % recovery (table 1). In comparison Savany and Cronenberger (1978) and Yamada and co-workers, (1984) reported purification factors in the same range i.e. of 600-fold and 380-fold, respectively for the rat gastric enzyme but, starting from rat fetal liver, a material with a specific activity approximately 6-fold higher than the gastric mucosa (unpublished result), Taguchi and co-workers, 1984) reached a purification factor of 3,000-fold and found a single band of 54 kDa on SDS-polyacrylamide gel electrophoresis (PAGE). Our final preparation submitted to SDS-PAGE under highly sensitive detection conditions (7 µg protein load per cm of gel and $AgNO_3$ staining) showed several bands among which the major ones corresponded to apparent M.W. of 95 and 45-50 kDa (the latter presumably corresponding to the enzyme monomer) and represented about 10 % of the total. However, in view of possible activity losses during the purification processes these calculations should be considered as approximative ones and higher purification factors might be required to completely reach homogeneity. This underlines the potential interest of monoclonal as compared to polyclonal antibodies from a specificity point of view.

PRODUCTION OF MONOCLONAL ANTIBODIES

The principle of the method developed by Köhler and Milstein (1975) is now well known : it involves obtaining from an immunised animal lymphoid cells that are immortalised by hybridisation with an established highly proliferating cell-line, and growing these hybrids in tissue culture so that antibody produced by individual clones can be detected. The finally selected clones can be utilised for in vivo"mass production" of antibody by i.p. injection to animals which develop antibody-rich ascites.

The problem of the mode of detection of antibodies in the cell cultures is a critical one in the development of monoclonal antibodies since in view of the large number of samples to be analysed a large-scale and not too much tedious method is required. In addition, when starting from a partially purified antigen, the sensitivity and selectivity of detection may be crucial. We have chosen to develop an immunoprecipitation method by which the mouse immunoglobulins directed towards the enzyme (from the semi-purified gastric preparation) are precipitated with the latter by a (sheep) anti-mouse immunoglobulin and the H.D. activity in the pellet detected by a sensitive radiochromatographic assay (Baudry and co-workers, 1973). This assay was sensitive enough to detect H.D. activity in 0.5 ug of the purified preparation and up to 50 samples can be run together in the same day. Preliminar studies with polyclonal antibodies raised in rabbits against our purified enzyme preparation had shown that the outlined method was applicable to antibody detection.

This screening method has the distinct advantage of detecting a large variety of antibodies, even non-precipitant ones, directed against any part of the H.D. molecule except the active site. The method has been successfully applied to the detection of antibodies at the various steps of monoclonal antibody production i.e. immunisation and production of hybridoma, clones or ascitic fluid (table 2). Three-month old BALB/c mice were immunised by s.c. injections of purified gastric H.D. (100 µg) coupled with a mitogenic derivative of bacterial lipopolysaccharide (Lange and co-workers, 1983) and emulsified in Freund's complete adjuvant. Boosters were performed at 2-week intervals using the same amount of H.D. preparation in Freund's incomplete adjuvant, antibodies being generally detected in the blood (1 % serum dilution) 2 weeks after the 2nd administration. Mice were bled 3 days following the last antigen administrations (50 µg i.p. and i.v.) and spleen cells were fused with non-secreting Sp_2/OAg myeloma cells using polyethylene glycol (Buttin and co-workers, 1978).

TABLE II   Immunoprecipitation of H.D. activity from the purified
gastric enzyme preparation at various steps of monoclonal antibody production

SAMPLE	IMMUNOPRECIPITATED H.D. ACTIVITY (dpm/h)
Mouse serum (1 % dilution)	
pre-immune	1,602 ± 155
immune	4,121 ± 333*
Hybridoma culture medium (undiluted)	
control	2,002 ± 111
HI 113-12	3,140 ± 120*
Clone culture medium (undiluted)	
control	1,729 ± 183
HI 113-12	3,322 ± 250*
Ascitic fluid (1 % dilution)	
control	527 ± 53
HI 113-12	10,133 ± 63*
Purified immunoglobulins (0.15 ug)	
control	510 ± 70
HI 113-12	4,131 ± 435*

Anti-H.D. antibodies detected in the presence of 1 µg of the partially purified gastric enzyme as described in Pollard and co-workers, (1983).
* $p < 0.005$ as compared to respective controls.

Hybridoma were selected on a hypoxanthine/azaserine culture medium and anti-H.D. producing cells were cloned by limit dilution. Among 2,000 hybridoma cell lines tested only one clear anti-H.D. antibody-producing clone (table 2) was selected and injected i.p. to BALB/c mice in order to produce ascites. Antibodies in undiluted culture media from positive hybridoma and clones (H.I. 113-12) were detected at the limit of sensitivity of the method (less than twice the corresponding control) because of 1) the limited antibody concentration in the culture medium ; 2) a non-specific precipitation of H.D. activity by culture medium constituents. In contrast the immunoprecipitation by the much more concentrated ascitic fluid (it was used at a 1 % dilution for the assay) was unambiguous (table 2). From this fluid, monoclonal anti-H.D. immunoglobulins were isolated by $(NH_4)_2 SO_4$ precipitation and ion-exchange chromatography and this purified preparation (Mab H.I. 113-12) was used for further immunochemical and immunohistochemical studies.

PROPERTIES AND SPECIFICITY PATTERN OF THE MONOCLONAL ANTIBODY (HI 113-12)

Although the homogeneous monoclonal antibody, being directed towards a single antigen, theoretically displays a high degree of selectivity it was important to establish its specificity pattern in view of possible cross-reactivity with

molecules distinct from the antigen (particularly with phylogenetically-related ones) as well as the possible existence of H.D. isoenzymes in various tissues (Savany and Cronenberger, 1982, Yamada and co-workers, 1984).
The recognition of the antigen by Mab H.I. 113-12 was first studied on Western blots of SDS polyacrylamide gel electrophoregrams of the purified gastric H.D preparation : of the multiple protein bands of the latter (of which a certain number were recognised by polyclonal antibodies previously raised in rabbits or in mice), only a single one, corresponding to an apparent MW of 45 kDa was distinctly labeled by Mab H.I. 113-12. For detection in this system, a second antibody (sheep anti-mouse immunoglobulin) and the sensitive streptavidin-biotin-peroxidase detection method were used.

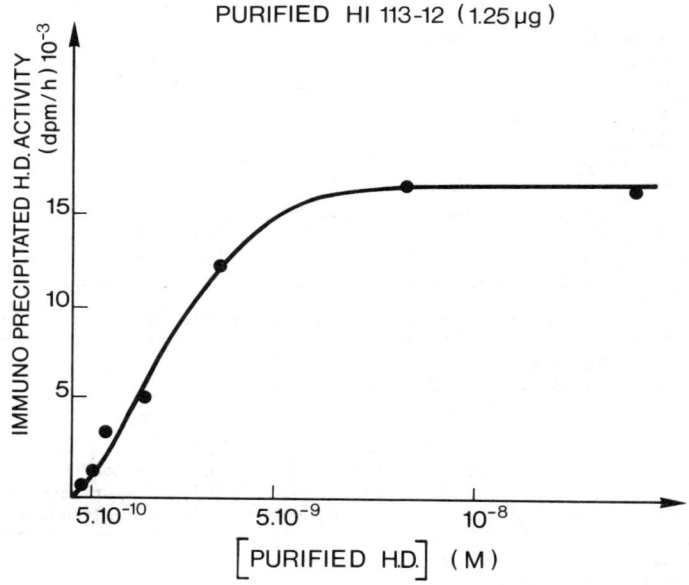

Fig. 1 Titration curve of Mab HI 113-12
Mab HI 113-12 (1.25 µg) incubated with the partially purified gastric enzyme in increasing concentrations and immunoprecipitation as described by Pollard and co-workers (1983).

Indeed the Mab H.I. 113-12 did not apparently recognise the H.D. active site since no inhibition of enzyme activity was ever observed in its presence.
Although the recognition of H.D. from the purified enzyme preparation was demonstrated by an immunoprecipitation assay similar to that used in the screening procedure (Table 3), no H.D. activity was precipitated when the second (anti-mouse) antibody was ommitted, indicating that the monoclonal antibody was not a precipitant one.

A maximal precipitation of 25 % of the total enzyme activity, occuring in the
presence of 0,5 ug the Mab HI 113-12 was observed, but these figures should be
considered as minimal ones since it may be that the catalytic activity of the
enzyme is somewhat impaired when the latter is insolubilised. From the titration
curve of Fig. 1 and taking into account a M.W. of 100 kDa for the enzyme and a
10 % purity of the preparation, an apparent dissociation constant of about   3
nM for the antibody can be calculated.

TABLE III   Biochemical specificity of the monoclonal antibody HI 113-12

PREPARATION	TOTAL H.D. (OR DECARBOXYLASE) ACTIVITY (dpm/h) x 10^3	SPECIFICALLY IMMUNO-PRECIPITATED $H.D_3$ ACTIVITY	
		(dpm/h) x 10^3	(% of total)
Purified gastric H.D.	6.2 ± 0.5	1.4 ± 0.1	24 ± 1
High Speed Supernatant from			
Rat gastric mucosa	3.9 ± 0.2	0.9 ± 0.1	24 ± 1
Rat hypothalamus	4.1 ± 0.3	1.0 ± 0.1	24 ± 1
Rat striatum	3.9 ± 0.4	1.0 ± 0.2	22 ± 4
Mouse mastocytoma	3.7 ± 0.1	0.6 ± 0.1	17 ± 1
Bacterial H.D. (from Cl. Welchii)	2.8 ± 0.2	non detectable	
Striatal Glutamic acid decarboxylase	3.6 ± 0.4	nd	
Striatal DOPA decarboxylase	2.7 ± 0.2	nd	

Decarboxylase activity specifically immunoprecipitated by Mab HI 113-12 (0.5 µg)
was   calculated by subtracting the activity precipitated under similar conditions in the presence of a control ascitic fluid (Pollard and co-workers, 1983).

The monoclonal antibody apparently recognised in the same manner (similar percentages of immunoprecipitation at similar dilutions) the H.D. activity from the
purified gastric preparation, and crude extracts from rat gastric mucosa, hypothalamus, striatum or mouse mastocytoma cells (table 3). In contrast neither the
bacterial H.D. from Cl. Welchii, an enzyme largely different from mammalian
H.D., nor glutamate and DOPA decarboxylase activities were significantly recognised. The latter observation is important since a polyclonal antibody against
purified H.D. has been reported to cross react with DOPA decarboxylase and its
possible cross-reaction with glutamate decarboxylase not assessed   (Watanabe
and co-workers, this Symposium).

IMMUNOHISTOCHEMICAL STUDIES WITH THE MONOCLONAL ANTIBODY

Our Mab HI 113-12 was used to localise H.D. immunoreactive structures in various
mammalian tissues, utilising either indirect fluorescent labelled   antibody
techniques or, more often, Sternberger's peroxidase-antiperoxidase (PAP) method

or the Avidin-biotin peroxidase complex technique. In all cases controls were run which consisted in either including a Mab directed against a protein different from H.D. or in ommitting the first antibody.

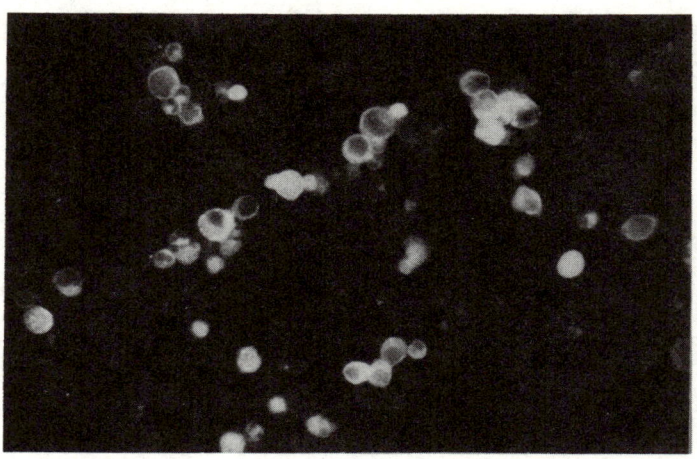

Fig. 2 Indirect immunofluorescence photomicrograph of mastocytoma cells (P 815, BDA_2 mices, kindly provided by Dr. Kinsky). X 400

Structures known to present a very high enzyme activity were clearly labelled with the anti-H.D. monoclonal antibody. This was, for example, the case for rat foetal liver on day 19 of gestation which was uniformally stained, as also shown with a polyclonal H.D. (Taguchi and co-workers, 1984).
In cultured mouse mastocytoma cells (P 815 from BDA_2 mice), from which the H.D. activity is clearly recognised by Mab HI 113-12 (table 3), a positive immunohistochemical response was located in the cytoplasm (fig. 2) ; however whereas some cells were stained, other were not, a difference which may reflect variable degrees of maturity with only some cells having fully expressed their H.D. activity.
In the rat stomach, another tissue with high H.D. activity, numerous H.D. immunoreactive mast-cells were found in the submucosa (Fig. 3) and in the superficial portion of the mucosa. Staining was also observed in some experiments at the level of cells located at the mid portion of gastric glands (not shown) but this was inconsistent and requires confirmation, particularly in view of discrepant results obtained with various polyclonal antibodies (see introduction).
In the rat brain some H.D immunoreactive structures could be visualised even without colchicine pretreatments. So far, H.D. perikarya were only found in the hypothalamus.

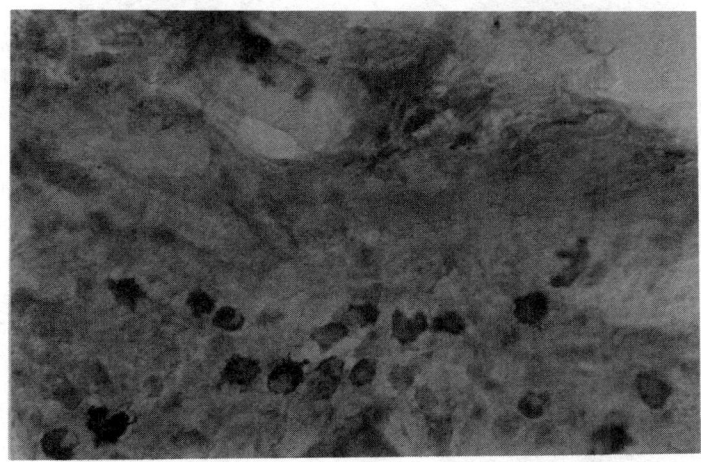

Fig. 3 Photomicrograph of transversal freeze microtome section (20 μm thickness) through the rat fundus after incubation with Mab HI 113-12 and immunostaining with the avidin-biotin peroxidase complex method. Note the presence of numerous H.D. immunoreactive cells (apparently gastric mast-cells) in the submucosa of the gland. X 400

A large group of H.D. cell-bodies were located in the posterior basal hypothalamus at the level of caudal magnocellular nucleus and around the arcuate nucleus (between A : 2800 and A : 3800 um according to Konig and Klippel stereotaxic atlas). This nucleus (Fig. 4A) is densely packed with large and fusiform cells which have large round nuclei and possess long processes. More caudally H.D. cells appeared in the nucleus mamillaris ventralis. More rostrally some H.D immunoreactive neurones were present in the supraoptic and paraventricular nuclei, at the dorsal tip of the third ventricle. Immunoreactive varicose fibers restricted to the rat hypothalamus were detected entering into or emanating from the median eminence, and a dense network of H.D. nerve-terminals which presents a rather large aspect and suround unlabelled cells was widely distributed in the arcuate nucleus.
This preliminary distribution of H.D.-containing neurones in rat brain, detected with our Mab HI 113-12 is in rather good agreement with findings obtained with polyclonal antibodies against either H.D. (Watanabe and co-workers, 1983, 1984 and this Symposium) or HA (Panula and co-workers, 1984 ; Steinbusch and Mulder, this Symposium).

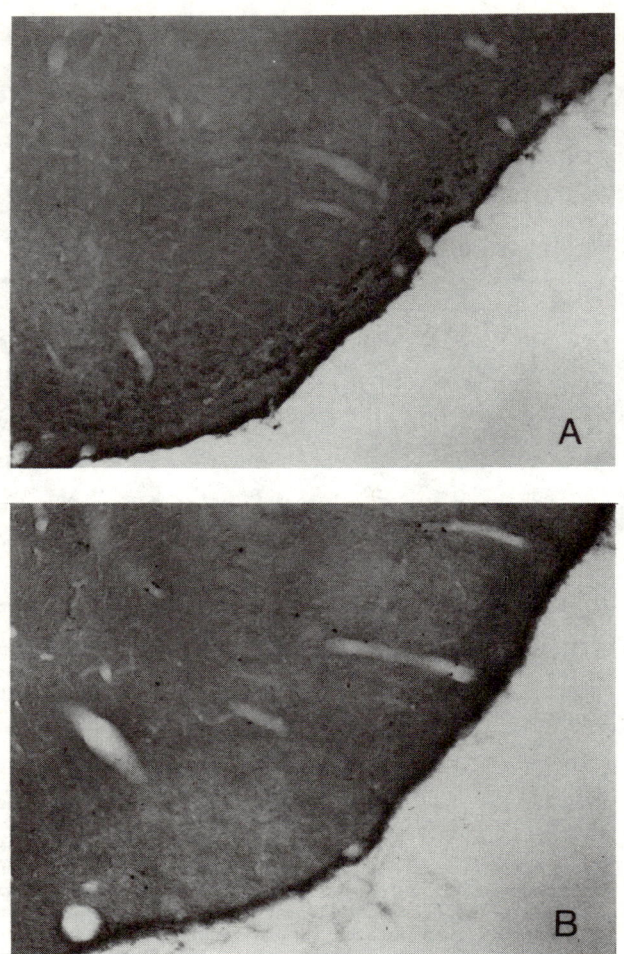

Fig. 4 A Photomicrograph of a frontal freeze microtome section (20 μM thickness) through the posterior hypothalamus of the rat, after incubation with Mab HI 113-12 and immunostaining with the PAP-method. Note the presence of a group of H.D.-immunoreactive neurons in the caudal magnocellular nucleus. X 100
Fig. 4 B Mab HI 113-12 ommitted.

Furthermore, this distribution is, at least in part, in good agreement with previous results obtained in our laboratory, indicating that electrolytic lesions located in the region of the mammillary bodies resulted in significant decreases in H.D. activity in several brain areas such as the anterior hypothalamus, striatum or cerebral cortex (Schwartz and co-workers, 1980, 1982a, 1982b ; Garbarg and co-workers, 1980a). In this study, an attempt at localising the areas from which emanate the ascending HA pathways ending in the telencephalon was realised (Garbarg and co-workers, 1980a). For this purpose selective lesions were performed at various anteriorities in the hypothalamus and upper brainstem and, for each animal, the volume and placement of the lesion were reconstituted by mapping the damaged areas. Then topographical data were correlated by a computer program with the decrease in H.D. in putative terminal areas in order to determine the efficient lesion areas. The pictures drawned by the computer included all the histaminergic cell-bodies so far described by immunochemical methods but also suggested their presence in the neighbouring mesencephalic reticular formation, the latter localisation not yet confirmed by immunohistochemical approaches.

A neurochemical confirmation of the localisation of perikarya in the region of mammillary bodies was found in the effects of locally administered kainic acid, (Table IV). This neurotoxin which ablates perikarya but spares axons induced significant unilateral decreases in H.D. activity in both the injected area and putative terminal areas like the cerebral cortex and striatum. This contrasts with the unchanged local H.D. activity when kainic acid is injected in a terminal area like the striatum (Unpublished data).

It should be mentionned that finally the presence of H.D.-synthetising perikarya in the hypothalamus was also suggested by the early recovery of the enzyme activity in this region after irreversible inactivation by α-fluoromethylhistidine (Garbarg and co-workers, 1980b).

TABLE IV Effects of a kainic acid microinjection into the mammillary bodies region on H.D. activities in injected and putative terminal brain areas

	H.D. ACTIVITY (dpm/µg protein/h) IN		
	MAMMILLARY BODIES	CEREBRAL CORTEX	STRIATUM
Controls	42.3 ± 3.3	8.1 ± 0.4	8.9 ± 0.5
Lesioned	29.5 ± 14**	6.7 ± 0.3*	6.5 ± 0.4**
Difference	(- 31 %)	(- 15 %)	(- 28 %)

* $p < 0.05$; ** $p < 0.005$

Rats were killed 10 days after unilateral infusion of kainic acid (1 µg) at the following coordinates from the atlas of König and Klippel (A 3.3 ; L 0.8 ; V 3.2). The injected area was punched out, telencephalic regions dissected out and H.D. activity determined with the radiochromatographic assay (Baudry and co-workers, 1973). Values of the injected side are compared to those of untreated animals (Means ± S.E.M. from 8-10 experiments).

CONCLUSIONS

The monoclonal antibody obtained against a semi-purified H.D. preparation (Pollard and co-workers, 1983) has already allowed us to confirm the presence of HA-synthetising perikarya in the mammillary region of the posterior hypothalamus previously suggested by our lesion studies and, recently, with polyclonal antibodies against either HA (Panula and co-workers, 1984) or H.D. (Watanabe and co-workers, 1983,1984 ; Steinbusch and Mulder, this Symposium). In addition, retrograde tracing experiments have recently shown the existence of an ascending pathway emanating from magnocellular neurons in the same region and directly innervating widespread regions of the neocortex (Vincent and co-workers, 1984). Although immunohistochemical studies indicated that at least some cells of the pathway were GABAergic, it might be assumed that the same pathway is also histaminergic. Indeed starting from the apparently diffuse projections of histaminergic neurons in brain, and taking into account a large variety of data like several analogies with monoaminergic systems, circadian turnover changes and the effects of H_1-antihistamines it was repeatedly proposed that the ascending histaminergic pathway should be considered as a part of the "reticular activating system" (Schwartz, 1977 ; Schwartz and co-workers, 1980c, 1982b, 1984). Hence the idea that ascending histaminergic neurons provide a widespread input to telencephalic areas like the cerebral cortex from the hypothalamus and provide them, through a direct pathway, with limbic, emotional and visceral information seems now reinforced by precise anatomical data . Interestingly this hypothesis is also reinforced by the recent discovery of Haas and Konnerth (1983), (see also Haas, this Symposium) that HA blocks a calcium-activated, potassium-conductance and thereby potentiates specific excitatory signals. This mode of action is consistent with the idea that "histaminergic neurons might contribute to set in a coordinate manner the overall excitability of various telencephalic areas" (Schwartz and co-workers, 1980).

ACKNOWLEDGEMENT

We are extremely grateful to Drs. C. Sotelo and M. Wassef for hospitality in their laboratory (U. 106 INSERM) as well as for very helpful advices and discussion during our histological work and to Dr. S. Kinsky (U. 23 INSERM) for giving us murine mastocytoma.

REFERENCES

Aures, D., and Håkanson, R. (1971).Histidine decarboxylase (mammalian). In H. Tabor and C.W. Tabor (Eds.), Methods in Enzymology, vol. 17B, Academic Press, New York. pp 667-677.

Aures, D., Håkanson, R., and Clark, W.G. (1970). Histidine decarboxylase and DOPA decarboxylase. In A. Lajtha (Ed.), Handbook of Neurochemistry, vol. 4, Plenum Press, New York. pp 165-187.

Barbin, G., Hirsch, J.C., Garbarg, M., and Schwartz, J.C. (1975). Decrease in histamine content and decarboxylase activities in an isolated area of the cerebral cortex of the cat. Brain Res., 92, 170-174.

Barbin, G., Garbarg, M., Schwartz, J.C., and Storm-Mathisen, J. (1976). Histamine synthetizing afferents to the hippocampal region. J. Neurochem., 26, 259-263.

Baudry, M., Martres, M.P., and Schwartz, J.C. (1973). The subcellular localization of histidine decarboxylase in various regions of rat brain. J. Neurochem., 21, 1301-1309.

Ben Ari, Y., Le Gal La Salle, G., Barbin, G., Schwartz, J.C., and Garbarg, M. (1977). Histamine synthesizing afferents within the amygdaloid complex and bed locus of the stria terminalis of the rat. Brain Res., 138, 285-294.
Brody, M.J., Håkanson, R., Owman, C., and Sundler, F. (1972). J. Histochem. Cytochem., 20, 945-950.
Buttin, G., Leguern, C., Phalente, L., Lin, E.C.C., Medrano, L., and Cazenave, P.A. (1978). Production of hybrides secreting monoclonal antiidiotypic antibodies by cell fusion on membrane filter. In F.M. Potter and N. Warner (Eds.), Current Topics in Microbiology and Immunology, vol. 81, Springer Verlag, New York. pp. 27-36.
Garbarg, M., Barbin, G., Feger, J., and Schwartz, J.C. (1974). Histaminergic pathways in rat brain evidenced by lesions of the MFB. Science, 186, 833-835.
Garbarg, M., Barbin, G., Bischoff, S., Pollard, H., and Schwartz, J.C. (1976). Dual localization of histamine in an ascending neuronal pathway and in non neuronal cell evidenced by lesions in the lateral hypothalamic area. Brain Res., 106, 333-348.
Garbarg, M., Barbin, G., Llorens, C., Palacios, J.M., Pollard, H., and Schwartz, J.C. (1980a). Recent developments in brain histamine research : pathways and receptors. In B. Essman (Ed.), Neurotransmitters, receptors and drug action, Spectrum Publ. Inc., New York. pp. 179-202.
Garbarg, M., Barbin, G., Rodergas, E., and Schwartz, J.C. (1980b). Inhibition of histamine synthesis in brain by α-fluoromethyl histidine, a new irreversible inhibitor : in vitro and in vivo studies. J. Neurochem., 35, 1045-1052.
Haas, H.L., and Wolf, P. (1977). Central action of histamine : micro electrophorectic studies. Brain Res., 122, 269-279.
Haas, H.L., and Konnerth, A. (1983). Histamine and noradrenaline decrease calcium-activated potassium conductance in hippocampal pyramidal cells. Nature, 302, 432-450.
Håkanson, R. (1963). Histidine decarboxylase in the fetal rat. Biochem. Pharmacol., 12, 1289-1296.
Hammar, L., Pahlman, S., and Hjerten, S. (1975). Chromatographic purification of a mammalian histidine decarboxylase on changed and non changed alkyl derivatives of agarose. Biochem. Biophys. Acta, 403, 554-562.
Hammar, L., and Hjerten, S. (1980). Purification and immunochemical analysis of histidine decarboxylase from murine mastocytoma. Agents & Actions, 10, 92-98.
Jarrott, B., Hjelle, J.T., and Spector, S. (1979). Association of histamine with cerebral microvessels in regions of bovine brain. Brain Res., 168, 323-330.
Karnyushina, I.L., Palacios, J.M., Barbin, G., Dux, E., Joo, F., and Schwartz, J.C. (1980). Studies on a capillary-rich fraction isolated from brain : histaminergic components and characterization of the histamine receptors linked to adenylate cyclase. J. Neurochem., 34, 1201-1208.
Köhler, G., and Milstein, C. (1975). Continuous cultures of fused cells secreting antibody of predefined specificity. Nature, 256, 495-497.
Kollonitsch, J., Patchett, A.A., Marburg, S., Maycock, A.L., Perkins, L.M., Doldouras, G.A., Duggan, D.E., and Aster, S.D (1978). Selective inhibitors of biosynthesis of aminergic neurotransmitters. Nature, 274, 906-908.
König, J.F.R., and Klippel, R.A. (1970). The rat brain, a stereotaxic atlas of the forebrain and lower parts of the brainstem. R.E. Krieger Publishing Co. inc..
Lange, M., Le Guern, C., and Cazenave, P.A. (1983). Covalent coupling of antigens to chemically activated lipopolysaccharide : a tool for in vivo and in vitro specific B cell stimulation. J. of Immunol. Meth., 63, 123-131.
Leslie, R., and Osborne, N. (1983). An immunohistochemical study to localise histaminergic neurones in invertebrate and vertebrate nervous systems. Neuroscience Letters, abstracts of the seventh European Neuroscience Congress, Hamburg, F.R.G.
Martres, M.P., Baudry, M., and Schwartz, J.C. (1975). Histamine synthesis in the developing rat brain : evidence for a multiple compartmentation. Brain Res., 83, 261-275.

Panula, P., Yang, H.Y.T., and Costa, E. (1984). Histamine containing neurons in the rat hypothalamus. Proc. Natl. Acad. Sci., U.S.A., 81, 2572-2576.

Pollard, H., Bischoff, S., Llorens-Cortes, H., and Schwartz, J.C. (1976). Histamine and histidine decarboxylase in discrete nuclei of rat hypothalamus and the evidence for mast-cells in the median eminence. Brain Res., 118, 509-513.

Pollard, H., Llorens, C., Barbin, G., Garbarg, M., and Schwartz, J.C. (1978). Histamine and histidine decarboxylase in brainstem nuclei : distribution and decrease after lesions. Brain Res., 157, 178-181.

Pollard, H., Pachot, I., Schwartz, J.C., Lange, M., Legrain, P., and Buttin, G. (1983). Production d'anticorps monoclonaux anti L-Histidine decarboxylase.C.R. Acad. Sci., Paris, 297, 553-556.

Sastry, B.S.R., and Phillis, J.W. (1976). Evidence for an ascending inhibitory histaminergic pathway to the cerebral cortex. Canad. J. Physiol. Pharmacol., 54, 782-786.

Savany, A., and Cronenberger, L. (1978). Purification et detection de plusieurs formes moléculaires de l'histidine decarboxylase de la muqueuse gastrique de rat. Biochemica Biophysica Acta, 526, 247-258.

Savany, A., and Cronenberger, L. (1982). Isolation and properties of multiple forms of histidine decarboxylase from rat gastric mucosa. Biochem. J., 205, 405-412.

Schwartz, J.C. (1975). Histamine as a transmitter in brain. Life Sci., 17, 503-518.

Schwartz, J.C. (1977). Histaminergic mechanisms in brain. Ann. Rev. Pharmacol. Toxicol., 17, 325-339.

Schwartz, J.C., Barbin, G., Baudry, M., Garbarg, M., Martres, M.P., Pollard, H., and Verdière, M. (1980). Metabolism and function of histamine in the brain. In W.B. Essman and L. Valzelli (Eds),Current developments in Psychopharmacology, vol. 5, pp. 173-261.

Schwartz, J.C., Barbin, G., Duchemin, A.M., Garbarg, M., Llorens, C., Pollard, H., Quach, T.T., and Rose, C. (1982a). Histamine receptors in the brain and their possible functions. In C.R. Ganellin and M.E. Parsons (Eds.), Pharmacology of histamine receptors, Wright PSG, Bristol, London, Boston. pp. 351-391.

Schwartz, J.C., Barbin, G., Duchemin, A.M., Garbarg, M., Pollard, H., Quach, T.T., and Rose, C. (1981). Functional role of histamine in the brain. In G.C. Palmer (Ed.), Neuropharmacology of Central and behavioral disorders. Academic Press, Inc., New York. pp. 539-572.

Schwartz, J.C., Garbarg, M., Lebrecht, W., Nowak, J., Pollard, H., Rodergas, E., Rose, C., Quach, T.T., Morgat, J.L., and Roy, J. (1982b). Histaminergic systems in brain : studies on localisation and actions. In B. Uvnas and K. Tasaka (Eds), Advances in the biosciences, vol. 33. Pergamon Press, Oxford and New York. pp. 71-80.

Schwartz, J.C., Garbarg, M., and Pollard, H. (1984). Histaminergic transmission in brain. In F.E. Bloom (Ed.), The handbook of Physiology, volume on the intrinsic regulatory system of the brain. American Physiological Society Publ. (in press).

Schwartz, J.C., Lampart, C., and Rose, C. (1970). Properties and regional distribution of histidine decarboxylase in rat brain. J. Neurochem., 17, 1527-1534.

Schwartz, J.C., Lampart, C., Rose, C., Rehault, M.C., Bischoff, S., and Pollard, H. (1971). Histamine formation in rat brain during development. J. Neurochem., 18, 1787-1789.

Schwartz, J.C., Pollard, H., and Quach, T.T. (1980c). Histamine as a neurotransmitter in mammalian brain : neurochemical evidence. J. Neurochem., 35, 26-33.

Taguchi, Y., Watanabe, T., Kubota, H., Hayayuki, H., and Wada, H. (1984). Purification of histidine decarboxylase from the liver of fetal rats and its immunochemical and immunohistochemical characterizations. J. Biol. Chem., 259, 5214-5221.

Tran, V.T., and Snyder, S.H. (1981). Histidine decarboxylase, purification from fetal rat liver, immunologic properties and histochemical localization in brain and stomach. The Journal of biological chemistry, 256, 680-686.
Vincent, S.R., Hokfelt, T., Skirboll, L.A., and Yenwu, J. (1983). Hypothalamic ϒ-aminobutyric acid neurons project to the neocortex. Science, 220, 1309-1310.
Watanabe, T., Nakamura, H., Liang, L.Y., Yamatodani, A., and Wada, H. (1979). Partial purification and characterization of L-histidine decarboxylase from fetal rats. Biochem. Pharmacol., 28, 1149-1155.
Watanabe, T., Yamada, M., Taguchi, Y., Kubota, H., Maeyama, K., Yamatodani, A., Fukui, H., Shiosaka, S., Tohyama, M., and Wada, H. (1982). Purification and properties of histidine decarboxylase isozymes and their pharmacological significance. In B. Uvnas and K. Tasaka (Eds), Advances in the Biosciences, vol. 33. Pergamon Press, Oxford and New York. pp. 93-106.
Watanabe, T., Taguchi, Y., Hayashi, H., Wada, H., H. Kubota, Terano, Y., Tanaka, J., Shiosaka, S., and Tohyama, M. (1983). Evidence for the presence of histaminergic nervous system in the brain : an immunochemical analysis. Neurosci.- Lett., 39, 249-254.
Watanabe, T., Taguchi, Y., Shiosaka, S., Tanaka, J., Kubota, H., Terano, Y., Tohyama, M., and Wada, H. (1984). Distribution of the histaminergic neuron system in the central neurons system of rats : A fluorescent immunohistochemical analysis with histidine decarboxylase as a marker. Brain Res., 295, 13-25.
Wilcox, B.J., and Seybold, V.S. (1982). Localization of neuronal histamine in rat brain. Neuroscience letters, 29, 105-110.
Yamada, M., Watanabe, T., Fukui, H., Taguchi, Y., and Wada, H. (1984). Comparison of histidine decarboxylases from rat stomach and brain with that from whole bodies of rat fetus. Agents and Actions, 14, 143-152.

LOCALIZATION AND PROJECTIONS OF HISTAMINE-IMMUNOREACTIVE NEURONS IN THE CENTRAL NERVOUS SYSTEM OF THE RAT

H. W. M. Steinbusch and A. H. Mulder

Department of Pharmacology, Free University Medical Faculty, van der Boechorststraat 7, 1081 BT Amsterdam, The Netherlands

ABSTRACT

An immunohistochemical method for the localization and distribution of histamine in the central nervous system was developed, using an antibody raised against histamine coupled to a carrier protein in conjunction with an optimal fixation procedure. The immunostaining appeared to be highly specific for histamine, showing no cross-reactivity to other biogenic amines and also highly sensitive, unveiling a diffuse distribution of histaminergic nerve fibers in the rat di- and telencephalon.

Histamine-immunoreactive cell bodies were strictly confined to the ventral part of the posterior hypothalamus and the region of the mammillary nuclei. They can be divided in two main cell groups with two major ascending projections and one minor descending projection. The ascending histaminergic fiber tracts innervate almost all regions of the di- and telencephalon with high concentrations in e.g. the eminentia mediana, the nucleus tractus diagonalis of Broca, the caudato-putamen complex and cortical structures. The arrangement of the histaminergic neuronal system viz. a compact cell group with a widespread distribution of fibers, resembles that of other monoaminergic , i.e. serotonergic and catecholaminergic systems.

KEYWORDS

histamine; histaminergic neurons; central nervous system; immunohistochemistry.

INTRODUCTION

Although for a long time histamine has been ascribed a neurotransmitter role in the mammalian CNS on the basis of an impressive amount of indirect - mainly neurochemical - evidence (Green, 1970; Snyder and Taylor, 1972; Schwartz, 1975; Schwartz, Pollard and Quach, 1980) appropriate histochemical methods to actually visualize histaminergic neurons have been lacking until recently. The formaldehyde-induced fluorescence (FIF) method, which has been used successfully to localize other monoaminergic systems, appears not to be applicable in the case of histamine (Björklund, Falck and Owman, 1972). Although by using ortho-phtaldialdehyde instead of formaldehyde, a method has been developed that makes it possible to visualize histamine in mast cells and onyx cells of the gastric mucosa (Buteau and Duitschaever, 1981), its sensitivity appears to be too low to be usable in studies on the localization of histaminergic neurons (Håkanson and others, 1976).

However, recently a major breakthrough has been achieved by utilizing immunohistochemical procedures. Histamine-producing cells contain a specific histidine-decarboxylase (HDC; EC 4.1.1.22) that is different from the L-aromatic aminoacid decarboxylase (EC 4.1.1.26), present in catecholaminergic as well as indolaminergic neurons (Schwartz, 1975; Schwartz, Pollard and Quach, 1980). Watanabe and coworkers (1983, 1984) succeeded to purify HDC from fetal rat liver, to raise antibodies against the enzyme and to localize immunohistochemically HDC-positive cell bodies and fibers in rat brain. Another immunohistochemical approach which has been applied successfully to localize other monoaminergic systems is to use antibodies directed against the monoamine neurotransmitter itself, following its coupling to a carrier protein (Steinbusch, Verhofstad and Joosten, 1978; Steinbusch and others, 1981; Steinbusch and Tilders, 1984). Here we briefly describe the preparation of antibodies to histamine conjugated with thyroglobulin and present data on the localization of histaminergic neurons in the rat CNS, obtained with these antisera.

METHODS

Histamine was coupled to thyroglobulin by the following procedure: 1 ml distilled water containing 10 mg histamine-HCl (Sigma), 30 mg thyroglobulin (Sigma) in 1 ml distilled water, 1 ml 3 M sodium-acetate buffer, pH 6.8, 1 ml 7.5% paraformaldehyde ($^w/v$) (Merck) and 60 ul 25% glutaraldehyde ($^v/v$ Merck) were mixed. The coupling reaction proceeded for 30 min at room temperature in a shaker in the dark, the pH being maintained at 6.8. The reaction was stopped by adding 15 ml of distilled water and 50 ml 1 N HCl. The reaction mixture was dialyzed against running tapwater for 3 days at 4°C in the dark. The precipitate was removed by centrifugation at 20.000xg and discarded. The protein concentration of the supernatant was measured according to the method of Lowry and others (1951). The coupling efficiency and the molar ratio were determined by measuring ultraviolet absorption spectra (between 250 and 450 nm) or, in some pilot experiments, by measuring the incorporation of ^{3}H-histamine in the conjugate.
For immunization adult rabbits (New Zealand strain) were injected subcutaneously with an emulsion consisting of 1 mg conjugate in 0.3 ml PBS and 0.6 ml complete Freund's adjuvant (Difco) at several sites around the neck and shoulders. At least three booster injections (with incomplete Freund's adjuvant) (Difco) were given intramuscularly with intervals of three weeks. Serum samples were collected from the marginal ear vein after 8 days and tested for their capacity to induce an immunohistochemical reaction.
The fixation procedure appeared to be very crucial. In our hands the best immunostaining was achieved by using antibodies to an immunogen which was prepared by utilizing formaldehyde/glutaraldehyde as the coupling reagent. Fixation with a mixture of 4% paraformaldehyde ($^w/v$), 0.05% glutaraldehyde ($^v/v$) and 0.2% picric acid ($^w/v$) in 0.1 M sodium phosphate buffer, pH 7.3, appeared to be the fixative of choice for histamine. Perfusion fixation was carried out as follows: Adult rats (bodyweight 140-180 g) were anesthetized with sodium-pentobarbital (100 mg/kg i.p.). A gauge needle was inserted through the left ventricle of the heart and a preperfusion with cold oxygenated Ca^{++}-free Tyrode solution, pH 7.4, for 1 min was followed by a perfusion with the above mentioned fixative. After 20 min perfusion, tissues were promptly removed and cut into 5-8 mm slabs in either frontal, sagittal or horizontal direction. The tissue slabs were postfixed with 4% paraformaldehyde and 0.2% picric acid for 90 minutes at 4°C. Following fixation, three methods were used to produce tissue sections, i.e. cryostat (4-10 um), freeze-microtome (16-30 um) or vibratome (30-100 um) sections.
Two types of immunostaining were used. The indirect immunofluorescence method was applied to cryostat sections, whereas the unlabelled peroxidase-antiperoxidase method was applied to thick freeze microtome and vibratome sections. A detailed description of the sectioning and immunostaining procedures for histamine and the production and application of the dopamine antiserum can be found elsewhere (Steinbusch and Tilders, 1984). The antibody to HDC was a generous gift of Dr Watanabe.

LOCALIZATION OF HISTAMINERGIC NEURONS IN THE RAT CNS

Specificity of the Immunohistochemical Method

The specificity of the immunohistochemical methods using antibodies directed against histamine coupled to carrier proteins, such as haemocyanin and thyroglobulin, will be discussed at length elsewhere (Steinbusch and Tilders,1984; Steinbusch and Mulder, in preparation). Briefly, immuno-inhibition

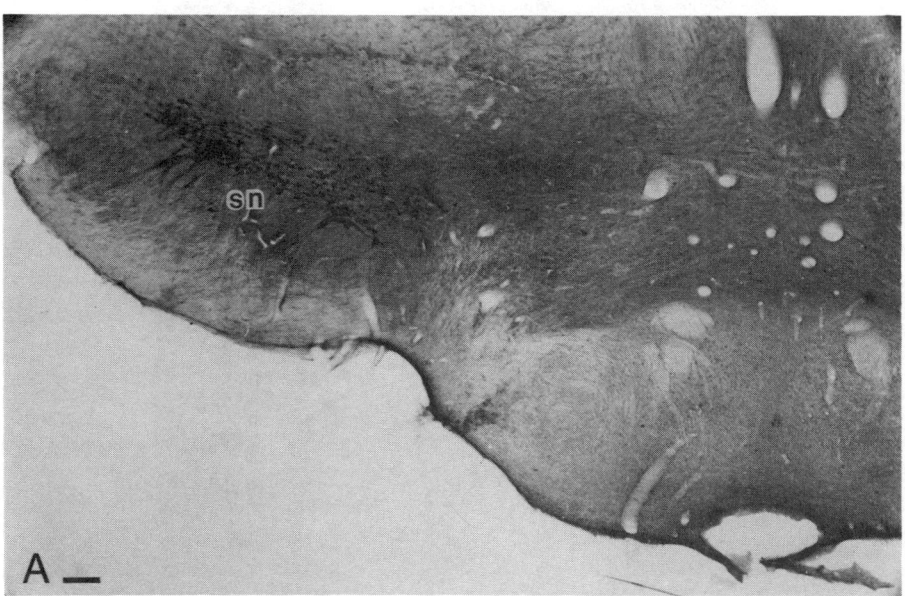

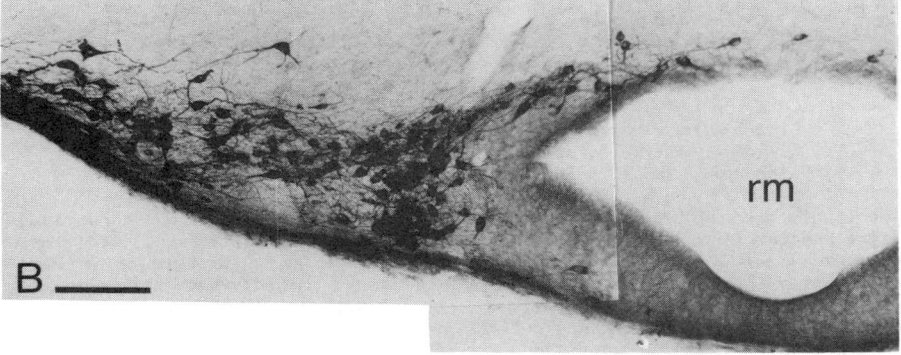

Fig. 1. Photomicrographs of transversal-Vibratome sections through the substantia nigra (sn)(A) and the recessus mammillaris (rm)(A,B) after incubation with an antibody to dopamine (A) and histamine (B). Note the presence of DA_i-cell bodies in the sn (A) and HA_i-perikarya in the mammillary region (B). Bars: 75 um.

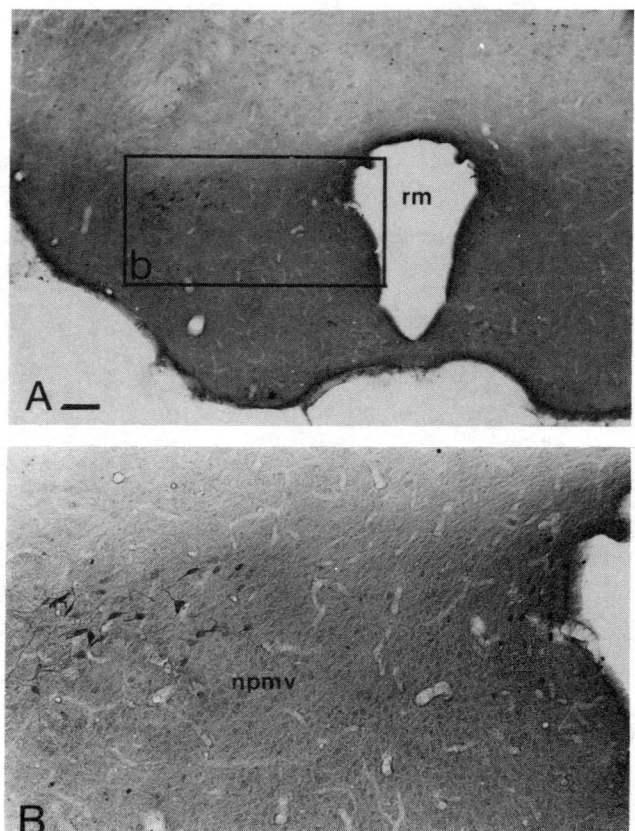

Fig. 2. Photomicrographs of a transversal-Vibratome section through the recessus mammillaris (rm) and the nucleus premammillaris ventralis (npmv) after incubation with an antibody to dopamine. DA-perikarya are situated at the dorsal tip of the rm and dorsolaterally to the npmv. Bars: 75 um.

experiments demonstrated the absence of cross-reactivity of the antiserum used in the present study towards other monoamines or their derivatives. In addition, no staining was found in a number of brain regions known to be rich in cell bodies with high concentrations of monoamines other than histamine or histidine-containing peptides (Figs. 1A,B; 2A,B). Further elimination of catecholaminergic and serotonergic fiber systems with the respective neurotoxins 6-hydroxydopamine and 5,7-dihydroxytryptamine did not affect histamine-immunoreactivity (Mulder, Smits and Steinbusch, this volume). With regard to the cell bodies, there is a complete overlap using HDC-or HA-immunoreactivity. Finally, the use of pre-immune serum resulted only in a faint background staining. Therefore, our antiserum appears to recognize specifically histamine as its antigenic factor in paraformaldehyde-glutaraldehyde-fixated nervous tissue.

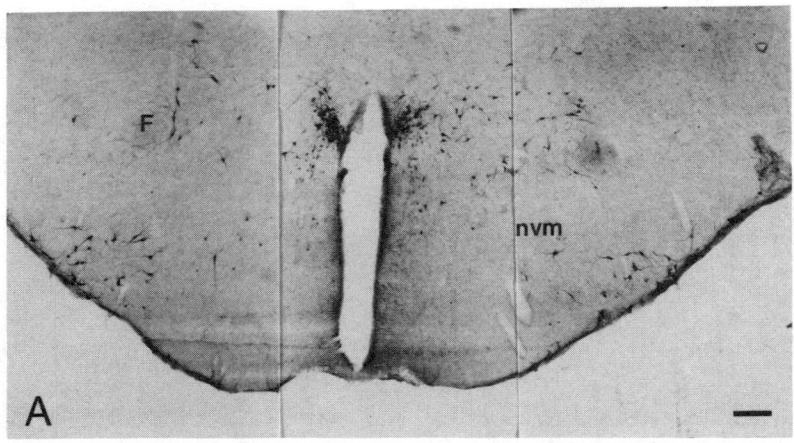
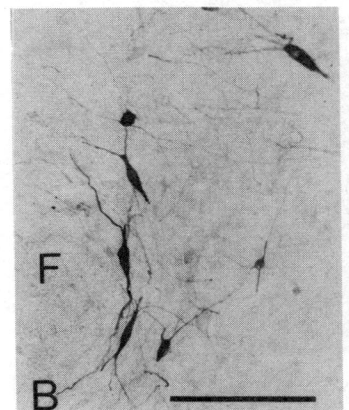
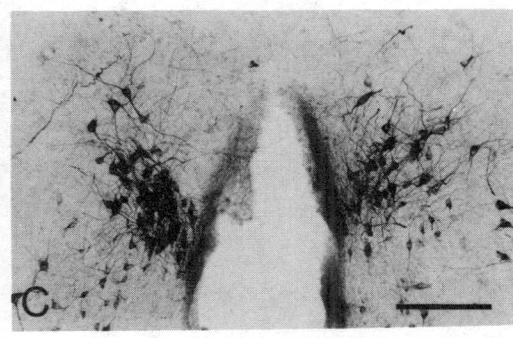

Fig. 3. Photomicrographs of a transversal-Vibratome section through the median hypothalamus after incubation with an antibody to histamine. Note the presence of HA_i-cell bodies at the dorsal tip of the third ventricle (A,B), medially to the fornix (F)(A,C) and ventrolaterally to the nucleus ventromedialis hypothalami (nvm)(A). Bars: 75 um.

Histamine-Immunoreactive Cell Bodies

Histamine-immunoreactive (HA_i)-cell bodies could be visualized in rats without any pharmacological manipulation. However, pretreatment with colchicine, resulted in a strong increase of the immunostaining intensity, enabling a distinct delineation of the histamine-positive perikarya and their dendritic arborizations. Similarly, pretreatment with the precursor L-histidine enhanced the immunostaining intensity, although to a lesser extent than did colchicine. The HA_i-perikarya were strictly confined to the region of the mammillary nuclei (Fig. 1B) and the ventral part of the posterior hypothalamus (Figs. 3A,B,C) They can be divided into two main groups: The most prominent group of HA_i-cell bodies was found between levels A 2800 and A 3800 (coordinates according to the atlas of König and Klippel). Caudally, they

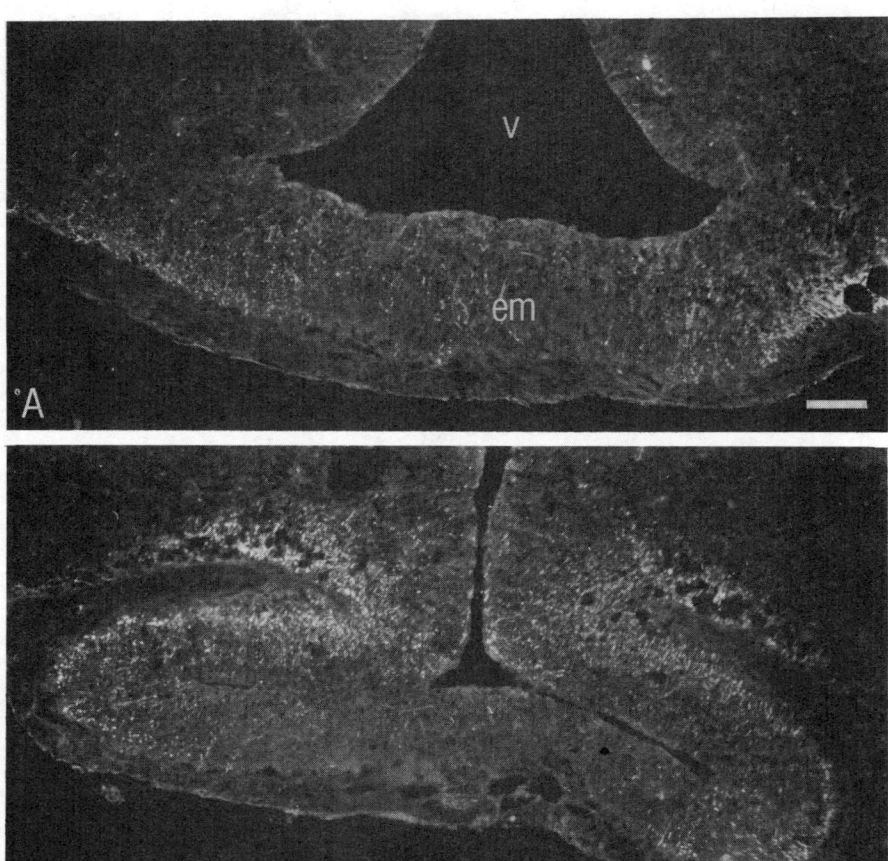

Fig. 4. Photomicrographs of transversal cryostat sections through the eminentia mediana (em) (A) and the infundibulum stalk (B) after incubation with an antibody to histamine. A: HA_i-fibers are demonstrated in the lateral aspects of the em, mostly in its external layer. B: HA_i-fibers are present in particular in the external layer of the dorsal labium. (v= ventricle). Bars: 75 um.

Fig. 5. Photomicrographs of transversal-Freeze-microtome sections through the cortex (A) and the regions of the nucleus lateralis septi (sl)(B), the nucleus hypothalamicus posterior (nhp)(C) and the nucleus raphe dorsalis (nrd)(D) after incubation with an antibody to histamine. Note in (A) the long HA_i-fibers in the entorhinal cortex, mainly situated the in upper laminae. B: A very high density of HA_i-varicose fibers was found in the sl, some of the fibers enter the fornix (F). C: A dense innervation of of mostly ventrically oriented HA_i-fibers demonstrated in the nhp. D: Some HA_i-fibers were found in the midline region of the nrd. Bars: 75 um.

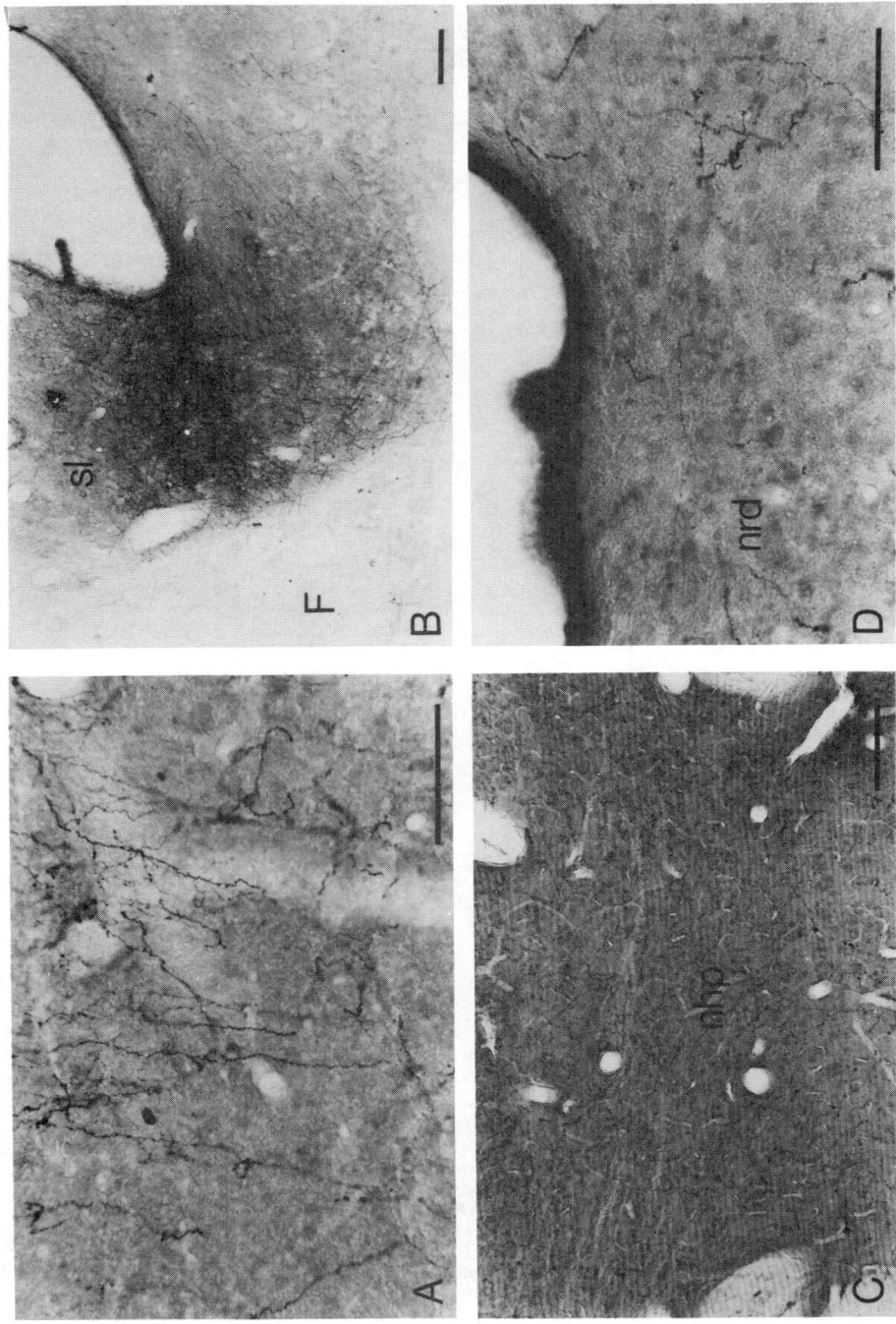

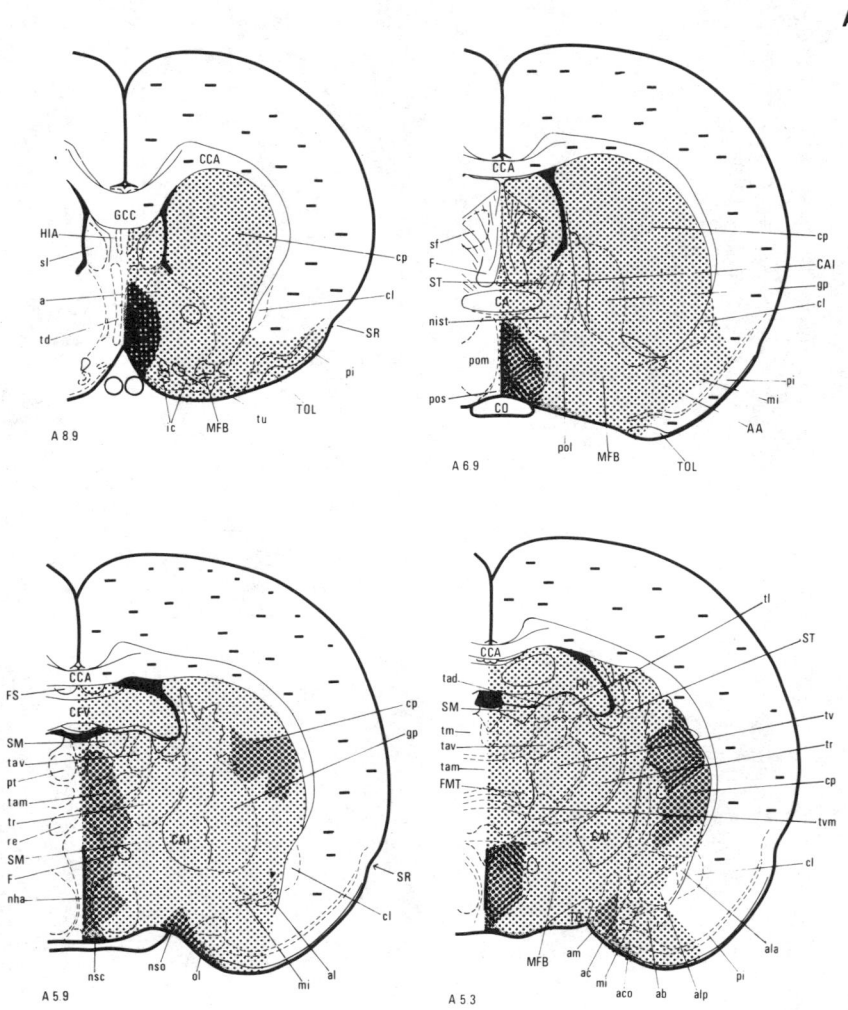

Fig. 6 A and B. Regional differences in the concentration of histamine-immunoreactivity in the di- and telencephalon of the rat. The variations in varicose fiber densities were estimated subjectively and have been pictured in different grey tones according to the scale shown in part B of this figure. The localization of histaminergic cell bodies is indicated by asterisks (which do not represent actual cell numbers).

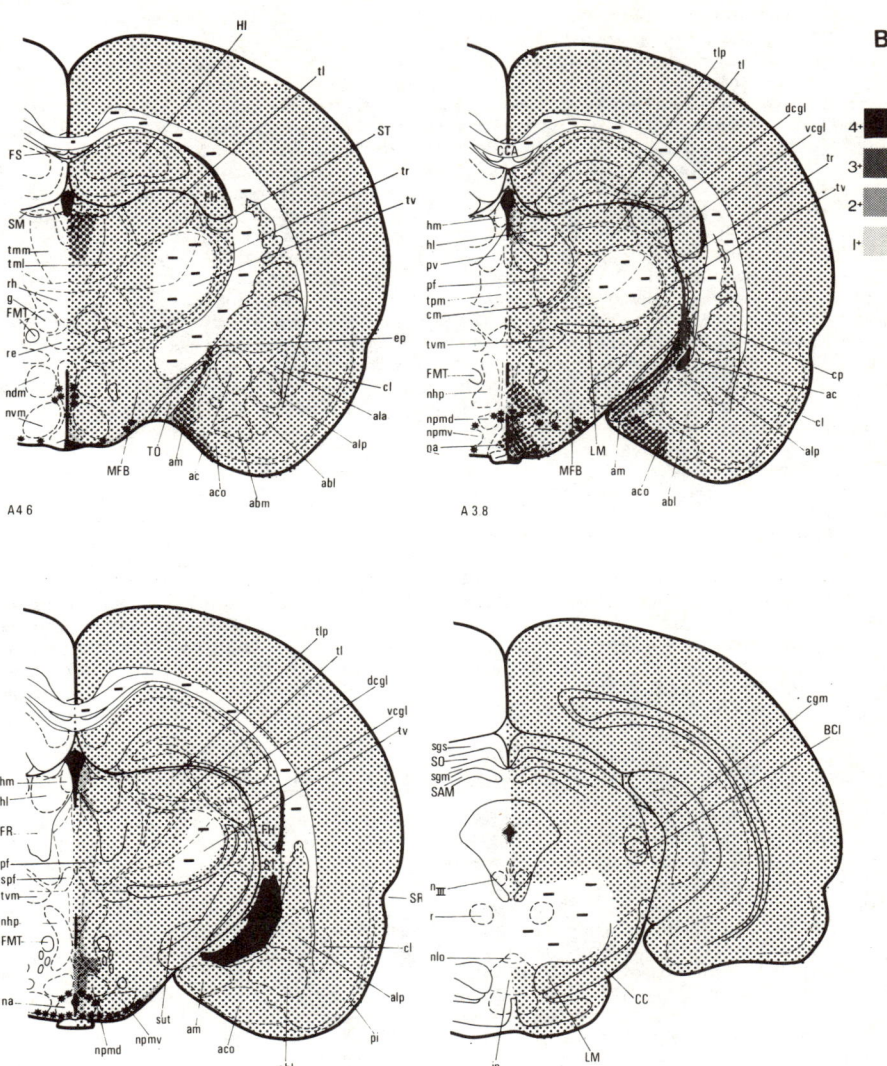

The abbreviations used in fig. 6 A and B have been taken
from the Handbook of Chemical Neuroanatomy, T. Hökfelt,
A. Björklund and M.J. Kuhar (Eds.), Elsevier, Amsterdam,
1984.

appear ventrolaterally to the nucleus mammillaris lateralis, immediately adjacent to the basal surface of the brain. Rostrally, this cell group extends to the recessus mammillaris, to form a narrow band of HA_i-perikarya ventral to and within the nucleus mammillaris lateralis (Fig. 1B).
The second group of HA_i-cell bodies is mainly situated between levels A 3400 and A 4400. This cell group is not as compact as the previous one. It is composed of HA_i-perikarya arising caudally at the dorsal tip of the recessus mammillaris. Rostrally, this group can be followed until the level of the third ventricle, where the HA_i-cell bodies are situated between the nuclei dorso- and ventromedialis hypothalami (Figs. 3A,B). In addition to these two cell groups, scattered HA_i-cell bodies were observed throughout the posterior hypothalamus (Figs. 3A,B). Caudally, at level A 2800, some HA_i-cell bodies were demonstrated in the dorsal part of the nucleus mammillaris medialis and lateralis, just ventrally to the fasciculus mammillothalamicus. Rostrally, at the posterior edge of the recessus mammillaris no cells were found. At level A 3400, we observed some HA_i-perikarya throughout the nucleus premammillaris ventralis. No HA_i-cells were seen in the nucleus arcuatus (Fig. 4A). At that same level, a few HA_i-cells were demonstrated in the nucleus premammillaris dorsalis. Rostrally between levels A 3800 and A 4400, these cells can be found in the nucleus hypothalamicus posterior and in the ventrolateral aspects of the hypothalamus, e.g. the region situated between the medial forebrain bundle (MFB) and the basal surface of the brain (Fig. 3A). Some HA_i-cells can be found within the MFB itself (Fig. 3A).
Apart from these HA_i-neurons, HA_i-mast cells were found at the basal surface of the hypothalamus, where they were especially prominent at the level of the eminentia mediana, immediately beneath the meninges.
Our findings are in general agreement with those of Watanabe and coworkers (1983, 1984), who used an antiserum to HDC and those of Panula, Yang and Costa (1984), who used an immunohistochemical method resembling ours, but with a different antibody to histamine. However, these data differ from those reported by Wilcox and Seybold (1982), who used an antibody raised against a complex between histamine and methylated bovine serum albumin and observed histamine-like immunoreactive cell bodies at the dorsal tip of the third ventricle. Unfortunately, these authors failed to give information about the coupling efficiency and specificity of their method.

Histaminergic Neuronal Projections and Areas of Termination

Our findings indicate that HA_i-varicose fibers innervate almost all regions of the rat CNS. They can even be found in the thick myelinated fiber bundles, such as the fornix (Fig. 5B) or the tractus cortico-spinalis. The HA_i-varicose fibers appeared most abundant in the di- and telencephalon, with their highest density in the eminentia mediana (Fig. 4A), the nucleus ventromedialis hypothalami and adjacent areas and the nucleus tractus diagonalis Broca and the contiguous nucleus lateralis septi (Fig. 5B). On the basis of preliminary data obtained in experiments examining the immunocytochemical localization of histamine together with the anterograde transport of lectins (Phaseolus vulgaris), three pathways can be traced: two ascending and one descending.
The dorsal ascending pathway arises from the HA_i-cell bodies situated in the region between levels A 3400 and A 4400, i.e. the HA_i-perikarya close to the third ventricle (Figs. 3A,C) and the dorsal tip of the recessus mammillaris. Its fibers do not enter the MFB but are situated dorsolaterally to it. The main areas of termination of this pathway are the caudatoputamen complex, the globus pallidus and the nucleus accumbens.
The ventral ascending pathway arises from the HA_i-cell bodies situated more ventrolaterally in the posterior hypothalamus, between levels A 2800 and A 3800, and its fibers enter the MFB. Rostrally, fibers leave the MFB to enter the fasciculus retroflexus, and distribute to the nucleus medialis habenulae and other thalamic structures. At this level some fibers enter the eminentia mediana (Fig. 4A) and run through the infundibulum (Fig. 4B) to the pars nervosa of the pituitary.

Further rostrally, fibers leave the MFB to enter the nucleus lateralis hypothalami, the nucleus suprachiasmaticus and the amygdala complex, by means of the striae terminalis. Finally, some HA_L-fibers were demonstrated, which reach the prefrontal-, frontal-, neo-, entorhinal- and hippocampal cortex (Fig. 5A) via the cingulum bundle.
A minor descending histaminergic pathway arises from the HA_i-cell group situated ventrolaterally to the nucleus mammillaris lateralis, between levels A 2800 and A 3400 (Fig. 1B). Its fibers are oriented dorsomedially and through the nucleus hypothalamicus posterior (Fig. 5C) and can be found in the medial part of the nucleus raphe dorsalis (Fig. 5D) and the surrounding periaquaductal central grey. From here the HA_i-fibers continue caudally through the ventromedial and lateral aspects of the substantium griseum. A few HA_i-fibers have been demonstrated in the dorsomedial part of the rhombencephalic formatio reticularis, the nucleus tractus spinalis nervi trigemini, the nucleus tractus solitarius. Some fibers were found in the ventrolateral aspects of the cerebellum.

CONCLUDING REMARKS

Until recently our knowledge of the distribution of putative histaminergic neurons in the CNS was based entirely on indirect evidence obtained from neurochemical studies, in particular the excellent work of Schwartz and colleagues, determining histamine levels and HDC-activity in small brain regions, before and after selective lesions placed at different levels in upper midbrain and hypothalamus (Brownstein and others, 1974; Garbarg and others, 1974, 1976; Barbin and others, 1976; Pollard and others, 1978; Schwartz, Pollard and Quach, 1980). It is worth noting the striking general agreement between the distribution of histaminergic neurons suspected on the basis of neurochemical findings and that revealed thus far in our immunohistochemical studies as well as those of others (Watanabe and others, 1983, 1984; Panula, Yang and Costa, 1984). Obviously, the immunohistochemical approach, as described in this paper, enables a more detailed localization of histaminergic neurons and their projections in the CNS. A complete immunohistochemical mapping of the histaminergic system(s) in the rat CNS is in progress in our laboratory.
The data obtained thus far suggest that the arrangement of the histaminergic neuronal system, viz. a compact cell group with a widespread distribution of fibers, resembles that of other monoaminergic systems, particularly the serotonergic dopaminergic and noradrenergic systems in the nucleus raphe dorsalis, substantia nigra and locus coeruleus, respectively (Figs. 1A,B). The widespread distribution of histaminergic fibers suggests that histamine, like the catecholamines and serotonin, may be involved in a large variety of physiological functions ruled by the CNS. Most prominent in this regard is the dense histaminergic innervation of the eminentia mediana, suggesting an involvement of histamine in the regulation of the anterior pituitary function. Further, the histaminergic innervation of the nuclei paraventricularis and suprachiasmaticus, suggests a functional link between the histaminergic systems and the magnocellular neurosecretory neurons producing the peptides vasopressin and oxytocin. Finally, the presence of histaminergic neurons -though small in number- in limbic structures, such as hippocampus and septum, might imply that they are involved in certain emotional and/or behavioral phenomena.

REFERENCES

Barbin, G., M. Garbarg, J.C. Schwartz and S. Storm-Mathisen (1976). Histamine-synthesizing afferents to the hippocampal region. J. Neurochem., 26, 259-263.
Björklund, A., B. Falck and Ch. Owman (1972). Fluorescence microscopic and microspectro-fluorometric techniques for the cellular localization and characterization of biogenic amines. Meth. of Invest. and Diagn. Endocrinol., 1, 318-368.
Brownstein, M.J., J.M. Saavedra, M. Palkovits and J. Axelrod (1974). Histamine

content of hypothalamic nuclei of the rat. Brain Res., 77, 151-156.
Buteau, C. and C.L. Duitschaever (1981). Stability of the o-phtaldialdehyde-histamine complex. Chromatography, 212, 23-27.
Garbarg, M., G. Barbin, J. Feger and J.-C. Schwartz (1974). Histaminergic pathway in rat brain evidenced by lesions of the medial forebrain bundle. Science, 186, 833-835.
Garbarg, M., G. Barbin, S. Bisschoff, H. Pollard and J.-C. Schwartz (1976). Dual localization of histamine in an ascending pathway and in non-neuronal cells evidenced by lesions in the lateral hypothalamic area. Brain Res., 106, 333-348.
Green, J.P. (1970). Histamine. In A. Lajtha (Ed.), Handbook of Neurochemistry, Vol. 4, Plenum Press, New York. pp. 221-250.
Håkanson, R., L.-J. Larsson, G. Liedberg and F. Sundler (1976). The histamine-storing enterochromaffin-like cells of the rat stomach. In R.E. Coupland and T. Fujita (Eds.),Chromaffin, Enterochromaffin and Related Cells, Elsevier, Amsterdam, p. 243-263.
Lowry, O.H., N.J. Rosebrough, A.L. Farr and R.J. Randall (1951). Protein measurement with the Folin phenol reagent. J. Biol. Chem., 193, 265-275.
Panula, P., H.-Y.F.T. Yang and E. Costa (1984). Histamine-containing neurons in the rat hypothalamus. Proc. Natl. Acad. Sci. USA, 81, 2572-2576.
Pollard, H., C.L. Llorens-Cortes, G. Barbin, M. Garbarg and J.-C. Schwartz (1978). Histamine and histidine decarboxylase in brain stem nuclei: distribution and decrease after lesions. Brain Res., 157, 178-181.
Schwartz, J.-C. (1975). Histamine as a neurotransmitter in brain. Life Sci., 17, 503-518.
Schwartz, J.-C., H. Pollard and T.T. Quach (1980). Histamine as a neurotransmitter in mammalian brain: neurochemical evidence. J. Neurochem., 35, 26-33.
Snyder, S.H. and K.M. Taylor (1974). Histamine in the brain: a neurotransmitter? In S.H. Snyder (Ed.), Perspective in Neuropharmacology: A tribute to Julius Axelrod, Oxford University Press, New York.
Steinbusch, H.W.M., A.A.J. Verhofstad and H.W.J. Joosten (1978). Localization of serotonin in the central nervous system by immunohistochemistry: description of a specific and sensitive technique and some applications. Neuroscience, 3, 811-:-819.
Steinbusch, H.W.M., A.A.J. Verhofstad, B. Penke, J. Varga and H.W.J. Joosten (1981). Immunohistochemical characterization of monoamine-containing neurons in the central nervous system by antibodies to serotonin and noradrenaline. A study in the rat and the lamprey (Lampetra fluviatilis). Acta Histochem., suppl. XXIV, 107-122.
Steinbusch, H.W.M. and A.H. Mulder (1984). Immunhistochemical localization of histamine neurons and mast cells in the rat brain. In A. Björklund, and T. Hökfelt (Eds.), The Handbook of Chemical Neuroanatomy, Vol. 2, Elsevier, Amsterdam, in press.
Steinbusch, H.W.M. and F.J.H. Tilders (1984). Localization of dopamine, noradrenalin, adrenalin, serotonin and histamine in the central nervous system. A light-microscopical immunohistochemical study. In J. Furness and M. Costa (Eds.), IBRO Handbook Series: Methods in the Neurosciences, Vol. 6, Wiley and Sons, Chichester, UK, in press.
Watanabe, T., Y. Taguchi, H. Hayashi, H. Wada, H. Kubota, Y. Terano, J. Tanaka, S. Shiosaka and M. Tohyama (1983). Evidence for the presence of histaminergic neuron system in the brain: an immunohistochemical analysis. Neurosci. Lett., 39, 249-254.Jb
Watanabe,T., Y. Taguchi, S. Shiosaka, J. Tanaka, H. Kubota, Y. Terano, M. Tohyama and H. Wada (1984). Distribution of the histaminergic neuron system in the central nervous system of rats; a fluorescent immunohistochemical analysis with histidine decarboxylase as a marker. Brain Res., 295, 13-25.
Wilcox, B.J. and V.S. Seybold (1982). Localization of neuronal histamine in rat brain. Neurosci. Lett., 29, 105-110.

MAST CELLS IN RAT BRAIN: CHARACTERIZATION, LOCALIZATION, AND HISTAMINE CONTENT

L. B. Hough**, R. C. Goldschmidt*, S. D. Glick**
and J. Padawer***

*Department of Pharmacology, Mount Sinai Medical School,
New York, NY 10029, USA
**Present Address: Department of Pharmacology and
Toxicology, Albany Medical College, Albany,
NY 12208, USA
***Department of Anatomy, Albert Einstein School of
Medicine, Bronx, NY 10461, USA

ABSTRACT

Mast cells (MCs) have been identified in rat brain, but their histologic characteristics, anatomical distribution, and relevance to brain histamine (HA) have remained obscure. Brain MCs stained characteristically with toluidine blue (TB) and Astrablau (AB) at low pH, and also fluoresced after exposure to o-phthalaldehyde (OPT), a cytochemical reagent for HA. Selective sequential staining showed that the identical cell population bound OPT, TB, and AB. MC numbers varied greatly between animals, but their localization was almost exclusively thalamic. Within thalamus, the relative anterior-posterior distribution was distinct and reproducible, with maximum MC numbers near the level of the lateral habenular nucleus. Quantitative analysis of this distribution showed that MC numbers from a single coronal section accurately predict the MC numbers in the entire thalamus of that brain, permitting the determination of both MC numbers and HA content from the same brain. Thalamic MC numbers were highly correlated with both the amount (ng) and the concentration (ng/g) of thalamic HA in both sexes. Slopes of these regression lines, indicative of the HA content of thalamic MCs, were 2.5 and 1.3 pg/cell in males and females, respectively. Thalamic HA levels were higher and more variable than previously reported, while nonthalamic HA levels were much less variable and in agreement with previous values. These results indicate that: a) rat brain MCs are almost exclusively thalamic, b) these cells resemble peritoneal MCs histologically, but with much less HA per cell, c) freezing the brain solid before and during dissection (as done presently for histologic purposes) seems necessary to detect biochemically a HA contribution by brain MCs, and d) thalamic MCs can contribute up to 92% of the HA in thalamus, and up to 50% of whole brain HA levels.

KEYWORDS

Mast cells; histamine; brain; histology; thalamus

INTRODUCTION

Mast cells (MCs) are ubiquitous connective tissue (CT) elements containing granules that stain metachromatically under normal conditions (Selye, 1965). They are known stores for large amounts of histamine (HA) which normally turns over only very slowly (Padawer, 1974; Padawer, 1979; Wingren and others, 1983). Traditionally, MCs have been viewed as absent in the central nervous system (CNS), except for perhaps sites such as area postrema, hypophysis, pineal, and dura (Olsson, 1968). It is now clear, however, that there are MCs in other areas of rat brain, but considerable confusion still exists over histologic criteria sufficient to identify them, biochemical indices (if any) to identify them, and the contribution they make to brain HA levels. Also, reliable data on numbers and distribution of CNS MCs are few. This report focuses on the identification of rat brain MCs, their quantitative distribution, and their relationship to HA.

HISTOLOGY OF RAT BRAIN MAST CELLS

MCs generally are identified by their metachromatic staining with certain basic dyes, a change in the color of the stain due to "polymerization" of dye molecules on crowded binding sites. With toluidine blue (TB), MCs take on a red-to-purple hue. Although TB or other stains have been used to identify brain MCs, metachromasia alone does not guarantee a MC (Padawer, 1957); other morphologic and histologic criteria (see below) must be included. Also, the specificity of basic dyes for MCs is greatly enhanced by staining at low pH (Padawer, 1963).

In rat brain, cells with characteristics of CT MCs have been described. Dropp (1972) used cresyl violet or TB, both at unspecified pH, to identify cells containing "intensely staining" granules in brains of kangaroo rats, gerbils, and albino rats (n=3 of each). His illustrations revealed cells whose size, shape, and morphology were similar to CT MCs, but staining of neuronal nuclei demonstrates the relatively high pH of these staining solutions. More than 80% of the MCs were within thalamus, all perivascular. Kruger (1974) identified MCs in rat CNS by staining with TB at pH 3.7 or with Astrablau, another stain specific for MCs at low pH (Bloom and Kelly, 1960). These cells, resembling CT MCs by light microscopy, were perivascular, and commonly seen in thalamus, olfactory lobe, and pia-arachnoid. Persinger (1977, 1980) identified MCs in rat brains as metachromatic cells with typical morphology after staining with unacidified thionine or TB. Again the MCs were perivascular and highly localized to thalamus. Despite unspecific staining procedures, all these studies seem to have correctly identified brain MCs.

Confusion over identification of CNS MCs is nevertheless a problem. For instance, a series of qualitative studies (Ibrahim, 1974) distinguished two types of granular perivascular cells in brain, termed type I and type II MCs. Type I, clearly identical with conventional CT MCs, had characteristic morphology and were concentrated in dorsal thalamus; they were seen in brains of small rodents and cats, but were absent from most other mammalian brains. Type II cells, described as lipid-rich MCs, were found in brains of all species examined. Because the latter are not clearly metachromatic and have granules of diverse size and shape (Ibrahim, 1974; Ibrahim and others, 1979), they are no longer viewed as MCs. They have been renamed "neurolipomastocytoid" cells, (Ibrahim and others, 1979) but may be pericytes (Edvinsson and others, 1977; Ibrahim, 1974; Kiernan, 1976;). Curiously, one laboratory observed MCs in rat brain only rarely (Kiernan, 1976); another (Edvinsson and others, 1977) found MCs in brain of several species, with a concentration in hypothalamus, with no mention of thalamus.

We studied several histologic characteristics of MCs in rat brain (Goldschmidt and others, 1984). These cells stained metachromatically with acidified (pH 2.3) TB. They were round to elongated, 9-15 µm in diameter, and identical in shape and staining to tongue MCs, which were 10-20 µm in diameter. As in earlier studies, these MCs were perivascular and highly concentrated within thalamus; they also stained characteristically with acidified (pH 1) Astrablau. Furthermore, identical distribution patterns of the cells were seen when brain sections were stained with ethanolic TB, photographed, destained, and restained with Astrablau (Goldschmidt and others, 1984). These results indicate that rat brain MCs are histogenous (i.e. CT "serosal") MCs, not mucosal MCs, the latter requiring special fixation and not staining at pH < 3 (Enerback, 1966).

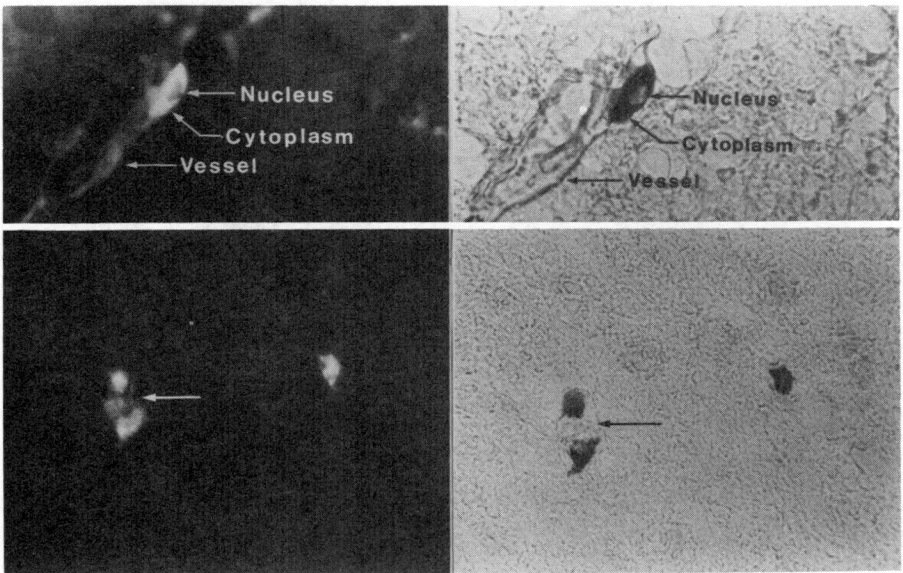

Fig. 1. Rat thalamic MCs. Frozen sections (10 μm) were exposed to OPT vapor, mounted, and photographed with a UV light source (left). The same cells were then simultaneously fixed and stained with ethanolic TB without moving the slide, and rephotographed with normal incandescent light (right). Lower arrows show a fluorescent vessel that did not react to TB. Ocular: 10x; Objective: 40x (above), 25x (below).

Contrary to early studies unable to demomstrate clearly the presence of HA in rat CNS MCs, (Hakanson, 1970; Ibrahim, 1974), we can now assert that HA is present in these cells. Edvinsson and colleagues (1977) reported that brain MCs fluoresced after exposure to o-phthalaldehyde (OPT), a cytochemical method for HA. Photographs of OPT-positive MCs in cerebral meninges were shown. Microspectrofluorimetry yielded identical spectral characteristics for the OPT adducts from brain MCs and for HA standards. We too found that granules from rat thalamic MCs fluoresce after OPT exposure (Goldschmidt and others, 1984 and Fig. 1). By photographing OPT-positive thalamic cells, then simultaneously fixing and staining the same cells with ethanolic TB, we were able to verify the correspondence of OPT-positive with TB-positive cells. Of 81 cells from 4 brains, 80% reacting to either treatment reacted to both. Cells not directly on the surface of the section reacted with TB (in solution), but not with OPT (in the vapor phase), and accounted for another 15% of the MCs. These results show that the same cells visualized by TB are also OPT-positive, and thus contain HA (Fig. 1).

In addition to CNS MCs, we sometimes observed OPT-fluorescence of CNS blood vessels (Fig. 1). If this vascular fluorescence represents HA (which remains uncertain), it could be due to diffusion or release from adjacent MCs, or be a true vascular HA pool (Jarrot and others, 1979; Karnushina and others, 1980; Robinson-White and Beaven, 1982).

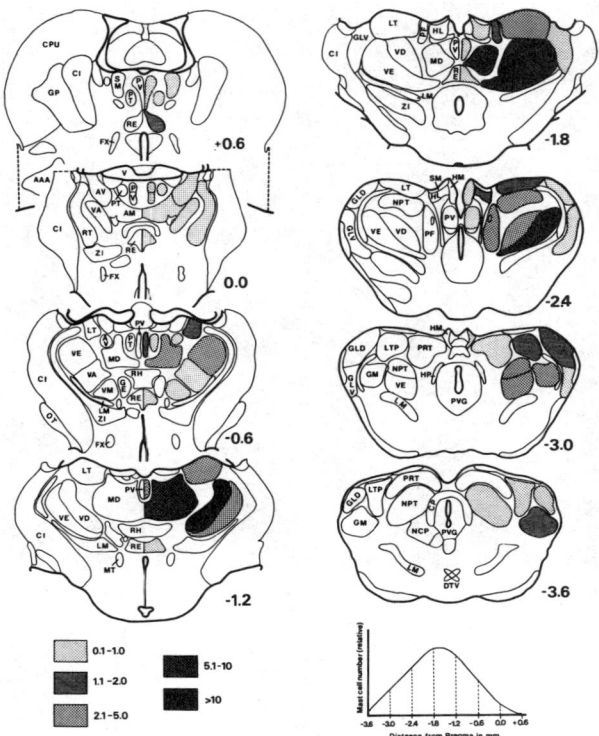

Fig. 2 Distribution of male rat thalamic MCs. The approximate number of MCs is shown for nuclei at the indicated A-P coordinate (mm, Pellegrino and others, 1979). Lower right: relative MC numbers for all thalamic nuclei at each coordinate.

QUANTITATIVE STUDIES OF RAT BRAIN MAST CELLS

We have made detailed studies of the number and anatomic localization of Sprague-Dawley rat brain MCs (Goldschmidt and others, 1984). Exclusive of cerebral meninges, hypophysis, and pineal (removed before sectioning), more than 98% of MCs in whole brains were found within thalamus (+0.8 to -3.6 mm from bregma). The few remaining cells were scattered throughout cortical and other areas, but none were in hypothalamus or basal ganglia. Consistent with other studies, brain MC numbers varied greatly among animals. Whole brain values for males ranged from 1,490 to 19,103 MCs per brain (mean+SEM: 6,966+2,217;n=9); female values ranged from 1,200 to 31,950 (7,854+3,231;n=9). Others found 632-1,205 (Dropp, 1976) or 3,328-10,144 (Persinger, 1977) MCs per brain. Kruger (1974) reported a mean of 1,700 MCs in the diencephalon of 7 rats.

Despite the enormous variation in absolute MC numbers, all brains we examined (Goldschmidt and others, 1984) showed a precise relative distribution within thalamus along the anterior-posterior (A-P) plane. Peak MC numbers occurred near the level of the lateral habenular nucleus (-1.7 mm), and declined to zero at the borders of the thalamus (Fig. 2). Persinger (1977), citing his unpublished work, mentioned a similar distribution. In our studies (Goldschmidt and others, 1984), 6 of 32 thalamic nuclei contained 70-75% of the MCs. They were, in decreasing order of MC numbers, the ventral (VE), medial dorsal (MD), ventral dorsal (VD), lateral (LT), paraventricular (PV), and reuniens (RE) nuclei (see Fig. 2). MC numbers in VE, MD, and VD were significantly greater than in all other nuclei in both sexes. Also, 89-95% of thalamic MCs were confined to 60% of thalamic volume, indicating that MCs are unevenly distributed within the thalamus. Figure 2 summarizes our studies of the nuclear and A-P distribution of brain MCs in adult male rats. The distinct shape of the A-P curve reflects the anatomical boundaries of MD, VE, and VD nuclei. Dropp (1972) reported a similar localization of CNS MCs in control kangaroo and albino rats (3 each).

Our data (Goldschmidt and others, 1984) also revealed that MCs were more numerous in brains of females than of males, and in left than right hemispheres. Cammermeyer (1972) mentioned, but did not quantify, an asymmetry in MC numbers in rodent and monkey area postrema. The sex and side differences in MC numbers, as well as their thalamic localization and great variation in numbers, may be clues to mechanisms underlying the accumulation of MCs in brain, as well as to their functional significance.

BIOCHEMICAL INDICES OF RAT BRAIN MAST CELLS

Studies of HA in brain suggest it is localized both within and outside neurons. As some biochemical characteristics of nonneuronal HA resemble those of MCs, it has been suggested that brain HA is present in both neurons and MCs. This "dual localization" hypothesis (Schwartz, 1975) has support from studies of ontogeny, lesions, subcellular fractionation, lesions, and enzyme inhibition.

Ontogenic studies of brain HA support a dual localization (Martres and others, 1975; Schwartz, 1975). Although most brain transmitters are found in the synaptosomal (P_2B) subcellular fraction, and show a postnatal increase in both transmitter levels and transmitter synthesis enzyme, rat brain HA levels (per gram of tissue) are highest at birth, are found in the nuclear (P_1) fraction, and exhibit a postnatal decline. By contrast, the activity of histidine decarboxylase (HD) is low at birth, and <u>increases</u> postnatally. Because peritoneal MCs contain high HA and low HD levels, this ontogenic pattern led to the suggestion that neonatal rat brain HA is mainly in MCs. Findings in support of this hypothesis are that neonatal rat brain contains more MCs than adult rat brain (Dropp, 1976; Ferrer and others, 1979), HA from peritoneal MCs sediments with the nuclear (P_1) fraction when homogenized with brain (Picatoste and others, 1977), and that P_1 HA levels and rat brain MC numbers show parallel changes during ontogeny (Ferrer and others 1979).

In adult brain, diverse studies indicate that HA exists in more than one compartment, but the evidence that all nonneuronal HA is in MCs is not as compelling. Subcellular fractionation of brain suggests multiple compartmentation of HA. By extrapolation from ontogeny studies, the P_1 fraction of adult animals has been assumed to represent the MC contribution to adult HA levels (Schwartz, 1975). Purified blood vessels from brain (a possible source of P_1 HA in adults) contain HA (Jarrot and others, 1979; Karnushina and others, 1980), but it is uncertain that this HA is in MCs (see Fig. 1 and below). Furthermore, because peritoneal MCs have a high HA/HD ratio, a high ratio in certain brain regions has been taken as evidence for the presence of MCs there in the absence of histological verification (Pollard and others, 1976).

Lesion studies also argue for multiple compartmentation. Medial forebrain bundle lesions that lower forebrain HD have less effect on HA levels, although synaptosomal HA is reduced (Garbarg and others, 1976). Neuronal degeneration could be accompanied by an abnormal influx of MCs. This has been observed after lesions of peripheral nerves (Enerback and others, 1965), as well as in some degenerative CNS lesions (e.g. multiple sclerosis, Olsson, 1974). MC influx could explain the apparent dual localization of HA in regions like cerebral cortex, where the lesion effects were measured, but which normally lacks MCs.

Studies with HD inhibitors also suggest more than one pool of brain HA. Alpha-fluoromethylhistidine (AFMH) irreversibly and totally inactivates brain HD, but only partially reduces HA levels, strong evidence for a portion of brain HA with substantially slower turnover. AFMH almost totally abolishes HA levels in W/W^v (MC-deficient) mice, but only reduces the levels in control animals by about one-half (Maeyama and others, 1983). This argues convincingly that MCs contribute to the stable HA pool. However, the MCs inferred to be present may be from surrounding dura or calvarial periosteum, not the brain itself, for liquid nitrogen was used to kill the animals in that study, a procedure recently shown (Orr, 1984) to degranulate "dural" MCs and increase "brain" HA levels. AFMH-resistant HA may be in brain MCs, but this deserves closer study.

In summary, the parallel between biochemical characteristics of neonatal brain HA and of peritoneal MCs indicates that MCs are a source of brain HA in neonatal rats. In adult rats, it is likely that some brain HA is extraneuronal, but MCs may not be the sole repository of nonneuronal HA. Although they may overlap, nonneuronal HA and MC HA may not be identical.

BIOCHEMICAL VS HISTOLOGIC STUDIES OF BRAIN MAST CELLS

If one postulates that <u>all</u> of the nonneuronal brain HA in adult rats is in MCs (the simplest version of the dual localization hypothesis), many inconsistencies arise. First, as discussed above, the enormous variability observed in brain MC numbers is not reflected in brain HA levels. Second, if brain and peritoneal MCs store equivalent amounts of HA per cell, a mere 200 MCs would suffice to account for all of the thalamic HA (Goldschmidt and others, 1984), a fact at variance with the findings of 600 to 30,000 MCs per brain. Finally, most histological studies of brain MCs found them largely concentrated in thalamus; the existence of brain MCs predicted by biochemical or lesion experiments has never pointed to such regional localization. The implications of these discrepancies are not trivial. For example, they imply that either a) the variation in MC numbers observed is somehow artifactual, b) brain MCs contain very little or no HA, or c) routine measurements of brain HA levels fail to detect the contribution made by MCs. <u>In short, the biochemical indices of MCs have not been reconciled with histological findings</u>.

To approach this problem, we developed a method to determine both the MC number and the HA content of the same rat thalamus. As noted above, although total MC numbers from rat brains vary enormously, their A-P distribution is very precise when expressed as a fraction of each brain's total MC number (Goldschmidt and others 1984; Goldschmidt and others, submitted). This distribution was so reproducible that the MC numbers observed in single coronal sections (from -0.4 to -3.0 mm) were highly predictive of total MC number in the same brain ($r=0.91$ to 0.99; $P<0.005$ to $P<0.0001$) for each sex. Thus, a highly reliable estimate of the total MC number from a thalamus was obtained by counting the MCs from a single section, noting the exact coordinate of that section, and multiplying by the slope of the correlation curve relating MCs per section (for that coordinate) to total MC number, with virtually the entire brain remaining for biochemical assays.

When MC numbers and HA levels were determined by this method, thalamic HA levels ranged from 89-1,138 ng/g in males (mean = 451 ± 60, n = 22) and 60-596 in females (mean = 264 ± 27, n=24), a significant sex difference. Nonthalamic HA (the remainder of the brain) showed no such variation (males: 41 ± 2.1, a range of 26-57; females: 45 ± 2, 28-67 ng/g). Furthermore, thalamic HA content (ng) as

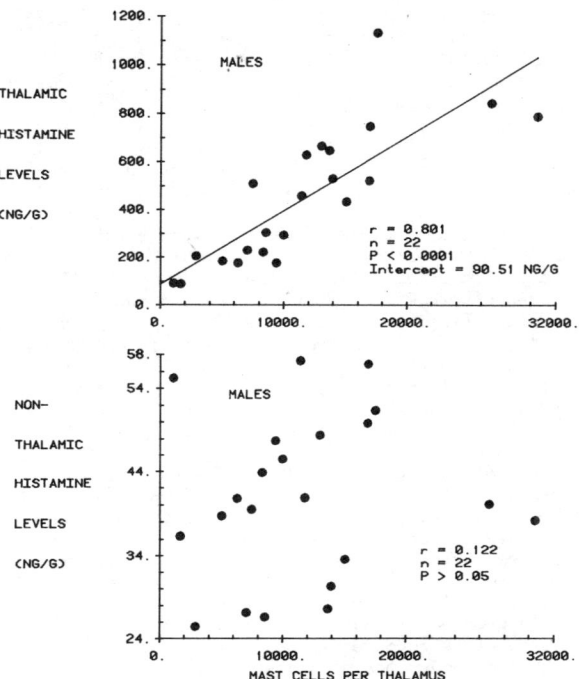

Fig. 3 Correlation of MC numbers and HA content. Total thalamic MC numbers (abscissa) were estimated from a single coronal section as described, and HA levels were determined (ordinate) in the thalamus (above) and remainder of the brain (below).

well as concentration (ng/g) were significantly correlated with estimated thalamic MC numbers in both sexes (ng vs MCs: males: r=0.843, n=22, P<0.0001; females: r=0.678, n=24, P<0.0005, data not shown; ng/g vs MCs for males, see Fig. 3; for females, r=0.654, P<0.0005, data not shown). The slopes of the fitted lines of HA (ng) vs MCs, indicative of the mean HA content per thalamic MC, were 2.52 and 1.27 pg/cell for males and females, respectively. Thalamic or body weights did not correlate with MC numbers, showing that these factors cannot explain the correlations. As expected, nonthalamic HA (ng or ng/g) was independent of thalamic MC number (see Fig. 3 for male ng/g).

These findings are strong evidence that thalamic MCs contain HA, in agreement with the histochemical studies presented above. They also permit estimates of the degree to which MCs can contribute to HA levels of thalamus and of whole brain. This is not feasible for individual animals, because the deviations from the ideal regression lines (top of Fig. 3) can be explained in more than one way. However, population approximations can be made. If nonMC HA is taken as relatively constant, i.e., if rat thalami contain 6-8 ng of nonMC HA (the intercept of the plot of MCs vs thalamic HA ng/g, not shown), then thalamic MCs contribute 81% (0-92%) and 54% (0-82%) of the HA in thalamus for males and females, respectively (Goldschmidt and others, submitted).

In this study, computed whole brain HA concentrations (thalamic + nonthalamic values per brain divided by total weight) were 57.8±3.4 and 53.7±2.7 ng/g for males and females, respectively, in good agreement with literature values (Hough and Green, 1984). Thalamic MC numbers also correlated with both whole brain amounts (ng) and levels (ng/g) of HA (ng vs MCs: males, r=0.694, P<0.002; females, r=0.591, P<0.002; ng/g vs MCs: males, r=0.626, P<0.002; females, r=0.591, P<0.002, data not shown). Similar calculations suggest that thalamic MCs contribute a mean of 20-30% of whole brain HA levels, but with a range of 0-50% for both sexes. In other words, up to one-half of rat whole brain HA levels can be contributed by MCs, depending on the number of MCs in any particular brain.

These data seem to resolve many discrepancies between biochemical and histological studies of rat CNS MCs. Our estimates of rat thalamic HA (the mean for males was 451 ng/g) contrast with previously reported values of 75 (Taylor and Snyder, 1972), 158 (Blanco and others,1973), 80 (Hough and Domino, 1979), and 122 (Oishi and others, 1983) ng/g. Previous studies also did not find such large variations in thalamic HA levels. Our new measurements are likely due to our method of tissue preparation, in which the brain was frozen solid before and during dissection (for histological purposes), whereas in the other studies, it was not. The y-intercept of our plot of thalamic HA (ng/g) vs MC number (90.5 ng/g, top of Fig. 3), predictive of the thalamic non-MC HA level, agrees well with the thalamic levels cited above. This suggests that brain must be kept completely frozen to detect any contribution by MCs to HA levels. Consistent with this, HA levels from the remainder of the brain (which contains very few MCs, but was subjected to the same freezing procedure) are in excellent agreement with previous data. Furthermore, swiss mouse brain HA levels were elevated by freezing the heads in liquid nitrogen before thawing for dissection, but no such increase was found in W/W^v mutants (Orr, 1984). The increased HA was suggested to be from CT surrounding the brain. Orr's finding (1984) also probably resolves a previous discrepancy: no difference was found between brain HA levels of normal littermate controls and W/W^v mice after room temperature decapitation (Orr & Pace, 1984; Hough and others) whereas mouse brain HA levels from controls (having MCs) were higher when the heads were first frozen then thawed. (Yamatodani and others, 1982). Thus, the reason why HA levels do not normally vary as much as brain MC numbers do is probably that brain MC HA is somehow rapidly metabolized or bound in a way no longer detectable by analytical procedures after room temperature decapitation.

The paradox that only about 200 MCs would account for all of thalamic HA also seems resolved: thalamic HA levels were previously assumed to be about 80 ng/g, when in fact they are over 400 ng/g (in males). It was also assumed that brain MCs contained 12-20 pg/cell as do peritoneal MCs when, in fact, our present data show brain MCs to contain only 1-3 pg/cell. This may also explain previous failures to identify HA in these cells histochemically. It must be recognized that our freezing procedure, which serendipitously revealed the MC HA component, may only yield part of the MC HA, so that we may be underestimating the HA content of thalamic MCs.

If rat CNS MCs contribute HA only to thalamus, then much work remains to understand the nature of the nonneuronal HA that may exist in other regions of rat brain. Vascular endothelium, perictyes, or perhaps as yet unsuspected cells could be storage sites for this HA.

Clearly, we do not yet fully understand the properties and functions of brain MCs. Their perivascular localization, enormous variation in number, and elusive HA content all seem clues to a fascinating, if unsolved, mystery.

ACKNOWLEDGEMENTS

Statistical analyses and graphics were performed on the PROPHET computer system, a national resource supported by the Division of Research Resources, NIH. This work was supported by NIDA grant DA-03816 (formerly DA-02923), U.S. P.H.S. Institutional NRSA GM-07163, and by the Norinsberg Foundation. We thank Dr. George Prell for helpful comments about the manuscript, and Mrs. Deborah Hackley for secretarial assistance.

REFERENCES

Bloom, J., and J.W. Kelly (1960). The copper phthalocyanin dye "Astrablau" and its staining properties, especially the staining of mast cells. Histochemie, 2, 48-57.
Cammermeyer, J. (1972). Mast cells in mammalian area postrema. Z. Anat. Entwick., 139, 71-92.
Dropp, J.J. (1972). Mast cells in the central nervous system of several rodents. Anat. Rec., 174, 227-238.
Dropp, J.J. (1976). Mast cells in mammalian brain. Acta Anat., 94, 1-21.
Edvinsson, L., J. Cervos-Navarro, L.I. Larsson, CH. Owman, and A.L. Ronnberg (1977). Regional distribution of mast cells containing histamine, dopamine, or 5-hydroxytryptamine in the mammalian brain. Neurology, 27, 878-883.
Enerback, L. (1966). Mast cells in rat gastrointestinal mucosa. Acta. path. microbiol. scandinav., 66, 289-302.
Enerback, L., Y. Olsson, and P. Sourander (1965). Mast cells in normal and sectioned peripheral nerve. Zeitschr. Zellforsch, 608, 596-608.
Ferrer, O., F. Picastoste, A. Garcia, J. Sabria, and I. Blanco (1979). Histamine and mast cells in developing rat brain. J. Neurochem, 32, 587-592.
Garbarg, M., G. Barbin, S., Bischoff, H. Pollard, and J.C. Schwartz (1976). Dual localization of histamine in an ascending neuronal pathway and in non-neuronal cells evidenced by lesions in the lateral hypothalamic area. Brain Res., 106, 333-348.
Garbarg, M., G. Barbin, E. Rodergras, and J.C. Schwartz (1980). Inhibition of histamine synthesis in brain by α-fluoromethyhistidine, a new irreversible inhibitor: in vitro and in vivo studies. J. Neurochem., 35, 1045-1052.
Goldschmidt, R.C., L.B. Hough, S.D. Glick, and J. Padawer (1984). Mast cells in rat thalamus: nuclear localization, sex difference, and left-right asymmetry. Brain Res., in press.
Hakanson, R. (1970). New aspects of the formation and function of histamine, 5-hydroxytryptamine, and dopamine in the gastric mucosa. Acta Physiol. Scand., Supp. 340, 1-31.
Hough, L.B., and J.P. Green (1984). Histamine and its receptors in the nervous system. In A. Lajtha (Ed.), Handbook of Neurochemistry, Vol. 6, Plenum Press, New York. pp.145-211.
Hough, L.B., J.K. Khandelwal, R.C. Goldschmidt, M. Diomande, and S.D. Glick (1984). Normal levels of histamine and tele-methylhistamine in mast cell-deficient mouse brain. Brain Res., 292, 133-138.
Ibrahim, M.Z.M. (1974). The mast cells of the mammalian central nervous system. J. Neurol. Sci., 21, 431-478.
Ibrahim, M.Z.M., E.A. Munib, and N. Bahuth (1979). The mast cells of the mammalian central nervous system. III. Ultrastructural characteristics in the adult rat brain. Acta Anat., 104, 134-154.
Jarrot, B., J.T. Hjelle, and S. Spector (1979). Association of histamine with cerebral microvessels in regions of bovine brain. Brain Res., 168, 323-330.
Karnushina, I.L., J.M. Palacios, G.Barbin, E. Dux, F. Joo, and J.C. Schwartz (1980). Studies on a capillary rich fraction isolated from brain: histaminic components and characterization of the histamine receptors linked to adenylate cyclase. J. Neurochem., 34, 1201-1208.
Kierman, J.A. (1976). A comparative survery of the mast cells of the mammalian brain. J. Anat., 121, 303-311.
Kruger, P.G. (1974). Demonstration of mast cells in the albino rat brain. Experientia, 30, 810-811.
Maeyama, K., T. Watanabe, A. Yamatodani, Y. Taguchi, H. Kambe, and H. Wada (1983). Effect of α-fluoromethylhistidine on the histamine content of the brain of

W/W^v mice devoid of mast cells: Turnover of brain histamine. J. Neurochem., 41, 128-134.

Martes, M.P., M. Baudry, and J.C. Schwartz (1975). Histamine synthesis in the developing rat brain: Evidence for a multiple compartmentation. Brain Res., 83, 265-275.

Olsson, Y. (1968). Mast cells in the nervous system. Int. Rev. Cytol., 24, 27-70.

Olsson, Y. (1974). Mast cells in placques of multiple sclerosis. Acta. Neurol. Scand., 50, 611-618.

Orr, E.L. (1984). Rat dural mast cells as a source of brain histamine. J. Neurochem., in press.

Orr, E.L., and K.R. Pace (1984). The significance of mast cells as a source of histamine in mouse brain. J. Neurochem., 42, 727-732.

Padawer, J. (1957). Studies on mammalian mast cells. Trans. N.Y. Acad. Sci., 19, 690-713.

Padawer, J. (1963). Quantitative studies with mast cells. Ann. New York Acad. Sci. - Mast Cells and Basophils, 103, 87-138.

Padawer, J. (1974). Mast cells: extended lifespan and lack of granule turnover under normal in-vivo conditions. Exp. Molec. Pathol., 20, 269-280.

Padawer, J. (1979). Mast cell structure: implications for normal physiology and degranulation. In J. Pepys and A.M. Edwards (Eds.), The Mast Cell - Its Role in Health and Disease, Pitman Medical, Turnbridge Wells. pp. 1-8.

Pellegrino, L.J., A.S. Pellegrino, and A.J. Cushman (1979). A Stereotaxic Atlas of the Rat Brain. Plenum Press, New York.

Persinger, M.A. (1977). Mast cells in the brain: Possibilities for physiological psychology. Physiol. Psychol., 5, 166-176.

Persinger, M.A. (1980). Handling factors not body marking influence thalamic mast cell numbers in preweaned albino rat. Behav. Neurol Biol., 30, 448-459.

Picastoste, F., I. Blanco, and J.M. Palacios (1977). The presence of two cellular pools of rat brain histamine. J. Neurochem., 29, 735-737.

Pollard, H., S. Bischoff, C. Llorens-Cortes, and J.C. Schwartz (1976). Histidine decarboxylase and histamine in discrete nuclei of rat hypothalamus and the evidence for mast cells in the median eminence. Brain Res., 118, 509-513.

Robinson-White, A., and M.A. Beaven (1982). Presence of histamine and histamine metabolizing enzymes in rat and guinea pig microvascular endothelial cells. J. Pharmacol. Exp. Ther., 223, 440-445.

Schwartz, J.C. (1975). Histamine as a transmitter in brain. Life Sci., 17, 503-518.

Selye, H. (1965). The Mast Cells. Butterworths, London.

Taylor, K.M., and S.H. Snyder (1972). Histamine in rat brain: Sensitive assay of endogenous levels, formation in vivo, and lowering by inhibitors of histidine decarboxylase. J. Pharmacol. Exp. Ther., 179, 619-633.

Wingren, U., A. Wasteson, and L. Enerback (1983). Storage and turnover of histamine, 5-hydroxytryptamine, and heparin in rat peritoneal mast cells in vivo. Int. Archs. Allergy Appl. Immun., 70, 193-199.

Yamatodani, A., K. Maeyama, T. Watanabe, H. Wada, and Y. Kitamura (1982). Tissue distribution of histamine in a mutant mouse deficient in mast cells: Clear evidence for the presence of non-mast cell histamine. Biochem. Pharmacol., 31, 305-308.

Histamine in the Brain: Release and Metabolism

HISTAMINE SYNTHESIS AND RELEASE IN CNS: CONTROL BY AUTORECEPTORS (H_3)

J-M. Arrang, M. Garbarg and J-C. Schwartz

Unité 109 de Neurobiologie, Centre Paul Broca de l'INSERM,
2ter rue d'Alésia, 75014 Paris, France

ABSTRACT

Regulation of histamine (HA) release was studied on brain slices prelabeled with ^{3}H-L-histidine and depolarised in a non-superfused system. Exogenous HA reduced the release of endogenously synthesised ^{3}H-HA via stimulation of a new class of receptors (H_3) pharmacologically distinct from the two classes previously characterised, the H_1-and H_2-receptors. The persistence of the inhibitory effect of exogenous HA after destruction of neuronal cell-bodies by kainate and on synaptosomal preparations left little doubt that H_3 receptors were directly located on HA-synthesising terminals. The maximal inhibitory effect of exogenous HA progressively diminished as the strength of the depolarising stimulus or the external Ca^{++} concentration were elevated. These results suggest that the inhibition of ^{3}H-HA release by H_3 autoreceptors is mediated by a restricted access of Ca^{++} and that its extent is influenced by the degree of autostimulation by endogenous HA as well as, possibly, by actual internal Ca^{++} concentration. Exogenous HA also reduced the stimulation of ^{3}H-HA synthesis from ^{3}H-L-histidine in depolarised brain slices. This effect was antagonised by impromidine and burimamide with potencies very similar to those found at H_3 receptors modulating HA release and was also observed in cortical synaptosomes. It is concluded that HA modulates its own release and its own synthesis in the brain by interacting with H_3-presynaptic autoreceptors whose pharmacology clearly differs from that of H_1- and H_2-receptors.

KEYWORDS

Brain slices ; Brain synaptosomes ; Synthesised ^{3}H-histamine ; Release regulation ; biosynthesis regulation ; H_3-presynaptic autoreceptors.

INTRODUCTION

A combination of biochemical, electrophysiological and lesion studies in rat brain have shown that histamine (HA) is synthesised in endings of neurones ascending through the lateral hypothalamic area and widely projecting in the telencephalon (reviewed by Schwartz and co-workers, 1980,1984). The various actions of HA on target-cells seem to be mediated in mammalian brain by the two classes of receptors (H_1 and H_2) previously characterised in peripheral organs (reviewed by Schwartz, 1979 ; Green, 1983 ; Hough and Green, 1984). Electrophysiological studies (Haas and Wolf, 1976,1977) and biochemical studies in le-

sioned animals (Garbarg and co-workers, 1978 ; Palacios, Wamsley and Kuhar, 1981) suggest that both H_1 and H_2-receptors are postsynaptically located, relatively to HA axon terminals.
Elevated extracellular K^+ concentration was largely used as a depolarising stimulus for release of various neurotransmitters and, in the case of either endogenous HA (Taylor and Snyder, 1973) or endogenously synthesised ^{3}H-HA (Verdière, Rose and Schwartz, 1975), results in a Ca^{++}-dependent HA release. It is well established that several neurotransmitters may control their own release from cerebral neurones by interacting with presynaptic autoreceptors (Langer, 1977 ; Starke, 1981). In order to assess the existence of such a self regulation process of HA release in brain, we developped a model in which slices of rat cerebral cortex were labeled by preincubation with ^{3}H-L-histidine (^{3}H-L-His) to allow for ^{3}H-HA synthesis and subsequently depolarised in a non-superfused system. The cerebral cortex was selected for this study as various approaches have shown that HA synthesis in this region occurs in terminals of histaminergic extrinsic neurons (Baudry, Martres and Schwartz, 1973 ; Garbarg and co-workers, 1974 ; Barbin and co-workers, 1975).

AUTOINHIBITION OF BRAIN HISTAMINE RELEASE : PHARMACOLOGICAL DEFINITION OF H_3-RECEPTORS

Depolarisation by 30 mM K^+ of cortical slices in the absence of any exogenous HA added resulted in the release of about 15 % of tissue ^{3}H-HA. However when nonradioactive exogenous HA was present in the medium, an inhibition of the K^+-induced ^{3}H-HA release was observed (Arrang, Garbarg and Schwartz, 1983). The inhibitory action of HA was concentration-dependent and saturable with a maximal inhibition of 60 % (Fig. 1).

TABLE 1 Comparison of potencies of chiral histamine derivatives on the inhibition of cortical ^{3}H-histamine release , the guinea pig ileum contraction (H_1-receptors) and atrial rate (H_2-receptors)

	S(-)	R(+)	R(-)	S(+)
G.P. Ileum (H_1)	0.7	0.7	0.3	0.3
G.P. Atrium (H_2)	1	0.4	51	7
Inhibition of ^{3}H-HA release	0.09	2.9	0.001	2.4

Results are expressed as relative potencies to HA, calculated as the ratio EC_{50} of HA/EC_{50} of agonist x 100. The EC_{50} value of HA was of 0.04 ± 0.01 µM. Relative potencies at H_1 and H_2 receptors are from Schunack and Gerhard (1982).

The inhibition of release was reversible since it was no longer observed when slices were rapidly washed after exposure to the amine and before depolarisation. The characters of saturability and reversibility of the inhibitory effect of HA suggest that it is a receptor mediated process. The EC_{50} value of HA was of 0.04 ± 0.01 µM when it was added 5 min before the K^+-stimulus, and it was only three-fold increased (0.13 ± 0.02 µM) when HA was added together with K^+. This indicates that HA in this response is about 100 times more potent than in the H_1 and H_2-receptor-mediated responses previously described in the brain. The inhibitory action of HA was only mimicked by its two Nα and Nα,Nα -methyl derivatives (Fig. 1), two agonists both at H_1 and H_2-receptors.

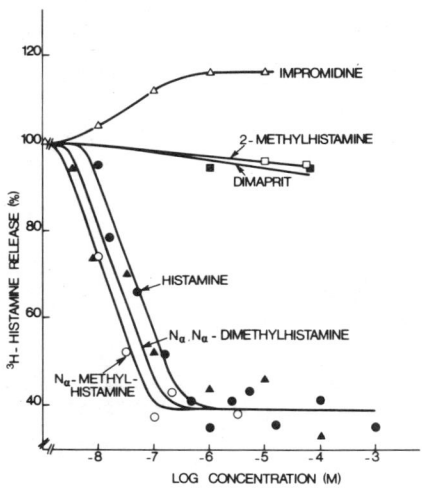

Fig. 1 Effect of exogenous histamine and various agonists on the K^+-evoked release of endogenously synthetised ^{3}H-histamine from slices of rat cerebral cortex.
Slices resuspended in modified Krebs-Ringer's bicarbonate medium, gassed with O_2/CO_2 (95:5) were preincubated with ^{3}H-L-His (0.3 µM) for 30 min and thereafter extensively washed. Aliquots of the slice suspension were then distributed in microtubes containing the solutions of HA or agonists. Five minutes later, the final concentration of K^+ was eventually raised to 30 mM K^+ and after 2 min, the incubations were stopped by rapid centrifugation. ^{3}H-HA present in tissue and medium was isolated by ion-exchange chromatography (Schwartz and co-workers, 1971). The spontaneous efflux of ^{3}H-HA (2 mM K^+) represented 3.0 ± 0.2 % of total ^{3}H-HA. In the absence of added agents, ^{3}H-HA release induced by 30 mM K^+ (expressed in percent of total ^{3}H-HA released over spontaneous efflux) represented 9.9 ± 0.8 %. Each point represents the results from 1-10 separate experiments with at least triplicate determinations. From Arrang, Garbarg and Schwartz, 1983.

In contrast, neither specific H_1 agonists such as 2-methyl-HA nor specific H_2 agonists such as dimaprit had any inhibitory effect. Autoinhibitory receptors show a strong stereoselectivity as shown with two HA derivatives including a chiral centre : α,Nα-dimethyl HA and Nα methyl-αchloromethyl HA (Schunack and Gerhard, 1982). Both compounds acted as weak agonists and the activity ratio of their respective enantiomers was higher than at H_1 and H_2 receptors. Moreover, at autoinhibitory receptors (+)-isomers of both structures (absolute configuration corresponding to S-configurated D-histidine) possessed greater activity, whereas at H_2-receptors (-)-isomers were more active (Table 1).

Impromidine, a selective and potent H_2 agonist, not only failed to mimick the inhibitory action of HA, but increased the K^+-evoked release of ^{3}H-HA (Fig. 1). This facilitatory action of impromidine suggested that it might have been acting as an antagonist at autoinhibitory receptors towards endogenous HA released together with ^{3}H-HA by the K^+ stimulus. Indeed, the inhibitory action of exogenous HA on release was antagonised in a competitive manner by impromidine (Arrang, Garbarg and Schwartz, 1983).

Burimamide also antagonised in a concentration-dependent manner the inhibition of release elicited by HA (Fig. 2).

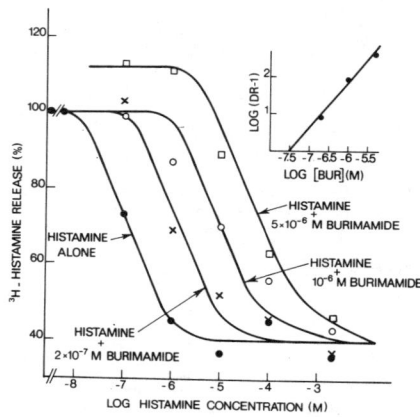

Fig. 2. Reversal by burimamide of the exogenous histamine-induced inhibition of K^+-evoked ^{3}H-histamine release.
Exogenous HA (in increasing concentrations) was added together with the depolarising solution i.e. after a 5 min preincubation with burimamide (in fixed concentration).
Inset : Schild plot of the data, dose ratios (DR) being determined from the EC_{50} values of HA. The slope and 95 % confidence limits for the regression of log (DR-1) on log [Bur] was 1.19 (0.47-1.92) and the correlation coefficient 0.990. The pA_2 value for burimamide was 7.5. From Arrang, Garbarg and Schwartz, 1983. Fig. 1 and 2 reprinted by permission from Nature, vol. 302, N° 5911, pp 832-837. Copyright (c) 1983 Macmillan Journals Limited.

The antagonism was always surmountable by increasing the HA concentration and the Schild plot analysis of the data was compatible with its competitive nature (inset of Fig. 2). Again, a facilitation of ^{3}H-HA release similar to that elicited by impromidine was observed in the presence of burimamide in high concentrations (Fig. 2). In contrast various H_1-antihistamines like mepyramine or chlorpheniramine were uneffective in concentrations at which they block H_1-receptors (Table 2).

TABLE 2 Comparison of potencies of histaminergic agents on the inhibition of cortical ^{3}H-histamine release, the guinea-pig ileum contraction (H_1-receptors) and atrial rate (H_2-receptors).

	INHIBITION OF ^{3}H-HA RELEASE	G.P. ILEUM (H_1)	G.P. ATRIUM (H_2)	
	ANTAGONIST ACTIVITY (Ki, μM)	ANTAGONIST ACTIVITY (Ki, μM)	ANTAGONIST ACTIVITY (Ki, μM)	AGONIST ACTIVITY (HA=100)
Mepyramine	> 3	0.0005		
D-Chlorpheniramine	> 0.06	0.0005		
Cimetidine	33		0.8	
Burimamide	0.07		8	
Norburimamide	0.8		115	
Ranitidine	> 1		0.06	
Tiotidine	> 12		0.02	
Impromidine	0.06		0.6*	4,810
R(-)sopromidine	0.06			740
S(+)sopromidine	0.04		2.3	
SKF 91486	0.09		22	

* When tested as HA antagonist on the cyclic AMP response of G.P. hippocampal slices.
Potential antagonists were added in at least four different concentrations 5 min before 1 μM HA and 30 mM K^+ and their IC_{50} value (concentration for which the inhibitory effect of exogenous HA was reduced by 50 %) determined using an iterative computer method. Apparent dissociation constants (Ki values) were calculated assuming a competitive antagonism according to the equation : Ki = $IC_{50}/(1 + S/EC_{50})$, S representing the concentration of exogenous HA (1 μM), the EC_{50} value of the amine being 0.13 ± 0.02 μM. The values defining the activity of compounds on the guinea-pig ileum and atrium are taken from the review of Ganellin (1982), except for sopromidine enantiomers (Schunack and Gerhard, 1982).

Also the two potent H_2-antihistamines, tiotidine and ranitidine were almost uneffective at autoinhibitory receptors, whereas burimamide and its lower homologue, norburimamide were about 100 times more potent than at H_2 receptors.
Impromidine acted as a potent antagonist at autoinhibitory receptors (Ki value = 0.06 ± 0.01 μM). A very similar potency as antagonist was found for both enantiomers of its chiral derivative, sopromidine , whose R isomer is a potent and selective H_2 agonist whereas S isomer is an H_2 antihistamine (Schunack and Gerhard, 1982). Another guanidine derivative, SKF 91486, a partial structure of impromidine, was 200 times more potent at autoinhibitory receptors than at H_2-receptors (Table 2).
Thus, from the potencies of agonists and the apparent dissociation constants of antagonists, as well as from the lack of effect of antagonists of other neurotransmitters, it can be concluded that the autoinhibition of HA release in brain

is mediated by a novel class of HA receptor that we recently proposed to term H_3 (Arrang, Garbarg and Schwartz, 1983).

LOCATION OF H_3 AUTOINHIBITORY RECEPTORS

The extent to which slices from various rat brain regions were labeled after preincubation in the presence of ^{3}H-L-His was in good agreement with the regional distribution of histaminergic neurone markers like endogenous HA content or L-histidine decarboxylase activity. The degree of K^+-evoked ^{3}H-HA release and of its inhibition by exogenous HA were of similar magnitude in cerebral cortex, striatum, hippocampus and hypothalamus in which both lesion and electrophysiological studies suggest that terminals of extrinsic histaminergic neurons are present.

More direct evidence for H_3-receptors being directly located on HA-synthesising axon-terminals and not on interneurones or nearby axon terminals impinging on the formers was provided by a series of additional experiments.

Hence the unchanged inhibitory effect of exogenous HA in brain slices in which the traffic of action potentials was blocked by tetrodotoxin tends to exclude the participation of interneurones. This is confirmed by the persistence of H_3-receptor mediated effect in striatal slices after a kainate treatment (Table 3) while this treatment abolishes the HA-induced cyclic AMP response mediated by H_1 and H_2 receptors but does not modify the L-Histidine decarboxylase activity, a presynaptic marker (Garbarg and co-workers, 1978).

TABLE 3   Auto-inhibition of ^{3}H-histamine release in rat striatum after unilateral injection of kainic acid

	CONTROL SIDE	LESION SIDE
GAD activity (pmole/µg protein/h)	169 ± 9	88 ± 2 [a]
Total ^{3}H-HA (dpm/µg protein)	6.3 ± 0.3	7.1 ± 0.5
^{3}H-HA release (% of total)		
30 mM K^+ [HA] = 0	10.5 ± 1.4	8.7 ± 1.2
30 mM K^+ [HA] = 1 µM	6.4 ± 1.1* (- 39 %)	4.7 ± 1.2* (- 46 %)

[a] $P < 0.001$ as compared with control side (48 % decrease)
* $P < 0.05$ as compared with 30 mM K^+ alone.

7-9 animals were sacrificed 9 days after infusion of 2.5 µg kainic acid in the left striatum. ^{3}H-HA release induced by 30 mM K^+ is expressed over the mean spontaneous efflux (2 mM K^+) i.e. 4.6 ± 0.7 % and 3.3 ± 0.6 % of total ^{3}H-HA for control and lesion side, respectively. Values between brackets indicate the change as compared with 30 mM K^+ alone. Means ± S.E.M. of at least 6 determinations from two separate experiments.

Moreover, experiments with rat brain cortex synaptosomes left little doubt that pharmacologically-identified H_3 receptors were directly located on HA-synthesising terminals. Thus, exogenous HA inhibited ^{3}H-HA release from depolarised synaptosomes, with an EC_{50} value (0.20 ± 0.05 μM) similar to that found with slices (Fig. 3a) and, on the two preparations, the effect was inhibited by impromidine, a competitive H_3-receptor antagonist with similar apparent Ki values e.g. 0.11 ± 0.03 μM and 0.06 ± 0.01 μM, respectively (Fig. 3b). In conclusion all these data support the hypothesis that HA modulates its own release from cerebral neurones by interacting with H_3 presynaptic autoreceptors.

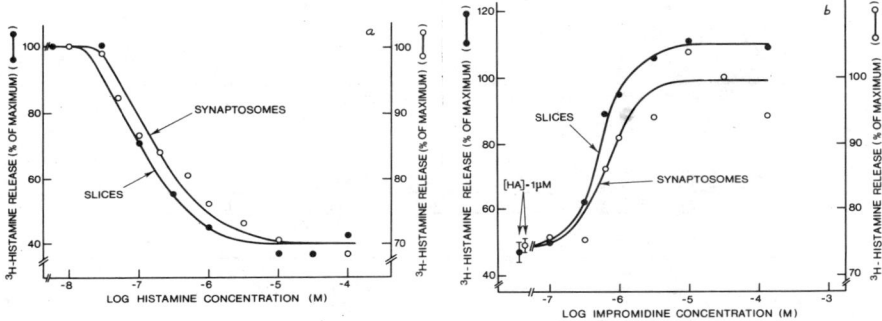

Fig. 3. Inhibition by exogenous histamine of ^{3}H-histamine release from slices and synaptosomes of rat cerebral cortex and its reversal by impromidine. Preincubations were performed in the presence of 0.3 μM ^{3}H-L-His. In the absence of added agents, ^{3}H-HA release induced by 30 mM K^+ represented 12.3 ± 1.6% for slices and 23.2 ± 1.7 % for synaptosomes. When required, exogenous HA (a) was added together with 30 mM K^+ and impromidine (b) 5 min before the simultaneous addition of HA and K^+. IC_{50} values of impromidine (b) were of 0.68 ± 0.16 μM and 0.57 ± 0.11 μM for synaptosomes and slices respectively. Each point represents the results from 1-14 separate experiments with at least triplicate determinations.

PUTATIVE MECHANISMS FOR THE PRESYNAPTIC MODULATION OF HA RELEASE

The maximal inhibitory effect of exogenous HA (100 μM) on ^{3}H-HA release strikingly varied with the conditions under which release was elicited : it progressively diminished as the strength of the depolarising stimulus was increased (Table 4) or as the external Ca^{++} concentration was elevated (Table 5).
Similar inverse relationships between the potency of presynaptic modulators and external Ca^{++} concentration, frequency of electrical stimulation or external K^+ concentration appear to exist for a variety of neurotransmitters. These effects were generally interpreted as reflecting a modulation of Ca^{++} influx by presynaptic receptors together with a saturation kinetic of the effect of intraneuronal Ca^{++} on stimulus-release coupling (Starke, 1977). Another contributing factor might be that with stronger depolarising stimuli or higher Ca^{++} concentrations a larger amount of HA is released leading to a higher degree of occupation of H_3 auto-receptors which therefore become less available to stimulation by exogenous HA.

TABLE 4 Autoinhibition of ^{3}H-histamine release from slices of rat cerebral cortex induced by potassium in increasing concentrations

CONDITIONS	PERCENT ^{3}H-HA RELEASE		DIFFERENCE
	[HA] = 0	[HA] = 100 μM	
20 mM K$^+$	2.3 ± 0.5	0.7 ± 0.2*	− 70 %
30 mM K$^+$	9.5 ± 1.9	5.5 ± 0.5*	− 42 %
55 mM K$^+$	36.3 ± 1.2	33.8 ± 1.4	− 7 %

* P < 0.05 as compared with the corresponding controls ([HA] = 0).

TABLE 5 Influence of calcium concentration on auto-inhibition of ^{3}H-histamine release from slices of rat cerebral cortex

CONDITIONS	PERCENT OF ^{3}H-HA RELEASE EVOKED BY			
	30 mM K$^+$		55 mM K$^+$	
	[HA] = 0	[HA] = 100 μM	[HA] = 0	[HA] = 100 μM
0.06 mM Ca^{++}	< 1.0		11.7 ± 0.5	6.5 ± 0.7** (− 45 %)
0.26 mM Ca^{++}	4.2 ± 0.5	2.2 ± 0.4** (− 48 %)	20.7 ± 1.3	15.2 ± 1.2** (− 27 %)
0.65 mM Ca^{++}	7.0 ± 0.3	3.2 ± 0.5** (− 55 %)	32.6 ± 0.3	25.0 ± 0.4** (− 23 %)
2.60 mM Ca^{++}	12.1 ± 1.1	6.9 ± 1.1** (− 43 %)	39.0 ± 0.7	34.7 ± 1.0* (− 11 %)
5.20 mM Ca^{++}	7.9 ± 0.3	6.1 ± 0.3** (− 22 %)	38.3 ± 0.7	34.1 ± 2.2 (− 11 %)

* P < 0.05 ; ** P < 0.01 as compared with K$^+$ alone.

Slices were allowed to synthesise ^{3}H-HA in a medium with 2.6 mM Ca^{++}. After 30 min incubation, the slices were extensively washed by successive transfer to medium with either 2.6 mM Ca^{++} (first five washings) or the final Ca^{++} concentration tested (last three washings), before application of depolarising stimuli (30 or 55 mM K$^+$), except before depolarisation with 30 mM K$^+$ in the presence of 0.26 mM Ca^{++} (every washing medium with 0.26 mM Ca^{++}).
Values for ^{3}H-HA release are given as percent of total over mean spontaneous efflux (2 mM K$^+$) which represented 3.8 ± 0.4 % at any calcium concentration.
Means ± S.E.M. of 3-14 determinations from 1-3 experiments.

The participation of the endogenous amine in the control of ^{3}H-HA release is clearly shown by the facilitatory effect of H_3-receptor antagonists like impromidine or burimamide (Fig. 1 and 2). The latter was not observed with synaptosomes from which the diffusion of the endogenous HA is likely to be easier, (Fig. 3b) but became particularly clear when the slices were loaded by preincubation with L-His in a concentration selected to allow a higher rate of HA synthesis by the non saturated enzyme L-histidine decarboxylase (Schwartz, Lampart and Rose, 1970 ; Verdière, Rose and Schwartz, 1974) whereas, conversely, the inhibitory action of exogenous HA became less apparent (Arrang, Garbarg and Schwartz, submitted).

However it is clear that there was not always a strict relationship between the amount of ^{3}H-HA released and the intensity of the braking effect since the HA-induced inhibition of release (elicited by 30 mM K$^+$) was less marked at 5.2 mM Ca^{++} (- 22 %) than at 2.6 mM Ca^{++} (- 43 %) in spite of a reduced non-inhibited ^{3}H-HA release (Table 5).

Hence it is more likely that, as assumed in the case of presynaptic receptors on other neuronal systems, the inhibition mediated by H_3-receptors results from a restricted access of Ca^{++} into depolarised histaminergic nerve-terminals and that its extent finally results from the interplay of various processes e.g. mainly actual internal Ca^{++} concentration and degree of auto-stimulation by endogenous HA.

AUTOINHIBITION OF BRAIN HISTAMINE SYNTHESIS MEDIATED BY H_3 AUTORECEPTORS

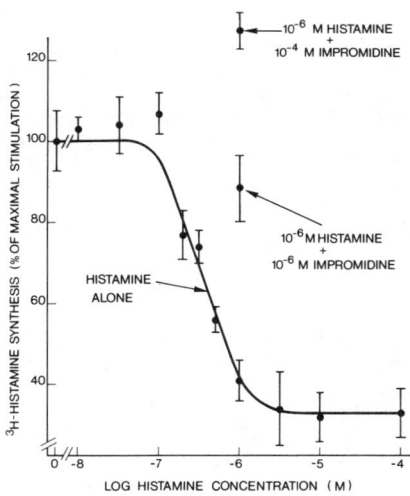

Fig. 4. Effect of histamine on the K$^+$-evoked stimulation of ^{3}H-histamine synthesis in slices of rat cerebral cortex and its reversal by impromidine.
The K$^+$-evoked stimulation of ^{3}H-HA synthesis (30 min incubation with 0.5 μM ^{3}H-L-His) was calculated as the difference between ^{3}H-HA synthesis in 30 mM K$^+$ (4.137 ± 291 dpm/mg protein) and 2 mM K$^+$ (2.079 ± 143 dpm/mg protein), respectively. The maximal inhibition by exogenous HA of 30 mM K$^+$-evoked stimulation was 68 ± 4 %.

As previously shown by Verdière, Rose and Schwartz (1975) with hypothalamic slices, depolarisation of slices from cerebral cortex in the presence of 30 mM K^+ for 30 min elicited a 100 % increase in synthesis of ^3H-HA from ^3H-L-His. However when nonradioactive exogenous HA was present in the medium, an inhibition of this K^+-induced response was observed. The inhibitory effect of HA was concentration-dependent and saturable (Fig. 4). As in the modulation of its release, HA in this response was about 100 times more potent than in H_1 or H_2 receptor-mediated responses in the brain (EC_{50} value = 0.38 ± 0.10 µM obtained by fitting the curve shown in Fig. 4 with an iterative computer least-squares method). A similar inhibition of synthesis was observed in cortical synaptosomes, indicating that it occurs at histaminergic nerve terminals.
Impromidine (Fig. 4) and burimamide acted as antagonists of HA with apparent dissociation constants very similar to that found at H_3 autoreceptors modulating HA release, whereas mepyramine and tiotidine were again uneffective.
These data strongly suggest that H_3 autoreceptors also modulate HA synthesis in brain. The control of amine synthesis via presynaptic autoreceptors is already documented for other cerebral neurotransmitters such as dopamine (Westfall and co-workers, 1976 ; Roth, 1979).
In the case of HA it is not clear at which biochemical level this control occurs. A direct retro-inhibition of the enzyme L-histidine decarboxylase by its product, HA was previously excluded whereas it was suggested that control of HA synthesis might occur at the step of L-his uptake into HA-synthesising cells (Verdière, Rose and Schwartz, 1975). However the latter uptake process cannot be easily studied because of the presumably small number of HA neurones in brain as compared with other cells in which active uptake of L-his occurs.

CONCLUSION

All the data support the hypothesis that HA modulates its own release from cerebral neurones by interacting with H_3 presynaptic autoreceptors, displaying a highly specific pharmacology and stereoselectivity. The activation of these autoreceptors seems to involve mechanisms bearing many similarities with those by which other neurotransmitters self-regulate their release. H_3 autoreceptors also mediate the modulation of HA biosynthesis in cerebral neurones. The development of compounds able to stimulate or to block these autoreceptors selectively might provide useful tools for elucidating the precise functions of histaminergic neurones in the brain.

REFERENCES

Arrang, J.M., Garbarg, M., and Schwartz, J.C. (1983). Autoinhibition of brain histamine release mediated by a novel class (H_3) of histamine receptor. Nature, 302, 832-837.
Barbin, G., Hirsch, J.C., Garbarg, M., and Schwartz, J.C. (1975). Decrease in histamine content and decarboxylase activities in an isolated area of the cerebral cortex of the cat. Brain Res., 92, 170-174.
Baudry, M., Martres, M.P., and Schwartz, J.C. (1973). The subcellular localisation of histidine decarboxylase in various regions of rat brain. J. Neurochem., 21, 1301-1309.
Ganellin, C.R. (1982). Chemistry and structure-activity relationships of drugs acting at histamine receptors. In C.R. Ganellin and M.E. Parsons (Eds.), Pharmacology of histamine receptors, Wright PSG, Bristol. Chap. 2, pp. 10-102.
Garbarg, M., Barbin, G., Feger, J., and Schwartz, J.C. (1974). Histaminergic pathway in rat brain evidenced by lesions of the medial forebrain bundle. Science, 186, 833-835.
Garbarg, M., Barbin, G., Palacios, J.M., and Schwartz, J.C. (1978). Effects of kainic acid on histaminergic systems in guinea pig hippocampus. Brain Res., 150, 638-641.

Green, J.P. (1983). Histamine receptors in brain. In L.L. Iversen, S.D. Iversen and S.H. Snyder (Eds), Handbook of psychopharmacology, vol. 17, Plenum Publishing Corporation, New York. pp. 385-420.

Haas, H.L. and Wolf, P. (1976). Possible histaminergic pathways in the cat and rat brain. Pflügers Arch., 362, 38.

Haas, H.L., and Wolf, P. (1977). Central actions of histamine microelectrophoretic studies. Brain Res., 122, 269-279.

Hough, L.B., and Green, J.P. (1984). Histamine and its receptors in the nervous system. In A. Lajtha (Ed.), Handbook of neurochemistry, vol. 6, Plenum Publishing Corporation, New York. pp. 145-211.

Langer, S.Z. (1977). Presynaptic receptors and their role in the regulation of transmitter release. Br. J. Pharmacol., 60, 481-497.

Palacios, J.M., Wamsley, J.K., and Kuhar, M.J. (1981). Gaba, benzodiazepine and histamine H_1 receptors in the guinea-pig cerebellum. Effects of kainic acid injections studied by autoradiographic methods. Brain Res., 214, 155-162.

Roth, R.H. (1979). Dopamine autoreceptors : pharmacology, function and comparison with post-synaptic dopamine receptors. In Communications in Psychopharmacology, Vol. 3, Pergamon Press, New York. pp 429-445.

Schunack, W. and Gerhard, G. (1982). Chiral agonists with stereoselective activity at histamine H_2-receptors. Arch. Pharmacol., 319 Suppl., abstr. 224.

Schwartz, J.C. (1979). Mini-review : histamine receptors in brain. Life Sci., 25, 895-912.

Schwartz, J.C., Garbarg, M., and Pollard, H. (1984). Histaminergic transmission in brain. In F.E. Bloom (Ed.), The handbook of physiology, volume on the intrinsic regulatory system of the brain. Am. Physiol. Society Publ. (in press).

Schwartz, J.C., Lampart, C., and Rose, C. (1970). Properties and regional distribution of histidine decarboxylase in rat brain. J. Neurochem., 17, 1527-1534.

Schwartz, J.C., Pollard, H., Bischoff, S., Rehault, M.C., and Verdière-Sahuque, M. (1971). Catabolism of ^{3}H-histamine in the rat brain after intracisternal administration. Eur. J. Pharmacol., 16, 326-335.

Schwartz, J.C., Pollard, H., and Quach, T.T. (1980). Histamine as a neurotransmitter in mammalian brain : Neurochemical evidence. J. Neurochem., 35, 26-33.

Starke, K. (1977). Regulation of noradrenaline release by presynaptic receptor systems. Rev. Physiol. Biochem. Pharmacol., vol. 77, 1-124.

Starke, K. (1981). Presynaptic receptors. Ann. Rev. Pharmac. Tox., 21, 7-30.

Taylor, K.M., and Snyder, S.H. (1973). The release of histamine from tissue slices of rat hypothalamus. J. Neurochem., 21, 1215-1223.

Verdière, M., Rose, C., and Schwartz, J.C. (1974). Synthesis and release of ^{3}H-histamine in slices from rat brain. Agents and Actions, 4, 184-185.

Verdière, M., Rose, C., and Schwartz, J.C. (1975). Synthesis and release of histamine studied on slices from rat hypothalamus. Eur. J. Pharmacol., 34, 157-168.

Westfall, T.C., Besson, M.J., Giorguieff, M.F., and Glowinski, J. (1976) The role of presynaptic receptors in the release and synthesis of ^{3}H-dopamine by slices of rat striatum. Naunyn Schmiedb. Arch. Pharm., 292, 279-287.

NEURONAL UPTAKE AND RELEASE OF HISTAMINE IN THE CENTRAL NERVOUS SYSTEM

A. H. Mulder, R. P. J. M. Smits and
H. W. M. Steinbusch

Department of Pharmacology, Free University Medical Faculty, van der Boechorststraat 7, 1081 BT Amsterdam, The Netherlands

ABSTRACT

Direct evidence for a neuronal uptake system for histamine, with characteristics similar to the specific and rapid high-affinity (re-)uptake mechanisms for other monoamine neurotransmitters, is lacking. However, radiolabelled histamine is taken up by brain slices and can subsequently be released by different depolarizing stimuli, viz. K^+-depolarization, electrical field stimulation and exposure to the alkaloid veratrine, in a calcium-dependent and tetrodotoxin-sensitive manner. These findings indicate that the depolarization-induced release of radiolabelled histamine originates from neurons and not from either mast cells or glial cells, but it is not yet certain that exclusively histaminergic neurons are involved. In view of some pharmacological data and recent experiments with brain slices from rats pretreated with the neurotoxins 6-hydroxydopamine or 5,7-dihydroxytryptamine, it is unlikely that noradrenergic and serotonergic neurons are involved in uptake and release of histamine.

KEYWORDS

CNS; brain slices; histaminergic neurons; histamine uptake; depolarization-induced-release; 6-hydroxydopamine; 5,7-dihydroxytryptamine.

Nerve terminals or axonal varicosities, the major sites of neurotransmitter biosynthesis and release, are potentially important targets of physiological regulatory mechanisms and pharmacological modulation. It is obvious that physiological neurotransmitter release is in the first place determined by the neuronal firing rate, which is subject to regulation via excitatory and inhibitory receptors, localized in the cell body/dendritic region of the neuron. In addition however, the neurotransmitter release process may be liable to local regulation via presynaptic receptor systems localized on or near the nerve terminals (Starke, 1981; Langer, 1981; Mulder and others, 1984). Furthermore, drugs may penetrate into nerve terminals and cause release of neurotransmitters, e.g. amphetamine-like drugs causing catecholamine release, or affect neurotransmitter release indirectly, e.g. reserpine-like drugs impeding vesicular storage of monoamine neurotransmitters or drugs inhibiting monoamine reuptake.
Since, generally speaking, direct measurement of neurotransmitter release in the CNS in vivo still is technically difficult and even in many cases not yet

possible, most studies on the release of central neurotransmitters, including regulatory mechanisms and pharmacological modulation, have been carried out in vitro thus far, using brain slices or synaptosomes. In many of these studies advantage is taken of the fact that, at low concentrations, a number of neurotransmitters are accumulated selectively into the appropriate nerve terminals by high-affinity uptake mechanisms. For instance, upon incubation of brain slices with 0.01-0.1 µM of tritiated noradrenaline (NA), dopamine (DA) or 5-hydroxytryptamine (5-HT), the respective endogenous stores of these monoamine neurotransmitters are labelled and their release can be measured conveniently even from very small samples (a few milligrams) of brain tissue. In order to simulate depolarization-induced neurotransmitter release, which normally results from neuronal firing, the tissue is usually exposed to either electrical field stimulation or high extracellular K^+ concentrations (Mulder, 1982).

Thus far, only a few studies have examined the release of neuronal histamine from brain tissue. Atack and Carlsson (1972) and Taylor and Snyder (1973) have reported that K^+-depolarization released endogenous histamine from slices prepared from mouse cerebral hemispheres and rat hypothalami, respectively, in a calcium-dependent manner. Furthermore, Verdière, Rose and Schwartz (1975) have shown that K^+-depolarization causes a calcium-dependent release of radiolabelled histamine, synthesized from ^{3}H-L-histidine, form rat hypothalamic slices. Using a similar procedure Arrang, Garbarg and Schwartz (1984) recently measured the K^+-induced and veratrine-induced release of newly-synthesized histamine from rat cerebral cortex slices and demonstrated that histamine inhibits its own release, apparently by activating a novel class (H3) of histamine receptors. In all probability the K^+-induced release of endogenous as well as newly-synthesized histamine emanates from histaminergic neurons and not from mast cells, since the latter do not possess voltage-dependent calcium channels in their cell membrane and, therefore, do not release histamine in response to depolarization (Douglas, 1974; Douglas and Kagayama, 1977). Moreover, incubation of brain slices with ^{3}H-L-histidine results in a preferential labelling of neuronal histamine because the L-histidine decarboxylase activity in mast cells appears to be very low compared to that in histaminergic neurons (Verdière, Rose and Schwartz, 1975).

However, the low levels of histamine and L-histidine decarboxylase activity in most brain regions outside the hypothalamus limit the feasibility of measuring the release of endogenous or newly-synthesized histamine from small samples of brain tissue, which, in addition, involves rather laborious assay and/or separation procedures. Therefore, the possibility to label histaminergic nerve terminals selectively with radioactive histamine of high specific activity, would considerably facilitate investigations on histamine release in the CNS, particularly in extra-hypothalamic brain regions.

Direct evidence for an uptake system for histamine, with characteristics similar to the specific and rapid high-affinity uptake mechanisms for the other monoamine neurotransmitters (Snyder and others, 1970), is lacking. Only one study has been reported (Tuomisto, Tuomisto and Walaszek, 1975) demonstrating a temperature-dependent and sodium-dependent uptake of radiolabelled histamine by rabbit hypothalamic slices. However, the uptake process measured in that study was very slow, taking several hours before reaching equilibrium and, moreover, the possibility that in addition to histaminergic neurons other cells, e.g. noradrenergic and serotonergic neurons, were involved could not be excluded. Nevertheless, since histaminergic neurons appear to be markedly similar to other monoaminergic neurons with regard to neurotransmitter biosynthesis, storage and release (Schwartz, Pollard and Quach, 1980), they would be rather exceptional in not possessing a specific (re-)uptake mechanism for their neurotransmitter. Difficulties in detecting such a mechanism may have to do with the relatively small number of histaminergic neurons (presumably only a small fraction of all monoaminergic neurons) and the contribution of mast cells to histamine uptake, so that specific neuronal uptake is too small, relative to non-specific uptake, to be measurable.

In a previous study from our laboratory (Subramanian and Mulder, 1976) it was shown that radiolabelled histamine is taken up by brain slices and can subsequently be released in a calcium-dependent manner by K^+-depolarization, at least suggesting the possibility of a specific uptake of this monoamine into presumed histaminergic neurons. Recently, we have extended this initial observation by showing that ^{3}H-histamine, previously taken up by brain slices, is also released by other depolarizing stimuli, viz. electrical pulses and exposure to the alkaloid veratrine, in a calcium-dependent and tetrodotoxin-sensitive manner (Mulder and others, 1983; Figs. 1 and 2). Electrical field stimulation of brain tissue in vitro at relatively low frequencies (1-20 Hz) is generally thought to approach most closely the physiological situation, in which the nerve terminal membrane is briefly depolarized upon invasion of an action potential. Elevation of the extracellular K^+-concentration results in a passive depolarization by reducing the electrochemical gradient of this ion over the nerve terminal membrane, whereas veratrum alkaloids depolarize the nerve terminal membrane by opening Na^+-channels. In spite of the differences in their primary mechanism of action, all of these stimuli ultimately increase the conductance of voltage-sensitive calcium channels in the nerve terminal membrane

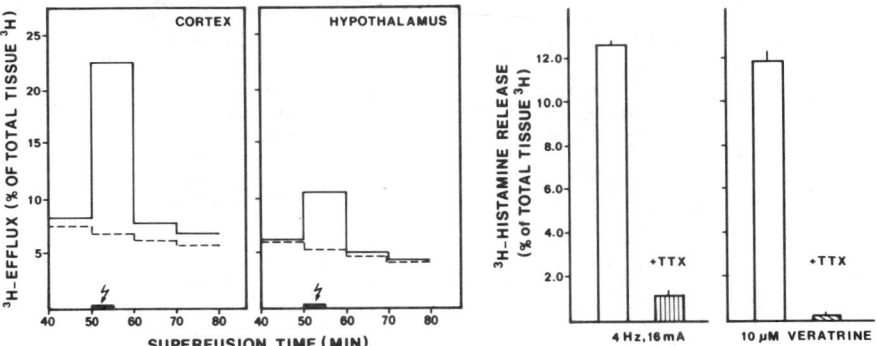

Fig. 1. Electrically-evoked release of tritium from superfused rat brain slices, previously labelled with ^{3}H-histamine, and its calcium-dependence. Small (0.3 x 0.3 x 2 mm) slices were incubated in 2.5 ml of oxygenated physiological medium, containing approx. 0.3 μM ^{3}H-histamine, at 37°C during 15 min. Then the slices were transferred to small superfusion chambers (0.20-0.25 ml volume; about 5 mg of tissue per chamber) and superfused with medium at 37°C. Electrical stimulation was carried out at 4 Hz, 16 mA with pulses of 2 ms duration, from t=50 to t=55 min, either in the presence (solid line) or absence (dashed line) of 1.2 mM Ca^{2+} in the medium. The data were taken from a typical experiment and represent means of duplicate determinations. The amount of tritium present in each superfusion chamber at t=50 min averaged about 4000 and 6000 d.p.m. for cortical and hypothalamic slices, respectively. From Mulder and others (1983), which should be consulted for further experimental details.

Fig. 2. Effect of tetrodotoxin (TTX, 0.3 μM) on ^{3}H-histamine release from rat cortical slices, induced by either electrical stimulation or exposure to 10 μM veratrine. Tetrodotoxin was present in the superfusion medium from 20 min before stimulation.

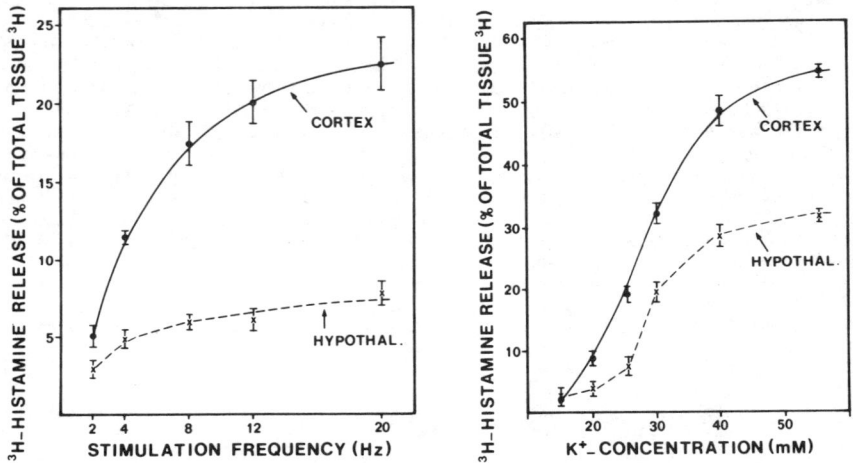

Fig. 3. Dependence of the electrically-evoked release of ^{3}H-histamine from rat brain slices on the frequency of stimulation. After labelling with ^{3}H-histamine the slices were superfused and exposed to electrical stimulation (16 mA, 2 ms pulse duration) at various frequencies, from t=50 to 55 min. From Mulder and others (1983).

Fig. 4. Dependence of K^+-induced ^{3}H-histamine release from rat brain slices on the K^+-concentration. After labelling with ^{3}H-histamine the slices were superfused and exposed to various K^+-concentrations from t=50 to t=55 min. From Mulder and others (1983).

thereby promoting the availability of Ca^{2+} for the stimulus-secretion coupling process (see e.g. Blaustein, 1975; Kostyuk, 1980; Schoffelmeer, Wemer and Mulder, 1981).
Figures 3 and 4 depict the dependence of ^{3}H-histamine release from cortical and hypothalamic slices, exposed to either electrical stimulation or K^+-depolarization, on the stimulation intensity in terms of frequency and K^+-concentration, respectively. Using a particular stimulation intensity, a higher percentage of total ^{3}H-histamine appears to be released from cortical than from hypothalamic slices. The reasons for this are not clear. One possible explanation is that in hypothalamic slices a substantial part of ^{3}H-histamine may be localized in mast cells (Subramanian and Mulder, 1976). An additional possibility could be that somehow the degree of depolarization needed to trigger the stimulus-secretion coupling process in nerve terminals releasing a particular neurotransmitter, differs between brain regions.

Only few mast cells are thought to occur in the brain, with the exception of the hypothalamus (Grzanna aand Shultz, 1982). Indeed, part of the ^{3}H-histamine taken up by hypothalamic slices appears to be localized in mast cells, since it could be released by compound 48/80, a specific mast cell histamine-releasing agent (Subramanian and Mulder, 1976). However, as mentioned above, it is unlikely that mast cells contribute to the depolarization-induced release of ^{3}H-histamine, because they have no voltage-sensitive calcium channels (Douglas, 1974).

Another group of cells that might be involved in uptake and release of ^{3}H-histamine, are glial cells. It has been shown that glial cells take up (putative) amino acid neurotransmitters and are able to release them upon K$^+$-depolarization or electrical stimulation. However, glial cells appear to require a considerably stronger depolarizing stimulus to induce amino acid release than amino acid-ergic nerve terminals and, moreover, glial release appears to display no or little calcium-dependence (see Orrego, 1979). We have demonstrated that depolarizing stimuli of relatively mild intensity (15-30 mM K$^+$ and electrical stimulation at 2-4 Hz and 16 mA) cause ^{3}H-histamine release from cortical and hypothalamic slices, which is completely calcium-dependent and, in the case of electrical stimulation, inhibited by the Na$^+$-channel blocker tetrodotoxin (Mulder and others, 1983; Figs. 1 and 2). Similarly, Subramanian (1982) reported that ^{3}H-histamine, previously taken up by rat hippocampal slices, is released by mild electrical stimulation in a calcium-dependent and tetrodotoxin-sensitive

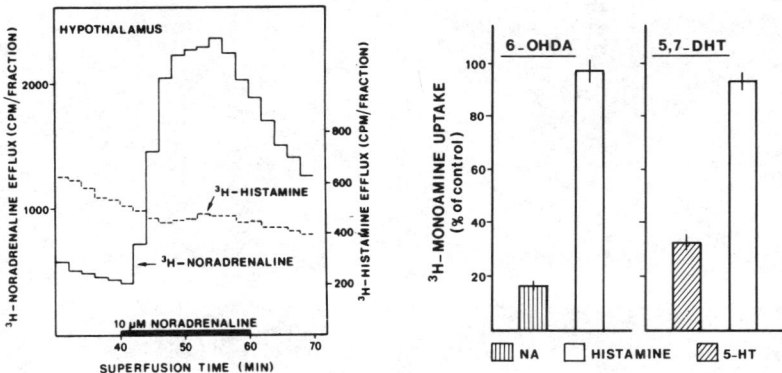

Fig. 5. Effect of superfusion with noradrenaline (NA) on the efflux of tritium from rat hypothalamic slices previously labelled with either ^{3}H-NA or ^{3}H-histamine. The slices were incubated in medium containing either 0.1 μM ^{3}H-NA or 1 μM ^{3}H-histamine, at 37°C for 15 min. Then the slices were superfused and exposed to 10 μM NA for 20 min (solid bar). From Subramanian and Mulder (1977).

Fig. 6. Uptake of tritiated monoamines by hippocampal slices obtained from rats lesioned with 6-hydroxy-dopamine or 5,7-dihydroxytryptamine. Rats received i.c.v. injections with the neurotoxins as described in the legend to Plate I and were used 10-14 days afterwards. Slices from 6-OHDA-lesioned rats and non-treated controls were incubated in 2.5 ml physiological medium containing either ^{3}H-NA (0.1 μM) or ^{3}H-histamine (0.3 μM) for 15 min, at 37°C. Slices from 5,7-DHT-lesioned rats and non-treated controls were incubated with either ^{3}H-5-HT (0.1 μM) or ^{3}H-histamine (0.3 μM). Then the slices were washed repeatedly with medium not containing radioactivity. The radioactivity retained by the slices was assayed after acid extraction and the protein content of the precipitate obtained after centrifugation of the acid tissue suspension was determined. Uptake was calculated as d.p.m. per mg of protein.

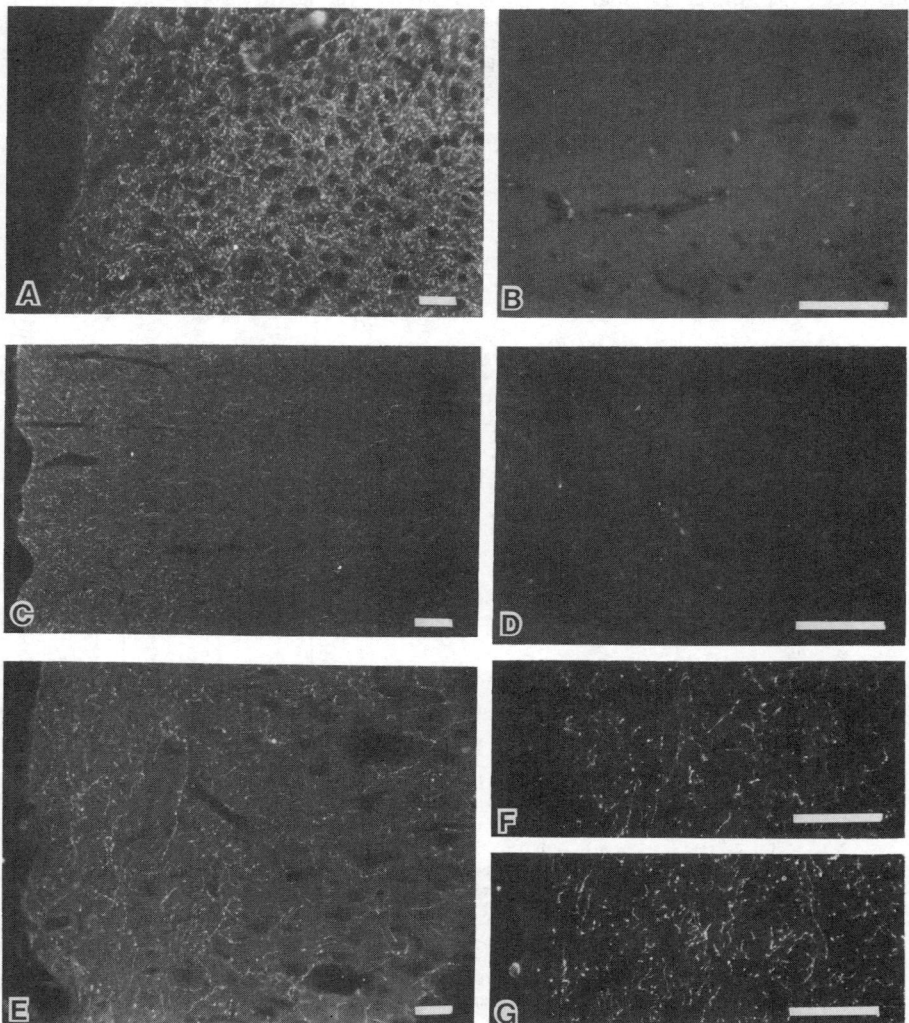

Plate I. Photomicrographs of transversal cryostat sections through the entorhinal cortex of normal (A, C, E) and 6-OH-dopamine- (B, F) or 5,7-diOH-tryptamine- (D, G) lesioned rats, after incubation with antisera to noradrenaline (A, B), serotonin (C, D) or histamine (E, F, G). Rats received i.c.v. injections (bilaterally) of 6-OHDA (100 μg/5 μl), or 5,7-DHT (50 μg/2.5 μl), rats receiving 5,7 DHT were pretreated with desipramine (25 mg/kg, i.p.) 2 hrs before the i.c.v. injections. The animals were decapitated 10 days afterwards. Note that the two neurotoxins selectively depleted noradrenaline and serotonin respectively, without affecting the histaminergic fibers. Bars: 75 μm.

manner. Therefore, it is unlikely that glial cells contribute to depolarization-induced ^{3}H-histamine release, although the possibility that during incubation of brain slices part of the radiolabelled amine is taken up by these cells cannot be excluded. This conclusion is further supported by our finding that ^{3}H-histamine is effectively released by veratrine (Mulder and others, 1983) since the membrane potential of glial cells, in contrast to that of nerve cells, is highly insensitive to veratrum alkaloids (Minchin, 1980).

Although ^{3}H-histamine released by depolarizing brain slices, previously labelled with the radioactive amine, apparently originates from neurons, it is not yet certain that exclusively histaminergic neurons are involved. One might suppose, for example, that other neurons, notably monoaminergic ones, take up, store and release (exogenous) histamine, similar to their own neurotransmitter. Indeed, a previous study (Subramanian and Mulder 1977) has shown that histamine may cause an increased efflux of radioactivity (consisting mainly of radiolabelled catecholamine metabolites) from brain slices previously labelled with radioactive catecholamines, although rather high concentrations (in the micromolar range) of histamine were needed to produce this effect. However, in the same study it was shown that tyramine or noradrenaline were unable to induce a significant increase in the efflux of tritium from hypothalamic slices labelled with ^{3}H-histamine, whereas the tritium efflux from slices labelled with ^{3}H-noradrenaline was strongly enhanced (Fig. 5). This argues against the possibility that histamine enters catecholaminergic neurons, subsequently (partially) displacing the catecholamine transmitter from its storage sites. Currently, further experiments are carried out in our laboratory to examine this question. Figure 6 summarizes data obtained from preliminary experiments with brain slices from rats pretreated with the neurotoxins 6-hydroxydopamine or 5,7-dihydroxytryptamine to destroy central catecholaminergic and serotonergic neurons, respectively. Using antisera directed against the respective monoamines (Steinbusch, Verhofstad and Joosten 1978; Steinbusch and Mulder, 1984) it was found that these neurotoxins did not affect histaminergic neurons to any significant extent (Plate I). In these experiments, the uptake of radiolabelled NA, 5-HT or histamine by hippocampal slices from lesioned rats was measured and compared to that found for non-treated controls. Figure 6 shows that a strong reduction of ^{3}H-NA uptake after 6-hydroxydopamine lesions, to less than 20% of controls, was not accompanied by a significant decrease of ^{3}H-histamine uptake. Similarly, 5,7-dihydroxytryptamine lesions resulting in a strongly reduced uptake of ^{3}H-5-HT did not significantly affect ^{3}H-histamine uptake. Therefore, these preliminary findings also suggest that (radiolabelled) histamine is not taken up to a significant extent by either noradrenergic or serotonergic neurons and support the hypothesis that the depolarization-induced release of this monoamine after its uptake by brain slices originates from histaminergic neurons.

REFERENCES

Arrang, J.M., M. Garbarg and J.C. Schwartz (1983). Auto-inhibition of brain histamine release mediated by a novel class (H3) of histamine receptor. Nature, 302, 832-837.
Atack, C. and A. Carlsson (1972). In vitro release of endogenous histamine, together with noradrenaline and 5-hydroxytryptamine from slices of mouse cerebral hemisphere. J. Pharm. Pharmac., 24, 990-992.
Blaustein, M.P. (1975). Effect of potassium, veratridine and scorpion venom on calcium accumulation and transmitter release by nerve terminals in vitro. J. Physiol. (London), 247, 617-655.
Douglas, W.W. (1974). Involvement of calcium in exocytosis and the exocytosis-vesiculation sequence. Biochem. Soc. Symp., 39, 1-38.
Douglas, W.W. and M. Kagayama (1977). Calcium and stimulus-secretion coupling in the mast cell: stimulant and inhibitory effects of calcium-rich media on exocytosis. J. Physiol. (London), 257, 433-448.

Grzanna, R. and L. Shultz (1982). The contribution of mast cells to the histamine content of the central nervous system: a regional analysis. Life Sci., 30, 1959-1964.
Kostyuk, P.G. (1980). Calcium ion channels in electrically excitable membranes. Neuroscience, 5, 945-959.
Langer, S.Z. (1981). Presynaptic regulation of the release of catecholamines. Pharmacol. Rev., 32, 337-362.
Minchin, M.C.W. (1980). Veratrum alkaloids as transmitter-releasing agents. J. Neurosci. Meth., 2, 111-121.
Mulder, A.H. (1982). An overview of subcellular localization, release and termination of action of amine, amino acid and peptide neurotransmitters in the central nervous system. In R.M. Buys, P. Pevet and D.F. Swaab (Eds.), "Chemical Transmission in the Brain", Progr. Brain Res., Vol. 55. Elsevier, Amsterdam, pp. 135-156.
Mulder, A.H., R.G.M. van Amsterdam, M. Wilbrink and A.N,M. Schoffelmeer (1983). Depolarization-induced release of ^{3}H-histamine by high potassium concentrations, electrical stimulation and veratrine from rat brain slices after incubation with the radiolabelled amine. Neurochem. Int., 3, 291-297.
Mulder, A.H., A.L. Frankenhuyzen, J.C. Stoof, J. Wemer and A.N.M. Schoffelmeer (1984). Catecholamine receptors, opiate receptors and presynaptic modulation of neurotransmitter release in the brain. In E. Usdin, A. Carlsson, A. Dahlström and J. Engel (Eds.), "Catecholamines", Part B: Neuropharmacology and Central nervous system. Theoretical aspects. Alan Liss, New York, pp. 47-58.
Orrego, F. (1979). Criteria for the identification of central neurotransmitters and their application to studies with some nerve tissue preparations in vitro. Neuroscience, 4, 1037-1057.
Schoffelmeer, A.N.M. and A.H. Mulder (1981). Comparison between electrically-evoked and potassium-induced ^{3}H-noradrenaline release from rat neocortex slices: role of calcium ions and transmitter pools. Neurochem. Int., 3, 129-136.
Schwartz, J.C., H. Pollard and T.T. Quach (1980). Histamine as a neurotransmitter in mammalian brain: neurochemical evidence. J. Neurochem., 35, 26-33.
Snyder, S.H., M.J. Kuhar, A.I. Green, J.T. Coyle and E.G. Shaskan (1970). Uptake and subcellular localization of neurotransmitters in the brain. Int. Rev. Neurobiol., 13, 127-158.
Starke, K. (1981). Presynaptic receptors. Ann.Rev.Pharmacol.Toxicol., 21, 7-30.
Steinbusch, H.W.M., A.A.J. Verhofstad and H.W.J. Joosten (1978). Localization of serotonin in the central nervous system by immunohistochemistry: description of a specific and sensitive technique and some applications. Neuroscience, 3, 811-819.
Steinbusch, H.W.M. and A.H. Mulder (1984). Immunocytochemical localization of histamine in neurons and mast cells in the rat brain. In A. Björklund and T. Hökfelt (Eds.) "Classical neurotransmitters", Handb. Chem. Neuroanatomy, Vol. 2. Elsevier, Amsterdam, in press.
Subramanian, N. (1982). Electrically-induced release of radiolabelled histamine from rat hippocampal slices: opposing roles for H_1- and H_2-receptors. Life Sci., 31, 557-562.
Subramanian, N. and A.H. Mulder (1976). Potassium-induced release of tritiated histamine from rat brain tissue slices. Eur. J. Pharmacol., 35, 203-206.
Subramanian, N. and A.H. Mulder (1977). Modulation by histamine of the efflux of radiolabelled catecholamines from rat brain slices. Eur. J. Pharmacol., 43, 143-152.
Taylor, K.M. and S.H. Snyder (1973). The release of histamine from tissue slices of rat hypothalamus. J. Neurochem., 19, 1343-1358.
Tuomisto, L., J. Tuomisto and E.J. Walaszek (1975). Uptake of histamine by rabbit hypothalamic slices. Med. Biol., 53, 40-46.
Verdière, M., C. Rose and J.C. Schwartz (1975). Synthesis and release of histamine studied on slices from rat hypothalamus. Eur. J. Pharmacol., 34, 157-168.

S-ADENOSYLMETHIONINE-DEPENDENT TRANSMETHYLATION OF HISTAMINE: PURIFICATION AND PARTIAL CHARACTERIZATION OF GUINEA PIG BRAIN AND RAT KIDNEY HISTAMINE N-METHYLTRANSFERASE

R. T. Borchardt and B. Matuszewska

Departments of Biochemistry and Pharmaceutical Chemistry,
The University of Kansas, Lawrence, KS 66045, USA

ABSTRACT

Histamine-N-methyltransferase (HMT, EC 2.1.1.8) catalyzes the transfer of a methyl group from S-adenosyl-L-methionine (AdoMet) to histamine resulting in the formation of 1-methylhistamine and S-adenosyl-L-homocysteine (AdoHcy). In this report we describe an affinity chromatography procedure for the purification of the guinea pig brain enzyme approximately 4400-fold in 12% yield and the rat kidney enzyme approximately 8420-fold in 44% yield. The basic steps in the purification included differential centrifugation, calcium phosphate adsorption, DEAE-cellulose chromatography and affinity chromatography on an AdoHcy-agarose matrix. The resulting proteins were homogeneous by SDS-polyacrylamide gel electrophoresis and they were stable for at least 3 months at $-80°$ C. The homogeneous proteins were characterized by determining their molecular weights (guinea pig brain, 29,000 Kdal; rat kidney, 31,500 Kdal), isoelectric points (guinea pig brain, 5.3; rat kidney, 5.4), pH optima (guinea pig brain, 7.5, 9.0; rat kidney, 8.5-9.0), the amino acid compositions and the kinetic parameters for known substrates (e.g., histamine, AdoMet) and inhibitors (L-AdoHcy, D-AdoHcy). The results of this study suggest that HMT isolated from a neuronal source (guinea pig brain) and a nonneuronal source (rat kidney) have similar physico-chemical and catalytic properties.

KEYWORDS

Histamine-N-methyltransferase, S-adenosylmethionine, S-adenosylhomocysteine, histamine, affinity chromatography.

INTRODUCTION

The metabolism of histamine in brain involves initial methylation followed by oxidation to yield 1-methylimidazole-4-acetic acid (Schayer, 1956; Schwartz and co-workers, 1971). The methylation of histamine is catalyzed by histamine N-methyltransferase (HMT, EC 2.1.1.8) (Borchardt, 1980). HMT catalyzes the transfer of a methyl group from S-adenosyl-L-methionine (AdoMet) to histamine resulting in the formation of 1-methyl-4(β-aminoethyl)imidazole (1-methylhistamine) and S-adenosyl-L-homocysteine (AdoHcy). Similar to most

AdoMet-dependent methyltransferases, HMT is sensitive to inhibition by the demethylated product L-AdoHcy (Borchardt, 1980; Baudry, Chast and Schwartz, 1973).

HMT has been purified to varying degrees using classical protein purification techniques. Brown, Tomchick and Axelrod (1959) have purified HMT approximately 36-fold from guinea pig brain, whereas Sellinger, Schatz and Ohlsson (1978) reported the purification of the rat brain enzyme 87-fold and the mouse brain enzyme 166-fold. Thithapandha and Cohn (1978) achieved a 200-fold purification of the guinea pig brain HMT, but the protein was not homogeneous. Recently, Bowsher, Verburg and Henry (1983) reported the purification of rat kidney HMT approximately 2,100-fold in 49% yield. The pivotal step in their purification of HMT was an affinity column procedure which involved the specific elution of the enzyme from DEAE-Sephacel by 1 mM histamine. The rat kidney enzyme is of particular interest because of its utility in the histamine radioenzymatic assay (Shaff and Beaven, 1979).

In this chapter we have described an affinity chromatography procedure for purification of HMT to homogeneity from guinea pig brain (Matuszewska and Borchardt, 1983) and from rat kidney (Matuszewska and Borchardt, 1984a). The pivotal step in our purification procedure is chromatography on an AdoHcy-agarose matrix with specific elution of HMT by AdoMet. In addition we have reviewed some of the physico-chemical and catalytic properties of the enzymes isolated from guinea pig brain and rat kidney.

MATERIALS AND METHODS

Chemicals were obtained from the following commercial suppliers: [methyl-^{14}C]-AdoMet, 44-56.2 mCi/mmol (New England Nuclear, Boston, MA); calcium phosphate gel (Calbiochem-Boehring Corp., La Jolla, CA); AdoHcy-agarose gel (BRL, Rockville, MD); acrylamide and N,N,N',N'-tetramethylethylene diamine (Eastman Kodak Co., Rochester, NY); AdoMet, histamine dihydrochloride, dithiothreitol (DTT), DEAE-cellulose, Sephadex G-25, Sephadex G-100, Trizma base (Sigma Chemical Co., St. Louis, MO); protein molecular weight markers (Pharmacia Fine Chemicals, Piscataway, NJ); and Bio-Lyte 3/10 (Bio-Rad Lab, Richmond, CA). Other chemicals were of reagent grade and were obtained commercially. Guinea pig brains were purchased from Pel-Freeze Biologicals, Inc., Rogers, AR. Standard buffers used for purification and assay of HMT were: Buffer A, 0.01 M sodium phosphate, pH 7.4 (1 mM DTT); Buffer B, 0.01 M sodium phosphate, pH 7.4 (1 mM DTT, 10% glycerol).

Enzyme Purification

The HMT's were purified from guinea pig brain (30 g) or rat kidney (28 g). Tissues were homogenized in four volumes of Buffer A. All subsequent steps were carried out at 4° C. The crude homogenates were centrifuged at 37,000 x g for 1 hr. The resulting supernatants were decanted and centrifuged at 225,000 x g for 12 hr to generate cytosolic fractions. The crude cytosolic HMT's were further purified using calcium phosphate gel adsorption and chromatography on DEAE-cellulose as basically described earlier by Thithapandha and Cohn (1978). This procedure was modified slightly to include the use of Buffer B starting with the DEAE-cellulose step.

Aliquots (guinea pig brain, 4.5 mg; rat kidney, 8.8 mg) of the DEAE-cellulose-purified HMT's in Buffer B were then applied to AdoHcy-agarose columns (1.5 x 3 cm, 5 ml bed volume) which had been equilibrated with Buffer B. The columns were washed with 5 ml of 0.12 M sodium phosphate buffer, pH 7.4 (1 mM DTT, 10% glycerol) to remove a major protein peak, followed by 100 ml of Buffer B. HMT activity was then eluted with 100 ml of Buffer B containing 0.2 M NaCl and 0.1 mM AdoMet. The columns were operated at a flow rate of 60 ml/hr. The

HMT-containing fractions were pooled, dialyzed against Buffer B, and then concentrated to a final volume of 1 ml. To remove trace amounts of AdoMet, the concentrated enzymes were applied to Sephadex G-25 columns (1 x 25 cm) and the columns eluted with Buffer B. The HMT-containing fractions were pooled and used as the enzyme source in all subsequent studies.

Enzyme Assay

HMT activity was determined using histamine and [methyl-^{14}C]-AdoMet as substrates according to the previously described assay (Borchardt and Wu, 1974). The [methyl-^{14}C]-1-methylhistamine was extracted from the incubation mixture with toluene-isoamyl-alcohol (1:1) and quantitated by liquid scintillation spectrometry. In the experiments to determine substrate kinetic patterns, either the histamine concentration was held constant at 2 mM and the AdoMet concentration varied from 11.6 µM to 83.6 µM or the AdoMet concentration was held constant at 100 µM and the histamine concentration varied from 10 µM to 100 µM. Processing of the kinetic data was carried out as described by Borchardt, Huber and Wu (1974). HMT activity was expressed in terms of nmoles of 1-methylhistamine formed/mg protein/min. Protein concentrations were determined by the method of Lowry and co-workers (1951) or from the amino acid composition determined after hydrolysis of the protein (see below).

Polyacrylamide Gel Electrophoresis

Purified HMT's were subjected to polyacrylamide gel electrophoresis using 7% crosslinked gels according to the procedure of Neville and Glossman (1974). The locations of the proteins were determined by staining with Coomassie blue. The location of the HMT activity was determined by slicing an unstained gel into 5 mm slices. The slices were extracted with Buffer B and the extracts assayed for HMT activity. In preparation for SDS-polyacrylamide gel electrophoresis, the enzymes were first incubated for 3 hr at 37° C with Buffer A, which contained 1% mercaptoethanol, 1% SDS and 8 M urea. The SDS-treated samples were dialyzed for 24 hr against Buffer A containing 0.1% mercaptoethanol and 0.1% SDS before electrophoresis was carried out using 7% polyacrylamide gels. Bromophenol blue was used as a tracking dye. The locations of proteins were determined by staining the gels with Coomassie blue. The pH gradient was checked by slicing the gels into 0.2 cm pieces, dissolving the pieces in hot water (1 ml), and measuring the pH's of the resulting solutions.

Amino Acid Analysis

The amino acid compositions of the HMT's were determined after hydrolysis in 6 M HCL in vacuo at 115° C for 24 and 72 hr. The hydrolyzed samples were analyzed according to the method of Spackman, Stein and Moore (1958) with a Glenco Amino Acid Analyzer equipped with a 3390 A Hewlett Packard Integrator. The amino acid compositions were calculated by averaging the 24 and 72 hr values for stable amino acids. Since the proportion of isoleucine and leucine increased with time, the 72 hr values for these amino acids were averaged. The serine and the threonine values were calculated by extrapolation back to zero time of hydrolysis. Results are expressed as residues/molecule of enzyme, assuming molecular weights of 29,000 for the guinea pig brain enzyme and 31,500 for the rat kidney enzyme. Half-cystine levels were determined as cysteic acid after performic acid oxidation (Hirs, 1967).

RESULTS AND DISCUSSION

Purification of Guinea Pig Brain and Rat Kidney HMT

In Table 1 is outlined the scheme developed for purification of guinea pig brain and rat kidney HMT's to homogeniety. The initial steps in the procedure are a modification of the methods described by Thithapandha and Cohn (1978). By differential centrifugation, calcium phosphate adsorption and chromatography on DEAE-cellulose, we were able to achieve a 154-fold purification of the guinea pig brain enzyme and 63-fold purification of the rat kidney enzyme. By including 10% glycerol in the buffer prior to DEAE-cellulose chromatography, significant stabilization of the enzyme was achieved, thus overcoming an HMT stability problem confronted by previous workers (Thithapandha and Cohn, 1978). HMT's were further purified approximately 29-fold for the guinea pig brain enzyme and 133-fold for the rat kidney enzyme by chromatography on an affinity matrix consisting of AdoHcy, which was covalently linked through the amino group of the homocysteinyl residue to agarose (Fig. 1). When the DEAE-cellulose-purified enzymes were applied to columns of the AdoHcy-agarose conjugate, the HMT activity was retained, while other proteins were eluted with 0.12 M sodium phosphate buffer, pH 7.4. HMT activity could be eluted using a buffer containing both a high salt concentration (0.2 M NaCl) and AdoMet (0.1 mM) (Fig. 2). After dialysis of the affinity-purified enzymes and chromatography on Sephadex G-25 to remove AdoMet, homogeneous HMT preparations were obtained having specific activities of 355 nmoles of product/mg protein/min for the guinea pig brain enzyme and 488 nmoles of product/mg protein/min for the rat kidney enzyme. These preparations were stable for at least 3 months at -80° C.

Recently, Bowster, Verburg and Henry (1983) reported another affinity chromatography based procedure for purification of rat kidney HMT. That procedure afforded a 2,100-fold purification of the enzyme in 49% yield. However, to stabilize the enzymatic activity, the Bowster, Verburg and Henry procedure required anaerobic conditions, avoidance of freeze-thawing the enzyme and maintaining a minimum ionic strength during the chromatography steps. The procedure described here seems less cumbersome, giving a higher fold purification in approximately the same yield as the Bowsher, Verburg and Henry procedure. With respect to the guinea pig brain enzyme, the procedure described here is the first to afford a stable, homogeneous form of the enzyme.

TABLE 1 Purification of HMT from Guinea Pig Brain and Rat Kidney[a]

Purification Step	HMT Units[b] Brain	Kidney	HMT Specific Activity[c] Brain	Kidney	Purification-fold Brain	Kidney	Recovery % Brain	Kidney
Crude Homogenate	277	161	0.08	0.06	1	1	100	100
225,000 x g Supernatant	116	106	0.54	0.14	6.7	2.4	42	66
Calcium Phosphate Negative Adsorption	108	98	1.04	0.32	13	6.2	39	61
DEAE-Cellulose Chromatography	61	92	12.4	3.49	154	63	22	57
AdoHcy-agarose + Sephadex G-25 Chromatography	33	71	355	488	4400	8420	12	44

[a] Guinea pig brains (30 g) or rat kidneys (28 g) were homogenized in 112 ml of sodium phosphate buffer, pH 7.4 (1 mM DTT). In general, protein concentrations were determined by the method of Lowry and co-workers (1951). After affinity-agarose + Sephadex G-25 chromatography, protein concentrations were calculated from the amino acid composition determined by hydrolysis of the protein for 72 hr.
[b] One HMT unit equals the amount of enzyme that can catalyze the formation of one nmol of [methyl-^{14}C]-1-methylhistamine.
[c] Specific activity expressed in nmoles of [methyl-^{14}C]-1-methylhistamine formed/mg/min.

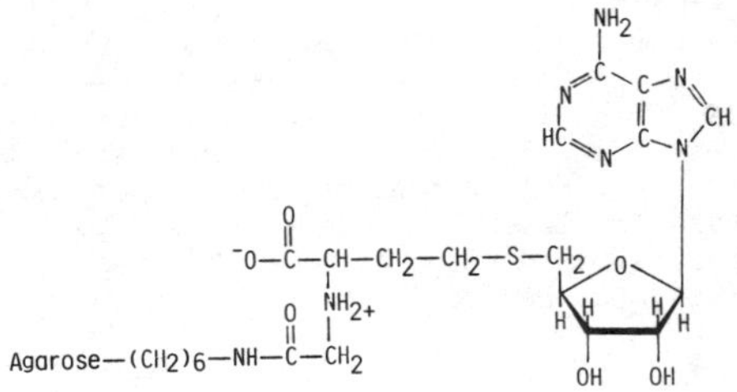

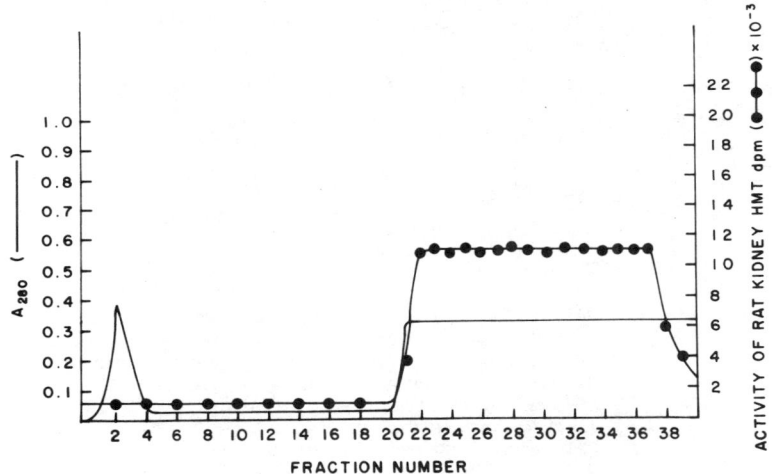

Fig. 1. AdoHcy-agarose affinity matrix used to purify guinea pig brain and rat kidney HMT's.

Fig. 2. Elution pattern of rat kidney HMT from AdoHcy - agarose column. An aliquot (8.8 mg) of the DEAE-cellulose purified HMT in Buffer B was applied to an AdoHcy-agarose column (1.5 x 3 cm). The column was eluted with 5 ml of 0.12 M sodium phosphate buffer, pH 7.4 (10% glycerol, 1 mM DTT) (fractions 1-4), 100 ml of Buffer B (fractions 4-20) and 100 ml of Buffer B containing 0.2 M NaCl and 0.1 mM AdoMet (fractions 20-40). HMT activity was detected with an assay using histamine and [methyl-^{14}C]-AdoMet. The increase in A_{280} starting with fraction 20 results from the AdoMet present in the eluting buffer.

Polyacrylamide gel electrophoresis of the purified guinea pig brain and the rat kidney HMT's each showed two protein bands, both bands exhibiting HMT activity (data not shown). If, however, the native enzymes were treated with SDS, then run on polyacrylamide gel electrophoresis, each showed single protein bands having molecular weights of 29,000 Kdal for the guinea pig brain enzyme and 31,500 Kdal for the rat kidney enzyme (Fig. 3). The two protein bands observed in the non-SDS treated samples apparently represent the monomer and a higher molecular weight aggregate of HMT. The molecular weights of the guinea pig brain and rat kidney HMT's were also determined using a calibrated Sephadex G-100 column and found to be 29,000 and 31,000, respectively (data not shown).

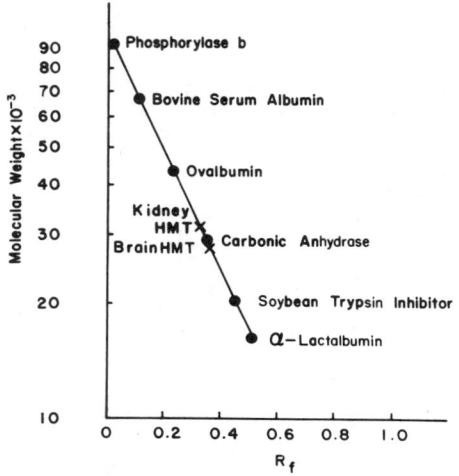

Fig. 3. Relationship of protein molecular weight to Rf value on SDS-polyacrylamide gel electrophoresis. Purified HMT or a standard protein was incubated for 3 hr at 37° C with Buffer A containing 1% mercaptoethanol, 1% SDS and 8 M urea. After dialysis of the sample, electrophoresis was carried out on 7% polyacrylamide gels according to the procedure of Neville and Glossman (1974). The gels were stained with Coomassie blue as described in the Materials and Methods Section. The following standard proteins (molecular weight) were used; phosphorylase b (94,000), bovine serum albumin (67,000), ovalbumin (43,000), carbonic anhydrase (30,000), soybean trypsin inhibitor (21,100) and α-lactalbumin (14,400).

Various molecular weights have been reported in the literature for HMT. Thithapandha and Cohn (1978) reported a molecular weight greater than 100,000 for guinea pig brain HMT, based on its elution from Sephadex G-100 and its mobility on polyacrylamide gel electrophoresis. In contrast, Sellinger, Schatz and Ohlsson (1978) determined molecular weights of 29,000 for both the rat and mouse brain HMT using gel filtration on Sephadex G-100.

The enzymes isolated by our procedure can apparently exist in aggregate forms, since when the purified protein samples were run on native polyacrylamide gels, each preparation of HMT showed two protein bands both having HMT activity. Such multiple forms of HMT have been reported earlier (Axelrod and Vessel, 1970; Suriyachan and Thithapandha, 1972). At this time we do not have an explanation for the differences in molecular weight for guinea pig HMT observed in our study versus that reported by Thithapandha and Cohn (1978). Perhaps the presence of glycerol in the buffers to stabilize the enzyme favors the monomer form over the aggregate form of the enzyme. The molecular weight of the rat kidney enzyme (31,500 Kdal) as determined in our study is similar to the value of 33,400 Kdal reported by Bowsher, Verburg and Henry (1983).

Properties of Guinea Pig Brain and Rat Kidney HMT

Isoelectric focusing of the purified HMT's showed single protein bands with pI's equal to 5.3 for the guinea pig brain enzyme and 5.4 for the rat kidney enzyme (Fig. 4). The amino acid composition of the HMT's were determined and the results are shown in Table 2. The HMT's had similar amino acid compositions consisting of all the common amino acids with relatively high contents of aspartic acid and glutamic acid. The pH optima for methylation of histamine was found to be 7.5 and 9.0 for the guinea pig enzyme and 8.5-9.0 for the rat kidney enzyme. With the guinea pig brain enzyme the Km's for histamine and AdoMet were 13.6 ± 0.7 μM and 6.1 ± 0.1 μM, respectively, and the Ki's for L-AdoHcy and D-AdoHcy were 24.5 ± 1.4 μM and 15.2 ± 0.4 μM, respectively. With the rat kidney enzyme the Km's for histamine and AdoMet were 12.4 ± 1.3 μM and 10.2 ± 0.5 μM, respectively, and the Ki's for L-AdoHcy and D-AdoHcy were 31.9 ± 3.4 μM and 32.0 ± 3.5 μM, respectively.

In general, the properties determined for these purified HMT's are similar to those reported earlier for crude preparations of the enzyme. Brown, Tomchick and Axelrod have previously reported a pH optimum of 7.2-7.4 for guinea pig brain HMT; whereas Bowsher, Verburg and Henry reported a pH optimum of 8.0-8.25 for the rat kidney enzyme. In the current study, we observed pH optima of 7.5 and 9.0 for the guinea pig brain enzyme and 8.5-9.0 for the rat kidney enzyme. Our observed Km value for histamine of 13.7 μM for the guinea pig brain enzyme is in the range of the Km values previously reported using less purified preparations (Taylor and Snyder, 1972; Baudry, Chast and Schwartz, 1973; Thithapanda and Cohn, 1978). The purified guinea pig brain enzyme showed a Km of 6.1 μM for AdoMet which is almost identical to the Km value of 6.0 μM reported by Baudry, Chast and Schwartz (1973); however, the Ki value for L-AdoHcy (24.5 μM) is slightly higher than the values of 18.1 μM and 4.0 μM reported by Borchardt, Huber and Wu (1974) and Baudry, Chast and Schwartz (1973), respectively.

The similarities in the molecular and catalytic properties of the guinea pig brain enzyme and the rat kidney enzyme reported in this study, support the hypothesis put forth by Bowsher, Verburg and Henry (1983) that the rat kidney and rat brain HMT's are the same proteins. The Bowsher, Verburg and Henry (1983) hypothesis was based primarily on the observation that these enzymes shared common antigenic determinants.

In summary, we have described here efficient procedures for isolation and purification of electrophoretically homogeneous HMT's from guinea pig brain and rat kidney. The purified enzymes were shown to be very stable (at least 3 months at -80° C). These purified HMT's should prove useful for analytical purposes such as histamine determinations (Shaff and Beaven, 1979) and for mechanistic studies (Borchardt, Wu and Wu, 1978; Matuszewska and Borchardt, 1984b).

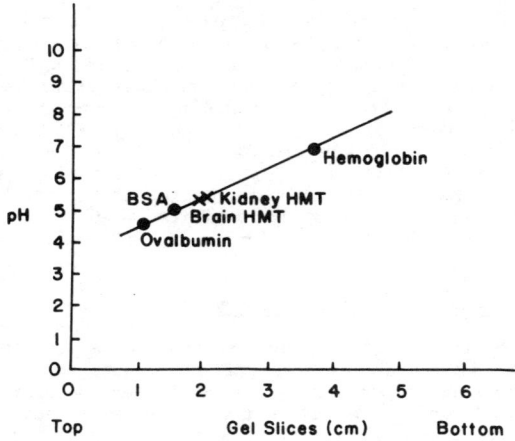

Fig. 4. Isoelectric focusing of purified HMT. Purified HMT's (100 µg) were subjected to electrophoresis for 5 hr at 150 V in 7.5% polyacrylamide gel with Bio-Lyte 3/10 to produce the pH gradient. The pH gradient was checked with standard proteins as shown or by slicing the gel into 0.2 cm pieces, dissolving the pieces in hot water (1 ml) and measuring the resulting pH's (data not shown). The standard proteins used were ovalbumin (pI = 4.6), bovine serum albumin BSA (pI = 4.9) and hemoglobin (pI = 6.8).

TABLE 2 Amino Acid Composition of Rat Kidney and Guinea Pig Brain HMT's[a]

Amino Acid Residue[b]	Number of Residues per Molecule of Enzyme	
	Rat Kidney HMT (MW 31,500)	Guinea Pig Brain HMT (MW 29,000)
Aspartic Acid	32	28
Threonine	18	18
Serine	18	18
Glutamic Acid	36	34
Glycine	21	22
Proline	14	14[d]
Alanine	21	23
Valine	18	16
Methionine	3	5
Isoleucine	12	13
Leucine	28	27
Tyrosine	10	8
Phenylalanine	14	11
Lysine	20	14
Histidine	10	6
Arginine	13	12
Half-cystine[c]	8	8

[a]Hydrolysis was carried out in 6 M HCl in vacuo at 115° C for 24 and 72 h. The hydrolyzed sample was analyzed in a Glenco amino acid analyzer.
[b]Thryptophan levels were not determined.
[c]Half cystine was determined as cysteic acid after performic acid oxidation (Hirs, 1967).
[d]This value represents a corrected estimate from that published earlier (Matuszewska and Borchardt, 1983).

ACKNOWLEDGEMENT

The authors acknowledge support of this work by a grant from the National Institutes of Health (GM-29332) and by the Center for Biomedical Research, The University of Kansas. The advice and assistance of Dr. Charles J. Decedue and the Enzyme Laboratory at The University of Kansas are gratefully acknowledged.

REFERENCES

Axelrod, J. and Vesell, E. S. (1970). Heterogenity of N- and O-methyltransferases. Mol. Pharmacol., 6, 78-84.
Baudry, M., Chast, F. and Schwartz, J. C. (1983). Studies on S-Adenosylhomocysteine inhibition of histamine transmethylation in brain. J. Neurochem., 20, 13-21.
Borchardt, R. T. (1980). N- and O-Methylation. In W. B. Jakoby (Ed.), Enzymatic Basis of Detoxication, Vol. 2, Academic Press, New York, pp. 43-62.
Borchardt, R. T. and Wu, Y. S. (1974). Potential inhibitors of S-adenosylmethionine-dependent methyltransferases. I. Modification of the amino acid portion of S-adenosylhomocysteine. J. Med. Chem., 17, 862-868.
Borchardt, R. T., Huber, J. A. and Wu, Y. S. (1974). Potential inhibitors of S-adenosylmethionine-dependent methyltransferases. 2. Modification of the base portion of S-adenosylhomocysteine. J. Med. Chem., 17, 868-873.
Borchardt, R. T., Wu, Y. S. and Wu, B. S. (1978). Affinity labeling of histamine N-methyltransferase by 2',3'-dialdehyde derivatives of S-adenosylhomocysteine and S-adenosylmethionine. Kinetics of inactivation. Biochemistry, 17, 4145-4153.
Borchardt, R. T., Wu, Y. S., Huber, J. A. and Wycpalek, A. F. (1976). Potential inhibitors of S-adenosylmethionine-dependent methyltransferases. 6. Structural modification of S-adenosylmethionine. J. Med. Chem., 19, 1104-1110.
Bowsher, R. R., Verburg, K. M. and Henry, D. P. (1983). Rat histamine N-methyltransferase: Quantification, tissue distribution, purification and immunologic properties. J. Biol. Chem., 258, 12215-12220.
Brown, D. D., Tomchick, R. and Axelrod, J. (1959). The distribution and properties of a histamine-methylating enzyme. J. Biol. Chem., 234, 2948-2950.
Hirs, C. H. W. (1967). Performic acid oxidation, in C.H.W. Hirs, Eds. Methods in Enzymology, Vol. 11, Academic Press, New York, p. 197-199.
Lowry, O. H., Rosebrough, N. J., Farr, A. L. and Randall, R. J. (1951). Protein measurement with the folin phenol reagent. J. Biol. Chem., 193, 265-275.
Matuszewska, B. and Borchardt, R. T. (1983). Guinea pig brain histamine N-methyltransferase: Purification and partial characterization. J. Neurochem., 41, 113-118.
Matuszewska, B. and Borchardt, R. T. (1984a). Rat kidney histamine N-methyltransferase: Purification and partial characterization. Anal. Biochem., submitted.
Matuszewska, B. and Borchardt, R. T. (1984b). Affinity labeling of histamine-N-methyltransferase by S-adenosylhomocysteine 2',3'-dialdehyde. Fed. Proc., 43, Abst. #750.
Neville, D. M. and Glossman, H. (1974). In S. Fleisher and L. Packer, Eds., Methods in Enzymology. Vol. 32, Academic Press, New York, p. 92.
Schayer, R. W. (1956). The metabolism of histamine in various species. Br. J. Pharmacol. Chemother., 11, 472-473.
Schwartz, J. C., Pollard, H., Bischoff, S., Rehault, M. C. and Verdiere-Sahuque, M. (1971). Catabolism of ^{3}H-histamine in the rat brain after intracisternal administration. Europ. J. Pharmacol., 16, 326-335.
Sellinger, O. Z., Schatz, R. A. and Ohlsson, W. G. (1978). Rat and mouse brain histamine N-methyltransferase: modulation by methylated indoleamines. J. Neurochem., 30, 437-445.

Shaff, R. E. and Beaven, M. A. (1979). Increased sensitivity of the enzymatic isotopic assay of histamine: measurement of histamine in plasma and serum. Anal. Biochem., 94, 425-430.

Spackman, D. M., Stein, W. H. and Moore, S. (1958). Automatic recording apparatus for use in the chromatography of amino acids. Anal. Chem., 30, 1190-1206.

Suriyachan, D. and Thithapandha, A. (1972). Distribution and heterogeneity of histamine N-methyltransferase. Biochem. Biophys. Res. Commun., 48, 1199-1207.

Thithapandha, A. and Cohn, V. H. (1978). Brain histamine N-methyltransferase purification, mechanism of action and inhibition by drugs. Biochem. Pharmacol., 27, 263-271.

SIMULTANEOUS DETERMINATION OF HISTAMINE AND TELE-METHYLHISTAMINE IN THE MAMMALIAN CENTRAL NERVOUS SYSTEM AND HISTAMINE TURNOVER MEASUREMENTS

K. Saeki, R. Oishi and M. Nishibori

Department of Pharmacology, Okayama University Medical School, Okayama 700, Japan

ABSTRACT

Histamine (HA) and tele-methylhistamine (t-MH) in the central nervous system were simultaneously assayed by a method of high-performance liquid chromatography with fluorescence detection. The turnover of neuronal HA in 9 brain regions and the spinal cord of the rat, guinea pig and mouse was measured, based on the pargyline-induced t-MH accumulation. The size of neuronal HA pool in each region was estimated from the α-fluoromethylhistidine-induced decrease in the HA levels. Species differences were observed in the regional HA turnover rate as well as in the percentage of neuronal HA to the total in each region. These results suggest that the activity level of the histaminergic (HAergic) system in each brain region differs with the species. Measuring HA turnover by the simultaneous assay of HA and t-MH in the brain facilitates a pertinent analysis of the effects of drugs on the HAergic neurons.

KEYWORDS

Histamine; tele-methylhistamine; high-performance liquid chromatography; pargyline; α-fluoromethylhistidine; histamine turnover; histamine half-life; neuronal histamine; brain; species difference.

INTRODUCTION

Neurochemical, pharmacological and physiological findings indicate that histamine (HA) acts as a neurotransmitter in the brain. HA may control vegetative and neuroendocrine functions, including body fluid homeostasis, body temperature, blood pressure and prolactin release, and also mechanisms related to behavior and arousal (Schwartz, 1977; Schwartz, Pollard and Quach, 1980; Hough and Green, 1984). The presence of cell bodies of histaminergic (HAergic) neurons in the posterior hypothalamic area and the widespread distribution of HAergic fibers throughout various brain regions, including the telencephalon, diencephalon and lower brain stem, were recently demonstrated in the rat brain, using fluorescent immunohistochemical techniques (Wilcox and Seybold, 1982; Watanabe and others, 1984).

Mast cells are present in the central nervous system (CNS) of various mammals (Hough and Green, 1984). These cells may account for one of the non-neuronal HA stores in the CNS. However, there is some argument as to the contribution of mast cells to the HA levels in the mouse brain, based on the data obtained in W/W^v mice which lack mast cells (Grzanna and Shultz, 1982; Maeyama and others, 1983; Hough and others, 1984; Orr and Pace, 1984). In addition to mast cells, microvascular endothelial cells contain HA and the enzymes for its catabolism (Karnushina and others, 1980; Robinson-White and Beaven, 1982). These cells may also contribute to non-neuronal HA pools.

Studies with histidine decarboxylase inhibitors showed the presence of at least two types of HA pools with different turnover rates in the mammalian brain (Schwartz, Lampart and Rose, 1972; Dismukes and Snyder, 1974; Garbarg and others, 1980). It is evident that most neuronal HA has a more rapid turnover than mast-cell HA which has a half-life of several days (Schayer, 1952; Dismukes and Snyder, 1974; Martres, Baudry and Schwartz, 1975; Verdière, Rose and Schwartz, 1977). However, at present there is no proof that all neuronal HA has a rapid turnover or that all non-neuronal HA is in pools with a slow turnover.

The mammalian brain lacks diamine oxidase, and HA in this tissue is almost quantitatively methylated by HA-N-methyltransferase to produce tele-methylhistamine (t-MH) (Schwartz and others, 1971; Schayer and Reilly, 1973). This enzyme appears to exist in cells other than HAergic neurons (Bischoff and Korf, 1978). t-MH is oxidized by type B monoamine oxidase, resulting in the formation of tele-methylimidazole acetic acid (Waldmeier, Feldtrauer and Maitre, 1977; Hough and Domino, 1979). There seems to be no re-uptake system for HA in HAergic neurons, yet all species cannot be included here (Hough and Green, 1984). Since the HA turnover in non-neuronal pools appears to be comparatively negligible, the accumulation of t-MH by pargyline, a monoamine oxidase inhibitor, can be assumed to relate almost exclusively to the HA turnover in the neuronal pool. Thus, this accumulation serves as an index of the activity of HAergic neurons (i.e. the release of HA from these neurons).

General theoretical surveys of the basis of measurements of the turnover of neurotransmitters by isotopic and non-isotopic methods have been made by Costa and Neff (1969). Using non-isotopic methods, the HA turnover rate in the brain can be estimated by determining the rate of either HA decrease or t-MH accumulation induced by the inhibition of histidine decarboxylase and monoamine oxidase, respectively. The former method was adopted by Dismukes and Snyder (1974) and Maeyama and others (1983).

Despite the merits of t-MH as an index of the brain HA turnover, this HA metabolite was not used for HA turnover measurements until recently, because of technical difficulties in its assay. Gas chromatography-mass spectrometry (GCMS) and high-performance liquid chromatography with fluorescence detection (HPLC-FD) have made feasible sensitive and specific determinations of tissue t-MH. Hough and others (1981) developed a GCMS method for t-MH assay and this was applied to measurements of the HA turnover in the rat whole brain (Hough, Khandelwal and Green, 1982). In this study, the rate of t-MH accumulation induced by pargyline was determined.

Using HPLC-FD (Tsuruta, Kohashi and Ohkura, 1981), we simultaneously assayed brain HA and t-MH (Oishi, Nishibori and Saeki, 1983a, 1983b) and estimated the HA turnover in various CNS regions of the rat (Oishi, Nishibori and Saeki, 1984). The steady-state levels of "neuronal" HA in the respective regions were estimated from the decrement in the regional HA levels induced by α-fluoromethylhistidine (α-FMH), a suicide inhibitor of histidine decarboxylase (Kollonitsch and others, 1978). Recently, we measured the turnover rate and half-life of "neuronal" HA in CNS regions of the guinea pig and mouse (Nishibori, Oishi and Saeki, 1984). The results obtained in these experiments will be presented below and a comparison made with the values obtained in the rat.

METHODS

Materials

HA dihydrochloride was obtained from Wako Chemicals (Osaka, Japan). t-MH dihydrochloride and pros-methylhistamine dihydrochloride were from Calbiochem-Behring Corp. (San Diego, CA) and pargyline hydrochloride was from Sigma Chemical Co. (St. Louis, MO). (S)-α-FMH monohydrochloride hemihydrate was a generous gift from Dr. J. Kollonitsch of Merck Sharp & Dohme Research Laboratories (Rahway, NJ). Other chemicals used were at least of a guaranteed reagent grade.

Animals

Male Sprague-Dawley rats weighing 250-300 g, female Hartley guinea pigs weighing 400-450 g and male ddY mice weighing 25-30 g (Shizuoka Laboratory Animal Center, Hamamatsu, Japan) were housed in groups in a room controlled at 22 ± 2°C. Food and water were provided ad libitum. Pargyline and α-FMH were injected i.p. in doses of 80 mg salt and 50 mg free base/kg, respectively.

Fixation of Brain Tissue

In most experiments, whole heads of rats, guinea pigs and mice were immersed in liquid nitrogen for 5, 5 and 2 s, respectively, immediately after decapitation. The brain was quickly removed, placed on ice and dissected into 9 regions, according to the procedure of Glowinski and Iversen (1966) with a slight modification (Oishi, Nishibori and Saeki, 1983b). The spinal cord (thoracic region T1-10) was also removed immediately after decapitation and without cooling in liquid nitrogen. The tissues were homogenized with more than 5 volumes of

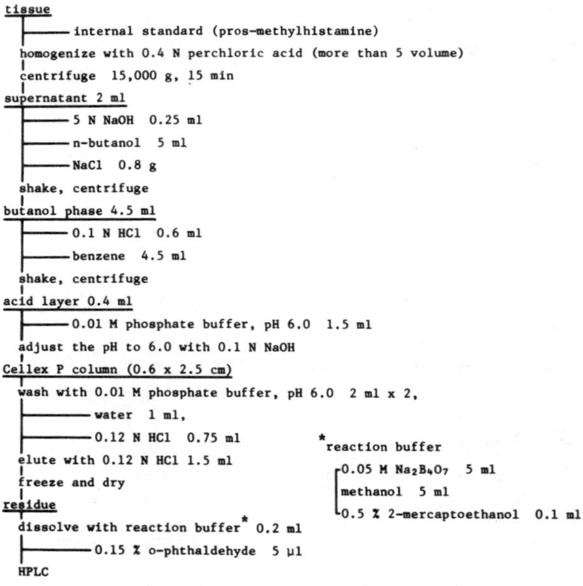

```
tissue
  ├── internal standard (pros-methylhistamine)
  homogenize with 0.4 N perchloric acid (more than 5 volume)
  centrifuge 15,000 g, 15 min
supernatant 2 ml
  ├── 5 N NaOH  0.25 ml
  ├── n-butanol  5 ml
  ├── NaCl  0.8 g
  shake, centrifuge
butanol phase 4.5 ml
  ├── 0.1 N HCl  0.6 ml
  ├── benzene  4.5 ml
  shake, centrifuge
acid layer 0.4 ml
  ├── 0.01 M phosphate buffer, pH 6.0  1.5 ml
  adjust the pH to 6.0 with 0.1 N NaOH
Cellex P column (0.6 x 2.5 cm)
  wash with 0.01 M phosphate buffer, pH 6.0  2 ml x 2,
    ├── water  1 ml,
    ├── 0.12 N HCl  0.75 ml         *reaction buffer
  elute with 0.12 N HCl 1.5 ml       ┌ 0.05 M Na₂B₄O₇  5 ml
  freeze and dry                     │ methanol  5 ml
residue                              └ 0.5 % 2-mercaptoethanol  0.1 ml
  dissolve with reaction buffer*  0.2 ml
  ├── 0.15 % o-phthaldehyde  5 μl
  HPLC
```

Fig. 1. Procedures used for simultaneous assay of HA and t-MH.

0.4 N perchloric acid with an appropriate amount (2-40 ng) of pros-methylhistamine as an internal standard. The homogenate was frozen and stored at -20°C until assay.

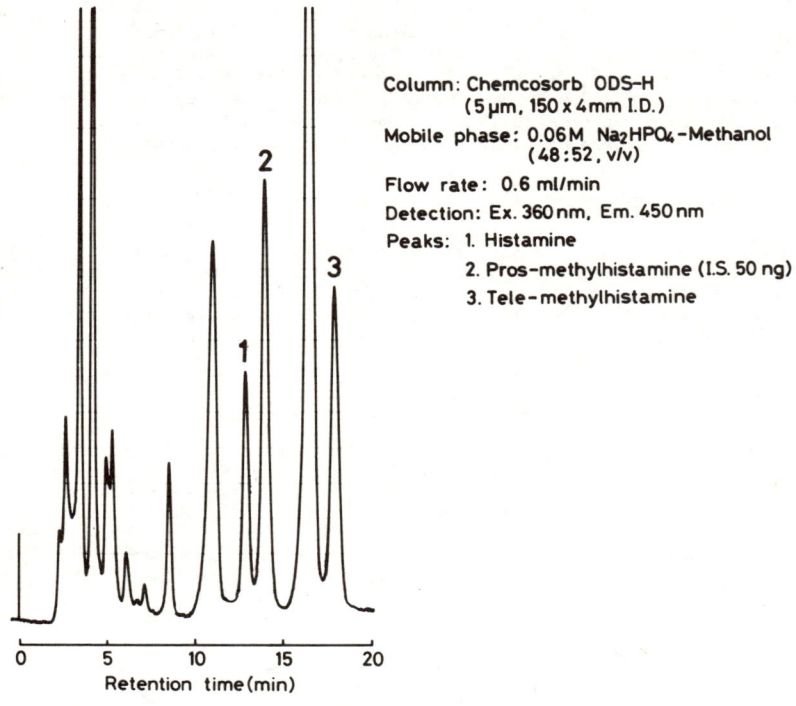

Fig. 2. Chromatogram of a mouse whole brain sample (excluding the cerebellum) obtained by HPLC-FD.

The influence of the method of fixation of brain tissue on the HA and t-MH levels was studied, as shown in Fig. 3. In these experiments, rats were killed by decapitation, whole body or focused microwave irradiation or immersion in liquid nitrogen. The condition of microwave irradiation and immersion in liquid nitrogen, and the time from killing the rat to placing the brain tissue in the 0.4 N perchloric acid solution are shown at the bottom of Fig. 3. The bodies of rats were left at room temperature until removal of the brain.

Determination of HA and t-MH

The HA and t-MH were simultaneously determined by a slight modification of the method of Tsuruta, Kohashi and Ohkura (1981) (Fig. 1). In brief, after centrifugation of the homogenate, these amines were extracted into n-butanol under NaCl-saturated alkaline conditions and transferred back to 0.1 N HCl by shaking with benzene. After adjusting the pH to 6.0, the HCl extracts were applied to Cellex-P columns. The columns were washed successively with 0.01 M phosphate buffer (pH 6.0) and water. The amines were eluted with 0.12 N HCl.[1] The amines eluted and lyophilized were subjected to the reaction with o-phthalaldehyde at pH 10.0 in the presence of 2-mercaptoethanol and fluorophores formed were injected onto HPLC. The HPLC-FD system was composed of a LC-3A pump (Shimadzu, Kyoto, Japan), a RF-530 fluorescence spectromonitor (Shimadzu) and a reserved phase column (150 × 4.0 mm I.D.) packed with Chemcosorb ODS-H (5 μm, spherical form; Chemco Scientific Co., Osaka, Japan) instead of LiChrosorb RP-18 (E. Merck, Darmstadt) as used in the original method.[2] The chromatogram of a mouse whole brain sample (excluding the cerebellum) obtained using our method is shown in Fig. 2.

Determination of the Percentage of "Neuronal" HA in Each Brain Region

The regional HA levels in the mammalian CNS were determined 4 hr after the treatment with α-FMH or saline. The percentage of rapidly depletable HA to the total in each brain region was calculated from the decrease in the HA levels

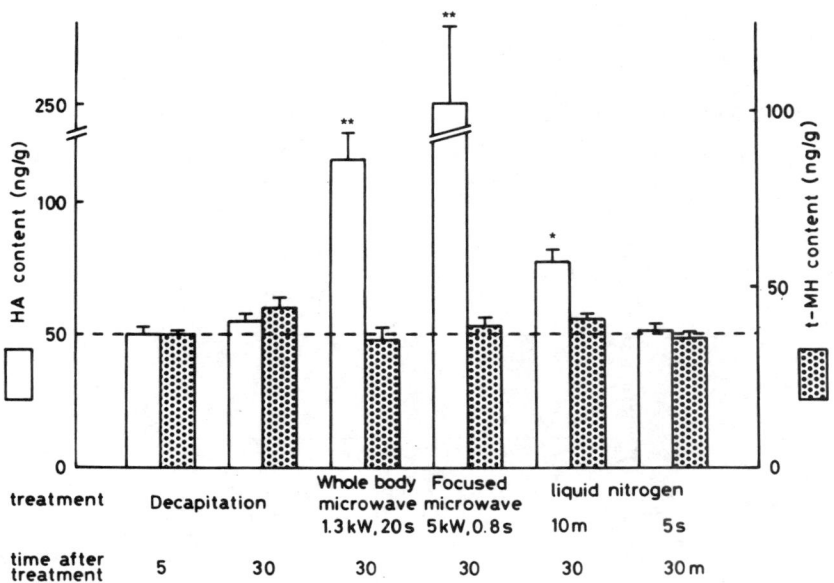

Fig. 3. HA and t-MH contents of the rat whole brain treated using various procedures. Each value represents the mean ± S.E.M. of 4-6 animals. Time in minute (m) or second (s). $^*p < 0.01$, $^{**}p < 0.001$ as compared with the corresponding value in the decapitation group (Student's t-test).

---

[1] According to the lot of Cellex-P, slight modifications from the values shown in Fig. 1 of the volume of each washing or eluting solution were occasionally necessary.

[2] According to delicate differences in the packed condition of each column, slight modifications of the ratio of 2 components of the mobile phase were occasionally necessary.

induced by α-FMH (Oishi, Nishibori and Saeki, 1984). Since the accumulation of t-MH during 4 hr after pargyline treatment was almost completely inhibited by the pretreatment with α-FMH (Oishi, Nishibori and Saeki, 1984), we tentatively assumed that rapidly depletable HA represents neuronal HA.

Estimation of Regional HA Turnover Rate

The HA methylation rate was estimated from the accumulation of t-MH during 2 (in guinea pigs and mice) or 4 (in rats) hr after pargyline treatment (see RESULTS). The HA turnover rate was assumed to be equal to the methylation rate. The "neuronal" HA content of each brain region was calculated from the regional total HA content and the percentage of rapidly depletable HA determined in the separate experiments. According to a one-compartment open-model (Costa and Neff, 1969), the rate constant (k) for neuronal HA methylation in each brain region was calculated as the t-MH accumulation rate (nmol/g·hr) divided by the neuronal HA content. The half-life (0.693/k) of neuronal HA was then estimated.

RESULTS

Relation of the Brain HA and t-MH Levels to the Methods of Tissue Fixation

When rat brains were fixed by either microwave irradiation or freezing in liquid

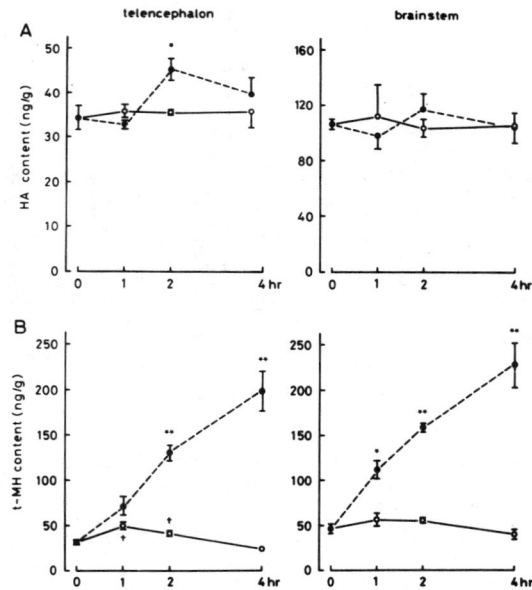

Fig. 4. Time course of effect of pargyline on the HA and t-MH contents of the telencephalon and brain stem of the rat. Pargyline (80 mg/kg, ●---●) was injected i.p. and control groups (o——o) were injected with saline. Each value represents the mean ± S.E.M. of 5 animals. *$p < 0.01$, **$p < 0.001$ as compared with the corresponding control values. †$p < 0.05$ as compared with 0 time (preinjection) value. (From Oishi, Nishibori and Saeki, 1984).

nitrogen, an erroneous increase in the HA levels was observed (Fig. 3).

Time Course of the Pargyline-Induced t-MH Accumulation in the Brain

The t-MH levels in both the telencephalon and brain stem of rats increased almost linearly up to 4 hr after pargyline treatment (Fig. 4). This made a striking contrast with the effect of pargyline on the HA levels. The whole brain t-MH levels in both guinea pigs and mice increased almost linearly up to 2 hr after pargyline treatment, and further increases in the t-MH levels thereafter were nil.

TABLE 1 Effect of Pargyline and α-FMH on the HA Levels in Various Brain Regions of the Guinea Pig and Mouse

	HA (ng/g)		
	Saline	Pargyline	α-FMH
Guinea-pig			
Cerebral cortex	25.5 ± 0.7	31.1 ± 3.0	11.4 ± 0.3^c
Hippocampus	30.3 ± 3.3	31.6 ± 4.5	9.0 ± 1.0^b
Amygdala	43.3 ± 2.4	51.2 ± 2.5	13.6 ± 0.8^c
Striatum	21.0 ± 1.9	29.4 ± 1.2^b	7.4 ± 0.7^c
Thalamus	45.8 ± 4.3	47.8 ± 6.6	18.5 ± 1.7^c
Hypothalamus	122.6 ± 13.1	119.4 ± 17.7	28.9 ± 4.9^c
Midbrain	25.4 ± 4.1	33.1 ± 2.7	8.3 ± 1.3^b
Pons- medulla oblongata	22.3 ± 1.3	21.4 ± 2.0	11.6 ± 0.7^c
Cerebellum	12.2 ± 1.0	11.1 ± 2.1	8.5 ± 0.7^b
Spinal cord	50.4 ± 7.7	58.9 ± 7.3	47.9 ± 5.9
Mouse			
Cerebral cortex	44.9 ± 4.4	46.0 ± 3.7	9.0 ± 0.9^c
Hippocampus	27.1 ± 2.9	33.4 ± 4.0	11.0 ± 1.8^c
Amygdala	41.9 ± 3.9	54.5 ± 3.1^a	13.9 ± 1.3^c
Striatum	33.2 ± 5.0	28.0 ± 4.2	10.9 ± 1.6^b
Thalamus	41.9 ± 4.4	42.4 ± 4.3	26.7 ± 2.8^a
Hypothalamus	91.8 ± 13.0	134.3 ± 16.5	13.6 ± 1.9^c
Midbrain	71.2 ± 5.6	76.3 ± 10.3	42.4 ± 7.2^b
Pons- medulla oblongata	28.4 ± 4.9	27.5 ± 3.3	19.0 ± 3.3
Cerebellum	11.3 ± 3.4	16.3 ± 3.8	11.9 ± 1.8
Spinal cord	39.6 ± 5.1	37.0 ± 6.1	36.2 ± 4.6

The animals were killed 2 hr after the intraperitoneal injection of saline or pargyline hydrochloride (80 mg/kg) and 4 hr after α-FMH (50 mg/kg). Each value represents the mean ± S.E.M. of 4-8 experiments. Significantly different from the corresponding saline control, $^a p < 0.05$; $^b p < 0.01$; $^c p < 0.001$. (From Nishibori, Oishi and Saeki, 1984).

Effects of Pargyline and α-FMH on the HA and t-MH Levels in Various CNS Regions of the Rat, Guinea Pig and Mouse

When examined 4 hr after the administration, pargyline significantly increased the t-MH levels in all CNS regions of rats except for the spinal cord, as compared with the levels in the saline treated control group (Oishi, Nishibori and Saeki, 1984). In this experiment, no significant difference in the HA levels in any region was observed between the saline- and pargyline-treated rats.

TABLE 2 Effect of Pargyline and α-FMH on the t-MH Levels in Various Brain Regions of the Guinea Pig and Mouse

	t-MH (ng/g)		
	Saline	Pargyline	α-FMH
Guinea-pig			
Cerebral cortex	54.9 ± 2.2	108.8 ± 12.0[b]	18.2 ± 2.1[c]
Hippocampus	114.6 ± 5.9	185.1 ± 12.4[c]	69.9 ± 11.5[a]
Amygdala	98.1 ± 7.4	185.4 ± 7.8[c]	50.5 ± 3.8[c]
Striatum	32.6 ± 2.7	84.1 ± 5.0[c]	6.6 ± 0.6[c]
Thalamus	88.5 ± 8.9	158.2 ± 16.8[b]	14.7 ± 1.5[c]
Hypothalamus	135.1 ± 19.9	236.1 ± 22.7[a]	44.5 ± 8.0[b]
Midbrain	29.6 ± 7.5	75.3 ± 8.7[b]	5.2 ± 1.3[a]
Pons-medulla oblongata	31.0 ± 3.8	71.5 ± 11.6[a]	9.1 ± 1.1[c]
Cerebellum	7.8 ± 1.4	21.2 ± 1.3[c]	3.7 ± 0.7[a]
Spinal cord	15.5 ± 2.4	20.2 ± 2.8	18.7 ± 1.5
Mouse			
Cerebral cortex	84.8 ± 5.7	173.6 ± 7.1[c]	26.3 ± 4.3[c]
Hippocampus	54.4 ± 6.7	107.5 ± 6.5[c]	18.1 ± 2.2[c]
Amygdala	123.3 ± 11.1	246.6 ± 9.6[c]	46.9 ± 4.2[c]
Striatum	58.5 ± 8.9	141.3 ± 10.6[c]	14.7 ± 2.2[b]
Thalamus	53.0 ± 11.1	162.5 ± 7.7[c]	22.1 ± 4.6[a]
Hypothalamus	163.9 ± 19.1	380.9 ± 30.9[c]	34.7 ± 4.1[c]
Midbrain	88.9 ± 12.4	200.4 ± 18.7[c]	17.5 ± 2.4[c]
Pons-medulla oblongata	34.1 ± 4.4	101.2 ± 11.2[c]	22.7 ± 2.9[a]
Cerebellum	10.4 ± 1.9	38.5 ± 6.3[b]	4.9 ± 0.8[a]
Spinal cord	32.9 ± 5.5	31.6 ± 10.0	28.9 ± 4.7

The same experiments as shown in Table 1. (From Nishibori, Oishi and Saeki, 1984).

Pargyline also significantly increased the t-MH levels in all CNS regions except for the spinal cord in both guinea pigs and mice. Except for the striatum of guinea pigs and the amygdala of mice, pargyline had no significant effect on the CNS HA levels in these species (Tables 1 and 2).

When tested 4 hr after the administration, α-FMH decreased both the HA and t-MH levels in most CNS regions of guinea pigs and mice (Tables 1 and 2). No significant changes in the HA and t-MH levels were observed in the spinal cord after α-FMH treatment. Similar results with α-FMH were obtained in rats (Oishi, Nishibori and Saeki, 1984).

Regional Differences in the HA Turnover Rate, the Percentage of Neuronal HA to the Total and the Half-Life of Neuronal HA in the CNS of the Rat, Guinea Pig and Mouse

The regional HA turnover rate was the highest in the hypothalamus in the 3 species studied. However, the rank order of the turnover rate in other brain regions varied with the individual species (Table 3).

Marked species differences were observed in the percentages of neuronal HA to the total in various brain regions. Except for the cerebral cortex and the pons-medulla oblongata, the percentages of neuronal HA in all regions of the guinea-

TABLE 3 Regional HA Turnover Rate, Percentage of Neuronal HA to the Total and Half-Life of Neuronal HA in the Guinea Pig, Mouse and Rat Brain

	Turnover rate (nmol/g·hr)	% of neuronal HA	Half-life (min)
Rat[a]			
Cerebral cortex	0.38	62.8	23.4
Hippocampus	0.19	44.9	14.1
Amygdala	0.35	48.4	19.0
Striatum	0.64	40.9	7.7
Thalamus	0.50	26.9	42.3
Hypothalamus	0.87	26.1	56.6
Midbrain	0.34	36.7	15.8
Pons- medulla oblongata	0.18	54.7	24.5
Cerebellum	0.02	15.9	10.2
Guinea pig[b]			
Cerebral cortex	0.22	55.2	24.4
Hippocampus	0.28	70.3	28.3
Amygdala	0.35	68.6	31.9
Striatum	0.21	64.6	24.8
Thalamus	0.28	59.6	36.7
Hypothalamus	0.40	76.4	86.9
Midbrain	0.18	67.2	35.1
Pons- medulla oblongata	0.16	48.0	24.8
Cerebellum	0.05	30.6	25.9
Mouse[b]			
Cerebral cortex	0.36	80.0	37.9
Hippocampus	0.21	59.3	28.4
Amygdala	0.49	66.8	21.2
Striatum	0.33	67.1	25.3
Thalamus	0.44	36.2	13.0
Hypothalamus	0.87	85.2	33.7
Midbrain	0.45	40.4	24.2
Pons- medulla oblongata	0.27	33.1	13.1
Cerebellum	0.11	—	—

[a]From Oishi, Nishibori and Saeki (1984). [b]From Nishibori, Oishi and Saeki (1984).

pig and the mouse brain were larger than the corresponding values in the rat brain. The difference was particularly marked in the hypothalamus.

Species differences were also observed in the regional half-life values for neuronal HA in the brain of these mammals. Compared with the guinea pig and the rat brain, the regional difference in the half-life of neuronal HA was less marked in the mouse brain, and the hypothalamus showed a half-life value similar to values obtained in other brain regions. In the rat and the guinea pig, the half-life of neuronal HA was the longest in the hypothalamus. In the guinea pig, the half-life value was notably larger in the hypothalamus than in other regions.

DISCUSSION

Since neuronal HA in the brain has a much more rapid turnover than most other amine neurotransmitters such as norepinephrine and dopamine (Bacopoulos and Bhatnagar, 1977), a rapid fixation of brain tissue was considered to be important to accurately determine the HA and t-MH levels. At present, the rapid cooling method in which the whole head of the animal is immersed in liquid nitrogen for several seconds seems to be the most appropriate. The fixation of brain by microwave irradiation or freezing in liquid nitrogen, although accomplished rapidly, cannot be recommended because of an erroneous increase in the HA levels. Other groups also observed similar phenomena in microwave-irradiated brains (e.g. Hough and Domino, 1977). As suggested by Oishi, Nishibori and Saeki (1983a), it is probable that freezing as well as microwave irradiation cause disintegration of mast cells in tissues surrounding the brain and brain tissue becomes contaminated with HA which leaks from the disrupted cells. Although the rapid "cooling" in liquid nitrogen may be required for the fixation of brain tissue in some special cases, a procedure comprising rapid removal of the brain and its subsequent cooling on ice seems to be adequate in most cases.

The curves for the t-MH accumulation in the telencephalon and brain stem of the rat were almost linear up to 4 hr after pargyline treatment. This is consistent with the result reported by Hough, Khandelwal and Green (1982) in the rat whole brain. However, the t-MH levels in the guinea pig and mouse whole brain increased almost linearly up to 2 hr after pargyline treatment. Due to such a species difference in the time course of the pargyline-induced t-MH accumulation, the HA methylation rate (HA turnover rate) in the rat brain was estimated from the accumulation during 4 hr after pargyline treatment, while that in the guinea-pig and mouse brain was estimated for 2 hr.

Despite the different assay methods for t-MH, the values for the HA turnover rate in various brain regions of the rat obtained in our laboratory (Oishi, Nishibori and Saeki, 1984) and those reported by Hough, Khandelwal and Green (1984) are very close. The values estimated from the t-MH accumulation approximate the values obtained in the rat whole brain by Pollard, Bischoff and Schwartz (1974), using an isotopic method. These results indicate the validity of the accumulation of endogenous t-MH, as a means to estimate the HA turnover in the brain. The regional HA turnover rate determined in our experiments paralleled the regional histidine decarboxylase activity (Schwartz, Lampart and Rose, 1970; Pollard, Bischoff and Schwartz, 1974; Garbarg and others, 1980) in the rank order.

To estimate regional half-life values for neuronal HA, we calculated the percentages of "neuronal" HA content to the total in various brain regions and the spinal cord, based on the α-FMH-induced decrease in the HA levels in the respective regions. As already indicated, our method may give a mere approximation of the size of neuronal HA pool in each CNS region. However, at present there appears to be no other method which is more appropriate to distinguish neuronal from non-neuronal HA. The regional half-life values for "neuronal" HA obtained by Oishi, Nishibori and Saeki (1984) in the rat brain are somewhat different from the values reported by Hough, Khandelwal and Green (1984), depending on the regions studied. This is probably because they assumed that the brain HA was in a single pool, when calculating the HA half-life. The HA half-life in the rat and the mouse whole brain was estimated by Pollard, Bischoff and Schwartz (1974) and Verdière, Rose, and Schwartz (1977), respectively, using an isotopic method. The values obtained in these studies are in good agreement with the present results, when corrected for the percentage of neuronal HA.

The half-life of neuronal HA may indicate the activity level (i.e. the rate of HA release) of individual HAergic fibers. The half-life was the longest in the hypothalamus in the rat and guinea pig and it was the second longest in this region in the mouse. The HAergic cell bodies are localized in the posterior hypothalamus in the rat (Wilcox and Seybold, 1982; Watanabe and others, 1984). Thus, in this region the rate of HA release may be lower than the rate of its synthesis, as postulated by Hough, Khandelwal and Green (1984).

The results of our experiments show that there are species differences in the regional HA turnover rate as well as in the proportion of neuronal to non-neuronal HA in each brain region. It is also suggested that the HA in the spinal cord of these animals is present largely, if not exclusively, in non-neuronal pool(s). Although the physiological functions of the HAergic system are still poorly understood, the species differences in the regional HA turnover rate and the regional half-life values for neuronal HA may reflect differences in the function of the HAergic system in each brain region of these species.

Using HPLC-FD, we most recently found that an acute administration of Δ^9-tetrahydrocannabinol decreases and that of morphine increases the turnover of neuronal HA in the mouse and rat brain. All these findings indicate that measurement of the brain HA turnover by simultaneously assaying HA and t-MH is useful for the study of effects of drug on the HAergic neurons in the brain.

REFERENCES

Bacopoulos, N. G., and R. K. Bhatnagar (1977). Correlation between tyrosine hydroxylase activity and catecholamine concentration or turnover in brain regions. J. Neurochem., 29, 639-643.
Bischoff, S., and J. Korf (1978). Different localization of histidine decarboxylase and histamine-N-methyltransferase in the rat brain. Brain Res., 141, 375-379.
Costa, E., and N. H. Neff (1969). Importance of turnover rate measurements to elucidate the function of neuronal monoamines. Topics mednl. Chem., 2, 65-95.
Dismukes, K., and S. H. Snyder (1974). Histamine turnover in rat brain. Brain Res., 78, 467-481.
Garbarg, M., G. Barbin, E. Rodergas, and J. C. Schwartz (1980). Inhibition of histamine synthesis in brain by α-fluoromethylhistidine, a new irreversible inhibitor: In vitro and in vivo studies. J. Neurochem., 35, 1045-1052.
Glowinski, J., and L. L. Iversen (1966). Regional studies of catecholamines in the rat brain — I. J. Neurochem., 13, 655-669.
Grzanna, R., and L. D. Schultz (1982). The contribution of mast cells to the histamine content of the central nervous system: A regional analysis. Life Sci. 30, 1959-1964.
Hough, L. B., and E. F. Domino (1977). Elevation of rat brain histamine content after focussed microwave irradiation. J. Neurochem., 29, 199-204.
Hough, L. B., and E. F. Domino (1979). Tele-methylhistamine oxidation by type B monoamine oxidase. J. Pharmac. exp. Ther., 208, 422-428.
Hough, L. B., and J. P. Green (1984). Histamine and its receptors in the nervous system. In Lajtha, A. (Ed.), Handbook of Neurochemistry, Vol. 6, Plenum Press, New York, pp. 145-211.
Hough, L. B., J. K. Khandelwal, R. C. Goldschmidt, M. Diomande, and S. D. Glick (1984). Normal levels of histamine and tele-methylhistamine in mast cell-deficient mouse brain. Brain Res., 292, 133-138.
Hough, L. B., J. K. Khandelwal, and J. P. Green (1982). Effects of pargyline on tele-methylhistamine and histamine in rat brain. Biochem. Pharmac., 31, 4074-4076.
Hough, L. B., J. K. Khandelwal, and J. P. Green (1984). Histamine turnover in regions of rat brain. Brain Res., 291, 103-109.
Hough, L. B., J. K. Khandelwal, A. Morrishow, and J. P. Green (1981). An improved GC-MS method to measure tele-methylhistamine. J. Pharmac. Meth., 5, 143-148.
Karnushina, I. L., J. M. Palacios, G. Barbin, E. Dux, F. Joó, and J. C. Schwartz (1980). Studies on a capillary-rich fraction isolated from brain: Histamine components and characterization of the histamine receptors linked to adenylate cyclase. J. Neurochem., 34, 1201-1208.
Kollonitsch, J., A. A. Patchett, S. Marburg, A. L. Maycock, L. M. Perkins, G. A. Doldouras, D. E. Duggan, and S. D. Aster (1978). Selective inhibitors of biosynthesis of aminergic neurotransmitters. Nature, 274, 906-908.

Maeyama, K., T. Watanabe, A. Yamatodani, Y. Taguchi, H. Kambe, and H. Wada (1983). Effect of α-fluoromethylhistidine on the histamine content of the brain of W/W^v mice devoid of mast cells: Turnover of brain histamine. J. Neurochem., 41, 128-134.

Martres, M. P., M. Baudry, and J. C. Schwartz (1975). Histamine synthesis in the developing rat brain: Evidence of a multiple compartmentation. Brain Res., 83, 261-275.

Nishibori, M., R. Oishi, and K. Saeki (1984). Histamine turnover in the brain of different mammalian species: Implications for neuronal histamine half-life. J. Neurochem., in press.

Oishi, R., M. Nishibori, and K. Saeki (1983a). The simultaneous assay of histamine and tele-methylhistamine in the rat brain after microwave irradiation and immersion in liquid nitrogen: contamination by extraencephalic mast-cell histamine. Brain Res., 261, 180-183.

Oishi, R., M. Nishibori, and K. Saeki (1983b). Regional distribution of histamine and tele-methylhistamine in the rat, mouse and guinea-pig brain. Brain Res., 280, 172-175.

Oishi, R., M. Nishibori, and K. Saeki (1984). Regional differences in the turnover of neuronal histamine in the rat brain. Life Sci., 34, 691-699.

Orr, E. L., and K. R. Pace (1984). The significance of mast cells as a source of histamine in the mouse brain. J. Neurochem., 42, 727-732.

Pollard, H., S. Bischoff, and J. C. Schwartz (1974). Turnover of histamine in rat brain and its decrease under barbiturate anesthesia. J. Pharmac. exp. Ther., 190, 88-99.

Robinson-White, A., and M. A. Beaven (1982). Presence of histamine and histamine-metabolizing enzyme in rat and guinea-pig microvascular endothelial cells. J. Pharmac. exp. Ther., 223, 440-445.

Schayer, R. W. (1952). Biogenesis of histamine. J. biol. Chem., 199, 245-250.

Schayer, R. W., and M. A. Reilly (1973). Formation and fate of histamine in rat and mouse brain. J. Pharmac. exp. Ther., 184, 33-40.

Schwartz, J. C. (1977). Histaminergic mechanisms in brain. A. Rev. Pharmac. Toxic., 17, 325-339.

Schwartz, J. C., C. Lampart, and C. Rose (1970). Properties and regional distribution of histidine decarboxylase in rat brain. J. Neurochem., 17, 1527-1534.

Schwartz, J. C., C. Lampart, and C. Rose (1972). Histamine formation in rat brain in vivo: Effects of histidine loads. J. Neurochem., 19, 801-810.

Schwartz, J. C., H. Pollard, S. Bischoff, M. C. Rehault, and M. Verdière-Sahuque (1971). Catabolism of ^{3}H-histamine in the rat brain after intracisternal administration. Eur. J. Pharmac., 16, 326-335.

Schwartz, J. C., H. Pollard, and T. T. Quach (1980). Histamine as a neurotransmitter in mammalian brain: Neurochemical evidence. J. Neurochem., 35, 26-33.

Tsuruta, Y., K. Kohashi, and Y. Ohkura (1981). Simultaneous determination of histamine and N^T-methylhistamine in human urine and rat brain by high-performance liquid chromatography with fluorescence detection. J. Chromatogr., 224, 105-110.

Verdière, M., C. Rose and J. C. Schwartz (1977). Turnover of cerebral histamine in a stressful situation. Brain Res., 129, 107-119.

Waldmeier, P. C., J. J. Feldtrauer, and L. Maitre (1977). Methylhistamine: Evidence for selective deamination by MAO type B in the rat brain in vivo. J. Neurochem., 29, 785-790.

Watanabe, T., Y. Taguchi, S. Shiosaka, J. Tanaka, H. Kubota, Y. Terano., M. Tohyama, and H. Wada (1984). Distribution of the histaminergic neuron system in the central nervous system of rats; A fluorescent immunohistochemical analysis with histidine decarboxylase as a marker. Brain Res., 295, 13-25.

Wilcox, B. J. and V. S. Seybold (1982). Localization of neuronal histamine in rat brain. Neurosci. Lett., 29, 105-110.

HISTAMINE TURNOVER IN REGIONS OF RAT BRAIN

J. P. Green and J. K. Khandelwal

Department of Pharmacology, Mount Sinai School of Medicine, Of the City University of New York, New York, NY 10029, USA

ABSTRACT

Turnover rates of histamine varied almost fifty-fold in different regions of rat brain, hypothalamus having the highest. The half-lives of histamine in the caudate nucleus and cortex were very brief, i.e., 11 min. The gas chromatographic-mass spectrometer method that is described can quantify as little as 1 ng of tele-methylhistamine and tele-methylimidazoleacetic acid in the same sample of brain or body fluid. The regional distribution in brain of these metabolites is similar to that of histamine, and the regional turnover rates of histamine correlate with the regional steady-state concentrations of histamine. The two metabolites were also measured in human cerebrospinal fluid, plasma and urine. pros-Methylhistamine could not be detected in either brain or the body fluids, but pros-methylimidazoleacetic acid was present.

KEYWORDS

Turnover, brain, histamine, tele-methylhistamine, tele-methylimidazoleacetic acid, pros-methylimidazoleacetic acid, gas chromatography-mass spectrometry.

INTRODUCTION

The hypothesis that histamine functions in brain (see Green, 1964) has been amply supported by evidence garnered over the past twenty years, and no evidence has been published to falsify the hypothesis (Garbarg and co-workers, 1980; Green, 1983; Green, Johnson and Weinstein, 1983; Hough and Green, 1984; Schwartz and co-workers, 1981, 1982): histamine has a non-uniform regional distribution in brain; it is stored in subcellular particles containing nerve endings; brain contains the enzyme, histidine decarboxylase, that synthesizes histamine, and the enzyme is specific for histidine; the enzyme, histamine methyltransferase, that metabolizes histamine and has no other known endogenous substrate is present in brain; lesions in brain produce a fall in the activity of the synthesizing enzyme distal to the lesions; histamine is released from brain slices by potassium in a calcium-dependent process; both histamine H_1-receptors and H_2-receptors are present in brain; neurons respond to histamine both in vitro and in vivo, and the responses are reduced by antagonists of histamine in concentrations that imply interactions with histamine receptors.

[Also interesting is that psychotropic drugs of different classes interact with histamine receptors (see Green, 1983).] All these observations support the assertion that histamine is a neuromediator or neuromodulator in brain. But that assertion had to be tempered until recently with two qualifications, both resting on inadequate methods: the histaminergic system had eluded visualization; and the metabolites of endogenous histamine could not be readily quantified, a lack that precluded many experiments that could probe the hypothesis of function. Both these deficiencies have been corrected. Immunocytochemistry has shown histaminergic nerve fibers in brain (Panula, Yang, and Costa, 1984; Wahlestedt and co-workers, 1984; Watanabe and co-workers, 1984; Wilcox and Seybold, 1982) and spinal cord (Wahlestedt and co-workers, 1984), projecting from cell bodies in the hypothalamus. Methods for measuring the major histamine metabolites in brain were developed (Hough, Stetson, and Domino, 1979; Hough and co-workers, 1981; Khandelwal and co-workers, 1982; Tsuruta, Kohashi, and Ohkura, 1981), and their applications yielded results supporting the hypothesis that histamine functions in brain (Hough, Khandelwal, and Green, 1984; Khandelwal, Hough, and Green, 1982; Khandelwal and co-workers, 1982; Khandelwal, Hough, and Green, 1984; Oishi, Nishibori, and Saeki, 1984).

The major, perhaps exclusive, metabolite of histamine in brain is tele-methylhistamine (or N^τ-methylhistamine; 1-methyl-4(β-aminoethyl)-imidazole; t-MH), which is oxidatively deaminated by monoamine oxidase to tele-methylimidazoleacetic acid (or t-MIAA) (Fig. 1). t-MH had early been measured in whole guinea pig brain (Fram and Green, 1968) and urine by a procedure (Fram and Green, 1965) that was more ordeal than method and encouraged little use. Since then, gas chromatography-mass spectrometry has been used to quantify both t-MH and t-MIAA (and related acids) in brain and body fluids (see below). High-performance liquid chromatography has also been devised to measure t-MH (Tsuruta, Kohashi, and Ohkura, 1981).

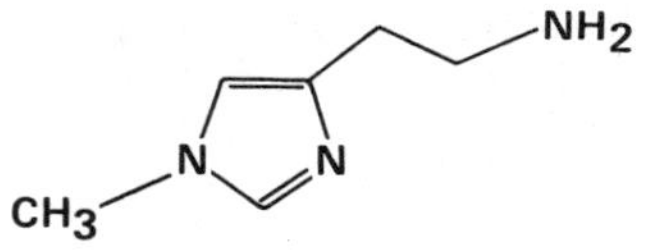

tele-**METHYLHISTAMINE**
or
N^τ-**METHLHISTAMINE**

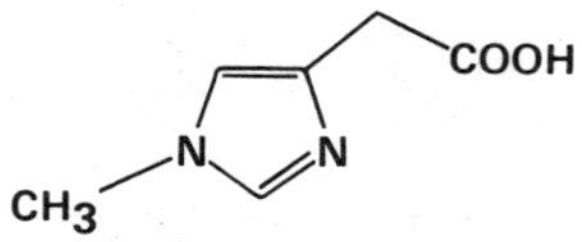

tele-**METHYLIMIDAZOLE ACETIC ACID**
or
N^τ-**METHYLIMIDAZOLE ACETIC ACID**

Fig. 1. The major metabolites of histamine in mammalian brain.

Both methods for measuring t-MH have been used to estimate the turnover of histamine in brain regions of rats. The animals were treated with pargyline, an irreversible inhibitor of monoamine oxidase, and the accumulation of t-MH was measured. The estimates of turnover are based on the assumptions that t-MH is the only major metabolite of histamine in rat brain and that t-MH derives solely from histamine in rat brain.

MEASUREMENT OF t-MH AND t-MIAA BY GAS CHROMATOGRAPHY-MASS SPECTROMETRY

A gas chromatographic-mass spectrometric (gc-ms) method to measure t-MH (Hough, Stetson, and Domino, 1979) was improved (Hough and co-workers, 1981), and then combined (Khandelwal, Hough, and Green, 1984) with the method devised to measure t-MIAA (Khandelwal and co-workers, 1982) so that both metabolites can be measured in the same sample of tissue or body fluid. In the combined method deuterated t-MH (d_3-t-MH) and deuterated t-MIAA (d_3-t-MIAA) are used as internal standards. t-MH is separated from t-MIAA by solvent extraction and then derivatized. The fraction containing t-MIAA is subjected to the additional step of ion-exchange chromatography before derivatization. t-MH is measured as the bis-heptafluorobutyryl derivative, t-MIAA as the n-butyl ester. The specificities of the methods were shown by various pocedures, including mass ion abundance ratios and by chemical ionization mass spectra. The methods accurately quantify amounts as low as 1 ng carried through the entire procedure.

The brain is weighed and homogenized in 4 volumes of ice-cold water for 20 s (Ultra-Turrax TP 18-10), from which 1 ml of the homogenate is removed for assay. The homogenate is diluted to 2 ml with water. The homogenate is heated in a boiling water bath for 10 min, cooled and centrifuged at 49,500 x $\underline{g}$ at 4°C for 20 min. The resulting supernatant is transferred to polypropylene tubes. To the supernatant (or to 3 ml of cerebrospinal fluid, 2 ml of plasma or 0.05 ml of urine) is added 10 ng each of d_3-t-MH and d_3-t-MIAA as internal standards.

Appropriate amounts of authentic t-MIAA and t-MH, mixed with the internal standards are processed in parallel to obtain standard curves. The samples are made alkaline by adding to each ml, 0.012 ml of 1 N NaOH and 0.1 ml of 50 mM Tris-acetate buffer, pH 9.0, mixed, and shaken for 30 min with 4 ml of n-butanol-chloroform (1:1) to extract t-MH into the organic phase. All subsequent centrifugation is done with a Sorvall GLC-2 centrifuge at 5,000 rpm. After centrifugation for 10 min, the aqueous phase is transferred to a fresh tube and shaken again with another aliquot of 4 ml of the butanol-chloroform mixture. The organic extracts are pooled and analyzed for t-MH; the aqueous phase is kept for t-MIAA analysis.

About 0.5 g of anhydrous sodium sulfate powder is added to the organic extract, which is vortexed and centrifuged for 5 min. The clear upper organic phase is transferred to a conical polypropylene tube containing 0.5 ml of 0.01 N HCl and 4 ml of heptane. After mechanical shaking for 5 min and centrifugation for 5 min, the organic phase is discarded by aspiration. The acidic aqueous phase is transferred to a silanized 1 ml reactivial. The samples are dried by vacuum centrifugation, and the residue analyzed for t-MH (see below).

For analysis of t-MIAA, the aqueous phase left behind after t-MH extraction is first subjected to ion-exchange chromatography on columns (Isolab, polypropylene QS-Q; internal diameter 1 cm) containing 2 ml of an ion exchange resin (acetate form, analytical grade Bio-Rad AG 1-X4 100-200 mesh). The columns are washed with 4 ml of deionized water, and the acids eluted by addition of 4 ml of 0.5 N acetic acid. To the eluate in 5-ml silanized screw cap vials is added 0.1 ml of 0.01 N HCl; the solution is taken to dryness at room temperature by vacuum centrifugation (Savant Instruments, Model SVC-100). The residue is rinsed with 0.2 ml of CH_3OH, transferred to 1-ml silanized reaction vials and dried.

To reactivials containing t-MH are added 25 ul toluene, 5 ul pyridine, 15 ul heptafluorobutyric anhydride; the vials are mixed by vortex. The vials exhibit two phases at this time; the reaction is allowed to proceed at room temperature for 10 min with intermittent mixing. The reaction is stopped by the addition of 0.2 ml saturated Tris buffer pH 8.0, and the vials are mixed until two clear layers are obtained. After centrifugation, the aqueous phases are removed and discarded. The vials are recapped, mixed, and centrifuged; the small aqueous phase that results is also discarded. Each vial receives a small amount of anhydrous granular Na_2SO_4 and is mixed and centrifuged. GC-MS analysis is carried out on a 6 ft by 2 mm silanized glass column containing 3% Poly 1-110 on Gas Chrom Q, 80-100 mesh (Applied Sci.) with helium (20 ml/min) as carrier at 200° C. The major fragment ions of the derivative are m/e 135 (base peak), m/e 291, and m/e 304 and the molecular ion is m/e 517. For quantification, m/e 304 of the derivative of endogenous or authentic t-MH is monitored along with m/e 307 of the derivative of the internal standard, d_3-t-MH.

For derivatization of t-MIAA, 0.1 ml of boron trifluoride-butanol is added to each vial. The mixture is vortexed and centrifuged. Samples are heated in a sand-bath at 90° C for 90 min with intermittent mixing and then cooled on ice. Each vial then receives 0.4 ml of toluene and 0.3 ml of saturated unbuffered Tris base, and the samples are vortexed and centrifuged for 1 min. After removal of the lower aqueous phase, 0.2 ml of water is added. The samples are again vortexed and centrifuged for 1 min each and the aqueous phase discarded. To each is added 0.1 ml of 0.1 N HCl. Samples are vortexed and centrifuged for 1 min, and the upper organic phase is aspirated. To the aqueous phase, 0.05 ml each of chloroform and unbuffered saturated Tris base are added, vortexed, and centrifuged for 1 min each. After removal of the upper aqueous phase, about 20 mg of anhydrous Na_2SO_4 are added to the chloroform layer. GC-MS analysis is carried out on a 3 foot by 2-mm silanized glass column containing mixed phase of 1% Poly A-135 and 2% Silar 5CP on Gas-chrom Q, 100-120 mesh with helium, 30 ml/min, as carrier gas at 200° C. The major fragment ions of the derivative are m/e 95 (base peak) and m/e 122, and the molecular ion is m/e 196. For quantification, m/e 95 of the derivative of endogenous or authentic t-MIAA (or p-MIAA) is monitored along with m/e 98 of the derivative of the internal standard, d_3-t-MIAA.

Electron impact (70 eV electron energy, 0.4 mA emission) and isobutane chemical ionization mass spectra are obtained on a Hewlett-Packard 5930A combined GC-MS system with a dual ion source. A Hewlett-Packard 5933A data system linked to a Tektronix display terminal (Model 4012) equipped with a hard copy unit (Model 4610) was used to acquire, reduce, and process the data including the determination of peak areas of the selected ion scans.

RESULTS AND DISCUSSION

TABLE 1 Concentration of t-MH, t-MIAA and p-MIAA in Whole Rat Brain and in Human Body Fluids

Substances	Brain (pmol/g)	CSF (pmol/ml)	Plasma (pmol/ml)	Urine (nmol/mg creatinine)
t-MH	445.8[a]	2.2[b]	13.4[b]	0.9[b]
t-MIAA[c]	373.2	22.8	84.6	20.8
p-MIAA[c]	110.3	80.8	73.6	73.0

[a]Hough and co-workers (1982)
[b]Khandelwal, Hough, and Green (1982)
[c]Khandelwal and co-workers (1982)

Table 1 shows the levels of t-MH in whole rat brain and human body fluids.

The method also measures pros-methylhistamine (i.e., p-MH) which yields the same fragment ions as does t-MH. No p-MH was detected in rat brain or human CSF, plasma or urine, even after treating rats with pargyline (Hough, Khandelwal, and Green, 1982, 1984).

Table 1 shows the concentrations of t-MIAA in rat brain and human fluids.

pros-Methylimidazoleacetic acid (i.e., p-MIAA), imidazoleacetic acid (i.e., IAA) and urocanic acid (molecular ion m/e 194) are also quantified by this method. The derivative of p-MIAA has the same fragment ions as the derivative of t-MIAA except lacking m/e 122. p-MIAA is found in rat brain and in human fluids (Table 1); its origins are obscure.

The derivative of IAA has a base peak of m/e 81; the molecular ion is 182. No IAA could be detected in rat brain, but it is present in human urine.

Treatment of rats with probenecid, 200 mg/kg of body weight, a dose that elevates brain levels of homovanillic acid and 5-hydroxyindoleacetic acid (Wilk, Watson, and Travis, 1975), did not raise brain levels of either t-MIAA or p-MIAA (Khandelwal, Hough, and Green, 1984); the finding on t-MIAA is in agreement with observations made after intracisternal injections of radioactive histamine (Schwartz and co-workers, 1971). The levels of 3, 4-dihydroxyphenylacetic acid in brain were similarly refractive to treatment with probenecid (Wilk, Watson, and Travis, 1975).

As shown in Table 2, the regional distribution of t-MH in rat brain is highly correlated with the distribution of both histamine (Hough and Domino, 1979a; Hough and co-workers, 1981; Hough, Khandelwal, and Green, 1984) and t-MIAA (Khandelwal, Hough, and Green, 1984).

TABLE 2 Regional Distribution of Histamine, Its Metabolites, and Histidine

Region	Histamine[a] (ng/g)	Histidine[a] (ng/g)	t-MH[b] (ng/g)	t-MIAA[c] (ng/g)
Cerebellum	26	19	11	21
Medulla-pons	25	16	10	56
Thalamus-midbrain	75	14	35	154
Hypothalamus	209	25	179	309
Striatum	56	20	36	132
Hippocampus	50	22	24	60
Cerebral cortex	39	9	30	74
Spinal cord	59[d]		6[e]	

[a]Taylor and Snyder (1972); a similar distribution was found by others, e.g., Schwartz and co-workers (1981) and Hough, Khandelwal, and Green (1984)
[b]Hough and Domino (1979a); a similar distribution was found by Hough and co-workers (1981), Hough, Khandelwal, and Green (1984), and Oishi, Nishibori and Saeki (1983)
[c]Khandelwal, Hough, and Green (1984)
[d]Schwartz and co-workers (1981)
[e]Oishi, Nishibori and Saeki (1983)

Whereas the regional distribution of histamine in brains of all mammalian species is very similar (see Green, 1970; Green, Johnson, and Weinstein, 1983; Oishi, Nishibori, and Saeki, 1983), the regional distribution of t-MH shows some variation among species as measured by HPLC (Oishi, Nishibori, and Saeki,

1983). Mouse and guinea pig resemble the rat in most respects, all showing high concentrations in the hypothalamus, but the guinea pig is distinguished by having in the hippocampus a concentration of t-MH about equal to that in hypothalamus (Oishi, Nishibori, and Saeki, 1983). It may be of interest to note that these slight differences among the species examined so far are in marked contrast to the great differences among species in the regional distribution of the histamine H_1-receptor, e.g., in rat and guinea pig (Chang, Tran, and Snyder, 1979; Hill and Young, 1980).

The most striking consistency that emerges from the regional distribution studies is that the hypothalamus is especially rich in histamine, its metabolites and the enzymes that form and metabolize histamine, at least in rat (Tables 2 and 3).

Treatments with pargyline lowered the levels of t-MIAA (Khandelwal, Hough, and Green, 1984) and raised the levels of t-MH in regions of rat brain, as measured by both GC-MS (Hough, Khandelwal, and Green, 1984) and by HPLC (Oishi, Nishibori, and Saeki, 1984).

TABLE 3 Regional Distribution of Enzymes Related to Histamine

Region	Histidine decarboxylase[a] (nmol/g·h)	Histamine methyltransferase[a] (nmol/g·h)	Monomine oxidase[b] (nmol/mg·h)
Cerebellum	3	370	5
Medulla-pons	5	470	6
Thalamus-midbrain	13	910	6
Hypothalamus	29	1,050	11
Striatum	10	920	7
Hippocampus	7	830	6
Cerebral cortex	6	820	7
Spinal cord	1		

[a]Taylor and Snyder (1972); a similar distribution was found by Schwartz and co-workers (1981)
[b]Hough and Domino (1979b): t-MH was the substrate

The rise in t-MH levels in brain regions of 11 to 12 week old male rats at 2 and 4 h after intraperitoneal administration of pargyline hydrochloride, 75 mg/kg of body weight, was approximately linear in all regions, and the slope of each regression line was used to estimate the turnover rates of histamine in each region. The turnover rates were correlated with the steady-state levels of histamine and t-MH (Hough, Khandelwal, and Green, 1984).

Another group, using HPLC to quantify t-MH, estimated turnover rate of histamine by measuring t-MH at 4 h after the intraperitoneal adminsitration of pargyline hydrochloride, 80 mg/kg (Oishi, Nishibori and Saeki, 1984). They too found that regional histamine turnover was correlated with steady-state histamine levels.

Table 4 shows the turnover rates of histamine as obtained by the two methods, in both of which a single compartment is assumed. The values obtained by the two methods are in very close agreement. The turnover rates varied over nearly a fifty-fold range among regions (Table 4), a greater range than the range of steady-state levels of histamine and t-MH among regions (Table 2).

TABLE 4 Turnover Rates (nmol/g·h) of Histamine in Rat Brain

Region	Hough, Khandelwal, and Green (1984)[a]	Oishi, Nishibori, and Saeki (1984)[b]
Cerebellum	0.029	0.026
Medulla-pons	0.113	0.199
Midbrain	0.302	0.381
Hypothalamus	1.329	0.979
Caudate nucleus	0.789	0.723
Cortex	0.447	0.431
Hippocampus	0.303	0.218
Thalamus	0.805	0.559

[a]From increase in t-MH at 2 and 4 h after treatment with pargyline hydrochloride, 75 mg/kg.
[b]From increase in t-MH at 4 h after treatment with pargyline hydrochloride, 80mg/kg.

Table 5 shows the rate constants and half-lives of histamine in regions of rat brain. The hypothalamus, which has a high concentration of histamine (Table 2), shows a low rate constant, which implies that a relatively small portion of the histamine in the hypothalamus is turning over. This finding is consistent with the presence of histamine-containing cell bodies in the hypothalamus, as shown by immunocytochemistry, (Panula, Young, and Costa, 1984; Wahlestedt and co-workers, 1984; Watanabe and co-workers, 1984; Wilcox and Seybold, 1982). The caudate nucleus and cortex have the highest rate constants and shortest half-lives of any of the brain regions (Table 5). It may be interesting that the half-lives of dopamine in the caudate nucleus and cerebral cortex are 47.8 and 70.5 min (Smith, Co, and Lane, 1978), far longer than the half-lives of histamine (Table 5).

TABLE 5 Rate Constants and Half-Lives of Histamine in Regions of Rat Brains[a]

Region	Rate constant[b] (h^{-1})	Half-life[c] (min)
Caudate nucleus	3.857	10.8
Cortex	3.704	11.4
Thalamus	2.401	17.4
Hippocampus	2.200	19.2
Midbrain	1.805	22.8
Hypothalamus	1.037	40.2
Medulla-pons	0.949	43.8
Cerebellum	0.296	140.4

[a]Hough, Khandelwal, and Green (1984)
[b]Rate constant (k) = turnover rate/histamine concentration
[c]Half-life (in hours) = 0.692/k

The kinetic values are based on a one-compartment model. There may be more than one pool of histamine in brain. If so, it is not likely to be mast cells, if the brain mast cells have properties even grossly similar to those of peritoneal mast cells. Early experiments with radioactive histamine failed to show metabolism of histamine by peritoneal mast cells of the rat (Furano and Green, 1964a) [which may, like mouse neoplastic mast cells, elaborate histamine into the surrounding medium (see Furano and Green, 1964b; Green, 1966a, b; Green and Day, 1963)]. Similarly, recent work (Goldschmidt, Khandelwal, and Hough, 1984a) failed to show histamine methyltransferase activity in rat peritoneal mast cells; and the low levels of t-MH (less than 0.2% of the histamine levels) that were found by GC-MS could have been sequestered from the plasma, since peritoneal mast cells take up, as well as synthesize, biogenic amines (Furano and Green, 1964a). Incubation of rat peritoneal mast cells with pargyline failed to increase the content of t-MH (Goldschmidt, Khandelwal, and Hough, 1984a). Since turnover rates of histamine derived from measurements of t-MH (to which mast cells contribute insignificantly) after treatment with pargyline (to which the low levels of t-MH in mast cells are unresponsive), it is most unlikely that brain mast cells contribute to the turnover measurements of histamine in regions of rat brain. Moreover, even if mast cells in brain differ from those in the peritoneum and vigorously methylate histamine, the histamine turnover measurments (Tables 4 and 5) can be confounded by mast cells only in thalamus where mast cells are exclusively localized in rat brain (Dropp, 1972; Goldschmidt and co-workers, 1984b; Persinger, 1979). All available evidence indicates that the histamine turnover that is being measured in brain (Tables 4 and 5) is neuronal histamine. What functions it subserves is now the compelling question.

ACKNOWLEDGEMENT

This work was supported by a grant from the National Institute of Mental Health (MH-31805).

REFERENCES

Chang, R. S. L., V. Y. Tran, and S. H. Snyder (1979). Heterogeneity of histamine H_1-receptors: species variations in [^{3}H]mepyramine binding of brain membranes. J. Neurochem., 32, 1653-1663.

Dropp J. J. (1972). Mast cells in the central nervous system of several rodents. Anat. Rec., 174, 227-238.

Fram, D. H. and J. P. Green (1965). The presence and measurement of methylhistamine in urine. J. Biol. Chem., 240, 2036-2042.

Fram, D. H. and J. P. Green (1968). Methylhistamine in guinea pig brain. J. Neurochem., 15, 597-602.

Furano, A.V. and J. P. Green (1964a). The uptake of biogenic amines by mast cells of the rat. J. Physiol., London, 170, 263-271.

Furano, A. V. and J. P. Green (1964b). The compartmentation and elimination of ^{14}C-histamine by neoplastic mast cells in culture. Biochem. Biophys. Acta., 86, 596-603.

Garbarg, M., G. Barbin, C. Llorens, J. M. Palacios, H. Pollard, and J. C. Schwartz (1980). Recent developments in brain histamine research: pathways and receptors. In W. B. Essman (Ed.), Neurotransmitters, Receptors and Drug Action, Spectrum, New York. Chap. 6, pp. 179-202.

Goldschmidt, R. C., J. K. Khandelwal, and L. B. Hough (1984a). Presence and measurement of tele-methylhistamine in mast cells. Agents Actions, 14, 174-178.

Goldschmidt, R. C., L. B. Hough, S. D. Glick, and J. Padawer (1984b). Characterization of mast cells in rat brain. Fed. Proc, 43, 958.

Green, J. P. (1964). Histamine and the nervous system. Fed. Proc., 23, 1095-1102.

Green, J. P. (1966a). Uptake and binding of histamine. Fed. Proc., 26, 211-218.

Green, J. P. (1966b). Synthesis, uptake, and binding of histamine and 5-hydroxytryptamine in mast cells. In U.S. v. Euler, S. Rosell, and B. Uvnas (Ed.), Mechanism of Release of Biogenic Amines, Pergamon, London. pp. 125-145.

Green, J. P. (1970). Histamine. In A. Lajtha (Ed.), Handbook of Neurochemistry, Vol. 4. Plenum, New York. Chap. 10, pp. 221-249.

Green, J. P. (1983). Histamine receptors in brain. In L. L. Iversen, S. D. Iversen, and S. H. Snyder (Ed.), Handbook of Psychopharmacology, New Series, Vol 17. Plenum, New York. Chap. 8, pp. 385-420.

Green, J. P. and M. Day (1963). Biosynthetic pathways in mastocytoma cells in culture and in vivo. Ann. N. Y. Acad. Sci., 103, 334-350.

Green, J. P., C. L. Johnson, and H. Weinstein (1983). Histamine as a neurotransmitter. In M. A. Lipton, A. DiMascia, and K. F. Killam (Ed.), Psychopharmacology - A Generation of Progress, Raven, New York. pp. 319-332.

Hill, S. J. and J. M. Young (1980). Histamine H_1-receptors in the brain of the guinea pig and the rat: differences in ligand binding properties and regional distribution. Brit. J. Pharmacol., 68, 687-696.

Hough, L. B. and E. F. Domino (1979a). tele-Methylhistamine distribution in rat brain. J. Neurochem., 32, 1865-1866.

Hough, L. B. and E. F. Domino (1979b). tele-Methylhistamine oxidation by type B monoamine oxidase. J. Pharmacol. exp. Ther., 208, 422-428.

Hough, L. B. and J. P. Green (1984). Histamine and its receptors in the nervous system. In A. Lajtha (Ed.), Handbook of Neurochemistry, Vol. 6, 2nd ed. Plenum, New York. Chap. 7, pp. 145-211.

Hough, L. B., J. K. Khandelwal, and J. P. Green (1982). Effect of pargyline on tele-methylhistamine and histamine in rat brain. Biochem. Pharmacol., 31, 4074-4076.

Hough, L. B., J. K. Khandelwal, and J. P. Green (1984). Histamine turnover in regions of rat brain. Brain Res., 291, 103-109.

Hough, L. B., J. K. Khandelwal, A. M. Morrishow, and J. P. Green (1981). An improved GCMS method to measure tele-methylhistamine. J. Pharmacol. Methods, 5, 143-148.

Hough, L. B., P. L. Stetson, and E. F. Domino (1979). Gas chromatography-mass spectrometric characteristics and assay of tele-methylhistamine. Anal. Biochem., 96, 56-63.

Khandelwal, J. K., L. B. Hough, and J. P. Green (1982). Histamine and some of its metabolites in human body fluids. Klin. Wochenschr., 60, 914-918.

Khandelwal, J. K., L. B. Hough, and J. P. Green (1984). Regional distribution of the histamine metabolite, tele-methylimidazoleacetic acid, in rat brain: effects of pargyline and probenecid. J. Neurochem., 42, 519-522.

Khandelwal, J. K., L. B. Hough, A. M. Morrishow, and J. P. Green (1982). Measurement of tele-methlyhistamine and histamine in human cerebrospinal fluid, urine, and plasma. Agents Actions, 12, 583-590.

Khandelwal, J. K., L. B. Hough, B. Pazhenchevsky, A. M. Morrishow, and J. P. Green (1982). Presence and measurement of methlyimidazoleacetic acids in brain and body fluids. J. Biol. Chem., 257, 12815-12819.

Oishi, R., M. Nishibori, and K. Saeki (1983). Regional distribution of histamine and tele-methlyhistamine in the rat, mouse, and guinea pig brain. Brain Res., 280, 172-175.

Oishi, R., M. Nishibori, and K. Saeki (1984). Regional differences in the turnover of neuronal histamine in the rat brain. Life Sci., 34, 691-699.

Panula, P., H. Y. T. Yang, and E. Costa (1984). Histamine-containing neurons in the rat hypothalamus. Proc. Nat. Acad. Sci. U.S.A., 81, 2572-2576.

Persinger, M. A. (1979). Brain mast cell numbers in the albino rat: sources of variability. Behav. Neurol. Biol., 25, 380-386.

Schwartz, J. C., H. Pollard, S. Bischoff, M. C. Rehault, and M. Verdiere-Sahuque (1971). Catabolism of ^{3}H-histamine in the rat brain after intracisternal administration. Eur. J. Pharmacol., 16, 326-336.

Schwartz, J. C., G. Barbin, A. M. Duchemin, M. Garbarg, H. Pollard, and T. Quach (1981). Functional role of histamine in brain. In G. C. Palmer (Ed.), Neuropharmacology of Central Nervous System and Behavioral Disorders, Academic, New York. pp. 539-570.

Schwartz, J. C., G. Barbin, A. M. Duchemin, M. Garbarg, C. Llorens, H. Pollard, T. Quach, and C. Rose (1982). Histamine receptors in brain and their possible functions. In C. R. Ganellin and M. E. Parsons (Ed.), Pharmacology of Histamine Receptors, Wright PSG, Bristol. Chap. 9, pp. 351-391.

Smith, J. E., C. Co, and J. D. Lane (1978). Turnover rates of serotonin norepinephrine and dopamine concurrently measured in seven rat brain regions. Progr. Neuro-Psycopharmacol., 2, 359-367.

Taylor, K. M. and S. H. Snyder (1972). Isotopic microassay of histamine, histidine, histidine decarboxylase, and histamine methyltransferase in brain tissue. J. Neurochem., 19, 1343-1358.

Tsuruta, Y., K. Kohashi, and Y. Ohkura (1981). Simultaneous determination of histamine and N -methylhistamine in human urine and rat brain by high-performance liquid chromatography with fluorescence detection. J. Chromatog., 224, 105-110.

Wahlestedt, C., G. Skagerberg, R. Håkanson, F. Sundler, H. Wada, and T. Watanabe (1984). European Histamine Research Soc., 13th meeting, abstracts, p. 45.

Watanabe, T., Y. Taguchi, S. Shiosaka, J. Tanaka, H. Kubota, Y. Terano, M. Tohyama, and H. Wada (1984). Distribution of the histaminergic neuron system in the central nervous system of rats; a fluorescent immunohistochemical analysis with histidine decarboxylase as a marker. Brain Res., 295, 13-25.

Wilcox, B. J. and V. S. Seybold (1982). Localization of neuronal histamine in rat brain. <u>Neurosci. Lett.</u>, <u>29</u>, 105-110.

Wilk S., E. Watson, and B. Travis (1976). Evaluation of dopamine metabolism in rat striatum by a gas chromatographic technique. <u>Eur. J. Pharmacol.</u>, <u>30</u>, 238-243.

HISTAMINE METABOLITES IN CEREBROSPINAL FLUID, THE RATIONALE FOR STUDYING THEM AND ANALYTICAL ASPECTS

C-G. Swahn and G. Sedvall

Laboratory of Clinical Neurochemistry Department of Psychiatry and Psychology, Karolinska Institutet, Stockholm, Sweden

ABSTRACT

Evidence for studying the role of histamine and histamine metabolism in mental disease, especially schizophrenia, is shortly reviewed. Methods for the determination of the histamine metabolites methylhistamine and methylimidazoleacetic acid in cerebrospinal fluid (CSF) were developed. Chemical properties of the imidazole ring relevant to the analytical aspects are summarized. The new methods were used to study histamine metabolites in CSF from healthy control persons and from patients with different clinical conditions such as schizophrenia, rheumatoid arthritis or subarachnoidal hemorrhage. Data in these cases are presented.

KEYWORDS

Gas chromatography-mass spectrometry, methylhistamine; methylimidazoleacetic acid; schizophrenia; rheumatoid arthritis; subarachnoidal hemorrhage.

INTRODUCTION

The report that a c-AMP system coupled to histamine H_2-receptors was blocked by antidepressant drugs (Green and Maayani, 1977, Kanof and Greengard 1978) raised the question if histamine may be involved in mental disease, a major research area in our laboratory. In fact, this is not a new idea and work that is related to this subject will shortly be reviewed. It seems as if the observations on the lack of allergic symptoms (reviewed by Ehrentheil 1957) and rheumatoid arthritis in schizophrenic patients (e.g. Mellsop et al., 1974) stimulated many studies on the role of histamine in schizophrenia. Some earlier work was inspired by the alleged similarity between brains from schizophrenic patients and brains from histamine poisoned rabbits (Buscaino, 1930). Finally, it is not unexpected that histamine has been proposed to be involved in schizophrenia as almost every physiologically powerful endogenous substance has been so.

One of the earlier studies is the determination of histamine in cerebrospinal fluid (CSF) from schizophrenic patients by Trabucchi (1942) who did not find any difference from controls. Another study, giving data on histamine in CSF from a few schizophrenic patients is by Autio and Ermala (1949). An approach which has been used frequently is the study of the cutaneous response to histamine in schizophrenic patients. Several studies have claimed a diminished sensitivity compared to healthy controls but the latest study (Rauscher, Nasrallah and Wyatt, 1980) which also reviews the literature, could not demonstrate such an insensitivity in schizophrenic patients. Another way to study histamine tolerance in schizophrenia has been to inject histamine subcutaneously in larger and larger doses until a predetermined response on the blood pressure was achieved. One such study (Lucy, 1954) found an increasing tolerance to histamine in parallell with the duration of the disease. Schizophrenic patients generally tolerated larger doses of histamine than patients with manic-depressive psychosis or syphilis.

Histamine in blood has been determined in schizophrenia in several investigations. Gooszen and Donker (1956) found that schizoprenic men had a higher concentration of histamine in blood than normal men, something also found by Stern and coworkers (1957). The histamine metabolising capacity of serum from schizophrenic patients was studied by Bernstein, Mazur and Walaszek (1960) who found that such patients had a higher histaminolytic activity than normal controls. Pfeifer and coworkers (1970) found instead that schizophrenic patients mostly had low concentration of histamine in blood. Blood histamine tended to normalize when the illness improved.

What is said above does not cover all publications on histamine in schizophrenia. Additional references are given by Rauscher, Nasrallah and Wyatt (1977). However, they represent sufficient evidence that it is necessary to study the role of histamine in schizophrenia by other approaches than those which have been used above. Often it is more relevant to study metabolites of a transmitter substance rather than the transmitter itself. It is generally thought that the study of CSF is an indirect way to study metabolism in the living brain. Therefore we set out to determine the histamine metabolites tele-methylhistamine (MeHA) and 1-methylimidazole-4-acetic acid (MeImAA) in CSF with gas chromatographic-mass spectrometric methods. A literature survey at the time when this work started (1976) showed the existence of a GC method (Tham, 1968) for the determination of urinary MeImAA. Nothing was known of the presence or amount of MeHA or MeImAA in CSF. Preliminary experiments with the methyl ester of MeImAA on different GC columns showed bad GC behaviour, tailing and absorption. In the first experiments it was not possible to detect less than 100 ng in the mass spectrometer. By injection of a high-boiling base into the column it was possible to get a detection limit of 3 ng but the tailing did not disappear. Attempts with the benzyl ester of MeImAA and a capillary column were also unsuccessful.

At this point it seems appropriate to summarize some chemical properties of the imidazole ring. It has an UV_{max} at 207 nm (logE = 3.7). Its pK_a as a base is 7.1 and as an acid is 14.2. Imidazole is resistant to boiling in strong acid or strong base. Treatment with an acid chloride and alkali (Schotten-Baumann conditions) opens the ring. Imidazole is generally resistant to oxidation by nitric acid, chromium trioxide or alkaline permanganate. Peroxidic reagents usually cause oxidation. Imidazole itself with hydrogen peroxide gives oxamide. Histamine has been reported to give aspartic acid via hydantoin acetic acid in the presence of ascorbic acid, cupric ions and presumably molecular oxygen (Chatterjee and coworkers 1975). Irradiation of a histidine derivative with light in the presence of a sensitizer, eg. riboflavine, gave at least 15 products (Tomita, Irie and Ukita, 1969). Histidine is one of the few amino acids which are oxidized at these conditions. Finally, histidine is believed to play an important role in hemoglobin, hydrolytic enzymes and some phosphorylating enzymes by its acid- and base- accepting and hydrogen bonding properties and by the reactivity of acylated imidazole derivatives. N-trimethylsilylimidazole is a silylating agent and N-heptafluoro-butyrylimidazole an acylating agent.

RESULTS AND DISCUSSION

The UV_{max} of imidazole made it improbable to use HPLC with UV detection to determine histamine metabolites. Some attempts to introduce a chromophore into ImAA or MeImAA were also unsuccessful. In retrospect it is also doubtful whether the sensitivity would have been enough to determine them in CSF. One way to obtain better gas chromatographic properties that has shown for example for histidine is to attach an electron-withdrawing group to the imidazole ring, such as an isobutoxycarbonyl group and to use a stationary phase solid support which is coarser than usual to decrease the surface area which is responsible for absorption (Hušek, 1979). This approach has also been used for GC-MS determination of histamine (Mita, Yasueda and Skida 1980). However, the introduction of an alkoxycarbonyl group requires that the ring nitrogens are not substituted and is thus not applicable for the determination of MeImAA or MeHA which are believed to be the most important histamine metabolites in the central nervous system. An important break-trough came in 1979 when Hough, Stetson and Domino showed that MeHA gives a bis-perfluoroacyl derivative with perfluorocarboxylic acid anhydrides in the presence of pyridine and used this reaction to determine MeHA in brain tissue by GC-MS. We used their method with some modifications, the most important one was the use of deuterated MeHA as an internal standard, to determine MeHA in CSF. This was published in 1981 (Swahn and Sedvall). The same year Keyzer and coworkers (1981) determined MeHA in urine and plasma by essentially the same method. They came to the same conclusion as we that the perfluoroacyl group on the imidazole ring is situated on carbon 2, by NMR spectrometry. In retrospect, that was expected as similar reactions had been shown previously with N-substituted imidazoles. The reaction fails when there is no substituent on a ring nitrogen. As the acyl group is located on carbon it is not easily removed and the derivative can be expected to have good stability under ordinary circumstances. Strong alkali would probably remove the perfluoroacyl group in the ring by the haloform reaction.

It was found that the concentration of MeHA in CSF generally was low, about 1 ng/ml (7 pmol/ml) and therefore we started to develope a method for determining MeImAA in CSF with similar derivatization, which showed to be possible after MeImAA had been converted to its methyl ester. It was necessary with a more extensive clean-up procedure than for MeHA but in the end it did work. Meanwhile two other groups had published procedures for determination of MeImAA by GC or GC-MS methods, Keyzer and coworkers (1982) for urine and Khandelwal and coworkers (1982) for urine, brain, plasma and CSF. In these cases the imidazole ring was not deactivated. Instead their success consisted in finding a suitable rather polar mixed phase or deactivating the glass and solid support with Carbowax. The method developed by us (Swahn and Sedvall, 1983) differs in several aspects from the methods mentioned above, for instance use of a deuterated standard and different derivatization and may therefore be complementary to these two. This method seems to give lower concentrations of MeImAA in CSF than the method of Khandelwal and coworkers although no strict comparison is possible as the samples are not the same but the levels are at least fairly comparable. It turned out that the concentration of MeImAA is also generally low, about 1 ng/ml (7 pmol/ml) or less.

The metabolites seem to be stable in CSF when the samples are frozen although an increase of MeHA occurred after storage for several years. The stock solutions of MeHA were aqueous solutions stored in a refrigerator at $+4°C$ and generated the same calibration curve for at least one year. However, at one occasion there was a sudden, almost complete disappearance of MeHA from a solution and the cause of that was probably bacterial growth as inspection of the solution revealed the presence of a slimy lump. Therefore it seems advisable to acidify the solutions to prevent bacterial growth.

As far as we can see few data on the concentration of histamine metabolites in CSF in various clinical conditions have been reported. Therefore we want to diverge somewhat from the title and present some new data, mosty unpublished. All the data are reported as mean $\pm$ standard deviation. The determinations were not all made on the same occasion and therefore the data must be interpreted cautiously. A systematic error of the magnitude of tenths of ng may be involved from run to run. Whenever possible two groups of conditions were compared in a single run. A few persons were found who had very deviating values which probably are not related to the disease. It is not known whether these persons had any allergic diseases.

MeHA was determined in schizophrenic patients, 0.59 ± 0.08 ng/ml (n=3) Parkinson´s disease, 0.72 ± 0.11 (n=2) and Huntington´s chorea, 0.60 ± 0.01 (n=4). The result for patients with coeliac disease on a gluten-free diet was 1.35 ± 0.05 (n=4) and for patients with chronic pain, before electric stimulation, 0.54 ± 0.20 (n=6).

MeImAA was determined in healthy controls, 0.55 ± 0.40 ng/ml (n=28, range= n.d. - 1.2), n.d. = not detectable and was put to 0 in the calculations. Schizophrenic patients had 0.49 ± 0.48 (n=10, n.d. -1.3, three recieved neuroleptics), patients with rheumatoid arthritis 0.53 ± 0.36 (n=10, n.d. -1.1), patients with subarachnoidal hemorrhage 0.92 ± 0.70 (n=9, n.d. -1.9), depressive patients before treatment 0.90 ± 0.59 (n=7, n.d. -1.4), two patients with Parkinson´s disease 0.1 and 0.2 and two patients with Huntington´s chorea 0.6 and 2.3 ng/ml. The last patient is deviating and is discussed further below. In addition, MeImAA was determined in serum from healthy control persons 10.5 ± 2.7 ng/ml (n=10) and schizophrenic patients 9.5 ± 2.4 ng/ml (n=10, three recieved neuroleptics). CSF from alcoholic persons was examined during intoxication and in a sober state, 0.97 ± 0.47 and 1.06 ± 0.34 ng/ml respectively (n=10). The general impression of these data is that no significant differences were seen between the different groups studied either in MeHA or MeImAA.

It may be asked if the low values are due to the fact that all samples were taken in the morning and higher concentrations would perhaps be found at another time of the day. Attempts to solve this problem were made in two ways. Groups of healthy control persons were studied in the morning 0.89 ± 0.22 ng/ml and in the evening 1.82 ± 0.94 ng/ml (n=10 in both cases). The difference is significant (p < 0.01) but might be unspecific as the metabolites of other transmitter substances were also elevated. The other way was to study the same person during a whole day or longer. The opportunities to do so are rather rare and are mostly restricted to surgical cases where the unphysiological conditions may obscure firm conclusions. Two such cases are shown in fig. 1 and 2.

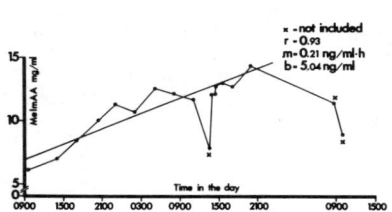

Fig. 1. Methylimidazoleacetic acid in ventricular cerebrospinal fluid from a patient with ventricular drainage.

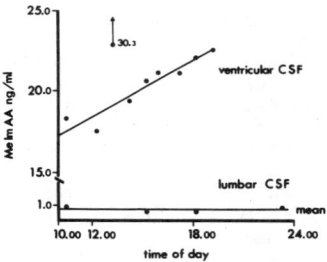

Fig. 2. Methylimidazoleacetic acid in lumbar and ventricular cerebrospinal fluid from a patient with hydrocephalus during replacement of a ventricular shunt.

There is a general rise of the concentration during the whole period under study which may indicate that the situation is abnormal. The data in fig. 1, which were obtained from a patient with ventricular drainage, together with information of the volumes collected, permit the calculation of the efflux of MeImAA to CSF. The mean value is 6.8 ng/h or 1.0 nmol/h which can be compared to homovanillic acid in the same case, 30 nmol/h.

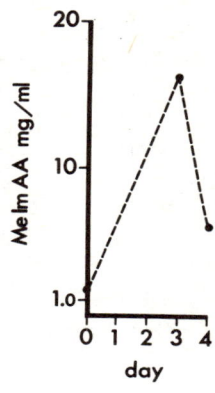

Fig. 3. Methylimidazoleacetic acid in lumbar cerebrospinal fluid from a patient with subarachnoidal hemorrhage.

Figure 3 shows MeImAA in lumbar CSF from a patient with subarachnoidal hemorrhage at three different occasions after the event and supports the idea that histamine could be liberated and metabolised in an abnormal way in some pathological cases. The peak concentration is also the highest one that we have seen up to date.

Figure 2 also shows the simultaneous sampling of lumbar and ventricular CSF which confirms that there is a rostro-caudal gradient of MeImAA, probably due to an active transport mechanism. This mechanism is not of the same kind as the one for homovanillic acid e.g. as it does not seem to be probenecid sensitive. Two patients with Huntingtons´s chorea obtained probenecid in connection with other experiments in a dose of 40 mg/kg intravenously during one hour before the first lumbar puncture which was followed by further three at three hours´ intervals. The result was 0.40, 0.23, 0.54 and 0.32 ng/ml for one patient and 7.40, 2.24, 3.19 and 2.93 ng/ml for the other patient which had previously been found to have a high concentration of MeImAA in CSF which thus persisted several months later. These data do not indicate a raise in the concentration of MeImAA whereas homovanillic acid showed the expected rise on both patients. This is in accordance with Schwartz and coworkers (1971) who showed that probenecid had no effect on the efflux of tritiated histamine metabolites from rat brain.

In summary, MeImAA and MeHA are present in CSF in low concentrations, which do not seem to correlate with the clinical conditions studied. Nevertheless this does not exclude that histamine may be involved in mental diseases as all the determinations were done on lumbar CSF. It is possible that the levels reflect more the activity of transport mechanisms than neuronal activity in brain. However, at the present time there is no other way to study the role of histamine in the living human brain.

ACKNOWLEDGEMENT

This research has been supported by the Swedish Medical Research Council, National Institute of Health, USA, Hässle-Ciba Geigy, Hoffman La Roche, Magnus Bergvalls Stiftelse and Karolinska institutet. Several different collegues collected the CSF used and they are gratefully acknowledged. The help from Mr. Milton Ampuero in the preparation of the figures and from Ms. Birgit Lönn in the preparation of the manuscript are thankfully appreciated.

REFERENCES

Autio, L. and Ermala, P. (1949). Ann. Med. Exptl. Biol. Fenniae, 27, 87-101.
Bernstein, J., Mazur, W.P. and Walaszek, E.J. (1960). Med. Exp., 2, 239-244.
Buscaino, V.M. (1930). L´encephale, 25, 48-56.
Chatterjee, I.B., Majumder, A.K., Nandi, B.K. and Subramanian, N. (1975). Ann. N. Y. Acad. Sci., 258, 24-47.
Ehrentheil, O.F. (1957). Arch. Neurol. Psychiatr., 77, 178-186.
Gooszen, J.A.H. and Donker, J. (1956). Acta Allerg., 10, 149-169.
Green, J.P. and Maayani, S. (1977). Nature, 269, 163-165.
Hough, L.B., Stetson, P.L. and Domino, E.F. (1979). Anal. Biochem., 96, 56-63.
Hušek, P. (1979). J. Chromatogr., 172, 468-470.
Kanof, P.D. and Greengard, P. (1978). Nature, 272, 329-333.

Keyser, J.J., Wolthers, B.G., Muskiet, F.A.J., Kauffman, H.F. and Groen, A. (1981). Clin. Chim. Acta, 113, 165-173.
Keyzer, J.J., Wolthers, B.G. Breukelman, H., Kauffman, H.F. and de Monchy, J.G.R. (1982). Clin. Chim. Acta, 121, 379-387.
Khandelwal, J.K., Hough, L.B., Pazhenchevsky, B., Morrishow, A.M. and Green, J.P. (1982) J. Biol. Chem., 257, 12815-12819.
Lucy, J.D. (1954) Arch. Neurol. Psychiat., 71, 629-639.
Mellsop, G.W., Koadlow, L., Syme, J. and Whittingham, S. (1974) Aust. NZ J. Med., 4, 247-252.
Mita, H., Yasueda, H. and Skida, T. (1980) J. Chromatogr., 221, 1-7.
Pfeiffer, C.C., Iliev, V., Goldstein, L., Jenney, E.H. and Schultz, R. (1970) Res. Comm. Chem. Pathol. Pharmacol., 1, 247-265.
Rauscher, F.P., Nasrallah, H.A. and Wyatt, R.J. (1977) Neuroreg. Psychiat. Disord. Proc. Conf., 1976, 416-424.
Rauscher, F.P., Nasrallah, H.A. and Wyatt, R.J. (1980). J. Clin. Psychiatry, 41, 44-51.
Schwartz, J -C., Pollard, H., Bischoff, S., Rehault, M.C and Verdiere-Sahuque, M. (1971). Eur. J. Pharmacol., 16, 326-335.
Stern, P., Huković, S., Madjerek, Z. and Karabaic, S. (1957) Arch. Int. Pharmacodyn., 109, 294-299.
Swahn, C -G. and Sedvall, G. (1981) J. Neurochem., 37, 461-166.
Swahn, C -G. and Sedvall, G. (1983) J. Neurochem., 40, 688-696.
Tham, R. (1966) J. Chromatogr., 23, 207-216.
Tomita, M., Irie, M. and Ukita, T. (1969) Biochem., 8, 5149-5160.
Trabucchi, C. (1942). Riv. Patol. Nerv. Ment., 59, 131-161.

Histamine in the Brain: Actions and Role

NEUROBIOLOGY OF A HISTAMINERGIC NEURON IN THE CNS OF THE MOLLUSK APLYSIA CALIFORNICA

D. Weinreich

Department of Pharmacology and Experimental Therapeutics, University of Maryland School of Medicine, Baltimore, MD 21201, USA

ABSTRACT

The invariant location and enormous size of neurons found in the nervous system of the mollusk Aplysia californica provide unique conveniences for the detection and direct characterization of neurotransmitter substances at the cellular level. Both pre- and post-synaptic neurons, once mapped, can be dissected for chemical analysis of substrates and enzymes or penetrated with multibarreled microelectrodes for examination of synaptically released or exogenously applied transmitter substances. To date, acetylcholine, serotonin, and dopamine are strongly implicated transmitter substances at identified molluscan synapses. The present chapter provides an in-depth assessment of the role of histamine as a neurotransmitter in the Aplysia nervous system.

KEYWORDS

Histaminergic synapses; multi-component post-synaptic potentials; γ-glutamylhistamine; histamine uptake and metabolism; histamine receptors; γ-glutamylhistamine synthetase inhibitors.

INTRODUCTION

Histamine is a biogenic amine present in the CNS of a variety of invertebrate species (Reite, 1972). Although it has generally been assumed that this imidazolamine may function as a synaptic neurotransmitter, its role in nervous function is still poorly understood. Efforts to establish physiological evidence supportive of a transmitter role for histamine require identification of neurons containing relatively high levels of histamine and their post-synaptic targets. To date, such neuronal circuits have only been clearly established within the CNS of mollusks (Leake and Walker, 1980).

There is a growing body of physiological and biochemical data suggesting that arthropod nervous systems may also utilize histamine as a neurotransmitter (Elias and Evans, 1983; Claiborne and Selverston, 1984). With the improvements in isolating individual neurons for chemical assay (Ono and McCaman, 1980) and the application of newly developed immunological methods for localizing histamine in nervous tissue (Wilcox and Seybold, 1982; Panula et al., 1984), there is every reason to expect that histamine-containing neuronal circuits will become established within the CNS of arthropoda and other phyla.

Molluscan nervous systems in general provide very attractive systems for correlative chemical and physiological studies (see Osborne 1977). The CNS of the marine mollusk, Aplysia californica, in particular, offers numerous advantages for transmitter identification studies. The unusually large size and invariant location of individual presynaptic nerve cells permit
contiguous electrophysiological experiments employing conventional intracellular recording techniques with biochemical measurements of the same identified neuron (Kehoe and Marder, 1976; Ono and McCaman, 1980). In addition, there is an abundance of correlative cellular electrophysiological, pharmacological, and biochemical data pertaining to established and putative neurotransmitters in this nervous system (see, Gerschenfeld, 1973; Ascher and Kehoe, 1975; Kehoe and Marder, 1976, Ono and McCaman, 1984).

Recently, individual identifiable neurons within the cerebral ganglion of Aplysia have been shown to contain unusually large concentrations of histamine (Weinreich, et al., 1975; Ono and McCaman, 1980). These same histamine-enriched neurons synthesize and store radiolabelled histamine and possess at least three orders of magnitude more histidine decarboxylase activity than any other Aplysia neuron examined (Weinreich and Yu, 1977). These observations provide the first direct evidence that histamine-containing neurons (HCNs) can be distinguished from other nerve cells within a heterogeneous CNS by their unique biochemical properties. The distinctive levels of histamine and histidine decarboxylase activity in the HCNs suggests, in a manner analogous to biochemical data available for other neurotransmitters in the same CNS, that the HCNs may utilize histamine as a synaptic neurotransmitter (Weinreich, 1977a). An important corollary of these findings is that the localization of HCNs offers the opportunity to define the physiological and pharmacological properties of histaminergic synapses.

1. PHYSIOLOGY AND PHARMACOLOGY OF HISTAMINERGIC TRANSMISSION.

Histamine's role in synaptic transmission has now been made more tenable because we have characterized numerous re-identified cerebral neurons showing monosynaptic responses following intracellular stimulation of the HCNs (Weinreich, 1977b; McCaman and McKenna, 1978, McCaman and Weinreich, 1982; 1984). The successful localization of a number of identified post-synaptic (follower) neurons receiving chemical monosynaptic potentials from the HCNs has allowed us to test the physiological and pharmacological correspondence between histamine and the HCN transmitter. Our results of an analysis of HCN-mediated slow synaptic hyperpolarizing responses indicate that histamine and the HCN transmitter produce similar post-synaptic ionic conductances and activate pharmacologically identical post-synaptic histamine receptors.

Both histamine and the HCN transmitter increased the conductance of the appropriate follower membrane. The increased membrane conductance was shown to be produced by potassium ions since the average estimated reversal potential values for both responses were similar (-84 mV) and close to the equilibrium potential for potassium (-80 mV). Moveover, changes in extracellular potassium ions shifted the reversal potentials in a manner predicted by the Nernst equation for a pure potassium response. These results show that exogenously applied histamine can mimic many of the effects produced by the natural transmitter.

The pharmacological properties of the receptors mediating slow hyperpolarizing histamine and synaptic responses were found to be similar. Bath application of cimetidine, a specific histamine recognition-site antagonist in Aplysia (Gruol and Weinreich, 1979a,b) completely abolished, in a reversible manner, only this type of histamine and synaptic response (see Fig. 11 in McCaman and Weinreich, 1982). This effect of cimetidine is specific since in similar concentrations it was ineffective on other classes of histamine and HCN-mediated post-synaptic responses. These results, in conjunction with the finding described above, constitute evidence satisfying the physiological and pharmacological identity-of-action criteria (Paton, 1958; Werman, 1966, 1980) commonly utilized to identify neurotransmitter substances.

2. MULTIPLE POST-SYNAPTIC POTENTIALS (p.s.p.s.) PRODUCED BY SINGLE HCNs.

A remarkable feature of the HCNs examined to date is the multiplicity of p.s.p responses they evoke in different post-synaptic neurons (Fig.1). Intracellular recordings from the 15 ipsilateral follower neurons that have been characterized as receiving monosynaptic connections from each HCN have already resulted in the identification of eight distinctive types of p.s.p.s. It is our belief that there are five basic p.s.p. components, which either individually or in combination, give rise to the various single- and multi-component histaminergic p.s.p.s. These basic components consist of three different depolarizing responses: a fast e.p.s.p. (E_f); a slow e.p.s.p. (E_s); and a very slow e.p.s.p. (E_{vs}); and two different hyper-polarizing responses: a fast i.p.s.p. (I_f) and a slow i.p.s.p. (I_s)(see Fig. 1). The p.s.p.s observed to date are (Fig.1): E_sPSP, I_sPSP, $E_f I_s$PSP, $I_f E_s$PSP, $E_f E_s$PSP, $I_f I_s$PSP, $E_f I_f I_s$, and $I_f E_f E_{vs}$PSP. The latter pair of three-component p.s.p.'s have only recently psp been observed (McCaman and Weinreich, 1984); in earlier studies they were believed to be only two-component p.s.p.s. As previously shown by Kehoe (1972c) it may, under some circumstances, be extremely difficult to detect the multi-component nature of some p.s.p.s particularly those that consist of superimposed fast inhibitory and fast excitatory components. The experiments on the multiple p.s.p.s. evoked by HCNs are still in progress. We need to define rigorously the identity of the

FIG. 1 HISTAMINERGIC POST-SYNAPTIC POTENTIALS (P.S.P.s)

COMPONENT P.S.P.	CONDUCTANCE	ANTAGONIST	OBSERVED RESPONSES	
E_f-Fast excitatory	↑gNa$^+$	---		E_sp.s.p.
E_s-Slow excitatory	↑gNa$^+$	2-(aminoethyl)-thiazole pyrilamine		I_sp.s.p.
E_{vs}-Very slow excitatory	↓gK$^+$	---		$E_f E_s$p.s.p.
E_s-Slow inhibitory	↑gK$^+$	cimetidine		$I_f E_{vs}$p.s.p.
I_f-Fast inhibitory	↑gCl$^-$	---		$I_f I_s$p.s.p.
				$E_f I_s$p.s.p.
				el.p.s.p.

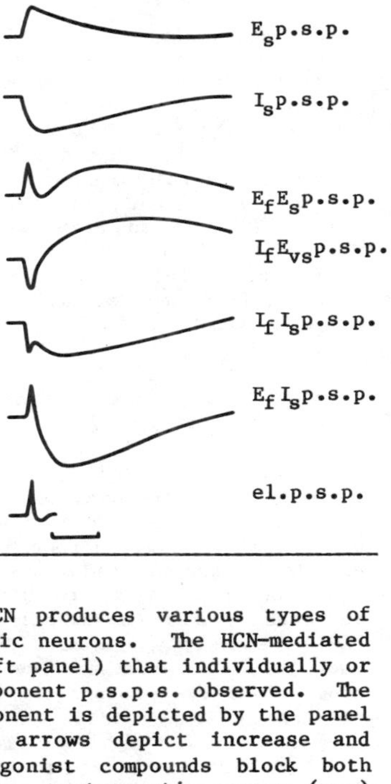

An action potential in a single presysnaptic HCN produces various types of unitary p.s.p.s. in different identified postsyantic neurons. The HCN-mediated p.s.p.s. are composed of five basic components (left panel) that individually or in combination give rise to single or multiple component p.s.p.s. observed. The ionic conductance associated with each p.s.p. component is depicted by the panel marked conductance. Upward and downward going arrows depict increase and decrease ionic conductance, respectively. Antagonist compounds block both synaptic and histamine-induced response in the same postsynaptic neuron (---) indicates specific recognition site antagonist not yet characterized. I_sp.s.p. (slow monophasic inhibitory post-synaptic potential), E_sp.s.p. (slow monophasic excitatory post-synaptic potential), $I_f E_s$p.s.p. (fast inhibitory post-synaptic potential-slow excitatory post-synaptic potential, $E_f I_s$p.s.p. (fast excitatory post-synaptic potential-slow inhibitory post-synaptic potential, $E_f E_s$p.s.p. (fast excitatory post-synaptic potential-slow excitatory post-synaptic potential, $I_f E_{vs}$p.s.p. (fast inhibitory post-synaptic potential-very slow inhibitory post-synaptic potential, el.p.s.p. (electrical post-synaptic potential). Data after McCaman and Weinreich (1982; 1984). Time bar - 1 sec.

ionic currents associated with several p.s.p. types. These results will enable us and other investigators to discern common vs. distinctive features of the post-synaptic actions of histamine and other known neurotransmitter substances within the same CNS.

Although the ionic mechanism underlying all the HCN-mediated p.s.p components are not yet complete, it is of interest to compare their basic components with those underlying cholinergic and serotoninergic p.s.p.s which have been previously described in the Aplysia CNS. The components we call E_f, I_f, and I_s seem to be completely analogous to the three basic components underlying cholinergic p.s.p.s and involving increased conductances to Na+ (Blankenship et al, 1971), Cl⁻ (Blankenship, et al., 1971; Kehoe, 1972a) and K+ (Kehoe, 1972b, c) respectively. As pointed out by Kehoe, the three basic components of the cholinergic responses could, when taken singly or in various combinations, give rise to seven possible distinct types of p.s.p.s; her studies revealed six of these. Our studies indicate that there are five basic components underlying HCN-induced responses so a greater variety of p.s.p.s may be anticipated; eight have already been revealed to date.

It is difficult to directly compare histaminergic vs. serotonergic synaptic responses. Central serotoninergic p.s.p.'s described to date in Aplysia are generally detected only after firing the presynaptic cells in bursts of 10 to 30 spikes. This results in compound p.s.p.'s consisting of slow waves of depolarization or hyperpolarization in which no discrete p.s.p.s could be recognized (Gerschenfeld and Paupardin-Tritsch, 1974b). Thus, only three types of central serotonin-mediated synaptic response have been described, i.e., and excitatory (probably similar to our $E_f E_s$ PSP), classical inhibitory (similar to our I_s PSP) and an atypical inhibitory response (Gerschenfeld and Paupardin-Tritsch, 1974a). On the other hand, the study of serotonin-evoked responses from various Aplysia neurons have identified six different types of responses (Gerschenfeld and Paupardin-Tritsch, 1974a) which may be compared to the basic histaminergic responses as follows: "A" (cf. E_f), "A^1" (cf. E_s), " α " (cf. E_{vs}), "B" (cf. I_s), "C" (cf. I_f) and "β". Only the last one seems to have no analogy with presently known histamine responses. This β response appears to be the basis of the "atypical" inhibitory synaptic response (Gerschenfeld and Paupardin-Tritsch, 1974a, b).

Some features shared by different central neurotransmitters in Aplysia are becoming more apparent. Thus, like cholinergic and serotonenergic neurons, HCNs are also "multiaction neurons" (Kandel and Gardner, 1972). They all mediate excitation on some followers, inhibition on other followers and mixed functions on still others. All mediate responses involving 'classical' increases in membrane premeability to Na$^+$, Cl$^-$, and K$^+$. The greater diversity of p.s.p.s mediated by HCNs may be more apparent than most other transmitters because they can be evoked by single action potentials. Thus, serotonin-evoked conductance mechanisms are quite diverse but presently characterized central synaptic connections of serotonergic neurons are generally too weak to permit study of discrete unitary PSPs. It seems quite likely that additional serotonergic connections will be discovered that will offer a diversity comparable to that observed for HCNs. It may also be that 'non-classical' conductance mechanisms, such as those underlying some of the HCN and serotoninergic p.s.p.s, may yet be uncovered for cholinergic p.s.p.s (e.g., Kehoe, 1975).

3. PHARMACOLOGY OF HISTAMINE RECEPTORS IN APLYSIA.

Histamine (HA) receptors have been divided into H_1-type or H_2-type based on the relative potency of HA agonists and antagonist compounds (Douglas, 1980). If the action of HA or H_1-type antagonists (e.g., 2-MeHA, PEA) is blocked by H_1 type antagonists (e.g., pyrilamine) the receptor is classified as H_1-type. Similarly, if the action of HA or H_2-type agonists (e.g., 4-MeHA, betazole) is blocked by H_2-type antagonists (e.g., cimetidine) the receptor is classified as H_2-type. Carpenter and Gaubatz (1975) have described depolarizing and hyperpolarizing responses evoked by HA applied ionophoretically to unidentified Aplysia neurons. Since these responses were blocked by the H_1 antagonist, pyrilamine, or the H_2 antagonist, burimamide, they concluded that the two types of HA receptors (H_1 or H_2) exist on Aplysia neurons. Similar conclusions have been reached utilizing H_1 and H_2 agonist and antagonist drugs ionophoretically applied onto vertebrate neurons in situ (Hass, 1974; 1981; Haas and Wolf, 1977; Sastry and Phillis, 1976; Geller, 1979). In the neurons of the land snail, Achatina fulica, however, the excitatory effects produced by exogenously applied HA was not antagonized by either pyrilamine or burimamide (Takeuchi et al., 1976), suggesting that different pharmacological classes of HA receptors may exist on snail neurons.

We have tested extensively a number of H_1 and H_2 agonist and antagonist compounds on HA receptors which mediate two ionically distinct hyperpolarizing responses on identified neurons of Aplysia. Our results (Gruol and Weinreich, 1979a, b) indicate that caution must be exercised when attempting to catergorize HA receptors pharmacologically with H_1 and H_2 reagents in this (and possibly other) nervous systems because: (1) at concentrations required to partially or totally block HA-induced hyperpolarizations, many antihistamine compounds, both H_1- and H_2-type, also depressed acetylcholine and dopamine-induced K^+ and Cl^- conductances in the same neuron and (2) the HA receptors mediating membrane hyperpolarization could not be classified as either H_1 or H_2 based upon commonly used criteria, since the H_2 antagonist cimetidine diminished equally the K^+ response to both H_1 and H_2 agonists, while H_1 antagonists were ineffective or nonselective. In addition, neither H_1 nor H_2 agonists or antagonists affectd the receptors for the Cl^- response. This lack of discrimination by H_1 and H_2 compounds implies that HA receptors in the Aplysia brain have different properties than vertebrate peripheral HA receptors. In light of the unique pharmacological features of acetylcholine, serotonin and dopamine receptors in this nervous system (see review by Ascher and Kehoe, 1975), it is perhaps not surprising that the pharmacological properties of the two HA receptors we have described preclude their classification as either H_1 or H_2.

Although we could not classify HA responses as H_1- or H_2-type, we were successful in characterizing one antihistamine compound, cimetidine, as being a very selective and useful antagonist at synaptic and extrasynaptic HA receptors in Aplysia CNS. This compound was shown to block post-synaptic increases in K^+ conductances produced by HA or H_2 agonists (but not K^+-conductances induced by several other biogenic amines) by a direct competition at HA recognition sites rather than on ionic channels. Furthermore, as described above, cimetidine selectively and reversibly blocked hyperpolarizing, K^+-mediated, synaptic responses elicited by HCN activation. Thus, we have shown that cimetidine in Aplysia CNS selectively antagonizes a specific type of post-synaptic HA receptor which mediates an increase in K^+ conductance. Given that there exists at least four additional basic p.s.p components (see Fig.1), the possibility also exists that as many as five pharmacologically distinct HA receptors may occur on Aplysia neurons. In this regard, it is interesting to note that certain HA-induced responses recorded intracellularly from mammalian hippocampal neurons in tissue slices are not blocked by bath applied H_1 or H_2 histamine receptor antagonists nor simulated by H_1 or H_2 receptor agonists (H. Hass, personal communication).

4. HISTAMINE METABOLISM IN APLYSIA CNS.

Our interest in elucidating the products of histamine degradation was based upon the following considerations: (1) to discern whether histamine metabolism may participate in the inactivation of synaptically released histamine; and (2) to identify histamine metabolite(s) and examine whether they may possess neuronal activity. The results we have accumulated concerning histamine metabolism were not only unanticipated but they have important implications for experiments to demonstrate release of endogenous histamine from activated HCNs.

An unexpected finding was that histamine in situ is metabolized almost exclusively (>90%) to a single product; a dipeptide which we have conclusively identified as γ-glutamylhistamine (GHA), Weinreich, 1979; Stein and Weinreich, 1982). The γ-glutamylation of histamine in Aplysia CNS represents a unique pathway for histamine metabolism in nervous tissue; in most other neuronal and non-neuronal tissues examined, histamine is either methylated and/or deaminated (Douglas, 1980). Gotoh and Schwartz (1980) have recently demonstrated GHA formation following intrasomatic injection of radiolabelled histamine into the HCNs. Their results not only confirmed our observations but demonstrated that HCNs may contain the biochemical machinery to metabolize histamine (see Stein and Weinreich, 1983).

We have tested whether GHA was an active metabolite by examining the effects of this peptide on neuronal histamine and glutamate receptors and at synaptic responses mediated by the HCNs. Bath applied GHA, to 10^{-3}M, had no discernable agonist or antagonist effects on three different types of histamine- and glutamate-induced responses and two multicomponent p.s.p.s ($E_f I_s$ PSP and $L_f E_{vs}$ PSP, see Fig.1). In addition GHA did not produce any noticeable changes in the resting membrane potential, input impedance, or spontaneous p.s.p and action potential activity. Thus, we believe that GHA is a physiologically inactive histamine metabolite.

In Aplysia ganglia extracts and in single neurons we have characterized a novel enzyme, GHA synthetase, which catalyzes the incorporation of histamine into a peptide linkage with L-glutamate (Stein and Weinreich, 1982a; 1983). GHA synthetase was found to have an absolute requirement for ATP and the enzyme revealed a narrow substrate specificity. Of the imidazole compounds examined, those having free ring and side-chain nitrogens were the best inhibitors of histamine utilization, decreasing GHA synthesis by 65%. When one or both of the side-chain amine hydrogens was replaced by a methyl or acetyl group, this inhibitory activity was abolished. Although both N π-methyl and N$^+$τ-methyl histamine, displayed inhibitory activity, they were only half as effetive as 2- and 4-methylhistamine. The length of the side-chain was found to be an important determinant of synthetase activity as well. Imidazole base itself has no inhibitory activity since it cannot form a peptide bond. Lengthening the side-chain by three methyl grouyps, as in 4(5)-aminopropyl imidazole, inhibits histamine utilization by 28%; further addition of an alkyl group results in only a 15% inhibition. Carnosine, homocarnosie and anserine, dipeptides structurally similar to GHA, had little effect on histamine utilization by the synthetase enzyme.

One of the most provocative results from these structure-activity-relation studies was the finding that the requirement for an imidazole ring was not absolute; indeed, aromatic or straight-chain hydrocarbon-containing amines having the requisite ethylamine structure were effective inhibitors of histamine utilization by the synthetase enzyme. Pyridylethylamine and butylamine bases caused a decrease in GHA synthesis by 82% and 57%, respectively. Several glutamate analogs and glutamate-containing peptides were tested to see whether they could be incorporated into peptide linkage with histamine. Of the compounds examined only L-glutamyl- γ -methyl ester and D-glutamate were incorporated into a peptide linkage with histamine, but only to a small extent (5%). In addition, D-glutamate showed a concentration-dependent inhibition of the synthetase enzyme. Presumably the D-glutamate binds to the glutamate-binding site but the synthetase does not recognize the D-amino acid as an active substrate.

γ-glutamylation of histamine could be catalyzed by several enzymes: glutamine synthetase; γ-glutamyl cysteine synthetase; and γ-glutamyltranspeptidase (see review by Meister and Tate, 1976). Utilizing numerous enzyme inhibitors, false substrates, and subcellular fractionation, (see Stein and Weinreich, 1982a) we could differentiate between the properties of GHA synthetase and those of other enzymes. Our results clearly demonstrate GHA formation in Aplysia is catalyzed by GHA synthetase and not by the above-mentioned three enzymes.

The final disposition of GHA in Aplysia is not yet known. It is possible that GHA is being excreted into the hemolymph. Alternatively, γ-glutamyltranspeptidase, which is present in Aplysia ganglia, could theoretically (Meiter, 1973, Orlowski, personal communication) slowly degrade GHA back to its components, histamine and glutamate.

5. INHIBITION OF HISTAMINE METABOLISM.

A major obstacle impeding the examination of histamine release is the ubiquitous presence of GHA synthetase in neural and non-neurnal cells (Stein and Weinreich, 1982a; 1983). Inhibition of GHA synthetase would allow insights not only about synaptically relesed histamine but it may reveal whether this enzyme participates in terminating the actions of histaminergic transmission. In collaboration with Dr. Owen W. Griffith, we have discovered that S-n-alkyl sulfoximines formed from analogs of methionine sulfoximines, i.e., buthionine, pentathionine, hexathionine etc. (Griffith, et al., 1979), inhibit γ-glutamylhistamine formation in-vitro and in-vivo. In-vitro inhibition was dependent upon ATP, length of S-alkyl chain but independent of glutathione concentration. DL hexathionine sulfoximine was the most potent analog tested (K_I=10 μ M); its D-isomer was essentially inactive. Preincubation of intact ganglia with 100 μ M hexathionine sulfoximine for 1 hr does not block radiolabelled histamine uptake but reduces histamine metabolism to 3% in a nearly irreversible manner. Further, this compound does not appear to interfere with histamine recognition sites because histamine-induced post-synaptic responses were unaffected. Thus, hexathionine sulfoximine may be a valuable tool to examine several aspects of histaminergic transmission.

6. ENDOGENOUS γ-GLUTAMYLHISTAMINE

Experimental evidence that GHA is the major metabolite of histamine in Aplysia nervous tissue is derived from three sources: (1) Ganglia incubated with radiolabelled HA in situ (Weinreich, 1979); or (2) ganglia and single cells incubated in vitro (Stein and Weinreich, 1982a; 1983) produce only this peptidoamine; (3) In addition, Gotoh and Schwartz (1980) have reported the presence of GHA following injection of labeled HA into the cell body of the labelled HCN. All these studies, however, relied on exogenous application of radiolabelled HA to produce the metabolite. No data had been compiled on the presence or concentration of the endogenous peptide in Aplysia ganglia.

We have measured endogenous GHA in ganglia of Aplysia californica (Stein and Weinreich, 1982b). The concentration of this HA metabolite in Aplysia nervous tissue ranged from 3-32 pmol/mg protein. Endogenous GHA was also measurable in connective tissue, penis muscle, and buccal muscle (2.5, 1.3 and .4 pmole/mg protein, respectively). Heart and "liver" did not possess detectable levels of GHA (<.1 pmole/mg protein). The level of GHA in ganglia is, therefore, about 100-fold less than that of its precursor, HA (Weinreich, 1977); however, it is approximately two orders of magnitude greater than the concentration ofγ -glutamylglutamine, γ-glutamylvaline, γ-glutamyglycine and other γ-glutamyl compounds identified in ox brain (Sano et al., 1966).

The apparent Vmax for GHA synthesis in vitro is 87 μ mol/g protein/h. The low endogenous level of GHA, compared with the much higher concentrations of both HA and glutamate, suggests that GHA synthesis occurs at a very low rate in the intact animal, or is strictly regulated. It is tempting to speculate that this synthetic machinery (that is GHA synthetase) is "turned-on" when steady-state HA levels increase as HA, synaptically released, is taken up into the cells. The low GHA concentration may be maintained by disposition of the peptide in a manner which has not yet been defined.

7. RE-UPTAKE OF HISTAMINE

From subcellular distribution studies (Stein and Weinreich, 1982a) we have determined that GHA synthetase appears to be a soluble enzyme (although we have not excluded the possibility that it may be located on extracellular or intracellular surfaces of plasma membranes). This observation indicates that histamine would first have to be transported from the extracellular compartment to its site of metabolism. Recently, Osborne et al. (1979) reported that isolated snail ganglia accumulated ^{14}C-histamine (tissue: medium ratios of about 4) and that this process could be characterized as a high-affinity, temperature and sodium-dependent uptake. In addition they reported that accumulated ^{14}C-histamine was released into the bathing medium by elevated extracellular K^+, in a calcium-dependent manner.

We have performed similar uptake experiments with _Aplysia_ ganglia. _Aplysia_ ganglia also accumulate radiolabelled histamine in the micromolar range and yield tissue: medium ratios (corrected for inulin space) ranging between 5-50. This uptake process temperature-and-sodium-dependent. However, identification of the accumulated radioactivity revealed that essentially _all_ the material was GHA. We attempted to demonstrate release of accumulated radioactivity by bathing ganglia in elevated extracellular K^+. Over the range of 20 to 100 mM (two to ten times the normal K^+) we could not detect any significant acceleration above the small leakage of radioactivity from ganglia preincubated with ^{3}H or ^{14}C-histamine.

During the course of these experiments we repeated some of the experiments reported by Osborne et al. (1979). We were interested to know whether histamine was also metabolized to GHA in snail brain and we were curious about the identity of the radioactivity released by K^+ (the identity of their accumulatd and released radioactivity was not reported). Using snail brain from _Helix aspera_ we observed that under the conditions described by Osborne et al. (1979), i.e., 20 min incubation with 10^{-7} M ^{14}C-histamine, essentially _all_ the accumulated radioactivity could be identified as GHA. Moreover, both the spontaneous and K^+-induced release of accumulated radioactivity was identified as ^{14}C-peptide. In an analogous series of experiments we examined the fate of radiolabelled histamine in _Limas maximus_ (a terrestrial slug which abounds in the author's garden). Again, a single radioactive metabolite was detected which could be identified as ^{14}C-GHA. These results reveal that γ-glutamylation of histamine may be a general feature of histamine metabolism in the nervous systems of gastropod mollusks.

The K^+-induced release of GHA from snail but not from _Aplysia_ ganglia remains an enigma. It would be interesting, and potentially useful for resolving this puzzle, to determine whether GHA alters the excitability of snail neurons.

8. SUMMARY

From the results described above we now have evidence to show that a restricted population of reidentifiable neurons possessing distinctive biochemical properties exist within the CNS of _Aplysia_. These neurons contain unusually large concentrations of histamine and selectively possess the histamine forming enzyme, histidine decarboxylase. These data provide the first direct evidence that histamine and histidine decarboxylase reside within nerve cells. They also satisfied two essential criteria commonly employed to establish the identification of neurotransmitter substances; namely, the demonstration of the presence of a puative neurotransmitter and its biosynthetic enzyme in presynaptic neurons.

Multidisciplinary research with _Aplysia_ neurons have satisfied two additional criteria that histamine maybe a neurotransmitter: (1) physiological identity-of-action between histamine and the HCN transmitter; and (2) pharmacological correspondence between the effects of histamine and the HCN transmitter on postsynpatic membranes. Histamine and the HCN transmitter produce similar postsynaptic effects-they both decrease the excitability in one class of postsynaptic neurons by increasing the post-synaptic membrane permeability to potassium ions, i.e., both histamine and the natural transmitter produce their effects through similar ionic mechanisms. Thus, in all aspects examined to date, histamine mimics the action of the natural transmitter.

The mechanism for inactivating synaptically released histamine remains to be determined. Exogenously applied histamine is rapidly metabolized by a specific and novel enzyme (glutamyl-histamine synthetase) to a single dipeptide product, glutamylhistamine. Our existing data suggests that metabolism of histamine is closely linked to its removal from the extracellular space. The recent characterization of hexathionine sulfoximine as a selective blocker of histamine metabolism but not of histamine uptake will provide new insights about the relative roles of metabolism vs. uptake in terminating the actions of synaptically released histamine. Thus, it will be very interesting to explore the effects of this reagent on the efficacy of histaminergic synaptic transmission in Aplysia.

Of the numerous criteria commonly used to identify neurotransmitter substances, the most decisive, and the technically most demanding criterion is the demonstration that the putative substance is released from presynaptic neurons in amounts proportional to activity of the presynaptic neuron and in a Ca^{++}-dependent manner.

Gershenfeld et al., (1978) demonstrated, by direct chemical assay, the Ca^{++}-dependent release of 5-HT following stimulation of single 5-HT-containing neurons in Aplysia. These observations culminated a long series of multidisciplinary experiments to establish 5-HT as a genuine neurotransmitter. The documented release of 5-HT from single neurons also established the feasibility of demonstrating transmitter release from identified Aplysia neurons. The impulse-dependent release of 5-HT, however, could only be demonstrated when 5-HT re-uptake was pharmacologically impaired. We believe that an analogous situation may exist when attempting to characterize HCN-evoked histamine release. As discussed previously we have evidence that histamine is taken up by Aplysia CNS tissue and it is rapidly metabolized by γ-glutamylhistamine synthetase to a dipeptide, γ-glutamylhistamine. We do not, as yet, know how closely linked histamine uptake is to metabolism. Our suspicion, based upon preliminary observations of the in situ actions of synthetase inhibitors, is that the two processes may be in close association with each other.

ACKNOWLEDGEMENT

I would like to express my gratitude to the National Science Foundation for their support of this work during the past ten years.

REFERENCES

Ascher, P. and Kehoe, J.S. (1975), In: Handbook of Psychopharmacology (Ed.), Iversen, L.L., Iversen, S.D. and Snyder, S.H. 4, 265-310, Plenum Press, New York.
Blankenship, J.E., Wachtel, H., and Kandel, E.R. (1971), J. Neurophysiol., 34, 76-92.
Carpenter, D.O. and Gaubatz, G.L. (1975), Nature(London), 254, 343-344.
Claiborne, B.J. and Selverston, A.I. (1984), J. Neurosci.4, 708-721.
Douglas, W.W. (1980), In: The Pharmacology Basis of Therapeutics, 6th ed.,Macmillan, New York.
Elias, M.S. and Evans, P.D. (1983), J. Neurochem. 41, 562-568.
Geller, H.M. (1979), Neuroscience Let., 14, 49-53.
Gerschenfeld, H.M. (1973), Physiol. Rev., 53, 1-119.
Gerschenfeld, H.M., Hamon, M., Paupardin-Tritsch, D. (1978), J. Physiol., 274, 265-278.

Gerschenfeld, H.M. and Paupardin-Tritsch, D. (1974a), J. Physiol., 243, 427-456.
Gerschenfeld, H.M. and Paupardin-Tritsch, D. (1974b), J. Physiol., 243, 457-481.
Gotoh, H. and Schwartz, J.H. (1980), Proc. 10th Meeting Neuroscience, 6, 502.
Griffith, O.W., Anderson, M.E. and Meister, A. (1979), J. Biol. Chem., 254, 1205-1210.
Gruol, D.L. and Weinreich, D. (1979a), Brain Res., 162, 281-301.
Gruol, D.L. and Weinreich, D. (1979b), Neuropharm., 18, 415-421,
Haas, H.L. (1974), Brain Res., 76, 363-366.
Haas, H.L. and Wolf, P. (1977), Brain Res., 122, 269-279.
Kandel, E.R. and Gardner, D. (1972), Neurotransmitters, Res. Publ. A.R.N.M.D., 50, 91-145.
Kehoe, J.S. (1972a), J. Physiol., 225, 85-114.
Kehoe, J.S. (1972b), J. Physiol., 225, 115-146.
Kehoe, J.S. (1972c), J. Physiol., 225, 147-172.
Kehoe, J.S. (1975), J. Physiol., 244, 23P-24P
Kehoe, J.S. and Marder, E. (1976), Ann. Rev. Pharmac. 16, 245-268
Leake, L.D. and Walker, R.J. (1980), Invertebrate Neuropharmacology. John Wiley and Sons, N.Y.
McCaman, R.E. and McKenna, D.G. (1978), Brain Res, 141, 165-171.
McCaman, R.E. and Weinreich, D. (1982), J. Physiol. 328, 485-506.
McCaman, R.E. and Weinreich, D. (1984), J. Neurophysiol. (in press)
Meister, A. (1973), Science, 180, 33-39.
Meister, A. and Tate, S.S. (1976), Ann. Rev. Biochem., 45, 559-604.
Ono, J. and McCaman, R.E. (1980), Neuroscience, 5, 835-840.
Ono, J.K. and McCaman, R.E. (1984) In: Model Neural Circuits and Behavior, ed Selverston, A.I. and Jensen, K., Plenum Press.
Osborne, N.N. (1977), Microchemical Analysis of Nervous Tissue, Pergamon Press, New York.
Osborne, N.N. Wolter, K.D., and Neuhoff, V. (1979), Biochem. Pharm., 28, 2799-2805.
Panula, P. H-Y T. Yang and Costa, E. (1984), Proc. Nat. Acad. Sci., 81, 2572-2576.
Paton, W.D. (1958), Ann Rev. Physiol., 20, 431-470.
Reite, O.B. (1972), Physiol. Rev., 52, 778-919.
Sano, I., Kakimoto, Y., Kanazawa, A., Wakajima, T. and Shimizu, H. (1966), J. Neurochem., 13, 711-719.
Sastry, B.S.R. and Phillis, J.W. (1976), Eur. J. Pharmacol., 38, 269-273.
Stein, C. and Weinreich, D. (1982a), J. Neurochem., 38, 204-214.
Stein, C. and Weinreich, D. (1982b), Proc. 12th meeting, Soc. Neurosci. 8, 988.
Stein, C. and Weinreich, D. (1983), Comp. Biochem. Physiol. 74, 79-83.
Takeuchi, H., Yokoi, I., and Horisaka, K. (1976), C.R. Acad. Science (Paris), 170, 1118-1126.
Weinreich, D. (1977a) In: Biochemistry of Characterized Neurons, Pergamon Press, N.Y.
Weinreich, D. (1977) Nature, 267, 854-856.
Weinreich, D. (1979), J. Neurochem., 32, 363-369.
Weinreich, D., Weiner, C., and McCaman, R. (1975), Brain Res., 84, 341-345.
Weinreich, D. and Yu, Y.-T. (1977), J. Neurochem., 28, 361-369.
Werman, R. (1966), Comp. Biochem. Physiol., 18, 745-766.
Werman, R. (1980), In: Receptors for Neurotransmitters and Peptides Hormones, Raven Press, New York.
Wilcox, B.J. and Seybold, V.S. (1982), Neurosci. Letters, 29, 105-110.

HISTAMINE ACTIONS IN THE MAMMALIAN CENTRAL NERVOUS SYSTEM

H. L. Haas

Neurochirurgische Universitätsklinik, 8091 Zürich, Switzerland

ABSTRACT

Microionophoretic investigations on histamine in the mammalian central nervous system are summarized. More recent investigations using the brain slice method have revealed the mechanism of a modulatory action: In the hippocampus histamine blocks a calcium activated potassium conductance and profoundly potentiates excitatory signals.

KEYWORDS

Histamine, microionophoresis, brain slices, modulation, calcium, potassium

INTRODUCTION

"Seeing is believing", this attitude is probably responsible for the neglect histamine has suffered for a long time. The more popular amines (acetylcholine, noradrenaline, dopamine, serotonin) whose cells of origin and projections have been clearly visualized in the past decades are no closer to meeting the strict criteria for the identification as transmitters in the central nervous system than histamine. Direct demonstration of histaminergic pathways is now also available (Pollard and colleagues, Steinbusch and Mulder, Watanabe and colleagues, this volume) and confirms the lesion studies of Garbarg and colleagues (1974). Advances of in vitro techniques have allowed a better insight in the basic mechanisms representing central histamine functions. These investigations give indications for a classical transmitter role - direct effects on membrane permeability of certain ions - but a typical modulator action seems to be predominant and has been much better characterized. This modulation is potentially very powerful ranging between suppression and maximal transmission of neuronal signals.

Microionophoresis of Histamine

This technique delivers a high concentration of histamine (or other substances) to the immediate environment of the tip of a multibarreled glasspipette. Pressure applied to the same pipettes has also succesfully been used to eject drugs in a highly localized manner. By these ways depressant actions of histamine have been found on many neurones all over the central nervous system. Motoneurones of the cat were hyperpolarized and synaptic potentials reduced (Phillis, Tebecis and York, 1968a). Engberg, Flatman and Kadzielawa (1976) showed an increase in membrane resistance and a reduction in spike afterhyperpolarization. The specificity and physiological relevance of these observations was however questioned by the authors. Similar actions of histamine and several of its metabolites occur on the big medial reticular formation neurones in the brain stem of unanaesthetized and decerebrate cats. Some related imidazole compounds seem to activate GABA receptors, most notably imidazoleacetic acid (Haas, Anderson and Hösli, 1973).

In cortical regions of rat, cat and guinea pig, most responsive neurones are depressed by ionophoretic histamine (Phillis, Tebecis and York, 1968b) an action which seems to be mediated by H2-receptors (Haas and Bucher, 1975; Phillis, Kostopoulos and Odutola, 1975; Haas and Wolf, 1977) but may also involve H1 receptors (Sastry and Phillis, 1976a). The H2 agonists 4-methylhistamine and impromidine exert also depressions and these are blocked by the H2 antagonists metiamide and cimetidine. Excitatory and dual actions occur but cannot be clearly related to H1 or H2 receptors. Metiamide seems to specifically block the histaminergic medial forebrain bundle neocortical pathway (Sastry and Phillis, 1976b; Haas and Wolf, 1977). The complex synaptic response following afferent stimulation (comprising histaminergic fibers) in the hippocampus is also modified by ionophoretic metiamide (Haas and Wolf, 1977). Furthermore, lesions in the medial forebrain bundle of guinea pigs lead to an increased sensitivity of cortical neurones to local histamine administration. This supersensitivity occurs in parallel with the fall in histidine decarboxylase activity (Haas and colleagues, 1978).

In the hypothalamus, ionophoresis of histamine often leads to excitation (Haas, 1974). A slow (several seconds) and rarely a faster time course (less than 1 sec) was described for those actions which may be related to H1 receptors (Renaud, 1976; Haas and Wolf, 1977; Carette, 1978). Depression of firing is also found and is blocked by H2 antagonists. The catabolites of histamine, 2-methylhistamine and 2-methylimidazoleacetic acid were much weaker than histamine: in the absence of a high affinity reuptake mechanism, methylation could be the major way of histamine inactivation (Green, 1970; Haas and Wolf, 1977). The excitation of identified neurosecretory neurones projecting to the neurohypophysis can explain the antidiuretic action of histamine (Haas, Wolf and Nussbaumer, 1975; Haas and Wolf, 1977; Haas and Geller, 1982).

Brain Slices in Vitro: Hypothalamus

Inspection of the 400 - 500 uM thick slices in a perfusion chamber with a stereomicroscope allows clear identification of most hypothalamic nuclei. Response patterns similar to those observed in vivo were found in several nuclei. Comparable results were also obtained from tissue cultures, where metiamide blocked inhibitory (H2) actions and promethazine blocked excitatory (H1) actions (Geller, 1981). Intracellular recordings from presumed neurosecretory neurones in the paraventricular and supraoptic nuclei have revealed strong excitation by bath applied histamine, presumably as a result of increased epsps. This indicates that the direct effect of histamine took place on neigbouring elements (Haas and Geller, 1982).

Hippocampus

The hippocampal slice is not only the most investigated brain slice, it is also quite suitable for studying the mechanism of action of histamine on the cellular and membrane level as histaminergic projections to this structure have been clearly identified (Garbarg and colleagues, 1974; Schwartz, Garbarg and Pollard, 1984). The manipulations of the ionic environment in a perfusion chamber allow an analysis hitherto unavailable on central neurones. In accordance with the in vivo studies, locally restricted application of histamine by ionophoresis or pressure injection depresses the spontaneous firing of the majority of CA 1 pyramidal and dentate granule cells. This is accompanied by a hyperpolarization and sometimes a moderate conductance change. The hyperpolarization appears to be postsynaptic and mediated by H2 receptors (Haas, 1981). Microdrops applied to the slice surface can also cause a slow depolarization without a conductance change. Extra- and intracellularly recorded epsps were found to be augmented by Segal (1980, 1981), who suggested that these effects are presynaptic and mediated by the H1 receptor. Experiments with bath applied histamine are described in the following sections.

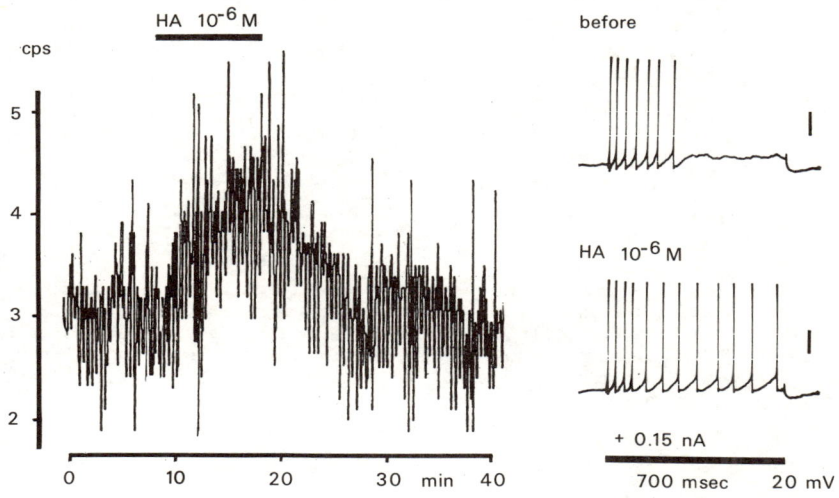

Fig. 1. Histamine blocks accommodation of firing and increases firing rate. Oscilloscope photographs on the right show responses of a CA 1 pyramidal cell to depolarizing current injection (+ 0.15 nA for 700 msec, bar below picture). In the presence of histamine (1 uM) firing continues through the whole pulse. The diagram on the left is a ratemeter record showing the number of action potentials per second (cps) versus time. Histamine (HA) was added to the perfusion fluid during the time indicated by the bar above the trace. About one half of the increase in frequency results from the increased response to the depolarizing pulses which were given every 10 sec, the other half represents increased spontaneous firing.

METHODS

Conventional techniques were used for preparation and incubation of transverse hippocampal slices from 48 Wistar rats in a perfusion chamber (Haas, Schaerer and Vosmansky, 1979). Microelectrodes for extracellular recording were filled with 1 M NaCl, those for intracellular recording with 2-4 M KCl, K-acetate or CsCl. Drugs were added to the perfusion medium usually for periods of at least 5 - 10 min. Although equilibration was achieved within 1 min in the chamber the same concentration at the receptor sites in the slice was probably not reached within 10 min. Stimulation and recording electrodes were placed on the appropriate locations on the slices under direct observation through a stereomicroscope. Signals were recorded with a bridge amplifier, viewed on a storage oscilloscope and analysed with the aid of a microprocessor.

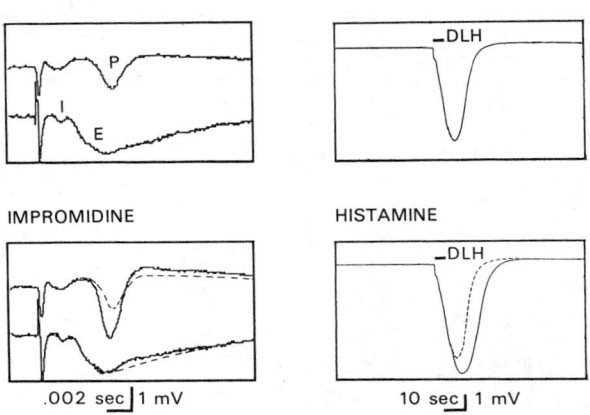

Fig. 2. H2 actions on extracellular epsp (E) population spike (P) and response to ionophoretic (10 nA, during bar) D,L-homocysteic acid (DLH). Upper records and broken lines in lower records are controls. Lower records show potentials in the presence of 1 uM impromidine and 10 uM histamine respectively. Left: Upper traces are recorded in pyramidal layer of CA 1, lower traces in stratum radiatum (I: input volley, E: epsp).

RESULTS

Resting Potential and Accommodation of Firing.

Micromolar concentrations of histamine and impromidine depolarized pyramidal cells in the CA 1 region slightly (2.5 +- 1.5 SD mV, n = 16) and increased their spontaneous firing rate (Fig. 1, left diagram). The response to low intensity depolarizing current injection usually displayed strong accommodation of the action potential frequency: In Fig. 1 (before) spike firing is only seen during the first 300 msec of a 700 msec, + 0.15 nA pulse, but occurs through the whole pulse when 1 uM histamine is present. This effect was observed in all 27 investigated neurones; in 9 of those careful examination showed that the effect was independent of changes in soma potential or conductance.

The firing caused by ionophoretic pulses of glutamic or D,L-homocysteic acids to the apical dendritic region was prolonged by histamine and impromidine (n = 7). This was often registered as an extracellular DC field representing the firing of several neurones (Fig. 2, right records). Furthermore, burst discharges in spontaneously epileptic slices (n = 2) were potentiated when histamine was added to their bathing fluid (Haas 1984, 1985).

Afterhyperpolarization (AHP)

Single action potentials or bursts of spikes in CA 1 pyramidal cells are followed by a two-component AHP (Figs. 3; 4C). The fast component is ascribed to the delayed rectifier potassium current while the long lasting component is due to a calcium activated potassium current (gK(Ca)). This late but not the early AHP is blocked by histamine and impromidine in micromolar concentrations. The block is completely reversed by adding the H2 antagonists metiamide or cimetidine (5 - 10 uM) to the medium. Neither mepyramine (H1 antagonist) nor propranolol (beta antagonist, which blocks a similar action of noradrenaline on the AHP) antagonized this effect (Madison and Nicoll, 1982; Haas and Konnerth, 1983).

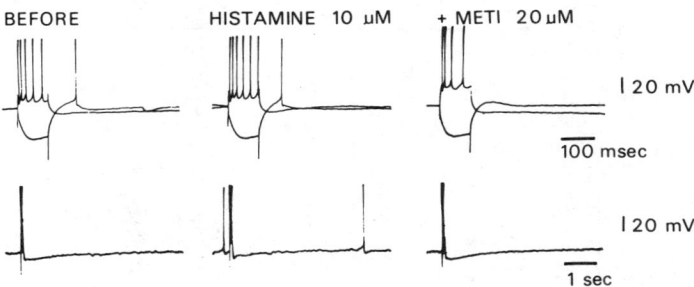

Fig. 3. Intracellular recordings from a CA 1 pyramidal cell before and during histamine action and after addition of metiamide. Upper records show responses to +- 1 nA lower records to + 1 nA, 100 msec current injection. Histamine blocks the late AHP after a burst of spikes (and the accommodation of firing) and this effect is (more than) fully reversed by metiamide.

The AHPs are also observed following slow (calcium) spikes in TTX poisoned preparations. The late component is blocked in this condition in the absence of a reduction in the calcium spike indicating that the block of gK(Ca) was not secondary to a reduction in calcium inflow. In fact an increase in calcium spike amplitude and the number of calcium spikes fired by a given depolarization was usually seen. In order to better analyse the calcium spike per se recording was performed with caesium chloride filled electrodes. Caesium ions diffusing into the cell quickly blocked the late AHP and revealed large calcium spikes. Now 10 uM histamine had no effect (Fig.4 A). Comparable data were also obtained when gK(Ca) was reduced by adding tetraethylammonium (10 uM) or barium ions (0.3 mM) to the perfusion fluid. The large calcium spikes recorded when restricting potassium currents were reduced were often followed by an afterdepolarization lasting for several 100 msec. This potential which presumably reflects a persistent calcium inflow was facilitated and prolonged by histamine.

Synaptic Potentials

Excitatory postsynaptic potentials (epsps) in CA 1 after stimulation of strata radiatum or oriens were found unchanged during perfusion with histamine (Fig. 2). This was investigated with intracellular and extracellular (field epsp) recording. However, the population spike, i.e. the compound action potential fired by a given stimulation and epsp, was always increased by histamine and impromidine. The relation between field epsp and population spike is illustrated in Fig. 6. In the CA 3 region, an increase of epsps by histamine has been observed (Segal, 1982; Tagami and colleagues, 1984).

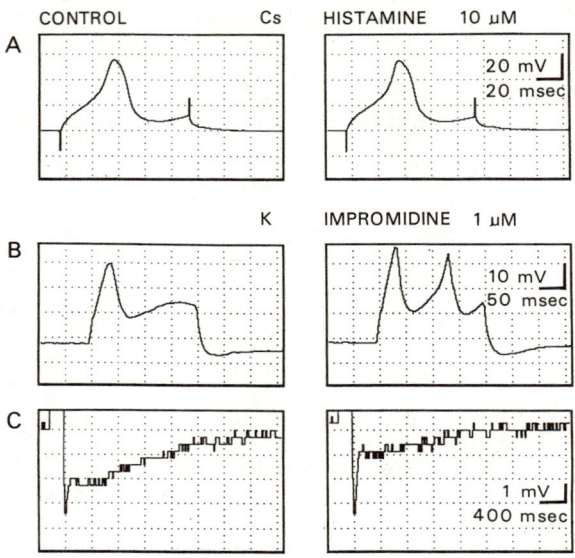

Fig. 4. Histamine and impromidine actions in a tetrodotoxin poisoned slice. Averaged (9 sweeps) intracellular records from 2 CA 1 pyramids. A: Calcium spike evoked by positive current injection (100 msec) recorded with a caesium chloride filled electrode. Intracellular caesium blocks potassium channels revealing a large calcium spike (58 mV) without late AHP. The addition of 10 uM histamine does not reduce the calcium spike and hence presumably calcium inflow; the spike is in fact slightly faster in onset and wider. B: Calcium spikes recorded with a potassium chloride filled electrode. The addition of 1 uM impromidine (H2 agonist) to the medium causes an increase of the calcium spikes and a block of accommodation: the same 200 msec pulse evokes now two slow spikes. C: Tails after the responses shown in B. Note different gain (x8) and time base (x8). The calcium spikes are (upward) out of scale, the first downward deflections are the early afterhyperpolarizations due to the delayed rectifier potassium current (unaffected). The late afterhyperpolarization is markedly reduced by 1 uM impromidine.

DISCUSSION

The widespread arborization of histaminergic (and other aminergic) projections to the forebrain suggest that they may regulate the functional state of target regions rather than transmit discrete signals. Such a function would be very well served by the modulatory action described here: A range of different excitatory signals are shown to be potentiated by histamine through activation of an H2 receptor. They include synaptically evoked population spikes, epileptiform bursts, responses to depolarization by current injection through

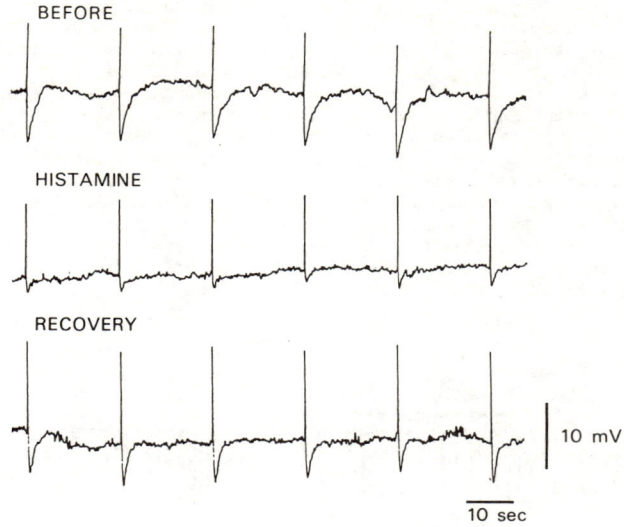

Fig. 5. Effect of histamine (1 uM) on the late afterhyperpolarization (AHP) in tetrodotoxin containing medium. Upstrokes are calcium spikes (elicited every 20 sec by depolarizing current injection), downward deflections are AHPs. Lowest trace obtained 20 min after withdrawal of histamine. Traces from pen recorder.

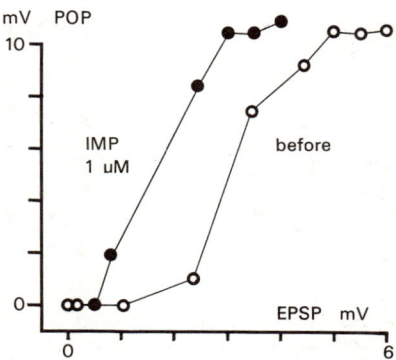

Fig. 6. Relationship between field epsp and population spike (POP) at varying stimulation strength in CA 1 (see Fig. 3). The epsp was unchanged (not shown) but the population spikes evoked by given epsps were enhanced by 1 uM impromidine (filled circles).

the recording electrode or by ionophoretic application of excitatory amino acids. All these actions could be explained by a block of gK(Ca), which was best illustrated by the long lasting AHP after excitatory signals. Strong and longer lasting depolarizations are selfrestricting by activation of gK(Ca). A release from this self-restriction by histamine may be described as an intrinisic disinhibition. Such an action would also increase signal to noise ratio by favoring larger potentials. No direct actions on calcium spikes were seen even in experiments optimizing their visibility. A voltage clamp study of CA 1 neurones however, has revealed a reduction in somatic calcium current by histamine (Pellmar, 1984). In low calcium high magnesium solutions an excitatory action of histamine (H2) is still present (Fig. 7) indicating that this effect is independent of extracellular calcium (Haas and colleagues, 1984): It may be a direct interaction with K channels or an influence on intracellular calcium level and sequestration. In each case cyclic AMP accumulation and, perhaps in the latter, phosphorylation of proteins leading to a larger calcium binding capacity may be involved (Haas, 1984, 1985).

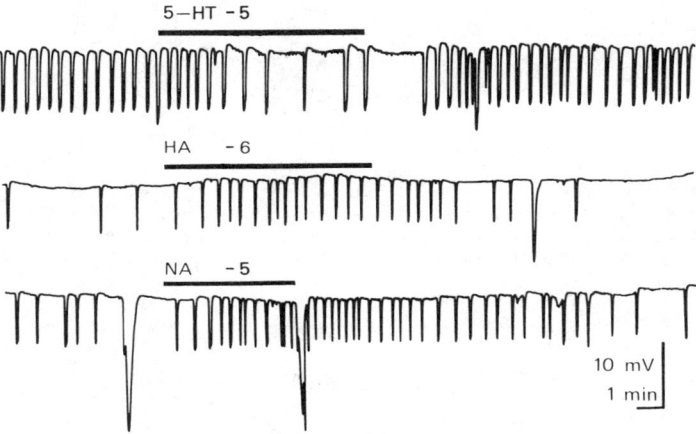

Fig. 7. Spontaneous field bursts (downward deflections), recorded in a low calcium high magnesium medium, are blocked by serotonin (5-HT, 10 uM) but accelerated by histamine (HA, 1 uM) and noradrenaline (NA, 10 uM). These effects parallel the actions on afterhyperpolarizations. (AHP-block = acceleration; AHP-enhancement = slowing) and argue for a mechanism of action which is independent of calcium inflow.

No direct data on presynaptic actions of histamine are available at present but the mechanisms described here on the postsynaptic level may well be operative in terminals and varicosities, where calcium inflow triggers release. Although a clearer picture of histamine's role in the central nervous system is emerging more information is needed to understand how it functions naturally. The mode of action of histamine (and the other amines) cannot be expected to serve very specific functions making it the transmitter of, for instance, thermoregulation or water balance. However, an involvement in many hypothalamic and forebrain functions is highly probable. Together with other systems ascending from the brain stem histamine neurones may participate in regulation of states of awareness, circadian and other rhythms, neuroendocrine and vegetative functions. The anatomical disposition and modulatory mechanism allow setting of the neuronal responsiveness and thus the functional state in target areas.

REFERENCES

Anderson, E. G., H. L. Haas, and L. Hösli (1973). Comparison of effects of noradrenaline and histamine with cyclic AMP on brain stem neurones. Brain Res., 49, 471-475.

Carette, B. (1978). Responses of preoptic-septal neurons to iontophoretically applied histamine. Brain Res., 145, 391-395.

Engberg, I., J. A. Flatman, and K. Kadzielawa (1976). Lack of specificity of motoneurone responses to microiontophoretically applied phenolic amines. Acta Physiol. Scand., 96, 137-139.

Etgen, A. M., and E. T. Browning (1984). Activators of cyclic AMP accumulation in rat hippocampal slices: action of vasoactive intestinal peptide (VIP). J. Neurosci., in press.

Garbarg, M., G. Barbin, J. Feger, and J. C. Schwartz (1974). Histaminergic pathway in rat brain evidenced by lesions of the medial forebrain bundle. Science, 186, 833-835.

Geller, H. M. (1981). Histamine actions on activity of cultured hypothalamic neurons: Evidence for mediation by H1- and H2-histamine receptors. Dev. Brain Res., 1, 89-101.

Green, J. P. (1970). Histamine. In A. Lajtha (Ed.), Handbook of Neurochemistry, Vol. 4 pp. 221-250.

Green, J. P. (1982). Histamine receptors in brain. In L. L. Iversen, S. D. Iversen, and S. H. Snyder (Eds.), Handbook of Psychopharmacology, Vol. 17, Plenum Press, New York, pp. 385-419.

Haas, H. L. (1974). Histamine: Action on single hypothalamic neurones. Brain Res., 76, 363-366.

Haas, H. L. (1981). Histamine hyperpolarizes hippocampal neurones in vitro. Neuroscience Lett., 22, 75-78.

Haas, H. L. (1984). Histamine potentiates neuronal excitation by blocking a calcium dependent potassium conductance. Agents and Actions, 14, 534-537.

Haas, H. L. (1985). Histamine may act through cyclic AMP on hippocampal neurones. Agents and Actions, 15, in press

Haas, H. L., E. G. Anderson, and L. Hösli (1973). Histamine and metabolites: Their effects and interactions with convulsants on brain stem neurones. Brain Res., 51, 269-278.

Haas, H. L., and U. M. Bucher (1975). Histamine H2-receptors on single central neurones. Nature, 255, 634-635.

Haas, H. L., and H. M. Geller (1982). Electrophysiology of histaminergic transmission in the brain. In B. Uvnäs, and K. Tasaka (Eds.), Advances in Histamine Research, Advances in the Biosciences, Vol. 33, Pergamon Press, pp. 81-91.

Haas, H. L., J. G. R. Jefferys, N. T. Slater, and D. O. Carpenter, (1984). Modulation of low calcium induced field bursts in the hippocampus by monoamines and cholinomimetics. Pflügers Arch., 400, 28-33.

Haas, H. L., and A. Konnerth (1983). Histamine and noradrenaline decrease calcium-activated potassium conductance in hippocampal pyramidal cells. Nature, 302, 432-450.

Haas, H. L., and P. Wolf (1977). Central actions of histamine, microelectrophoretic studies. Brain Res., 122, 269-279.

Haas, H. L., P. Wolf, and J. -C. Nussbaumer (1975). Histamine: action on supraoptic and other hypothalamic neurones in the cat. Brain Res., 88, 166-170.

Haas, H. L., B. Schaerer, and M. Vosmansky (1979). A simple perfusion chamber for the study for nervous tissue slice in vitro. J. Neuroscience Meth., 1, 323-325.

Haas, H. L., P. Wolf, J. M. Palacios, M. Garbarg, G. Barbin, and J. C. Schwartz (1978). Hypersensitivity to histamine in the guinea-pig brain: Microiontophoretic and biochemical studies. Brain Res., 156, 275-291.

Hough, L. B., and J. P. Green (1984). Histamine and its receptors in the nervous system. In A. Lajtha (Ed.), Handbook of Neurochemistry, Vol. 6, 2rd ed. Plenum Publishing Corporation, New York. pp. 145-210.

Madison, D. V., and R. A. Nicoll (1982). Noradrenaline blocks accommodation of pyramidal cell discharge in the hippocampus. Nature, 299, 636-638.

Palacios, J. M., M. Garbarg, G. Barbin, and J. C. Schwartz (1978). Pharmacological characterization of histamine receptors mediating the stimulation of cyclic AMP accumulation in slices from guinea pig hippocampus. Mol. Pharmacol., 14, 971-982.

Pellmar, T. C. (1984). Histamine decreases calcium inward current in guinea-pig hippocampal CA1 pyramidal cells. J. Physiol., in Press.

Phillis, J. W., G. K. Kostopoulos, and A. Odutola (1975). On the specificity of histamine H2-receptor antagonists in the rat cerebral cortex. Can. J. Physiol. Pharmac., 53, 1205-1209.

Phillis, J. W., A. K. Tebecis, and D. H. York (1968a). Depression of spinal motoneurones by noradrenaline, 5-hydroxytryptamine and histamine. Eur. J. Pharmac., 4, 471-475.

Phillis, J. W., A. K. Tebecis, and D. H. York (1968b). Histamine and some antihistamines: their actions on cerebral cortical neurones. Br. J. Pharmac., 33, 426-440.

Renaud, L. P. (1976). Histamine microiontophoresis on identified hypothalamic neuons: 3 Patterns of response in the ventromedial nucleus of the rat. Brain Res., 115, 339-344.

Roberts, F., and C. R. Calcutt (1984). Histamine and the hypothalamus. Neuroscience, 9, 721-739.

Sastry, B. S. R., and J. W. Phillis (1976a). Depression of rat cerebral cortical neurones by H1 and H2 histamine receptors agonists. Eur. J. Pharmac., 38, 269-273.

Sastry, B .S. R., and J. W. Phillis (1976b). Evidence for an ascending inhibitory histaminergic pathway to the cerebral cortex. Can. J. Physiol. Pharmac., 54, 782-786.

Satayavivad, U., and E. Kirsten (1977). Iontophoretic studies of histamine and histamine antagonists in the feline vestibular nuclei. Eur. J. Pharmac., 41, 17-26.

Schwartz, J. C. (1979). Histamine receptors in brain. Life Sciences, 25, 895-912.

Schwartz, J. C., M. Garbarg, and H. Pollard (1984). Histaminergic transmission in brain. Handbook of Physiology, in Press.

Segal, M. (1980). Histamine produces a calcium-sensitive depolarization of hippocampal pyramidal cells in vitro. Neuroscience Lett., 19, 67.

Segal, M. (1981). Histamine modulates reactivity of hippocampal CA 3 neurons to afferent stimulation in vitro. Brain Res., 213, 443-448.

Sweatman, P., and R. M. Jell (1977). Dopamine and histamine sensitivity of rostral hypothalamic neurones in the cat: Possible involvement in thermoregulation. Brain Res., 127, 173-178.

Tagami, H., A. Sunami, M. Akagi, and K. Tasaka (1984). Effect of histamine on the hippocampal neurons in guinea-pig. Agents and Actions, 14, 538-542.

PHYSIOLOGICAL FUNCTIONS OF HISTAMINE IN THE BRAIN

H. Wada*, T. Watanabe*, A. Yamatodani*,
K. Maeyama*, N. Itoi*, R. Cacabelos*, M. Seo**,
S. Kiyono**, K. Nagai*** and H. Nakagawa***

*Department of Pharmacology II, Osaka University School of
Medicine, Osaka, Japan
**Institute for Developmental Research, Aichi Prefectural
Colony, Aichi, Japan
***Institute for Protein Chemistry, Osaka University,
Suita, Japan

ABSTRACT

From the distribution of the histaminergic neuron system in rat brain, elucidated in our laboratory (Watanabe and others, in this symposium), it seems clear that histamine plays some important physiological roles as a neurotransmitter or neuromodulator in the brain. We studied for its roles using two specific tools, α-fluoromethylhistidine (FMH) and W/W^v mice. Acute or chronic administration of FMH to W/W^v mice or to rats did not result in any detectable changes in gross behaviour. However, careful observation revealed that a single i. p. injection of FMH into rats caused a significant decrease in the arousal time with concomitant increase of slow wave sleep. On microinfusion of histamine into the suprachiasmatic nuclei, rats became active and took more food during the light period, indicating some disturbance of their circadian rhythm. These results were strongly supported by the finding that the content of histamine in the posterior hypothalamus, which contains cell bodies of histaminergic neurons, exhibited a circadian rhythm. Depletion of histamine in the brain by treatment with FMH blocked the increase of the plasma ACTH, vasopressin and oxytocin induced by bilateral adrenalectomy. All these results suggest that the histaminergic neuron system does not have independent and/or separate functions in the CNS, but acts as a kind of neuromodulator in controlling the CNS as a whole.

KEYWORDS

Histamine; histidine decarboxylase; α-fluoromethylhistidine; W/W^v mice; circadian rhythm; sleep-wakefulness; food intake; neuroendocrine function; locomotor activity.

INTRODUCTION

There are many works reporting that histamine influences the circadian rhythms such as sleep-wakefulness and food intake, thirst, cardiovascular functions including control of blood pressure, sexual behavior, neuroendocrine functions and so on (Donoso and Alvarez, 1984; Green, 1983; Hough and Green, 1984; Roberts and Calcutt, 1983; Schwartz and co-workers, 1977, 1980, 1982; Taylor, 1982). These reports suggest that histamine may be involved in fundamental physiological functions. We are examining this problem using histidine decarboxylase (HDC, L-histidine carboxylase, E.C.4.1.1.22) as a probe. In the last 8 years, mammalian HDC has been extensively studied in our laboratory (Fukui, Watanabe and Wada, 1980; Taguchi and others, 1984; Wada and co-workers, 1984; Watanabe and others, 1979, 1982; Watanabe and Wada, 1983; Yamada and others, 1984). It was most extensively purified from fetal rat liver, and some of its enzymatic and immunochemical properties were investigated. The results of these studies can be summarized as follows.

(1) In general, the content of HDC is very low, and HDC is very labile during purification procedures. The finding of the stabilizing effects of polyethylene glycol in purification steps and the effectiveness of carnosine-affinity column chromatography contributed very much to its purification to homogeneity.

(2) Using antibody against purified HDC, it was originally demonstrated that there were two kinds of HDC's, mast cell type and non-mast cell type. The existence of two types was deduced from the finding that the precipitin line of the antibody against fetal liver (mast cell type) formed a spur with the precipitin line against the partially purified brain enzyme (non-mast cell type). This antibody also inhibited mast cell type HDC much more strongly than non-mast cell type HDC.

(3) However, a recently obtained antibody, although obtained using enzyme from the same source for immunization, had a strong inhibitory action on not only mast cell type HDC, but also non-mast cell type HDC. With this new antibody, the precipitin lines against rat fetal liver HDC, and HDC's from adult brain and stomach, fused without spar formation. In other words, results depended on the antibody used, and the new antibody showed a strong binding affinity towards both brain and fetal HDC.

The new antibody was used to elucidate the histaminergic neuron system in rat brain by a fluorescent immunohistochemical technique (Hayashi and others, 1984; Takeda and others 1984a, 1984b,1984c; Watanabe and others, 1983, 1984). A tentative diagram of the projection of histaminergic neuron system in rat brain is shown in Fig. 1. Recently, essentially similar results were obtained using anti-histamine antibody in several laboratories (Panula, Yang and Costa 1984; Steinbusch and Mulder, 1984; Wilcox and Seybold, 1982) or [^{3}H]-mepyramine as a probe (Palacios, Wamsley and Kuhar, 1981).

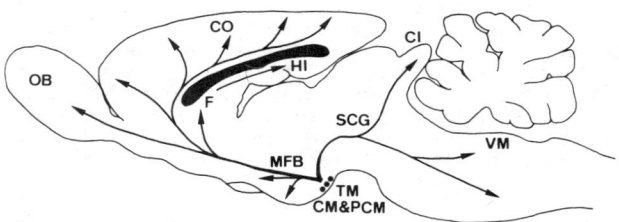

Fig. 1. Diagram of projection of the histaminergic neuron system from the TM, CM and PCM to various regions of rat brain. OB, olfactory bulb; CO, cortex; HI, hippocampus; CI, colliculus inferior; VM, n. vestibularis medialis; SCG, central grey matter; MFB, medial forebrain bundle; F, fornix; TM, CM, and PCM, tuberal, caudal, and postmammillary caudal magnocellular nuclei, respectively.

From the distribution of the histaminergic neuron system in rat brain described above, it is believed that histamine plays a role as a neurotransmitter or neuromodulator, just like noradrenaline, dopamine and serotonin. Schwartz and his collaborators studied on the localization of histaminergic neuronal pathways extensively without using a histochemical method (Ben-Ari and others, 1977; Garbarg and others, 1974a; Schwartz and coworkers, 1982). They measured the histamine levels and HDC activities in various telencephalic areas and observed the highest levels of histamine and HDC activity in the mammillary body (Pollard and others, 1976). They observed a substantial decrease in the histamine level and HDC activity after lesions of the lateral hypothalamic area interrupting the medial forebrain bundle. From the effects of a variety of lesions they proposed a scheme for the anatomical disposition of the histaminergic neuron system. They concluded that the most probable location of histamine cell bodies for the ascending pathway is the mesencephalic reticular formation and posterior mammillary bodies. It is noteworthy that the proposed pathways in rat brain are essentially in agreement with our results obtained by an immunohistochemical technique. Schwartz's group did much works on the physiological functions of histamine in the brain based on their proposed histaminergic neuron system(Schwartz and co-workers, 1977, 1980, 1982).

TOOLS TO STUDY THE PHYSIOLOGICAL FUNCTIONS OF HISTAMINE IN THE BRAIN

We are using two very useful tools in our laboratory to study the physiological functions of histamine in the brain, α-fluoromethylhistidine (FMH) and W/W^v mice which are devoid of mast cells. The results obtained so far in our laboratory can be summarized as follows.

Effect of FMH on HDC

FMH (with the structure shown on right) is a kind of suicide inhibitor which was developed by Kollonitsch and co-workers (1978). The mechanism of action of this inhibitor was studied extensively in our laboratory, with the following results.

In vitro studies (Kubota and others, 1984; Wada and co-workers, 1984). (1) FMH is decarboxylated at 1/36 the rate of histidine. (2) It inhibits HDC irreversibly (suicide substrate of HDC). (3) It shows saturation kinetics of inactivation. (4) It inactivates holo-HDC, but not apo-HDC. (5) Its inhibitory effect is prevented by the substrate, L-histidine, but not by D-histidine. (6) During preincubation with FMH, [ring-2-^{14}C]-FMH is incorporated into HDC, but [carboxyl--^{14}C]-FMH is not. (7) One molecule of FMH is incorporated into an HDC monomer (54K) per three decarboxylations.

In vivo studies (Maeyama and others, 1982, 1983) (1) When injected i.p. once at a dose of 50 mg/kg, FMH inactivates HDC specifically within 30 min. This result is in agreement with those of Garbarg and others (1980). (2) FMH causes rapid decrease in non-mast cell histamine, but not in mast cell histamine.

Studies on W/W^v Mice

Characteristics of W/W^v mice. W/W^v mice have a defect in the fifth chromosome and have been known as mice with macrocytic anemia. Kitamura, Go and Hatanaka (1978) found that the number of mast cells in the skin of W/W^v mice is less than 2 % congenic normal mice (+/+) and that W/W^v mice have no detectable mast cells in their tissues. These workers also showed that implantation of bone marrow of +/+ mice into W/W^v mice restored tissue mast cells, indicating that mast cells originate in the bone marrow (Kitamura, Go and Hatanaka, 1978). We compared the histamine contents of various tissues of W/W^v and +/+ mice and showed that the brain and stomach of W/W^v mice contained 44 and 34 %, respectively, of those of +/+ mice, suggesting that these tissues contain non-mast cell histamine (Yamatodani and others, 1982). Recently there have been several reports that there is no difference in the histamine contents of the brain of W/W^v and +/+ mice (Grzanna and Schultz, 1983; Hough and others, 1984; Orr and Pace, 1984).

Therefore, we re-examined the histamine contents and confirmed our previous results, as shown in Table 1. The difference was found in most areas except the cortex. Especially, the hypophysis and meninges (choroid plexus, data not shown) contain much more histamine in +/+ mice than in W/W^V mice. It is likely that the area rich in mast cells contains more histamine.

TABEL 1   Regional Distributions of Histamine in the Brain of W/W^V and +/+ Mice

	W/W^V	+/+	%Ratio
Whole Brain	0.27 ± 0.01	0.43 ± 0.02	61.2% (#2)
Cerebral Cortex	0.27 ± 0.02	0.28 ± 0.01	95.7% (#1)
Hypothalamus	1.47 ± 0.07	1.84 ± 0.12	80.2% (#3)
Globus Pallidus	0.41 ± 0.06	0.52 ± 0.05	79.2% (#1)
Thalamus	0.40 ± 0.04	0.55 ± 0.03	73.1% (#4)
Pons-Medulla	0.13 ± 0.01	0.22 ± 0.01	59.3% (#4)
Cerebellum	0.06 ± 0.01	0.15 ± 0.04	41.2% (#4)
Olfactory Bulb	0.14 ± 0.01	0.36 ± 0.08	39.0% (#4)
Hippocampus	0.22 ± 0.02	0.64 ± 0.09	34.5% (#4)
Hypophysis*	0.35 ± 0.05	2.65 ± 0.16	13.1% (#4)
Meninges**	0.15 ± 0.03	87.7 ± 12.4	0.2% (#4)

Mean + SEM, nmole/g (except *pmole/tissue, **pmole/cm^2)
Significance of difference: #1, n.s.; #2 P<0.01; #3, P<0.025; #4, P<0.005, by Student's t-test.

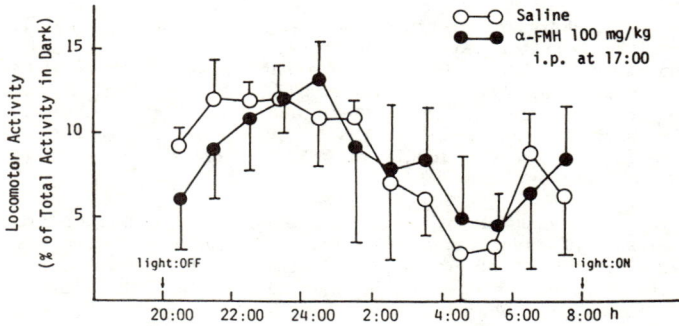

Fig. 2. Spontaneous locomotor activity of W/W^V mice during dark time. Each experiment was done with 4 mice. Activity was calculated as means + S.D. of counts per hr. Total counts of W/W^V mice treated with FMH and saline were 31500 ± 6700 and 26800 ± 6300, respectively. Each of total count was taken as 100 %.

PHYSIOLOGICAL FUNCTIONS OF THE HISTAMINERGIC NEURON SYSTEM

Effects of FMH on Spontaneous Locomotor Activity and Body Temperature

Based on the background information described above we studied the physiological significance of histaminergic neurons. We expected that i.p. administration of

FMH should cause some behavioral changes in mice, because it decreases the histamine level in the brain to almost zero. To study this we used $\overline{W/W^v}$ mice. As shown in Fig. 2, the spontaneous locomotor activity of groups of $\overline{4}$ mice was measured using an Animex activity meter, which is an automatic recorder of animal movements. However, we could not detect any difference between the activities of mice injected with FMH and with saline.

During this experiment, we also could not detect any abnormalities in behaviour of the animals. Table 2 summarises results on multidimensional behavior after i.p. administration of FMH (25 mg/kg) to male ddY mice. According to a modification of Irwin's methods, the observation was carried out 2 and 4 hrs after the FMH treatment. No remarkable changes in behaviour were observed. As positive controls several psychotropic drugs were administered.

TABLE 2 Multidimentional Observation in Mice by Modified Irwin Methods

Behaviour	Score (1 3 5 7 8 9)[a)]				
	⍺-FMH i.p. 25mg/kg	Chor-promazine P.o. 10 mg/kg	Diazepam P.o. 10 mg/kg	Amitri-ptyline P.o. 100mg/kg	Metam-phetamine P.o. 10 mg/kg
Body position	3 incr.	3 decr.	3 decr.	3 decr.	5 incr.
Catalepsy	1	5	1	1	1
Transfer arousal	1	3 decr.	1	1	1
Pelvic elevation	1	3 decr.	3 decr.	1	1
Tremore	1	1	3	1	1
Twitch	1	1	1	1	1
Convulsion	1	1	1	1	1
Tail elevation	1	5 decr.	1	3 decr.	1
Traction test	1	3	7	3	1
Abdominal tone	1	3 decr.	1	1	3 incr.
Positional struggle	1	3 decr.	1	1	3 incr.
Eye lid	1	7	3	1	1
Exophthalmos	1	1	1	1	9
Piloerection	1	1	3	1	3
Hypothermia	1	5	1	1	1
Salivation	1	1	1	1	7
Lacrimation	1	1	1	1	1
Diarrhea	1	1	1	1	1
Skin color	1	5	1	3	1
Pupil size	1	1	1	8 incr.	5 incr.

a): no effect; 1 - severe effect; 9. Behavior was observed 2h after administration (n=5). incr.: increase and decr.: decrease in comparison with the normal mice.

Bouclier and others (1983a,1983b) also reported that chronic infusion of FMH to rats caused marked depletion of histamine, but no gross changes associated with this depletion, including changes in body weight, body temperature and acidity of the stomach juice.

Effects of FMH and Diphenhydramine on Sleep-Wakefulness Cycle

Recently, polygraphic recordings revealed that i.p. administration of FMH to rats affected sleep-wakefulness cycle. Intraperitoneal administration of FMH (100 mg/kg) at 11:30 a.m. produced biphasic change in the sleep-wakefulness cycle; initial arousal, followed by a decrease of wakefulness (Fig. 3a). On the other hand, as shown in Fig. 3(b), increase of the slow wave sleep during night period (18:00-06:00 hr) was observed. The paradoxical sleep (Fig. 3c)increased long after drug injection, i.e., the next morning (05:00-11:00 hr). The H_1-antagonist diphenhydramine had an essentially similar effect. I.p. administration of diphenhydramine at a dose of 40 mg/kg resulted in immediate increase of wakefulness (12:00-16:00) followed by a decrease during night (23:00-06:00), whereas slow wave sleep and paradoxical sleep increased during night (23:00-06:00 and 22:00-04:00, respectively). These results seem to support the histamine arousal theory of Monnier, Sauer and Haff (1971).

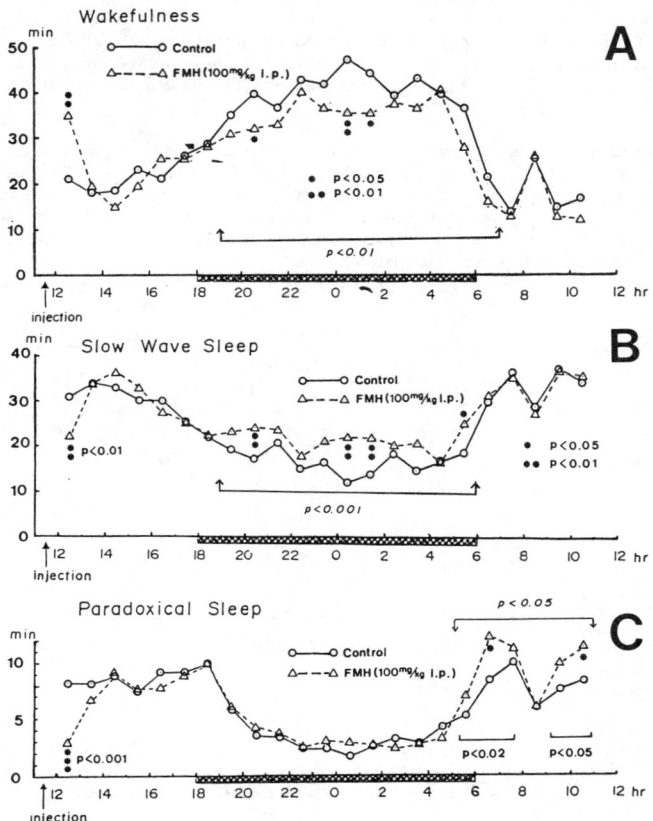

Fig. 3 Effect of FMH on wakefulness(A), slow wave sleep(B) and paradoxal sleep(C). Ordinate: time (min), abscissa: time of the day. The night period was indicated by a hatched horizotal column. Hourly mean values are plotted for the control (filled circles and thick straight lines) and FMH (open cicles and thick broken lines) groups. Statistical p values are calculated for each corresponding period.

Changes in Food Intake Induced by Infusion of Histamine into the Suprachiasmatic Nucleus and Demonstration of Circadian Change of Histamine Content in the Posterior Hypothalamus of Rats

The change in the circadian rhythm of food intake after infusion of histamine into the suprachiasmatic nucleus was investigated. Results are shown in Fig. 4. A cannula was implanted into in the suprachiasmatic nucleus on day −7, and histamine was infused on day 0 when the animals had recovered from the operation. Total food intake was slightly inhibited in the early period of the infusion but quickly recovered. So, on the whole, total food intake was not influenced. However, the food intake during the light period (08:00-20:00) was clearly increased by the infusion, and did not recover within a week. These results suggest that histamine plays some role in the generation of the circadian rhythm of rats.

Physiological functions of histamine in the brain   231

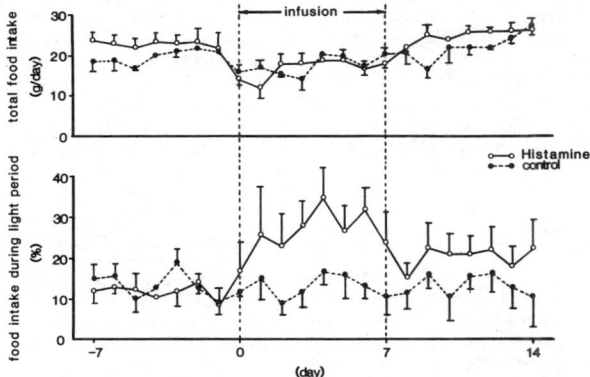

Fig. 4. Effect of histamine infusion into the suprachiasmatic nucleus on the feeding behavior in rats. Histamine (175 ng/h) or saline was infused into the suprachilasmatic nucleus with the rats of 1 μl/h for 7 days using an intracranial catheter and Alzet osmotic minipump under 12 hr light and 12 h dark condition. Ordinates indicate total daily food intake (g) and the percentage of food intake during the light period (=food intake during 12 h light period (g)/total daily food intake x 100). Data are expressed as means $\pm$ S.E. Each group of 5 animals was used for histamine or saline infusion.

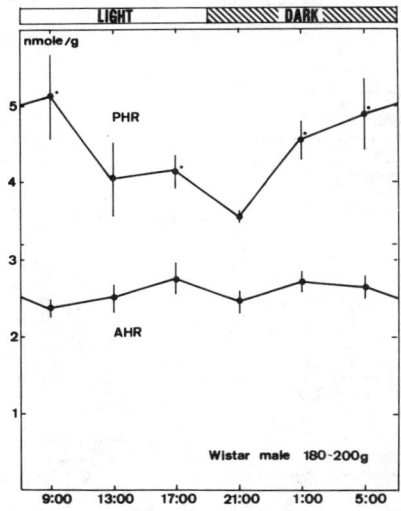

Fig. 5 Circadian changes of histamine levels in the anterior and posterior hypothalamic regions of rats. Male Wistar rats (150-200 gr) were kept in plastic cages (2 rats/cage) for 10 days under the artificial light and dark period (7:00-19:00). The rats were killed by decapitation under safety illumination. The brain was quickly removed and posterior and anterior hypothalamic area without median eminence and arcuate nucleus were dissected. Each point represents means $\pm$ S.E. (n=6-8).

These results were strongly supported by the finding that the content of histamine in the posterior hypothalamus exhibited a circadian rhythm, decreasing during the light period and increasing during the dark period, as shown in Fig. 5. Several workers have reported a circadian rhythm of histamine in the hypothalamus (Garbarg, Julien and Schwartz, 1974b; Orr and Quay, 1975a, 1975b; Mazurkiewicz-Kwilecki and Prell, 1980; Tuomisto and Tuomisto, 1982). But, this is the first demonstration that there is a circadian rhythm in the posterior hypothalamus with less rhythm in the anterior hypothalamus. Fluctuation in hypothalamic HDC was reported by Orr and Quay (1975a), and Tuomisto and Tuomisto (1982).

Effect of FMH on the Plasma Levels of ACTH, Vasopression and Oxytocin

Recently, we found that bilateral adrenalectomy caused marked but transient increase of histamine in the hypothalamo-hypophyseal system of rats (Cacabelos and others 1983, Proceedings of Jpn. Neurochem. Soc.). To determine the roles of histamine in the neuroendocrine system, we submitted female Wistar rats to long-term administration of FMH at a dose of 100 mg/kg/day i.p. and studied how this drug alters the plasma ACTH, oxytocin and vasopressin before and after bilateral adrenalectomy (Fig 6). After administration of FMH for 5 days, the basal plasma levels of these peptides were not significantly different from those of control rats. Seven days after bilateral adrenalectomy, plasma ACTH, oxytocin and vasopressin in the non-treated rats were increased to 1,107%, 139% and 114 %, respectively. However, the plasma peptides did not increase in rats receiving FMH throughout the experiment, and even tended to decrease. These findings strongly suggest that histamine modulates neuroendocrine functions at hypothalamic level, especially when the negative-feedback mechanism of the corticotropinergic system is broken.

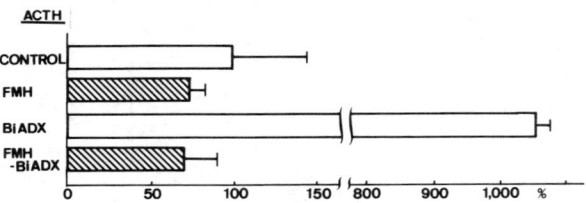

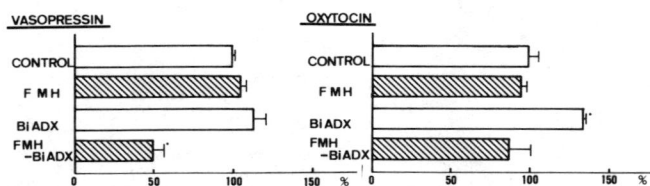

Fig 6 Effects of FMH and bilateral adrenalectomy on plasma ACTH, oxytocin and vasopressin in rats (n=3-5, female Wistar rats, 150-200g). The mean value of control is taken as 100%. FMH: (100 mg/kg/day, ip) for 5 days. BiIADX: 7 days after bilateral adrenalectomy. FMH-BiADX: 7 days after bilateral adrenalectomy, and FMH was administered from 5 days before the operation throughout the experiment at a dose of 100 mg/kg/day.

HYPOTHESIS FOR THE FUNCTION OF MONOAMINERGIC NEURONS IN THE BRAIN

All the results described here indicate that histamine acts as neuromodulator in controlling several activities of the central nervous system. It seems probable that the aminergic neuron system has no independent or separate functions on respective neuron in the CNS. A tentative hypothesis on the action of the CNS is presented in Fig. 7. The scheme is all based on the idea that the most important materials in living matter are Na^+ and Cl^-. In the nervous system, excitation is caused by influx of Na^+ which is controlled by acidic amino acids such as glutamic acid (Glu) or aspartic acid (Asp). On the other hand, inhibition is caused by the influx of Cl^- which is often controlled by neutral amino acids such as GABA, glycine (Gly) or taurine (Tau). Most monoaminergic neurons, such as dopaminergic (DA), noradrenalinergic (NA), serotoninergic (5-HT) and histaminergic (HA) neurons, may modulate such nervous functions by causing influx of Ca^{++} (or increase in the intracellular level of free Ca^{++}) or change of cyclic AMP level in the cell. These monoaminergic neurons may act in coordination to set up higher activities of the CNS, and it is readily conceivable that they are in close contact with several peptide neurons.

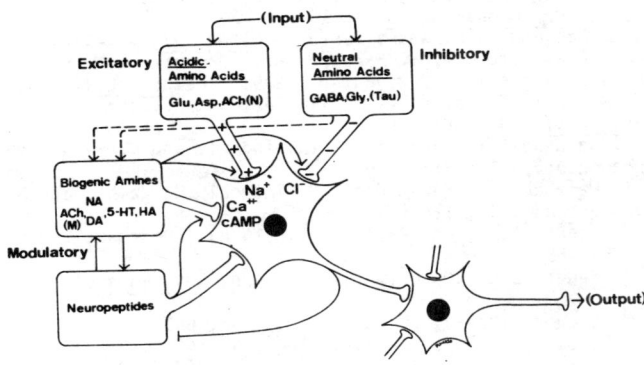

Fig. 7 A chemical basis of neuronal transmission

ACKNOWLEGEMENTS

We thank Dr. J. Kollonitsch, Merck Sharp & Dohme Research Laboratories, Rahway, USA for supply of FMH and Dr. H. Nakamura, Dainippon Pharmaceutical. Co., Osaka for carrying out the studies in Table 2. We thank Mrs. K. Tsuji for typing.

REFERENCES[1]

Ben-Ari, Y., G. LaSalle Legale, G. Barbin, J.C. Schwartz, and M. Garbarg (1977). Brain Res., 138, 285-294
Bouclier, M., M.J. Jung, and F. Gerhardt (1983a). Experientia, 39, 1303-1305.
Bouclier, M., M.J. Jung, and F. Gerhardt (1983b). Biochem. Pharmacol., 32, 1553-1556.
Donoso, A.O., and E.O. Alvarez (1984). Trends Pharmacol. Sci., 5, 98-100.
Fukui, B., Watanabe, and H. Wada (1980). Biochem. Biophys. Res. Commun., 93, 333-339.
Garbarg, M., G. Barbin, J. Feger, and J.C. Schwartz (1974a). Science, 186, 833-835.
Garbarg, M., G. Julien, and J.C. Schwartz (1974b). Life Sci., 14, 539-543.
Garbarg, M., G. Barbin, E. Rodergas, and J.C. Schwartz (1980). J. Neurochem., 1045-1052.
Grzanna, R. and L.D. Schultz (1982). Life Sci., 30, 1959-1954.
Green, J.P. (1983). In L. Iversen, S.D. Iversen, and S.H. Snyder (Ed.), Handbook of Psychopharmacology, Vol. 17. Plenum, New York, pp. 385-420.
Hayashi, H., H. Takagi, N. Takeda, Y. Kubota, M. Tohyama, T. Watanabe, and H. Wada (1984). J. Com. Neurol., in press.
Hough, L.B., J.K. Khandelwal, R.C. Goldschmidt, M. Diomande, and S.D. Glick (1984). Brain. Res., 292, 133-138.
Hough, L.B., and J.P. Green (1984). In A. Lajtha (Ed.), Handbook of Neurochemistry, Vol. 6, Plenum, New York. pp. 145-211.
Irwin, S. (1968). Psychopharmacologia, 13, 222-257.
Kitamura, Y., S. Go, and K. Hatanaka (1978). Blood, 52, 447-452.
Kollonitsch, J., A.A. Patchett, S. Marburg, A.L. Maycock, L.M. Perkins, G.A. Doldouras, D.E. Duggan, and S.A. Aster (1978). Nature, 2741, 906-908.
Kubota, H., H. Hayashi, T. Watanabe, Y. Taguchi, and H. Wada (1984). Biochem. Pharmacol., 33, 883-900.
Maeyama, K., T. Watanabe, Y. Taguchi, A. Yamatodani, and H. Wada (1982). Biochem. Pharmacol., 31, 2367-2370.
Maeyama, K., T. Watanabe, A. Yamatodani, Y. Taguchi, H. Kambe, and H. Wada (1983). J. Neurochem. 41, 128-134.
Mazurkiewicz-Kwilecki, I.M., and Prell, G.D. (1980). Pharmacol. Biochem. Behav., 12, 549-553.
Monnier, M., R. Sauer, and A.M. Haff (1971). Ann. Rev. Physiol., 12, 265-305.
Orr, E., and W.B. Quay (1975a). Endocrinology, 96, 941-945.
Orr, E., and W.B. Quay (1975b). Endocrinology, 97, 481-484.
Orr, E., and K.R. Pace (1984). J. Neurochem., 42, 727-732.
Palacios, J.M., J.K. Wamsley, M.J. Kuhar (1981). Neuroscience, 6, 15-37.
Panula, P., H-YT. Yang, E. Costa (1984). Proc. Nat. Acad. Sci. USA., 81, 2572-2576.
Pollard, H., S. Bischoff, C. Llorens-Cortes, and J.C. Schwartz (1976). Brain Res., 118, 509-513.
Roberts, F., and C.R. Calcutt (1983). Neuroscience, 9, 721-739.
Schwartz, J.C. (1977). Annu. Rev. Pharmacol., 17, 325-339.
Schwartz, J.C., H. Pollard, and T.T. Quach (1980). J. Neurochem., 35, 26-33.
Schwartz, J.C., G. Barbin, A.M. Duchemin, M. Garbarg, C. Llorens, H. Pollard, T.T. Quach, and C. Rose (1982). In C.R. Ganellin, and M.E. Parsons (Ed.). Pharmacology of Histamine Receptors. Wright PSG, Bristol, London, Boston. pp. 351-191.
Steinbusch, H.W.M., and A.H. Mulder (1984). In A. Bjorklund, and T. Hokfelt (Ed.). The Handbook of Chemical Neuroanatomy, Vol. 2. Elsevier, Amsterdam, in press.

Taguchi, Y., T. Watanabe, H. Kubota, H. Hayashi, and H. Wada (1984). J. Biol. Chem., 259, 5214-5221.
Takeda, N., S. Inagaki, Y. Taguchi, M. Tohyama, T. Watanabe, and H. Wada (1984a). Brain Res., in press.
Takeda, N., M. Morita, T. Watanabe, H. Wada, M. Tohyama, T. Kubo, and T. Matsunaga (1984b). Neurochem. Res., in press.
Takeda, N., S. Inagaki, S. Shiosaka, T. Taguchi, W.H. Oertel, M. Tohyama, T. Watanabe, and H. Wada (1984c). Proc. Nat. Acad. Sci. USA, in press.
Taylor, J.E. (1982). Neurochem. Intern., 4, 89-96.
Tuomisto, L., and J. Tuomisto (1982). Med. Biol., 60, 204-209.
Wada, H., T. Watanabe, K. Maeyama, Y. Taguchi, and H. Wada (1984). In A.E. Evangelopoulos (Ed.). Chemical and Biological Aspects of Viamin B_6 Catalysis, Part A, Alan R. Liss, New York. pp. 245-254.
Watanabe, T., T. Nakamura, L.Y. Liang. A. Yamatodani, and H. Wada (1979). Biochem. Pharmacol., 28, 1149-1155.
Watanabe, T., M. Yamada, Y. Taguchi, H. Kubota, K. Maeyama, A. Yamatodani, H. Fukui, S. Shiosaka, M. Tohyama and H. Wada (1982). In B. Uvnas, and K. Tasaka (Ed.). Advances in Histamine Research, Pergamon, Oxford, New York. pp. 93-106.
Watanabe, T., and H. Wada (1983). In S. Partvez, T. Nagatsu, I. Nagatsu, and H. Pravez (Ed.). Methods in Biogenic Amine Research, Elsevier, Amsterdam. pp. 689-720.
Watanabe, T., Y. Taguchi, H. Hayashi, J. Tanaka, S. Shiosaka, M. Tohyama, H. Kubota, Y. Terano, and H. Wada (1983). Neurosci. Lett., 39, 249-254.
Watanabe, T., Y. Taguchi, S. Shiosaka, J. Tanaka, H. Kubota, Y. Terano, M. Tohyama, and H. Wada (1984). Brain Res., 295, 13-25.
Wilcox, B.J., and V.S. Seybold (1982). Neurosci. Lett., 29, 105-110.
Yamada, M., T. Watanabe, H. Fukui, Y. Taguchi, and H. Wada (1984). Agents Actions, 14, 143-152.
Yamatodani, A., K. Maeyama, T. Watanabe, and H. Wada (1982). Biochem. Pharmacol., 31, 305-309.

[1]These references do not include all the papers relevant to physiological functions of histamine in the CNS.

HISTAMINE RECEPTORS, CYCLIC NUCLEOTIDES AND PSYCHOTROPIC DRUGS

E. Richelson

Departments of Psychiatry and Pharmacology, Mayo Clinic and Foundation, Rochester, MN 55905, USA

ABSTRACT

This chapter will briefly review the evidence for cyclic AMP and cyclic GMP as second mesesengers of histamine receptors; discuss some mechanisms of receptor-effector coupling associated with these second messengers; and present data for the interactions of psychotropic drugs (antidepressants and neuroleptics) with histamine receptors of brain.

KEYWORDS

Cyclic AMP; cyclic GMP; histamine H_1; histamine H_2; murine neuroblastoma clone N1E-115; human brain; antidepressants; neuroleptics.

INTRODUCTION

For many years it has been known that histamine receptors in nervous tissue have cyclic nucleotides, cyclic AMP and cyclic GMP, as "second messengers." A second messenger is the chemical inside the cell which is thought to effect the intracellular changes brough about by the first messenger of the neuron, the neurotransmitter, acting at the outside of the cell. Either the histamine H_1 or the histamine H_2 receptor when stimulated causes a rise in the intracellular level of cyclic AMP; but it may be that only the histamine H_1 receptor can mediate an increase in the intracellular concentration of cyclic GMP. These cyclic nucleotide responses have been very useful as assays for histamine receptors of nervous tissue to determine the affinities of psychotropic drugs for these receptors. On a more fundamental level, researchers have been studying these responses to determine the mechanisms involved in the coupling of these receptors to the effectors which ultimately cause the synthesis of the cyclic nucleotides.

HISTAMINE RECEPTORS AND CYCLIC NUCLEOTIDES

Using slices of rabbit cerebellum, Kakiuchi and Rall (1968) first demonstrated that histamine elevates intracellular levels of cyclic AMP in nervous tissue. Since the initial work, histamine-mediated cyclic AMP synthesis has been shown to occur in several different brain regions and in several different species of animal. There appear, however, to be species differences in the ability of histamine to evoke cyclic AMP in certain brain regions.

With the availability of selective agonists and antagonists of histamine receptors, researchers defined what receptors were involved in the cyclic AMP response. In brain slices (Chasin and co-workers, 1973; Palacios and co-workers, 1978) or relatively intact dissociated brain tissue (Kanba and Richelson, 1983) both histamine receptors are involved with cyclic AMP production. However, in homogenates of brain tissue (Hegstrand, Kanof and Greengard, 1976; Green and Maayani, 1977), only the histamine H_2 receptor mediates cyclic AMP synthesis.

There has been some uncertainty about whether the histamine H_1 receptor can alone mediate cyclic AMP synthesis or whether it does so only indirectly in combination with a second receptor, such as the histamine H_2 receptor (Palacios and co-workers, 1978; Daly and co-workers, 1980). Chasin and co-workers (1973) using guinea pig brain slices found that in the cerebral cortex, histamine-mediated cyclic AMP synthesis is completely abolished by a selective histamine H_1 antagonist which only partially blocks the response to histamine in the hippocampus. These results suggest that the histamine H_1 receptor in the guinea pig cerebral cortex can directly mediate cyclic AMP synthesis. However, in parts of the brain where both types of histamine receptors exist, such as in the hippocampus of the guinea pig, there is good evidence to suggest that the cyclic AMP response mediated by the histamine H_1 receptor is dependent on activation of the histamine H_2 receptor (Palacios and co-workers, 1978). Schwartz and co-workers (1982) have reported that removal of extracellular calcium ions strongly reduces the cyclic AMP response resulting from activation of the histamine H_1 receptor but removal of this ion has no effect on the response mediated by the histamine H_2 receptor. Based on these data, this group of researchers has suggested that calcium ion translocation presumed to occur with histamine H_1 receptor activation is a likely coupling signal between activation of this receptor and the cyclic AMP response. However, using dissociated cells of the guinea pig hippocampus (S. Kanba and E. Richelson, unpublished data), we have found no calcium ion dependency of the cyclic AMP responses to selective histamine receptor antagonists.

As mentioned above in homogenates of brain tissue, only the histamine H_2 receptor can mediate cyclic AMP synthesis. That is, the histamine H_2 receptor is coupled to adenylate cyclase, the enzyme which synthesizes cyclic AMP from ATP. It is likely that the coupling of the histamine H_2 receptor to adenylate cyclase and the subsequent activation of this enzyme involve mechanisms identical to those hypothesized to occur for many other receptors such as the β-adrenergic, prostaglandin E and dopamine (D-1) receptors (Rodbell, 1980). Histamine H_2-stimulated adenylate cyclase activity is dependent on the presence of GTP and thus this activity likely involves the formation of a ternary complex consisting of histamine, its receptor and a nucleotide regulatory component (or nucleotide binding protein, N). After binding GTP, the ternary complex then binds to adenylate cyclase and activates it. In addition, there appear to be two types of nucleotide regulatory components, one that is stimulatory, N_s, and one that is inhibitory, N_i. No histamine receptor has been shown to couple to N_i.

Although it was shown many years ago that histamine elevates cyclic GMP levels in rabbit cerebral cortex (Kuo and co-workers, 1972), there have been few studies on histamine-mediated cyclic GMP synthesis by brain tissue and the type of histamine receptor mediating this response in brain has never been identified. However, based on studies with the bovine superior cervical ganglion (Study and Greengard, 1978) and with murine neuroblastoma cells (Richelson, 1978a), it is very likely that the histamine H_1 receptor in brain mediates this cyclic GMP response.

Table 1 Receptors of Murine Neuroblastoma Clone N1E-115 and their Effects on Cyclic Nucleotides

RECEPTOR	CYCLIC NUCLEOTIDES	
	cyclic AMP	cyclic GMP
ADENOSINE	+[a]	0
ANGIOTENSIN II	?	+
BRADYKININ	?	+
GLUCAGON	+	0
HISTAMINE H_1	0	+
MUSCARINIC M_1	0	+
MUSCARINIC M_2	-	0
NEUROTENSIN	0	+
δ-OPIOID	-	0
PROSTAGLANDIN E	+	+
SECRETIN/VIP	+	0
THROMBIN	?	+

[a] + = stimulates; - = inhibits; 0 = no effect; ? = unknown effect

Receptor-mediated cyclic GMP synthesis is mechanistically very different from receptor-mediated cyclic AMP synthesis. There are two main observations that suggest this. First, receptor-mediated cyclic GMP synthesis requires intact cells since, unlike cyclic AMP responses, it has never been shown to occur with cellular homogenates. Second, receptor-mediated cyclic GMP synthesis has an absolute dependence on extracellular calcium ions, a requirement not usually found for cyclic AMP responses. These and other observations (Richelson and El-Fakahany, 1981) have led to the hypothesis that receptor-mediated cyclic GMP synthesis results from an influx of calcium ions which stimulate guanylate cyclase, the enzyme converting GTP into cyclic GMP.

Using clone N1E-115 cells of murine neuroblastoma C-1300 (Amano, Richelson and Nirenberg, 1972), we tested the hypothesis that there is a receptor-mediated increase in intracellular calcium ions (Snider, McKinney, Forray and Richelson, 1984). This clone, which possibly is the most widely studied of all neuroblastoma clones, is an ideal model system for studying many different putative neuro-

Table 2 Effects of Inhibitors of Arachidonic Acid Metabolism on Histamine H_1-Mediated Cyclic [^{3}H]GMP Formation in Intact Murine Neuroblastoma Cells[a]

	CYCLIC [^{3}H]GMP[b]	
	dpm/10^6 cells	percent control
CONTROL	55400	
+ Quinacrine (phospholipase inihibitor)		
40 µM	44300	80
120 µM	25400	46
200 µM	13300	24
CONTROL	48300	
+ ETYA[c] (lipoxygenase inhibitor)		
5 µM	44600	92
15 µM	30500	63
30 µM	19900	41

[a] Data from Snider, McKinney, Forray and Richelson (1984)
[b] Increase above basal after 0.1 mM histamine for 45 sec
[c] 5,8,11,14-eicosatetraynoic acid

transmitter receptors from both a functional and biochemical standpoint. It contains more than 10 different receptors which affect intracellular levels of cyclic nucleotides (Table 1). In addition, some of these receptors have been studied electrophysiologically and found to alter the transmembrane potential. More specifically, activation of the histamine H_1 (Oakes, Taylor and Richelson, 1983), muscarinic (Wastek, Lopez and Richelson, 1982), bradykinin, angiotensin II, neurotensin or thrombin (S. G. Oakes, S. Taylor and E. Richelson, unpublished observations) receptor on these cells results in a hyperpolarization of the transmembrane potential. The time course for the development of this electrical change (peak at about 7 sec), its duration (about 30 sec), and the magnitude of this change (about -10 mv) are very similar for all the receptors studied. In addition, the time course for this electrical change is consistent with the time course for receptor-mediated cyclic GMP synthesis (peak at about 30-60 sec). These facts suggest that cyclic GMP is involved in this receptor-mediated hyperpolarization of N1E-115 cells.

We sought to gather direct evidence to test the hypothesis that neurotransmitter receptor-mediated cyclic GMP formation occurs as the result of an increase in intracellular calcium ions. One of the most satisfactory tools for directly monitoring changes in intracellular calcium in living cells is the bioluminescent protein aequorin, which changes the intensity of its light emission in response to variations in intracellular calcium within the physiological range (Blinks and co-workers, 1982). A population of murine neuroblastoma cells was "loaded" with aequorin by making them reversibly hyperpermeable by incubation with EGTA. Immediately after the loading procedure, cells do not respond to agonists in the cyclic GMP assay. However, cells loaded with aequorin and placed back in complete culture medium overnight, completely recover their responsiveness to agonists while retaining large amounts of active aequorin.

We found no evidence for an increase in intracellular calcium ions upon activation of either the histamine H_1 or muscarinic receptor of clone N1E-115 cells (Snider, McKinney, Forray and Richelson, 1984) and therefore we discarded the hypothesis for the direct role of these ions in the cyclic GMP response.

With a clue from our studies showing that α-thrombin mediates cyclic GMP synthesis in these cells (Snider and Richelson, 1983; Snider, McKinney, Fenton and Richelson and Richelson, 1984) in a manner similar to histamine, we obtained evidence to support a new hypothesis that putative neurotransmitters such as histamine mediate cyclic GMP synthesis by stimulating the release of arachidonic acid (possibly by activating phospholipase A_2) followed by the metabolism of arachidonic acid by lipoxygenase(s) to a product that stimulates guanylate cyclase (Snider, McKinney, Forray and Richelson, 1984; McKinney and Richelson, 1984). In platelets thrombin causes a well-characterized stimulation of phospholipase A_2 activity which results in the release of arachidonic acid (Lapetina, Billah and Cuatrecasas, 1981). In support of our new hypothesis are the data showing that histamine H_1 receptor-mediated cyclic GMP synthesis by clone N1E-115 cells is

Table 3 Histamine H_1 Receptor-Mediated Release of [^{3}H]Arachidonic Acid from Intact Murine Neuroblastoma Cells[a]

	NET[b] [^{3}H]ARACHIDONIC ACID RELEASED	
	dpm/10^6 cells	percent control
CONTROL (0.1 μM Histamine, 30 sec)	5110	
+ Pyrilamine (1 μM)	1800	35
+ Quinacrine (350 μM)	150	3

[a]From Snider, McKinney, Forray and Richelson, 1984
[b]Increase above basal

antagonized by agents which inhibit phospholipase A_2 (quinacrine) and lipoxygenase(s) (ETYA) (Table 2) and that activation of this receptor stimulates a quinacrine-sensitive release of arachidonic acid (Table 3) (Snider, McKinney, Forray and Richelson, 1984).

RADIOLIGAND BINDING ASSAYS FOR HISTAMINE RECEPTORS

In addition to the cyclic nucleotide responses, radioligand binding has been used to study histamine receptors. It is clear from the published data that to date only the histamine H_1 receptor can be identified by this technique.

Direct binding to the histamine H_1 receptor has been achieved with the use of radiolabelled pyrilamine (mepyramine), a selective histamine H_1 antagonist. [^{3}H]pyrilamine binds in brains of many different species and in smooth muscle to a single class of sites with an equilibrium dissociation constant (K_D) of around 1 nM (Hill, Emson and Young, 1978; Hill, Young and Marrian, 1977; Taylor, Yaksh and Richelson, 1982).

As a result of findings discussed below, the tricyclic antidepressant doxepin has become commercially available for use as a radioligand for studying the histamine H_1 receptor. However, we have found that [^{3}H]doxepin has more than one high-affinity binding site in rat (Taylor and Richelson, 1982) and human (Kanba and Richelson, 1984) brain homogenates, a fact that complicates somewhat its use as a radioligand for the histamine H_1 receptor.

An advantage of a radioligand binding assay over a biological assay of a receptor is that the number of binding sites can be determined only with the binding assay (Richelson, 1984). Therefore, with a binding assay for the histamine H_1 receptor it is possible to map the brain for the density of this receptor. We did this for human brain using [^{3}H]doxepin as the radioligand (Kanba and Richelson, 1984) and found that the histamine H_1 receptor of human brain has a regional distribution which is different from those of animal brains, a result found previously by Chang and co-workers (1979). In our studies, the highest binding was

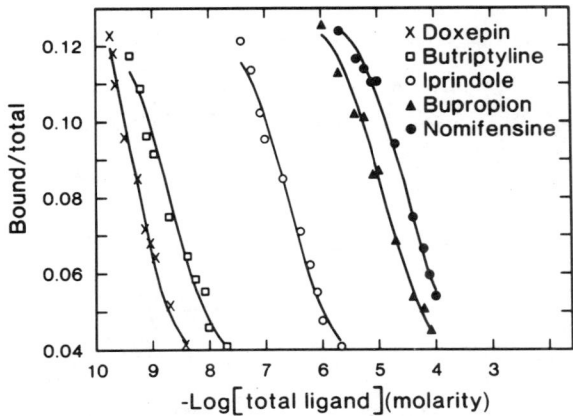

Fig. 1. Competition by antidepressants for [^{3}H]doxepin binding in human brain. From Richelson and Nelson (1984a) with permission from the publisher.

found in the neo-cortex (temporal > frontal > parietal > occipital). Binding in the limbic structures of orbital cortex, cingulate cortex, and amygdala were about as high as that found in the temporal cortex. In guinea pig brain, the highest binding is in the cerebellum; in rat brain, in the hypothalamus (Chang and co-workers, 1979).

Radioactively labeled histamine H_2 receptor antagonists have been used in binding assays to identify this receptor. However, the pharmacological specificity and the regional distribution of this binding is not consistent with what is known for the histamine H_2 receptor.

In our laboratory we attempted to identify the histamine H_2 receptor in brain with the use of [^{3}H]trimipramine, a tricyclic antidepressant with potent inhibitory effects in the cyclic AMP assay for the histamine H_2 receptor in homogenates of the guinea pig hippocampus. However, we found that this radioligand did not bind to the histamine H_2 receptor (Kanba and Richelson, 1983).

INTERACTIONS OF PSYCHOTROPIC DRUGS WITH HISTAMINE RECEPTORS

The first tricyclic antidepressant, imipramine hydrochloride, was originally synthesized as a histamine H_1 antagonist. However, it took about 20 years after this compound was shown to be effective as an antidepressant to learn just how potent this drug and others like it were as antihistaminics. Using intact murine neuroblastoma cells and histamine-mediated cyclic GMP synthesis, we showed that some of the tricyclic antidepressants (notably, doxepin, amitriptyline and trimipramine) are among the most potent histamine H_1 antagonists known (Richelson, 1978b; 1979). We studied many of these compounds in different assays using the receptor from several different non-human species and confirmed these results (Figge, Leonard and Richelson, 1979; Taylor and Richelson, 1980; Taylor, Yaksh and Richelson, 1982; Taylor and Richelson, 1982).

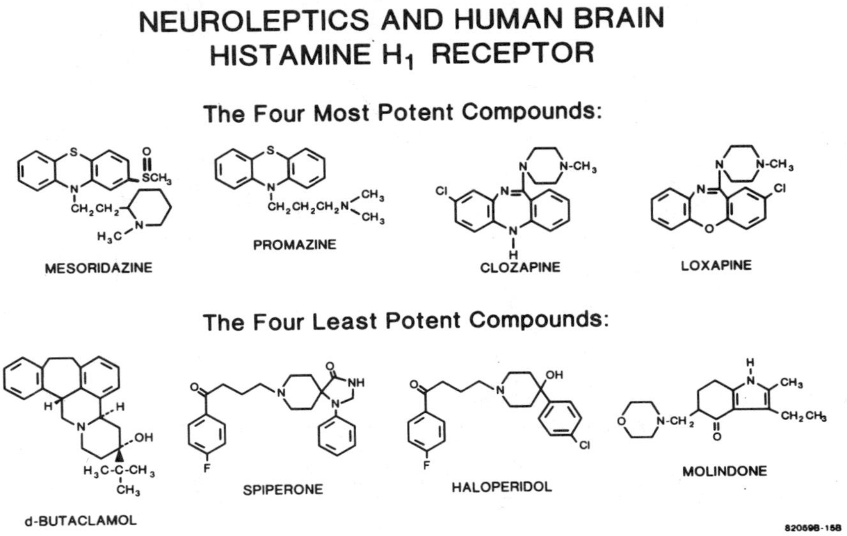

NEUROLEPTICS AND HUMAN BRAIN HISTAMINE H_1 RECEPTOR

The Four Most Potent Compounds:

MESORIDAZINE   PROMAZINE   CLOZAPINE   LOXAPINE

The Four Least Potent Compounds:

d-BUTACLAMOL   SPIPERONE   HALOPERIDOL   MOLINDONE

Fig. 2. Structures of the four most potent and the four least potent neuroleptics at the human brain histamine H_1 receptor.

In recent years we have been using normal human brain tissue obtained at autopsy as the source of receptors for our radioligand binding assays (for example, see Fig. 1). In studies of many antidepressants (Table 4) (Richelson and Nelson, 1984a), neuroleptics (Table 5 and Fig. 2) (Richelson and Nelson, 1984b) and histamine H_1 antagonists, we found that antidepressants remain among the most potent histamine H_1 antagonists available for clinical use. Furthermore, of all the known pharmacological effects of 25 antidepressants that we studied (Table 4), including blockade of synaptosomal uptake of biogenic amines (Richelson and Pfenning, 1984), in general, histamine H_1 receptor blockade is their most potent effect.

Some neuroleptics (in particular, mesoridazine, promazine, clozapine and loxapine; Fig. 2 and Table 5) are quite potent as antagonists of the human brain histamine H_1 receptor, but none that we have studied has higher affinity than the antidepressants at the top of the list of Table 4. Interestingly, the most potent neuroleptics at this receptor are tricyclic compounds (Fig. 2) with close structural analogy to the antidepressants with highest affinity for the histamine H_1 receptor.

Table 4 Antidepressants: Equilibrium Dissociation Constants (K_D's) for the Histamine H_1 Receptor of Human Brain Frontal Cortex[a]

ANTIDEPRESSANTS	K_D(nM)
Doxepin	0.24
Trimipramine	0.27
Mianserin	0.40
Amitriptyline	1.1
Butriptyline	1.1
Maprotiline	2.0
Dothiepin	3.6
Nortriptyline	10
Imipramine	11
Oxaprotiline	21
Amoxapine	25
Protriptyline	25
Clomipramine	31
Desipramine	110
Iprindole	130
Trazodone	350
Citalopram	470
Zimelidine	4000
Nisoxetine	4200
Fluoxetine	6200
Bupropion	6600
Clovoxamine	16000
Viloxazine	18000
Nomifensine	21000
Fluvoxamine	109000
ANTIHISTAMINES (H_1)	
Pyrilamine	5
Mequitazine	6[b]
Diphenhydramine	14
d-Chlorpheniramine	15

[a]Data from Richelson and Nelson (1984a)
[b]Data from Kanba and Richelson (1984)

For several years there have been data in the literature to indicate that antidepressants of all types are very potent antagonists of the brain's histamine H_2 receptor (Green and Maayani, 1977; Kanof and Greengard, 1978). This finding led to the hypothesis that the mechanism of action of antidepressants is the result of blockade of this receptor (Kanof and Greengard, 1978). However, more recently, it has become apparent that potent antagonism of the histamine H_2 receptor by antidepressants as well as by neuroleptics occurs only when this receptor is assayed in tissue homogenates and does not occur when this receptor is assayed in intact cell preparations (Tuong, Garbarg and Schwartz, 1980; Kanba and Richelson, 1983). Since the latter case is more analagous to what occurs clinically, we have concluded that antidepressants and neuroleptics are relatively weak antagonists of the histamine H_2 receptor (Table 6).

What is the clinical relevance of histamine receptor blockade by psychotropic drugs? It has been suggested by us (Richelson, 1978b; 1979) and others (Palacios and co-workers, 1978; Uzan and Le Fur, 1979) that histamine H_1 receptor antagonism by a drug is directly related to its propensity to cause sedation and drowsiness in patients. In addition, we have suggested (Richelson, 1979) that blockade of the histamine H_1 receptor in brain is also responsible for the

Table 5 Neuroleptics: Equilibrium Dissociation Constants (K_D's) for the Histamine H_1 Receptor of Human Brain Frontal Cortex[a]

NEUROLEPTICS	K_D(nM)
Mesoridazine	1.8
Promazine	2.0
Clozapine	2.8
Loxapine	4.9
cis-Thiothixene	6
Perphenazine	8
Chlorpromazine	9
Thioridazine	16
Prochlorperazine	19
Fluphenazine	21
Trifluoperazine	62
d-Butaclamol	390
Spiperone	480
Haloperidol	1900
Molindone	124000

[a]Data from Richelson and Nelson (1984b)

well-known appetite stimulating effect of psychotherapeutic drugs. Data for antidepressants at the human brain H_1 receptor (Table 4) can be useful to the clinician who wants to choose a sedating drug for a patient with an agitated depression. In addition, these data can help the clinician choose another drug of lower affinity for the histamine H_1 receptor for a patient who is bothered by a side effect associated with histamine H_1 receptor blockade.

Because of the impressive potency of doxepin at the histamine H_1 receptor, this drug has been receiving widespread use in the United States for the treatment of allergic and dermatological problems (Richelson, 1983).

There are good data to show that the tricyclic antidepressants trimipramine and doxepin have efficacy for treating duodenal ulcer (Richelson, 1983). Interestingly, these two drugs are the most potent of the antidepressants studied at the histamine H_2 receptor of guinea pig brain (Table 5). However, even doxepin, the most potent compound, is only about one-third as potent as cimetidine. The most widely studied antidepressant in duodenal ulcer is trimipramine which has been used at dosages of 25 and 50 mg per day to treat this peptic ulcer disease, far below the recommended dosage range for treating depression (150-300 mg). At this low dosage because of its low affinity, it is not likely to be blocking the histamine H_2 receptor. In fact clnical studies indicate that trimipramine does not block histamine-stimulated increases in gastric acid secretion (Richelson, 1983). Thus, the efficacy of tricyclic antidepressants for treating duodenal ulcer very likely does not depend on histamine H_2 receptor blockade.

Table 6 Antidepressants and Neuroleptics: Equilibrium Dissociation Constants (K_D's) for the Histamine H_2 Receptor of Guinea Pig Hippocampus[a]

ANTIDEPRESSANTS	K_D(nM)
Doxepin	1400
Amitriptyline	1900
Trimipramine	2400
Mianserin	2800
Imipramine	3300
Protriptyline	3700
Maprotiline	4600
Amoxapine	8000
Iprindole	8100
Desipramine	12000
Trazodone	15000
Nortriptyline	16000
Nomifensine	30000
NEUROLEPTICS	
Levomepromazine	2900
Chlorpromazine	3000
Thiothixene	4700
Clozapine	5200
Haloperidol	29000
Molindone	70000
ANTIHISTAMINES (H_2)	
Tiotidine	32
Ranitidine	120
Cimetidine	460

[a]Data from Kanba and Richelson (1983)

ACKNOWLEDGEMENTS

The writing of this paper and the research from our laboratory presented here have been supported by the Mayo Foundation and grant MH27692 from the U.S.P.H.S.

REFERENCES

Amano, T., E. Richelson and M. Nirenberg (1972). Neurotransmitter synthesis by neuroblastoma clones. Proc. Nat. Acad. Sci. USA., 69, 258-263.
Blinks, J., W. Wier, P. Hess and F. Prendergast (1982). Measurement of Ca^{2+} concentrations in living cells. Prog. Biophys. Mol. Biol., 40, 1-114.
Chang, R. S. L, V. T. Tran, and S. H. Snyder (1979). Heterogeneity of histamine H_1-receptors: Species variations in [^{3}H]mepyramine binding of brain membranes. J. Neurochem., 32, 1653-1663.

Chasin, M., F. Mamrak, S. G. Samaniego and S. M. Hess (1973). Characteristics of the catecholamine and histamine receptor sites mediating accumulation of cyclic adenosine 3',5'-monophosphate in guinea pig brain. J. Neurochem., 21, 1415-1427.

Daly, J. W., E. McNeal, C. Partington, M. Neuwirth and C. R. Creveling (1980). Accumulations of cyclic AMP in adenine-labeled cell-free preparations from guinea pig cerebral cortex: Role of α-adrenergic and H_1-histaminergic receptors. J. Neurochem., 35, 326-337.

Figge, J. P., P. Leonard and E. Richelson (1979). Tricyclic antidepressants: Potent blockade of histamine H_1 receptors of guinea pig ileum. Eur. J. Pharm., 58, 479-483.

Green, J. P and S. Maayani (1977). Tricyclic antidepressant drugs block histamine H_2 receptor in brain. Nature, 269, 163-165.

Hegstrand, L. R., P. D. Kanoff and P. Greengard (1976). Histamine-sensitive adenylate cyclase in mammalian brain. Nature, 260, 163-165.

Hill, S. J., P. C. Emson and J. M. Young (1978). The binding of [^{3}H]mepyramine to histamine H_1 receptors in guinea-pig brain. J. Neurochem., 31, 997-1004.

Hill, S. J., J. M. Young and D. H. Marrian (1977). Specific binding of [^{3}H]mepyramine to histamine H_1 receptors in intestinal smooth muscle. Nature, 270, 361-363.

Kakiuchi, S. and T. W. Rall (1968). The influence of chemical agents on the accumulation of adenosine 3',5'-phosphate in slices of rabbit cerebellum. Mol. Pharmacol., 4, 367-378.

Kanba, S. and E. Richelson (1983). Antidepressants are weak competitive antagonists of histamine H_2 receptors in dissociated brain tissue. Eur. J. Pharmacol., 94, 313-318.

Kanba, S. and E. Richelson (1984). Histamine H_1 receptors in human brain labelled with [^{3}H]doxepin. Brain Res., 304, 1-7.

Kanof, P. D. and P. Greengard (1978). Brain histamine receptors as targets for antidepressant drugs. Nature, 212, 329-333.

Kuo, J. F., T. P. Lee, P. L. Reyes, K. G. Walton, T. E. Donnely and P. Greengard (1972). Cyclic nucleotide-dependent protein kinases. J. Biol. Chem., 247, 16-22.

Lapetina, E. G., M. M. Billah and P. Cuatrecasas (1981). The initial action of thrombin on platelets. J. Biol. Chem., 256, 5037-5040.

McKinney, M. and E. Richelson (1984). The coupling of the neuronal muscarinic receptor to responses. Ann. Rev. Pharmacol. Toxicol., 24, 121-146.

Oakes, S.G., S. Taylor and E. Richelson (1983). Demonstration of a histamine (H_1) receptor-mediated cyclic GMP-related hyperpolarization of the membrane of murine neuroblastoma cells. Fed. Proc., 42, 906.

Palacios, J. M., M. Barbarg, G. Barbin and J. C. Schwartz (1978). Pharmacological characterization of histamine receptors mediating the stimulation of cyclic AMP accumulation in slices from guinea-pig hippocampus. Mol. Pharm., 14, 971-982.

Richelson, E. (1978a). Histamine H_1 receptor-mediated guanosine 3'5'-monophosphate formation by cultured mouse neuroblastoma cells. Science, 201, 69-71.

Richelson, E. (1978b). Tricyclic antidepressants block histamine H_1 receptors of mouse neuroblastoma cells. Nature, 274, 176-177.

Richelson, E. 1979). Tricyclic antidepressants and histamine H_1 receptors. Mayo Clin. Proc., 54, 669-674.

Richelson, E. (1983). Novel uses for tricyclic antidepressants. Mod. Med., 51, 74-86.

Richelson, E. (1984). Studying neurotransmitter receptors: binding and biological assay. In J. Marwaha and W. Anderson (Eds.), Neuroreceptors in Health Disease, S. Karger, Basel, pp. 4-19.

Richelson, E. and E. El-Fakahany (1981). Commentary: The molecular basis of neurotransmission at the muscarinic receptor. Biochem. Pharmacol., 30, 2887-2891.

Richelson, E. and A. Nelson (1984a). Antagonism by antidepressants of neurotransmitter receptors of normal human brain in vitro. J. Pharm. Exp. Therap., 230, 94-102.

Richelson, E. and A. Nelson (1984b). Antagonism by neuroleptics of neurotransmitter receptors of normal human brain in vitro. Eur. J. Pharm., in press.
Richelson, E. and M. Pfenning (1984). Blockade by antidepressants and related compounds of biogenic amine uptake into rat brain synaptosomes: most antidepressants selectively block norepinephrine uptake. Eur. J. Pharm., in press.
Rodbell, M. (1980). The role of hormone receptors and GTP-regulatory proteins in membrane transduction. Nature, 284, 17-22.
Schwartz, J. C., G. Barbin, A. M. Duchemin, M. Garbarg, C. Llorens, H. Pollard, T. T. Quach and C. Rose (1982). Histamine receptors in the brain and their possible functions. In C. R. Ganellin and M. E. Parsons (Eds.), Pharmacology of Histamine Receptors, Wright PSG, Bristol, Chap. 9, pp. 351-391.
Snider, R. M., M. McKinney, J. W. Fenton and E. Richelson (1984). Activation of cyclic nucleotide formation in murine neuroblastoma N1E-115 cells by modified human thrombins. J. Biol. Chem., 230, 9078-9081.
Snider, R., M., M. McKinney, C. Forray and E. Richelson (1984). Neurotransmitter receptors mediate cyclic GMP formation by involvement of arachidonic acid and lipoxygenase. Proc. Nat. Acad. Sci. USA, 81, 3905-3909.
Snider, R. M. and E. Richelson (1983). Thrombin stimulates cyclic GMP formation in murine neuroblastoma cells (clone N1E-115). Science, 221, 566-568.
Study, R. E. and P. Greengard (1978). Regulation by histamine of cyclic nucleotide levels in sympathetic ganglia. J. Pharm. Exp. Therap., 207, 767-778.
Taylor, J. E. and E. Richelson (1980). High-affinity binding of tricyclic antidepressants to histamine H_1 receptors: Fact and artifact. Eur. J. Pharm., 67, 41-46.
Taylor, J. E. and E. Richelson (1982). High affinity binding of [^{3}H]doxepin to histamine H_1 receptors in brain. Eur. J. Pharmacol., 78, 279-285.
Taylor, J. E., T. L. Yaksh and E. Richelson (1982). Histamine H_1 receptors in the brain and spinal cord of the cat. Brain Res., 243, 391-394.
Tuong, M. D. T., M. Garbarg and J. C. Schwartz (1980). Pharmacological specificity of brain histamine H_2-receptors differs in intact cells and cell-free preparations. Nature, 287, 548-551.
Uzan, A., G. Le Fur and C. Malgouris (1979). Are antihistamines sedative via a blockade of brain H_1 receptors? J. Pharm. Pharmacol., 31, 701-702.
Wastek, G. J, J. R. Lopez and E. Richelson (1981). Demonstration of a muscarinic receptor-mediated cyclic GMP-dependent hyperpolarization of the membrane potential of mouse neuroblastoma cells using [^{3}H]tetraphenylphosphonium. Mol. Pharm., 19, 15-20.

Actions and Role of Histamine in the Gastrointestinal Tract

ACTIONS AND THE ROLE OF HISTAMINE IN THE GASTROINTESTINAL TRACT

B. I. Hirschowitz

Division of Gastroenterology, University of Alabama in
Birmingham, Birmingham, Alabama 35294, USA

While an ever-widening range of actions and effects of histamine are being described, and this meeting bears eloquent testimony to that, the principal and perhaps best studied role of histamine has been related to gastric acid secretion. A dozen or so years ago, James Black and his colleagues answered the decades-old riddle of why antihistamines did not antagonize the effect of histamine on the stomach. Since then, many progressively more potent tools in the form of specific H_1 and H_2 agonists and antagonists have been developed; better pharmacologic techniques and newer models, including isolated organs, glands and cells have been put to use in studying histamine and the gut. Because of the phenomenal success of H_2 antagonists in the treatment of peptic ulcer, it is not surprising that gastric acid secretion and the stomach have received major attention, and this session of the congress deals largely with the stomach.

From all present evidence, histamine and its active analogs act directly on the parietal cell through H_2 receptors to stimulate acid in all species. Histamine also stimulates pepsin in a number of species, including man, but in dogs and cats, histamine both stimulates and inhibits pepsin secretion via H_2 receptors. In a few instances there is an H_1-mediated inhibition of acid secretion. Species-dependent differences are quite common and will have to be reconciled in telling the story.

Before acid secretion is initiated by histamine, there is a major change in the microscopic anatomy of the parietal cell, comprising a large gain in surface microvilli at the expense of vesicles. The effects of histamine on the parietal cell also include stimulation of secretion of other electrolytes (Cl^-, Na^+, K^+) and intrinsic factor (IF) in mammals. Not all mammals secrete IF from parietal cells. In submammalian species, histamine stimulates pepsinogen secretion as well as acid from the unitary oxyntic cell. It would appear that cAMP production, changes in parietal cell morphology, and secretion of acid and other secretants of the oxyntic/parietal cell all follow from histamine interaction with a single recognition site.

The use of different models has left several questions open. Thus while the parietal cell clearly has histamine H_2 receptors that are different from those of acetylcholine (ACh) or gastrin, H_2 antagonists block the actions of all stimuli of acid secretion in intact animals, indicating an intermediate messenger role for histamine in the action of non-histamine stimuli. The inhibition by atropine of gastrin and, to a lesser extent, histamine stimulation of secretion in intact animals and the interactions between histamine and ACh and gastrin (some potentiating, some additive) on parietal cells as well as in intact animals, has not been fully explained or localized to precellular, receptor or post-receptor sites. At least some of the results can be explained by the presence of histamine-containing cells in the mucosa, and some by different messengers (Ca^{2+} and cAMP) for different agonists. The pathway or mechanism of the probable trophic effect of histamine on gastric mucosa is unknown. The lack of effect of the methyl xanthines alone or on histamine-stimulated acid responses in the dog differs from several other species. However, prostaglandin E_2 is also most potent in inhibiting histamine-stimulated acid secretion in the dog, presumably by an effect on adenylcyclase. Somatostatin is a much less effective inhibitor of histamine stimulation than of cholinergic or vagal stimulation. All of these findings remind us that the role and actions of histamine in the stomach remain incompletely understood.

Histamine actions in the GI tract also include lesser secretory effects on salivary and pancreatic cells, via H_2 receptors. Histamine stimulates Cl^- secretion from enterocytes via both direct cellular and myenteric neuronal H_1 effects.

Gastric blood flow is also increased by histamine via H_1 receptors; an intermediate role for histamine in increases of gastric blood flow due to other secretagogues has not yet been shown. Mesenteric blood flow (H_1) and permeability (H_2), portal vein vasoconstriction (H_1) and hepatic artery dilatation (H_1) are important concomitant actions of histamine in the intact animal.

Gastric muscle, like the well-known effect of histamine on ileal muscle, contracts via H_1 receptors; gastric muscle contraction is relaxed via H_2 receptors. The effect on gastric emptying is not yet established by appropriate studies. Gallbladder muscle is contracted by histamine via H_1 and relaxed via H_2 receptors, and histamine may modulate the effects of CCK on gallbladder contraction.

Despite the extensive range of actions of histamine on various organs, there is only one practical application of the H_2 antagonists - the suppression of gastric acid secretion for the treatment of peptic ulcer and hypersecretory states. The H_1 antagonists have not found any real role in treating GI disorders.

RECEPTORS REGULATING ACID SECRETORY FUNCTION IN CANINE FUNDIC MUCOSA: A REDUCTIONIST APPROACH

A. H. Soll

Center for Ulcer Research and Education, Department of Medicine, UCLA School of Medicine and Medical and Research Services, Wadsworth VA Hospital Center, Los Angeles, CA 90073, USA

ABSTRACT

Despite the central role for histamine in the regulation of gastric acid secretion, details regarding histamine stores within the gastric mucosa and effects on parietal cell function remain controversial. These questions have been addressed in studies with cells dispersed by enzymes from canine fundic mucosa. Cells were separated by elutration and parietal cell function monitored indirectly using the accumulation of the weak base aminopyrine. The parietal cell was found to have pharmacologically typical H_2 and muscarinic receptors. Gastrin-17 (G17) stimulated parietal cell function; interaction with specific receptors on the parietal cell was confirmed using biologically active ^{125}I-[Leu^{15}]-G17. Histamine-containing cells were enriched using elutriation followed by density gradient separation. Morphologically typical mast cells appeared to fully account for the histamine content of these dispersed canine fundic cells. Neither acetylcholine nor gastrin were found to release histamine from these dispersed cells; the conclusion that these histamine cells lack gastrin and muscarinic receptors was supported by direct binding with ^{125}I-[Leu^{15}]-G17 and [^{3}H]-quinuclindinyl benzylate. Gastrin and muscarinic receptors were, however, present on cells in addition to parietal cells. Gastrin receptors were found in a small cell fraction from the elutriator rotor, and were found to correlate with the presence of somatostatin cells in density gradients of this elutriator fraction. Gastrin was found to stimulate and cholinergic agents were found to inhibit somatostatin release from these cells in short term culture. Thus it appears that gastrin and muscarinic receptors regulating secretory function are present on paracrine cells, as well as final effector cells. The physiological significance of these various receptors remains to be established, as does the identity of the chemotransmitters directly regulating release of histamine from canine fundic mucosal stores.

KEYWORDS

Isolated parietal cells; canine fundic mucosal histamine cells; gastrin; acetylcholine; receptors; gastric acid secretion; somatostatin cells;

INTRODUCTION

A unique link exists between histamine and gastric acid secretion. Examining phylogeny, histamine is not found in the gut of species more primative than the hagfish that lack a stomach capable of secreting acid. Higher in the phylogenetic tree, histamine appears in the upper portion of the gut conincident with the development of the capacity for acid secretion (Reite, 1972). This observation underlines the close association that exists between histamine and gastric acid secretion; however, the nature of this relationship has remained controversal over the seventy years since the discovery of histamine in the body and of its effects as an acid secretagogue.

Three pathways deliver the chemical messengers that regulate acid secretion: neurocrine (neurotransmiters released from postganglionic nerves innervating the fundic mucosa); endocrine (hormones such as gastrin delivered by blood); and paracrine (transmitters that diffuse across the intercellular compartment from local tissue stores). Many chemical transmitters that are stored in cells within the fundic mucosa, including histamine, somatostatin, and glucagon, are candidates for paracrine regulation. All three of these pathways are physiologically important (Grossman, 1981; Feldman, 1983). In particular, the paracrine pathway has been difficult to study. In fact, despite the close assocation of histamine and acid secretion, the role of histamine in the regulation of acid secretion was hotly debated (Code, 1965; Johnson, 1971) until Black and coworkers introduced the H_2 receptor antagonists in 1972 (Black, 1972). These H_2 antagonists blocked not only the action of histamine on acid secretion, but also stimulation by food, gastrin, and vagal stimuli thereby establishing that histamine played an essential role in the regulation of acid secretion (Black, 1972; Grossman, 1974; Gibson, 1974).

Interrelationships Between Pathways.

The complexity of the regulation of acid secretion reflects not only the fact that three pathways are involved, but also an interdependence between these pathways in all phases of acid secretion. This interdependence is clearly evident in the ability of specific histamine H_2 and muscarinic receptor antagonists to inhibit basal acid secretion and the response to most stimuli. For example, the cephalic phase of acid secretion (that occurs with the smell, sight or thought of food) that is mediated by vagal delivery of acetylcholine to the fundic mucosa is blocked by H_2 receptor antagonists, indicating a dependence upon endogenous histamine. Although the release of gastrin with a protein meal appears to largely account for the acid secretory response, both H_2 receptor antagonists and anticholinergic agents inhibit this gastric phase indicating dependency upon input from the neurocrine and paracrine pathways. Basal acid secretion is inhibited by both anticholinergic agents and H_2 receptor blockers, suggesting that the "resting" parietal cell receives both cholinergic and histamine input. Thus, a marked interdependency exists between the three pathways stimulating acid secretion.

The mechanism or mechanisms underlying this interplay between the various stimuli awaits elucidation. A basic element requiring definition is the target cell(s) mediating the effects of gastrin and acetylcholine on acid secretion. Code (1965), building upon earlier observations by MacIntosh, hypothesized that histamine was the final chemostimulator at the parietal cell for all pathways stimulating acid secretion. This view was reinforced by the findings that gastrin and acetylcholine influenced histamine formation in the rat gastric mucosa and by the demonstration that H_2 receptor antagonists blocked the acid secretory response to all stimuli. This model thus hypothesized that receptors for gastrin and acetylcholine resided on the histamine cell and that the parietal cell had receptors only for histamine. However, this view failed to account for findings such as the ability of anticholinergic agents to block histamine action and the interdependency between cholinergic pathways and gastrin. These factors led the late Morton I. Grossman (Grossman, 1974) to hypothesize that the parietal cell has separate specific receptors for histamine, gastrin and acetylcholine, with the interdependency between the pathways reflecting interaction at the parietal cell itself. The controversy thus centered about whether gastric secretagogues stimulated acid secretion by acting in parallel on the parietal cell, or in series with their final effects being mediated by release of histamine.

Resolution of these physiological questions requires 3 major steps: localization of the receptors mediating the actions of histamine, cholinergic agents and gastrin; identification of cells storing histamine in the fundic mucosa; and elucidation of the factors regulating histamine formation and release. Studies in intact mucosa are complicated by the heterogeneous cell population in the fundic mucosa and the presence of acetylcholine and histamine in the mucosa in the vicinity of the parietal cell. Cell separation techniques provide one approach to elucidating the receptors regulating acid secretory function. With isolation by enzyme treatment, the parietal cell can be removed from these background influences, thus allowing the effects of individual agents to be studied alone or in combination. The remainder of this review focuses on studies with isolated canine fundic cells aimed at elucidating the receptor interactions mediating acid secretion.

ISOLATION OF PARIETAL CELLS

Cells are dispersed from the fundic mucosa by treatment with enzymes. A variety of specific approaches have been developed, including rabbit gastric glands prepared with crude collagenase (Berglindh, 1976), parietal cells dispersed from canine (Soll, 1978a), rat (Lewin, 1974; Ecknauer, 1981), guinea pig (Batzri, 1981; Sewing, 1983), or amphibian (Michelangeli, 1978) gastric mucosa using sequential treatment with collagenase and EDTA or pronase. Several procedures have been used to enrich parietal cells, including velocity separation at either unit gravity or in an elutriator rotor and density gradient separation (see Soll, 1981a for more detailed review).

STUDIES OF PARIETAL CELL FUNCTION

With dispersion, parietal cells lose their polar orientation as a component of an epithelium, and thus H^+ ion secreted at the apical surface are neutralized by the concomitant secretion of bicarbonate ions. Indirect indices provide evidence of functional responses. With stimulation, isolated parietal cells undergo a morphologic transformation similar to that observed in vivo (Berglindh, 1976; Soll, 1981a); tubulovesicles which fill the cytoplasm in the basal state transform into secretory caniculi. Since the secretion of acid is a highly energy-dependent process, oxygen consumption and glucose oxidation both provide a reflection of the overall degree of cell activation. The accumulation of weak bases, such as ^{14}C-aminopyrine (AP), provides indirect evidence for the secretion of acid by isolated parietal cells (Berglindh, 1980a; Soll, 1980a). AP, with its pKa of 5.0, is largely unionized at cytoplasmic pH and freely diffuses across plasma membranes. Once AP has entered an acidic compartment, such as the tubulovesicles and secretory caniculi of the stimulated parietal cell, it becomes ionized and is thus locked in by the surrounding plasma membranes. Using fluorescent micorscopy, another weak base, acridine orange, has been shown to accumulate within vesicles of stimulated rabbit gastric glands (Berglindh, 1980a). It is important to emphasize that AP accumulation provides an index of the quantity of acid sequestered by parietal cells, rather than of the actual rate of acid secreted.

PARIETAL CELL RECEPTORS

Histamine, gastrin and cholinergic agents each stimulate oxygen consumption, AP accumulation, and glucose oxidation by canine parietal cells (Soll, 1978a, Soll, 1980a; 1981a). Histamine and cholinergic agents have been shown to stimulate parietal cell function in rabbit gastric glands (Berglindh, 1976; Chew, 1980), and parietal cells dispersed from the rat (Ecknauer, 1981; Dial, 1981), guinea pig (Batzri and Dyer, 1981) and frog (Michelangeli, 1976).

Several studies lead to the conclusion that histamine action on dispersed parietal cells is mediated by an H_2 receptor. H_2 blockers competitively inhibit histamine stimulation of oxygen consumption and AP accumulation by rabbit gastric glands (Berglindh, 1977a; Chew, 1980) and isolated canine, guinea pig, and rat parietal cells (Soll, 1978a, 1980a; Batzri 1981; Dial, 1981). For example, cimetidine in increasing concentrations produced a progressive parallel shift of the dose-response for histamine stimulation of AP accumulation in canine parietal cells (Soll, 1980a). The dissociation constant calculated from these data using a Schild plot is 1 µM and thus similiar to those found in guinea pig atrium and rat uterus. Anticholinergic agents in concentrations that markedly inhibit the response to cholinomimetics, fail to shift the dose-response to histamine.

Anticholinergic agents inhibit carbachol action on oxygen consumption and AP accumulation (Berglindh, 1977a; Soll, 1978a, 1980a; Batzri, 1981; Ecknauer, 1981). Atropine at concentrations between 3.2 nM and 100 nM produced a progressive, parallel rightward shift of the dose-response for carbachol stimulation of AP accumulation by isolated canine parietal cells, whereas cimetidine (10 µM) did not alter this dose-response relation (Soll, 1980a). The dissociation constant determined from this atropine effect was 1 nM, a value typical of muscarinic receptors in other tissues. Thus the isolated parietal cell after enzyme dispersion retains pharmacologically typical muscarinic and H_2 receptors.

The presence of gastrin receptors on the parietal cell remains controversal. With isolated canine parietal cells, gastrin produced a small, but definite increase in both oxygen consumption (Soll, 1978a) and AP accumulation (Soll, 1980a). These responses were not blocked by either H_2 antagonists or anticholinergic agents, indicating interaction at a separate receptor site. This gastrin effect was found in elutriator fractions enriched in parietal cells, but depleted in histamine cells, thus making it unlikely that gastrin action was mediated by release of histamine. Direct effects of gastrin on parietal cells isolated from species other than dog are less than dramatic. Pentagastrin did not stimulate oxygen consumption by parietal cells isolated from amphibian mucosa (Michelangeli, 1976), and only about one-third of parietal cell preparations from guinea pig responded to gastrin (Batzri,1981). Gastrin has only a small direct effect stimulating rabbit parietal cells (Chew, 1982). However, in the presence of isobutyl methyl xanthine, gastrin did produce an incremental increase in AP accumulation that was largely inhibited by cimetidine (Berglindh, 1980b; Chew, 1982). The mechanisms accounting for these observations remain uncertain, but gastrin has been reported to release histamine from rabbit gastric glands, as discussed latter.

The strongest evidence for the existence of a specific gastrin receptor on canine parietal cells comes from studies using a biologically active ^{125}I-[Leu^{15}]-G17 as a probe for the gastrin receptor (Soll, 1984a). ^{125}I-[Leu^{15}]-G17 has been used to study the gastrin receptor in a crude homogenate of rat fundic mucosa (Takeuchi, 1979). In our studies of the gastrin receptor on parietal cells, we also found it necessary to use [Leu^{15}]-gastrin for iodination, since oxidative damage presumably of methionine in the 15 position of native gastrin rendered specific receptor interactions inconsistent. In fractions containing 50 to 70% parietal cells 8 to 12% of the ^{125}I-[Leu^{15}]-G17 bound per million cells, with about 85% of the binding specific as determined by the difference of binding in the presence and absence of excess unlabelled gastrin. At 37°C, binding was rapid and reversible. In cell separation studies using the elutriator rotor, ^{125}I-[Leu^{15}]-G17 binding correlated with the distribution of parietal cells, indicating that parietal cells accounted for the majority of the gastrin binding to canine fundic mucosal cells. Step density gradients were performed on the parietal cell enriched elutriator fractions to provide enriched of greater than 85% parietal or chief cells respectively; ^{125}I-[Leu^{15}]-G17 binding correlated positively with the parietal cell content (r=0.96) and negatively with the chief cell content (r=-0.97) of these fractions. These data leave little question that the parietal cell, and probably not the chief cell, has a specific gastrin receptor. However, in the elutriator separation, there was indication of gastrin binding to one or more additional cell types that present in the small cell elutriator fractions (SCEF), as discussed subsequently. Gastrin binding was found to correlate with gastrin stimulation of parietal cell function (Soll, 1984a). Proglumide inhibited gastrin binding and the inhibition of binding was proportional with inhibition of gastrin stimulation of parietal cell function.

POTENTIATING INTERACTIONS BETWEEN SECRETAGOGUES

As discussed above, anticholinergic agents and H_2 histamine antagonists were found to be specific for the actions on the isolated parietal cell function of acetylcholine and carbachol, respectively. These findings are thus at odds with the in vivo observations that these inhibitors block all forms of acid secretion. This apparent contradiction may reflect the existence of potentiating interactions between secretagogues at the parietal cell, itself. Data obtained with studies of both oxygen consumption (Soll, 1978b) and AP accumulation (Soll, 1982) indicate that potentiating interactions occur between histamine and carbachol, but not between carbachol and gastrin, in that the responses to these former two combinations are significantly greater than the sum of the individual responses. A three-way interaction may, in addition, exist between histamine, carbachol, and gastrin (Soll, 1982). Interactions between cholinergic agents and histamine (Berglindh, 1977b) and possibly between gastrin and histamine (Chew, 1982) have been found in rabbit gastric glands. In the presence of these potentiating interactions, the actions of cimetidine and atropine display an apparent nonspecificity reminiscent of that found in vivo. Thus, for example, when gastrin action on isolated parietal cells was enhanced by potentiating interaction with histamine, cimetidine caused an apparent inhibition of the response to gastrin, which presumably reflected withdrawal of histamine's enhancement of gastrin°s action (Soll, 1978b, 1982).

ACTIVATION OF PARIETAL CELL FUNCTION

Both calcium and cyclic AMP are involved in the activation of the parietal cell. These second messengers, however, appear to be specific for acetylcholine and histamine, respectively, thus providing further support for the view that they act directly on parietal cell receptors. Despite the controversies resulting from studies with intact mucosa, work with isolated parietal cells and glands has consistently indicated that histamine stimulates parietal cell cyclic AMP production and/or adenylate cyclase (Batzri, 1978; Major, 1978; Sonnenberg, 1978; Wollin, 1979; Chew, 1980; Thompson, 1981; Manegeat, 1982; Schepp, 1983). In contrast, neither gastrin nor carbachol enhanced cyclic AMP production (Soll, 1979a). In cell separation studies, histamine stimulation of cyclic AMP correlated with the distribution of parietal cells (Major, 1978; Wollin, 1979). In studies with canine and rabbit preparations, the enhancement by histamine of cyclic AMP production appeared linked to stimulation of parietal cell function (Soll, 1979a; Chew, 1980). Species differences are of note in that both the functional and cyclic AMP responses to histamine are of much greater magnitude in rabbit parietal cells when directly compared to canine parietal cells (Soll, 1981a). Recent studies in guinea pig (reviewed by Sewing elsewhere in this volume) indicate a dissociation between histamine effects on cyclic AMP and stimulation of parietal cell function; causality in this interrelationship clearly requires further study.

In many cell types, increases in cytosol calcium appear to mediate cell activation by chemical transmitters. Such increases in cytosol calcium can be achieved by either enhanced influx of extracellular calcium or mobilization of intracellular calcium. The studies available at present indicate that cholinergic stimulation of parietal cell function is coupled to enhanced influx of extracellular calcium. The experiments supporting this conclusion include a dependency of cholinergic stimulation on extracellular calcium (Berglindh, 1980b,

Soll, 1981b). Furthermore, lanthanum, which blocks calcium fluxes across plasma membranes, also caused marked impairment of cholinergic action (Soll, 1981b). Lastly, carbachol stimulation is associated with enhanced $^{45}Ca^{++}$ influx into parietal cells, which, in turn, is closely correlated with cholinergic stimulation of oxygen consumption and AP accumulation (Soll, 1981b). In contrast to these findings, histamine stimulation of parietal cell function was only modestly impaired by removal of extracellular calcium and was not blocked by lanthanum nor associated with enhanced influx of $^{45}Ca^{++}$. Gastrin action showed an intermediate dependency upon the concentration of extracellular calcium, and treatment with lanthanum caused modest impairment of gastrin responsiveness. However, stimulation by gastrin was not found to be associated with enhanced calcium influx, and although gastrin action may be linked to mobilization of intracellular calcium, studies available with cells preloaded with $^{45}Ca^{++}$ did not confirm this hypothesis (Soll, 1981b).

Studies with isolated canine parietal cells support the hypothesis that histamine, gastrin, and acetylcholine modulate acid secretion by directly interacting with receptors on the parietal cell. Potentiating interactions may be an important mechanism underlying the interdependency between secretagogues in vivo. This discussion has not thus far considered the possibility that cholinergic and gastrin receptors may exist on other cells within the mucosa that also participate in the regulation of secretory function. These other cells with a potential regulatory role are endocrine, paracrine or even neurocrine cells that release transmitters such as histamine or somatostatin. Thus, integration between the pathways regulating acid secretion may occur by mechanisms in addition to potentiating interactions between secretagogues at the parietal cell itself. Recent studies have provided evidence that receptors for gastrin and acetylcholine exist on cells other than parietal cells; these studies will be reviewed in the following sections. Before considering muscarinic and gastric receptors on non parietal cells the cells storing histamine in the gastric mucosa will be considered.

HISTAMINE CELLS OF THE FUNDIC MUCOSA

High concentrations of histamine is present in the fundic mucosa, but the cells storing this histamine remain subject of much controversy fueled by major differences in these histamine stores between species. In the rat, histamine is stored in an enterochromaffin-like (ECL) cell (Thunberg, 1967; Aures, 1968a; Hakanson, 1970a). These cells lie within the epithelium deep in the gastric glands and not in the lamina propria. The identification of these cells as the site of histamine storage was based upon their parallel distribution with histidine decarboxylase activity and by their fluoreaction upon exposure to orthophthalaldehyde (Thunberg, 1967). These cells also concentrate tritium label after exposure to $(5-^3H)$-hydroxytryptophan (Rubin, 1979a) and L-[^{3}H]-histidine (Rubin, 1979b), thus indicating that these cells possess both APUD (amine precursor uptake and decarboxylation) and both form and store histamine. Histidine decarboxylase activity in the rat fundic mucosa is high, being considerably greater than found in other species. In the rat, gastrin stimulates the formation of histamine by inducing the activity of histidine decarboxylase. Acetylcholine and food, presumably by virtue of inducing the release of gastrin, have similar effects (Kahlson, 1968; Hakanson, 1970). Histamine release in the rat fundic mucosa may be stimulated by gastrin, but such effects have been demonstrated only by monitoring a decrease in histamine content of the fundic mucosa following gastrin treatment (Kahlson, 1968). Despite the considerable evidence suggesting that gastrin interacts with the histamine cell in the rat fundic mucosa, the existence of a causal link between this release of histamine by gastrin and gastrin stimulation of acid secretion remains controversial (Johnson, 1971; Hakanson, 1973).

In contrast to these findings in the rat fundic mucosa, in dog, man and pig, histamine appears to be stored in a mast-like cell (Aures, 1968b; Hakanson,

1969; Steer, 1976; Lorenz, 1968b). The term mast-like is used because these mast cells in the fundic mucosa were reported to have atypical staining properties and to be resistant to histamine release by Compound 48/80 (Lorenz, 1968a). In these species, orthophthalaldehyde induced fluorescence is not found over epithelial cells, but rather only over mast-like cells in the lamina propria, thus providing a sharp contrast to the rat fundic mucosa. Levels of histidine decarboxylase activity are low in these other species (Aures, 1968b; Hakanson, 1969), although some conflicting data exists on this latter point. No firm evidence has been presented to establish that either feeding or gastrin induces histamine formation.

There are some data to indicate that stimulation of acid secretion by pentagastrin causes the release of histamine from dog and human gastric mucosa, although these studies remain indirect and lack necessary controls. In duodenal ulcer patients, (Mann, 1982) following the infusion of pentagastrin, the histamine content of fundic mucosal biopsies decreased. Although initial studies indicated that pentagastrin treatment caused similar effects in dog (Thirlby, 1982), these findings were not confirmed in more detailed studies performed subsequently (S. Redfern, M. Feldman, personal communication). Peden and coworkers (1982) found that although pentagastrin increased the gastric juice histamine output in normal subjects, the histamine H_2-agonist, impromidine, increased histamine output to a greater extent. Lorenz (1976) reported data suggesting a similar increase in gastric juice histamine in dogs following treatment with the histamine analogue betazole. Several factors may influence histamine content and output from the fundic mucosa in response to stimulation; caution must be exercised in interpreting apparent effects as a reflection of action at specific receptors on the mast cell or as mediating stimulation of acid secretory responses until adequate controls are provided.

Isolation of Histamine Cells from the Canine Fundic Mucosa

Histamine is present in dispersed canine fundic mucosal cells and in the elutriator separation, histamine was found to be present in a cell of small size (Soll, 1979b). The fractions with peak histamine content still had several cell types present and therefore cells were further separated using a linear density gradient formed from a solution of bovine serum albumin and Ficoll. The histamine content of cells was maximal in fractions of high density and correlated with morphologically typical mast cells. The mast cells were enriched to about 75% in the fractions of highest density in this gradient (Soll, 1979b). In these separations of canine fundic mucosal cells, there was no indication of histamine in the portions of the gradients that contained endocrine markers (glucagon and somatostatin) (Soll, 1984b) or endocrine-like cell markers (serotonin and DOPA decarboxylase, Beaven, 1982). Despite the degree of enrichment of histamine cells, only trace activities of histidine decarboxylase was found in cell extracts of these fractions. However, using intact cells, histamine formation was detected by both a $^{14}CO_2$ release assay and by isotope dilution (Beaven, 1982). However, even with intact cells the formation of histamine was low, leaving open the question as to whether histamine was formed primarily in immature mast cells (Beaven, 1983), possibly before their migration into the fundic mucosa or whether these invitro studies underestimated histamine formation rates by cells in vivo.

Isolation of Histamine Cells from Rat Fundic Mucosa.

When similiar techniques to those described above were applied to the rat fundic mucosa, histamine was found in cells of very light density (Soll, 1981c). The cellular content of histamine and the activities of histidine decarboxylase and DOPA decarboxylase all had similar distributions in the density gradient of rat fundic cells. Cells with granules typical of ECL cells were present in the same region of the density gradient as was histamine. The degree of enrichment of ECL cells was modest, with a maximal content of about 12%. These studies were consistent with the previous work with intact mucosa that in the rat--but not canine--fundic mucosa histamine is present in an endocrine-like cell possessing high activities of histidine decarboxylase.

RECEPTORS ON NONPARIETAL CELLS IN THE CANINE FUNDIC MUCOSA

This brief overview of histamine cells in the fundic mucosa provides background information necessary for addressing the question of whether cells in addition to the parietal cell possess receptors for gastrin, acetylcholine or other transmitters. Histamine cells are good candidates for mediating effects of the endocrine or neurocrine pathways, but paracrine cells that store other biogenic amines or peptide hormones are also likely candidates.

Gastrin Receptors on Nonparietal Cells

In the studies of ^{125}I-[Leu^{15}]-G17 binding to canine fundic mucosal cells separated by elutriation, specific gastrin binding was found to the small cell elutriator fraction, as well as to parietal cells (Soll, 1984a). The SCEF has histamine cells, as noted, plus a variety of other cell types including endocrine and endocrine-like cells as noted above. In density gradients of the SCEF, a discrete distribution of ^{125}I-[Leu^{15}]-G17 binding was found in fractions of intermediate density; this profile was negatively correlated with the distribution of mast cells, thus indicating that canine fundic mucosal mast cells do not have gastrin receptors (Soll, 1984c). However, the distribution of ^{125}I-[Leu^{15}]-G17 binding did correlate with that for somatostatin-like immunoreactivity (SLI), suggesting the possibility that somatostatin cells in the fundic mucosa may have gastrin receptors (Soll, 1984c).

Evidence that gastrin receptors regulate SLI release was directly sought by studying somatostatin cells isolated from the canine fundic mucosa and cultured for 48 hours (Soll, 1984b). Cells in this preparation have a low basal release of SLI, but show 5- to 100-fold increases in SLI release in response to stimulation. The chemical transmitters that have thus far been shown to stimulate SLI release are epinephrine, acting at a β-receptor, cyclic AMP analogues, and gastrin. Furthermore, these canine somatostatin cells in short-term culture demonstrate remarkable potentiation of the secretory response when exposed to combinations of gastrin and either epinephrine or dibutyryl cyclic AMP. These data suggest that gastrin, in addition to acting as a stimulatory receptor on the parietal cell, may also activate an inhibitory pathway mediated by the release of somatostatin.

Cholinergic Receptors on Nonparietal Cells

As noted earlier, muscarinic ligands bind to many cell types within the fundic mucosa. These findings are not surprising since cholinergic agents stimulate pepsinogen, bicarbonate and mucus secretion probably acting directly at chief and mucous cell cholinergic receptors, respectively. An important question is whether muscarinic receptors on nonparietal cell serve as modulators of the acid secretory response. In our studies with somatostatin cells, we have found muscarinic receptors on SLI cells, that serve to inhibit--rather than stimulate--SLI release (Yamada, 1984). This carbachol effect is blocked by atropine, with the apparent dissociation constant about 1 nM, a value typical of muscarinic receptor sites. This cholinergic effect has a double negative effect; by blocking release of somatostatin, cholinergic agents attenuate the acid inhibitory mechanisms mediated by this peptide, thereby potentially enhancing the secretory response.

An important question concerns whether cholinergic receptors directly modulate histamine release from fundic mucosal histamine stores. In our studies of (^{3}H)-QNB binding to canine fundic cells, we found receptors in all of the elutriator fractions examined (Culp, 1983). However, in a density gradient performed on the small cell elutriator fraction, QNB binding was inversely correlated with histamine content (A. H. Soll, J. Park, D. Culp, M. A. Beaven, manuscript in preparation).

REGULATION OF HISTAMINE RELEASE FROM FUNDIC MUCOSAL STORES

To study factors regulating the release of histamine from canine fundic mucosal mast cells, we have placed the small cell elutriator fraction in short term suspension culture for 24 hours. Mast cells remain viable over this time and account for 30 to 60% of the cells surviving after this time period (Soll, Park and Beaven, unpublished studies). These mast cells demonstrate stimulation of histamine release by the calcium ionophore A23187 (1 uM) and antibody to rat IgE; there was no response to treatment with gastrin or cholinomimetics, alone or in combination. These latter negative findings, thus agree with the apparent absence of muscarinic and gastrin receptors in the region of the SCEF density gradient that contains the histamine cells. These potential validity of these negative conclusions is reenforced by that findings that gastrin receptors are present on other cells within the preparations and that these mast cells are capable of responding to other agents. However, negative findings must be interpreted with caution, since it is possible that specific mast cell receptors may be unstable under these conditions. Furthermore, it is not known whether mast cells isolated by these techniques are typical perivascular mast cells or a population of cells specialized for their functions in the fundic mucosa.

Gastrin and acetylcholine have been demonstrated to activate histamine release from rabbit gastric glands (Bergqvist, 1980) and from amphibian fundic mucosa (Rangachari, 1975), a topic considered elsewhere in this volume by Professor Obrink. These findings thus contrast with the studies with canine fundic mast cells discussed above. In light of this apparent difference it is important to firmly establish the identity of the cell(s) storing histamine in th fundic mucosa of these species. Conclusions regarding the regulation of histamine release based upon studies in rat and possibly in rabbit and frog, species in which histamine is stored in endocrine-like cells, may not be valid for regulation of histamine formation and release in species in which fundic mucosal histamine is stored in only mast cells.

OVERVIEW

Our present data obtained from studies with canine fundic cells indicate a complex model wherein both gastrin and acetylcholine have at least dual sets of receptors that are potentially involved in regulating acid-secretory function. Gastrin interacts with receptors on the parietal cell and on the somatostatin cell, and via these receptors has opposing acid-stimulatory and acid-inhibitory actions. This wiring appears to be a short circuit, but, several elements may modulate these opposing effects of gastrin on different cell types thereby coordinating the regulatory process. Acetylcholine is probably a major modulating element, increasing the acid secretory response to gastrin by simultaneously enhancing gastrin stimulation of parietal cell function and attenuating gastrin activation of the inhibitory mechanisms mediated by release of somatostatin. Administrating an anticholinergic agent would shift gastrin action toward acid-inhibitory effects by removing both endogenous muscarinic inhibition of somatostatin release and muscarinic stimulation at the parietal cell itself. The antisecretory efficacy of H_2 antagonists against gastrin may reflect inhibition of histamine enhancement of gastrin action at the parietal cell, while leaving unimpaired the acid-inhibitory effects of gastrin mediated by release of somatostatin. The profound effects of H_2 antagonists on gastrin action may also reflect a component of gastrin action due to histamine release, but this effect may be species variable and awaits direct confirmation.

The apparent complexity of proposed regulatory mechanisms of acid secretion has increased dramatically with the acquisition of a relatively small amount of knowledge. As further knowledge is gained, the importance of the various elements may become clear and a unifying hypothesis can be formulated based upon information gained from studies with more integrated systems. The regulation of histamine formation and release requires a great deal of additional study to clarify the interplay between the major pathways regulating acid secretion. There is no doubt that current models and knowledge will rapidly evolve, but the concept that the pathways mediating acid secretion both converge in parallel at the parietal cell and act in series, by modulating the release of paracrine transmitters, is attractive and likely to persist.

REFERENCES

Aures, D., R. Hakanson, and A. Schauer (1968a). Histidine decarboxylase and DOPA decarboxylase in the rat stomach. Properties and cellular localization. Eur. J. Pharmacol. 3, 217-34.

Aures, D., R. Hakanson, C.H. Owman, and B. Sporrong (1968b). Cellular stores of histamine and monoamines in the dog stomach. Life Sci 7, 1147-53.

Batzri, S., and J.D. Gardner (1978). Cellular cyclic AMP indispersed mucosal cells from guinea pig stomach. Biochim. Biophys. Acta. 541, 181-9.

Batzri, S. (1981). Interaction of histamine with specific membrane receptors on gastric mucosal cells. Biochem. Pharmacol. 30, 3013-3016.

Beaven, M.A., A.H. Soll, and K.J. Lewin (1982). Histamine synthesis by intact mast cells from canine fundic mucosa and liver. Gastroenterology. 82, 254-62.

Beaven, M.A., D.L. Aiken, E. WoldeMussie, and A.H. Soll (1983). Changes in histamine synthetic activity, histamine content, and responsiveness to compound 48/80 during maturation of rat peritoneal mast cells. J. Pharmacol. Exp. Therap. 224, 620-626.

Berglindh, T., H.F. Helander, and K.J. Obrink (1976). Effects of secretagogues on oxygen consumption, aminopyrine accumulation, and morphology in isolated gastric glands. Acta. Physiol. Scand. 97, 401-14.

Berglindh, T. (1977a). Potentiation by carbachol and aminophylline of histamine- and dbcAMP-induced parietal cells activity in isolated gastric glands. Acta. Physiol. Scand. 99, 75-84.

Berglindh, T. (1977b). Effects of common inhibitors of gastric acid secretion on secretagogue-induced respiration and aminopyrine accumulation in isolated gastric glands. Biochim. Biophys. Acta. 464, 217-33.

Berglindh, T., D.R. Dibona, S. Ito, and G. Sachs (1980a). Probes of parietal cell function. Am. J. Physiol. 238, (Gastrointest Liver Physiol. 1), G165-G176.

Berglindh, T., G. Sachs, and N. Takeguchi (1980b). Ca^+-dependent secretagogue stimulation in isolated rabbit gastric glands. Am. J. Physiol. 239, G90-4.

Bergqvist, E., M. Waller, L. Hammar, and K.J. Obrink (1980). Histamine as the secretory mediator in isolated gastric glands. In I. Shulz, G. Sachs, J.G. Forte, K.J. Ullrich, (eds.), Hydrogen Ion Transport in Epithelia, Elsevier/North-Holland Biomedical Press, Amsterdam. pp. 429-437.

Black, J.W., W.A.M. Duncan, C.J. Durant, C.R. Ganellin, and M.E. Parsons (1972). Definition and antagonism of histamine H_2-receptors. Nature (Lond.). 236, 385-90.

Chew, C.S., S.J. Hersey, G. Sachs, and T. Berglindh (1980). Histamine responsiveness of isolated gastric glands. Am. J. Physiol. 238 (Gastrointest Liver Physiol 1), G312-20.

Chew, C.S., and S.J. Hersey (1982). Gastrin stimulation of isolated gastric glands. Am. J. Physiol. 242,(Gastrointest Liver Physiol), G504-G512.

Code, C.F. (1965). Histamine and gastric secretion: a later look, 1955-1965. Fed. Proc. 24, 1311-21.

Culp, D.J., J.M. Wolosin, A.H. Soll, and J.G. Forte (1983). Muscarinic receptors and guanylate cyclase in mammalian gastric glandular cells. Am. J. Physiol. 245, (Gastrointest. Liver Physiol. 8), G641-G646.

Dial, E., W.J. Thompson, and G.C. Rosenfeld (1981). Isolated parietal cells: histamine response and pharmacology. J. Pharm. Exp. Ther. 219, 585-90.

Ecknauer, R., E. Dial, W.J. Thompson, L.R. Johnson, and G.C. Rosenfeld (1981). Isolated rat gastric parietal cells: Cholinergic response and pharmacology. Life. Sci. 28, 609-621.
Feldman, M. (1983). Gastric secretion. In M. Sleisenger, and J.S. Fordtran, (eds.), Gastrointestinal Diseases. Saunders, Philadelphia. Third Edition, pp. 541-558.
Gibson, R., B.I. Hirschowitz, and G. Hutchison (1974). Actions of metiamide, an H_2-histamine receptor antagonist, on gastric H^+ and pepsin secretion in dogs. Gastroenterology. 67, 93-99.
Grossman, M.I., and S.J. Konturek (1974). Inhibition of acid secretion in dog by metiamide, a histamine antagonist acting on H_2 receptors. Gastroenterology. 66, 517-21.
Grossman, M.I. (1982). Regulation of gastric acid secretion. In L.R. Johnson (ed.), Physiology of the Digestive Tract. Raven Press, New York. pp. 659-71.
Hakanson, R., B. Lilja, and C.H. Owman (1969). Cellular localization of the histamine and monoamines in the gastric mucosa of man. Histochemie. 18, 74-86.
Hakanson, R., and G. Liedberg (1970). The role of endogenous gastrin in the activation of gastric histidine decarboxylase in the rat. Effect of antrectomy and vagal denervation. Eur. J. Pharmacol. 12, 94-103.
Hakanson, R., G. Liedberg, C.H. Owman, and F. Sundler (1973). The cellular localization of gastric histamine and its implications for the concept of histamine as a physiological stimulant of gastric acid secretion. In C. Maslinski (ed.), Histamine: Mechanisms regulating the biogenic amine levels in tissues with special regard to histamine. Dowden, Hutchinson, and Ross, Inc., Stroudsbury, Penn. pp.209-22.
Johnson, L.R. (1971). Control of gastric secretion: No room for histamine. Gastroenterology. 61, 106-18.
Kahlson G., and E. Rosengren (1968). New approaches to the physiology of histamine. Physiol. Rev. 48, 155-96.
Lewin, M., A.M. Cheret, A. Soumarmon, and J. Girodet (1974). Methode pour l'isolement et le tri des cellules de la muqueuse fundique de rat. Biol. Gastroenterol. 7, 139-44.
Lorenz, W., A. Schauer, S.T. Heitland, R. Calvoer, and E. Werle (1969). Biochemical and histochemical studies on the distribution of histamine in the digestive tract of man, dog and other mammals. Naunyn-Schmiedebergs. Arch. Pharmak. 265, 81-100.
Lorenz, W., H. Troidl, H. Barth, H. Rohde, S. Schulz, H. Becker, P. Dormann, A. Schmal, J. Dusche, and R. Meyer (1976). Stimulus-secretion coupling in the human and canine stomach: role of histamine. In R.M. Case, and H. Goebell (eds.), Stimulus-Secretion Coupling in the Gastrointestinal Tract. MTP Press Limited. pp.177-191.
Major, J.S., and P Scholes (1978). The localization of a histamine H_2-receptor adenylate cyclase system in canine parietal cells and its inhibition by prostaglandins. Agents and Actions. 8, 324-31.
Mangeat, P., C. Gespach, G. Marchis-Mouren, and G. Rosselin (1982). Differential effects of histamine, vasoactive intestinal polypeptide, prostaglandin E_2 and somatostatin on cyclic AMP-dependent protein kinase activation in gastric glands isolated from the guinea pig fundus and antrum. Regul. Peptides. 3, 155-168.
Michelangeli, F. (1978). Acid secretion and intracellular pH in isolated oxyntic cells. J. Membrane. Biol. 38, 31-50.
Rangachari, P.K. (1975). Histamine release by gastric stimulants. Nature. 253, 53-55.
Reite, O.B. (1972). Comparative physiology of histamine. Physiol. Rev. 52, 778-819.
Rubin, W., and B. Schwartz (1979a). An electron microscopic radioautographic identification of the "enterochromaffin-like" APUD cells in murine oxyntic glands. Gastroenterology. 76, 437-49.
Rubin, W., and B. Schwartz (1979b). Electron microscopic radioautographic

identification of the ECL cell as the histamine-synthetizing endocrine cell in the rat stomach. Gastroenterology. 77, 456-67.

Schepp, W., H-K. Heim, and H-J. Ruoff (1983). Comparison of the effect of PGE_2 and somatostatin on histamine stimulated ^{14}C-aminopyrine uptake and cyclic AMP formation in isolated rat gastric mucosal cells. Agents and Actions. 13, 200-206.

Sewing, K-F., P. Harms, G. Schulz, and H. Hannemann (1983). Effect of substituted benzimidazoles on acid secretion in isolated and enriched guinea pig parietal cells. Gut. 24, 557-560.

Soll, A.H. (1978a). The actions of secretagogues on oxygen uptake by isolated mammalian parietal cells. J. Clin. Invest. 61, 370-380.

Soll, A.H. (1978b). The interaction of histamine with gastrin and carbamylcholine on oxygen uptake by isolated mammalian parietal cells. J. Clin. Invest. 61, 381-9.

Soll, A.H., and A. Wollin (1979a). Histamine and cyclic AMP in isolated canine parietal cells. Am. J. Physiol. 237, E444-E50.

Soll, A.H., K. Lewin, and M.A. Beaven (1979b). Isolation of histamine-containing cells from canine fundic mucosa. Gastroenterology. 77, 1283-90.

Soll, A.H. (1980a). Secretagogue stimulation of $[^{14}C]$-aminopyrine accumulation by isolated canine parietal cells. Am. J. Physiol. 238, (Gastrointest Liver Physiol 1), G366-75.

Soll, A.H. (1980b). Specific inhibition by prostaglandins E_2 and I_2 of histamine-stimulated ^{14}C-aminopyrine accumulation and cyclic AMP generation by isolated canine parietal cells. J. Clin. Invest. 65, 1222-9.

Soll, A.H., and B.J.R. Whittle (1981a). Prostacyclin analogues inhibit canine parietal cell activity and cyclic AMP formation. Prostaglandins. 21, 353-365.

Soll, A.H. (1981b). Extracellular calcium and cholinergic stimulation of isolated canine parietal cells. J. Clin. Invest. 68, 270-278.

Soll, A.H., K.J. Lewin, and M.A. Beaven (1981c). Isolation of histamine-containing cells from rat gastric mucosa: Biochemical and morphological differences from mast cells. Gastroenterology. 80, 717-727.

Soll, A.H. (1982). Potentiating interactions of gastric stimulants on $[^{14}C]$-aminopyrine accumulation by isolated canine parietal cells. Gastroenterology. 83, 216-223.

Soll, A.H., D.A. Amirian, L.P. Thomas, J. Park, M.A. Beaven, and T. Yamada (1984a). Gastrin receptors on isolated canine parietal cells. J. Clin. Invest. 73, 1434-1447.

Soll, A.H., T. Yamada, J. Park, and L.P. Thomas (1984b). Release of somatostatin-like immunoreactivity from canine fundic mucosal cells in primary culture. Submitted for Publication.

Soll, A.H., D.A. Amirian, L.P. Thomas, J. Park, M.A. Beaven, and T. Yamada (1984c). Gastrin receptors on non parietal cells isolated from canine fundic mucosa. Am J Physiol, in press.

Sonnenberg, A., W. Hunziker, H.R. Koelz, J.A. Fischer, and A.L. Blum (1978). Stimulation of endogenous cyclic AMP (cAMP) in isolated gastric cells by histamine and prostaglandin. Acta. Physiol. Scand. (Special Suppl), 307-17.

Steer, H.W. (1976). Mast cells of the human stomach. J. Anat. 121, 385-97.

Takeuchi, K., G.R. Speir, and L.R. Johnson (1979). Mucosal gastrin receptor. I. Assay standardization and fulfillment of receptor criteria. Am. J. Physiol. 237, E284-E294.

Thirlby, R., M. Feldman, M. Tharp, and C. Richardson (1982). Effect of pentagastrin on gastric mucosal histamine in dogs. Gastroenterology. 82, 1196.

Thompson, W.J., L.K. Chang, and G.C. Rosenfeld (1981). Histamine regulation of adenylyl cyclase of enriched rat gastric parietal cells. Am. J. Physiol. 240, (Gastrointest Liver Physiol 3), G76-G84.

Thunberg, R. (1967). Localization of cells containing and forming histamine in the gastric mucosa of the rat. Exp. Cell. Res. 47, 108-15.

Wollin, A., A.H. Soll, and I.M. Samloff (1979). Actions of histamine, secretin, and PGE_2 on cyclic AMP production by isolated canine fundic mucosal cells. Am. J. Physiol. 237, E437-E43.

HISTAMINE H_2 RECEPTORS AND GASTRIC CELLS

C. Gespach and S. Emami

Unité INSERM U.55, Hôpital Saint-Antoine, 184 rue du
Faubourg, Saint-Antoine, Paris 12°, France

ABSTRACT

Gastric histamine H_2 receptor activity (H_2R) has been analyzed in man and laboratory animals (rat, guinea pig, rabbit) and after the malignant transformation of the human gastric mucosa. In these models, we have investigated:
1) the pharmacological properties of H_2R in human or guinea pig gastric glands and in the human gastric cancer cell line HGT-1; 2) the tissular (fundus, antrum, duodenum) and cellular localization (parietal, mucous, peptic cells) of H_2R;
3) the regulation by somatostatin and vasoactive intestinal peptide (VIP) of H_2R;
4) the desensitization of H_2R; 5) H_2R in fetal and developing gastric glands in man or rat.

Histamine H_2 receptor activity has been evaluated by biochemical parameters (cellular cAMP production, adenylate cyclase and cAMP-dependent protein kinase activation, binding studies) and by biological parameters (acid secretion, ultrastructural transformation of the acid-secreting parietal cell).

The conclusions drawn from this investigation are that: a) gastric H_2R are expressed during the fetal life or after the malignant transformation in man; b) their tissular or cellular localization, their pharmacological properties and their regulation by peptide hormones are different according to animal species; c) H_2R can be blocked or antagonized by competitive (cimetidine) or noncompetitive inhibitors (somatostatin, VIP, AH 22216, SKF 93479); d) the HGT-1 cell line appears as a good model to further characterize gastric H_2 receptors in their subcellular localization, chemical structure and autoregulation (desensitization).

KEY WORDS

Normal, cancerous gastric cells; histamine H_2 receptors; pharmacology; ontogeny; desensitization; electron microscopy; morphology; somatostatin; VIP; human.

INTRODUCTION

Histamine has been suspected to play a central role on gastric secretion as a final mediator of the action of other secretagogues such as gastrin and cholinergic agents. Several data indicated that numerous other substances, including peptide hormones, neurotransmitters and prostaglandins may also interfere with histaminergic pathways in the gastric mucosa. The aim of the present paper was to analyze the biochemical basis for the various types of physiological and pathophysiological regulation of histamine H_2 receptor activity in gastric cells.

1. CLASSIFICATION OF HISTAMINE H_1, H_2 and H_3 RECEPTORS

Ash and Schild (1966) proposed that the pharmacological activity of histamine is mediated by at least two different classes of receptors since the H_1 antihistamine mepyramine, which inhibited histamine-induced contractions of the guinea pig ileum or bronchial constriction, was ineffective against histamine stimulation of gastric acid secretion.

Histamine H_2 receptors have been identified by Black (1972) after the discovery of a new class of histamine blocking drugs bearing an imidazole ring. Burimamide was shown to antagonize the actions of histamine on acid secretion or rat uterine contractility. In various tissues, histamine H_1 and H_2 receptors have been shown to mediate biological actions via calcium ions/cGMP levels or via cAMP as intracellular mediators, respectively (Schultz, 1973; Clyman, 1975; Tepperman, 1979).

In the brain, histamine has a neurotransmitter role and at very low doses inhibits its own release from depolarized slices of rat cerebral cortex (Arrang, 1983). Since the potencies of various selective histamine agonists or antagonists in this system are different from those previously characterized as H_1 or H_2 receptors, it has been suggested that this histamine auto-inhibitory process operates via a third class of histamine receptors, classified as H_3 receptors.

2. HISTAMINE EFFECTS ON THE STOMACH

In the submucosal arterioles of the corpus and antrum of the stomach, there is evidence showing that the vasodilator effects of histamine involved both H_1 and H_2 receptors in producing systemic hypotension (Black, 1972; Charbon, 1980; Harvey, 1980; Koo, 1983; Salvati, 1983). In the rat stomach, topical histamine increased microvascular permeability to macromolecules from venules in the muscularis externa via H_1 receptors (Nagata, 1983). Secretion of acid by histamine has been studied extensively in animals and humans (Popielski, 1920; Grossman, 1967). The effect of histamine on pepsin secretion is rather controversial. Hirschowitz (1977, 1981) found that histamine may have stimulant and inhibitory actions on the canine peptic cell, both effects mediated by one type of histamine receptors (H_2). In agreement, Ayalon (1982) described the stimulation of electrogenic ion transport by histamine H_2 receptors in enriched canine gastric chief cells. In the isolated whole stomach of the rat, Bunce (1981) presented evidences that cimetidine produced a dose-related inhibition of the pepsin output induced by histamine. However, Konturek (1974) suggested that the inhibition of pepsin secretion by H_2 receptor antagonists was secondary to changes in acid secretion, and Koelz (1982) indicated that pepsinogen secretion by the gastric chief cell is regulated by cholinergic and adrenergic mechanisms, but not by histamine. Histaminergic influence, via stimulation of H_2 receptors has been presented for the release of gastric somatostatin in dog (Schusdziarra, 1981) and man (Hanssen, 1983), or intrinsic factor in guinea pig and rabbit stomach (Batzri, 1982a).

3. MEASUREMENT OF GASTRIC H_2 RECEPTOR ACTIVITY

Interaction of histamine on gastric mucosal cells has been evaluated by binding studies using radiaoctive histamine (Salganik, 1976; Lewin, 1979; Batzri, 1981a, 1982b, 1982c, 1982d), cimetidine (Rosenfeld, 1980; Warrander, 1983) or tiotidine (Gajtkowski, 1983). However, labelling the gastric H_2 receptor with those ligands gave unsatisfactory results in regard to the inhibition constant values obtained, to the importance of the non-specific components, and to the lack of correlation with biological activities (Batzri, 1982c, 1982d; Warrander, 1983; Gaktowski, 1983). In frog gastric mucosa (Kasbekar, 1969), in isolated gastric glands from the rabbit (Chew, 1980) or in enriched parietal cells from guinea pig and dog gastric mucosa (Albinus, 1981), histamine is taken up and partially metabolized to N-methylhistamine. Again, differences in affinity of histamine agonists or antagonists on acid secretion or cAMP production indicate that the histamine uptake differs from the biological activity of the histamine H_2 receptor (Chew, 1980).

Occupancy of the H_2 receptor by histamine resulted in a cascade of biochemical events including adenylate cyclase (Perrier, 1970) and cAMP-dependent protein kinase activation (Wollin, 1975), oxygen consumption (Berglindh, 1976a, 1976b) and aminopyrine uptake (Berglindh, 1977) as indirect indexes of gastric acid secretion.

In the absence of cAMP-phosphodiesterase inhibitor, exogenous histamine produced substained (20 min) stimulation of basal cAMP levels in intact gastric glands or cells isolated from human (Gespach, 1983;a), guinea pig (Gespach, 1983b) and rabbit stomach (Chew, 1980). In dog (Soll, 1979a) and rat stomach (Gespach, 1980a), the stimulatory effect of histamine on the cAMP generating system was markedly potentiated or evidenced after addition of phosphodiesterase inhibitors, indicating that the cAMP degradating enzyme could be an important regulator of the histamine receptor activity during prolonged exposition of gastric cells to histamine.

Ultrastructural changes accompanying the onset of gastric acid secretion have been viewed by scanning and transmission electron microscopy after dibutyryl cAMP or histamine (Rosa, 1963; Berglindh, 1976b; Logsdon, 1982; Anteunis, 1984). Morphometric studies indicated that ultrastructural changes occured in rat gastric parietal cells according to the circadian rhythm (Jacobs, 1980) or altered feeding regimen (Jacobs, 1982). In agreement, Ainge (1981) indicated that parietal cells, instead of showing secretory changes appeared like a resting cell, even after feeding in dogs treated with the H_2 receptor antagonist ranitidine.

4. PHARMACOLOGY OF GASTRIC H_2 RECEPTORS

Figure 1 shows the pharmacological analysis of the effect of histamine and its H_1 or H_2 agonists and antagonists in human and guinea pig fundic glands (Gespach, 1983a). In the two models, H_1 agonists (AET, PEA) or antagonist (DPH) are much less potent than the H_2 agonists (I, 4-MH) or antagonists (RA, OX, C) investigated. The results indicate that the H_1, H_2 agonists and antagonists interact with a common set of H_2 receptors, as shown in gastric cells isolated from laboratory animals (Rosenfeld, 1980; Chew, 1980; Hersey, 1981; Batzri, 1982b, 1982c, 1982d) or in other tissues bearing H_2 receptors (Gespach, 1982a, 1982b).

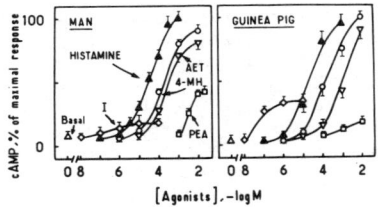 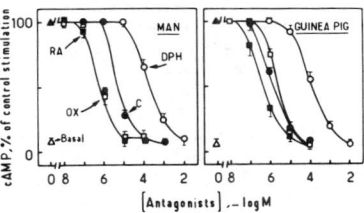

Fig.1. Dose-response curves for histamine and its H_1 or H_2 selective agonists (left) or antagonists (right) on H_2 receptor activity in human or guinea pig fundic glands. Glands were incubated with the indicated concentrations of histamine, impromidine (I), 4-methylhistamine (4-MH), 2-(2-aminoethyl) thiazole (AET), 2-(2-pyridyl)- ethylamine (PEA); cimetidine (C), oxmetidine (OX), ranitidine (RA) or diphenhydramine (DPH).

However, important differences were noticed for the relative potencies of I and OX in the two models (Table), indicating that informations on the pharmacological properties of the gastric H_2 receptor obtained in laboratory animals are difficult to transfer systematically to man. In contrast, the human gastric cancer cell line HGT-1, originating from a tumor localized in the fundus (Laboisse, 1982) possesses histamine H_2 receptors (Emami, 1982) with similar pharmacological properties to those characterized in normal human fundic glands (Table).

Table: Comparison of the relative potencies of histamine H_1 or H_2 agonists and antagonists on H_2 receptor activity in guinea pig, human fundic glands and in the human gastric cancer cell line HGT-1.

Models	Agonists					Antagonists			
	I	H	4-MH	AET	PEA	RA	OX	C	DPH
Guinea pig	200	1	0.09	0.18	0.18	5	0.8	1	0.01
Human	30	1	0.21	0.1	0.01	7	6.8	1	0.02
HGT-1 cells	50	1	0.16	0.02	0.01	9	9	1	0.05

The relative potency of each agonist or antagonist was established as the ratio: EC_{50} for histamine/EC_{50} for agonist; or IC_{50} for cimetidine/IC_{50} for antagonist.

As proposed by Emami (1982, 1983a, 1983b) this cell line can be a good model to study drugs used therapeutically during the treatment of patients for gastric ulcer. For example, the pharmacological properties of AH 22216 (Menez, 1983), SKF 93479 and cimetidine (Emami, 1985) in HGT-1 cells are in agreement with the kinetics and the inhibitory potencies of the antagonists inhibiting histamine-induced gastric acid secretion in vivo, in the conscious Heidenhain pouch dog (Stables, 1983) or in vitro in dispersed mucosal cells from the rabbit fundus (Gespach, 1983c).

5. TISSULAR, CELLULAR AND HISTOLOGICAL DISTRIBUTION OF GASTRIC H_2 RECEPTORS

Histamine-sensitive adenylate cyclase has been localized in the gastric fundic mucosa in dog (Dozois, 1977). Similar findings have been reported in fundic or antral glands isolated from man (Dupont, 1980) or rat (Gespach, 1980b). In dog (Scholes, 1976) and in isolated mucosa cells from rat corpus (Sonnenberg, 1978) histamine stimulation of the H_2 receptor has been localized in parietal cells. In gastric glands isolated from the guinea pig, histamine was about 10 times more potent in fundus ($EC_{50}= 10^{-5}$ M) than in antrum ($EC_{50}= 9 \times 10^{-5}$ M) and did not produce any cAMP stimulation in enterocytes isolated from the upper part of the duodenum (Gespach, 1983b). In both parts of the guinea pig stomach, histamine interacts with typical H_2 receptor mediating adenylate cyclase and cAMP-dependent protein kinase activation (Mangeat, 1982). In gastric cells isolated by pronase digestion from the guinea pig, histamine stimulated cAMP production via typical H_2 receptors in three fundic cell fractions ($EC_{50}= 1.6-2 \times 10^{-4}$ M) enriched in parietal (94%), peptic (63%) and mucous cells (87%), as well as in antral cells ($EC_{50}=4 \times 10^{-4}$ M) that are devoided of parietal cells (Gespach, 1982c). In agreement, histological distribution of the adenylate cyclase, using serial tissue sections of the rabbit gastric mucosa, indicated histamine stimulation from the surface mucous neck cell layer, to the chief cell sections at the base of the glands (Kaksumata, 1976). A recent study (Rutten, 1981) showed that surface epithelial cells isolated from the fundic piglet mucosa contain an histamine-sensitive cAMP system that has 10-fold lower activity than that of the parietal cell-rich fraction (H_2 receptor-sensitive). However, these authors showed that the activation of adenylate cyclase by histamine in surface cells could be blocked by the H_1 antagonist promethazine but not by the H_2 blocker cimetidine. This difference could be explained by the loss of the specificity of the histamine H_2 receptor during cellular or adenylate cyclase preparations (Ruoff, 1979). The presence of H_2 receptors in nonparietal cells in gastric mucosa (Rutten, 1981; Gespach 1982c, 1983b) correlates with the in vivo regulation by histamine of pepsin (Hirschowitz, 1977, 1981) and somatostatin (Schusdziarra, 1981; Hanssen, 1983) since in both cases, stimulation or inhibition are H_2 receptor-mediated effects.

6. INTERACTION OF SECRETAGOGUES OR SECRETORY INHIBITORS ON GASTRIC H_2 RECEPTOR ACTIVITY

Gastric secretory inhibitors (prostaglandins, somatostatin, vasoactive intestinal peptide: VIP) have been shown to inhibit histamine H_2 receptor activities and acid secretion (Robert, 1967; Barbezat, 1971; Barros D'Sa, 1975; Kulkarni, 1979). Prostaglandins (E type) and prostacyclin (PGI_2) inhibited both H_2 receptor adenylate cyclase system (Major, 1978) and histamine-stimulated aminopyrine accumulation in parietal cells (Soll, 1980).

In fundic and antral glands (Gespach, 1982d), somatostatin has been found in endocrine D-cells (Polak, 1975) at the vicinity of the parietal cell (Larsson, 1979). Somatostatins- 14 and -28 suppressed cAMP stimulation by histamine as well by its H_1 or H_2 agonists in rat (Gespach, 1980a) and guinea pig fundic glands (Gespach, 1983b). In these two models, the inhibition was partial, noncompetitive and highly selective since no effect of somatostatin was found on basal or cAMP production induced by secretin, VIP, PGE_2, in either fundic or antral glands or by histamine in guinea pig antral glands. In the guinea pig, somatostatin also reduced histamine-induced cAMP-dependent protein kinase activation (Mangeat, 1982; Gespach, 1983d) or aminopyrine uptake (Batzri, 1981b; Chew, 1983). In human fundic glands, somatostatin noncompetitively inhibits cAMP stimulation by catecholamines but does not affect VIP or histamine stimulations (Boige, 1984). Other mechanisms of action of somatostatin on gastric secretion such as cytosolic phosphoprotein phosphatase (Reyl, 1981) or carbonic anhydrase in oxyntic cells (Shapiro, 1981) are also possible.

VIP is a neurotransmitter which has been localized in gastrointestinal nerves (Larsson, 1976). In the guinea pig, this peptide stimulated cAMP production and cAMP-dependent protein kinase activity in mucopeptic cells (Mangeat, 1982; Gespach, 1983d) present in fundic or antral glands. Pretreatment of fundic glands by VIP resulted in a remarkable suppression of histamine-induced ultrastructural changes related acid secretion in the guinea pig (Anteunis, 1984), suggesting that VIP is an inhibitor of gastric acid secretion stimulated by histamine in the guinea pig.

Potentiating actions of the secretagogues carbamylcholine and gastrin have been demonstrated on histamine-induced oxygen uptake by isolated canine parietal cells (Soll, 1978) and on histamine-stimulated aminopyrine uptake by guinea pig gastric mucosal cells (Batzri, 1981c) indicating the occurence of separate receptors for histaminergic, cholinergic and gastrinic regulations on the parietal cell.

7. METABOLISM AND LOCALIZATION OF HISTAMINE IN THE STOMACH

Histamine and the enzyme forming or degradating the bioamine (histidine decarboxylase, histamine methyltransferase) are detected in appreciable amounts in extracts of the gastric mucosa (Thunberg, 1967; Fischer, 1981; Beaven, 1982; Savany, 1982). In the rat, gastric mucosal histamine is stored in two populations of histaminocytes (Lemmi, 1984) having morphologic and biochemical characteristics of endocrine-like cells (Thunberg, 1967; Soll, 1981). In other species, such as dog and human, histamine has been found only in mucosal mast cells (Lorenz, 1969; Hakanson, 1969; Soll, 1979b). An histamine-like gastrosecretagogue, resulting from a chemical complex between an imidazolic component and a tripeptide has been also isolated from the porcine gastric antral mucosa (Vatier, 1982). Histamine-containing mucosal cells occur in the lamina propria, in close proximity to parietal cells, and copurify with the acid-secreting cells during separation by Percoll of isolated gastric mucosal cells from man and rat (Ruoff, 1984). It is threfore conceivable that gastric histamine receptors are exposed to histamine released by histaminocytes during cell preparation or separation, producing alteration (desensitization) in H_2 receptor activity.

8. DESENSITIZATION OF GASTRIC H_2 RECEPTORS

Desensitization of cells to hormone and neurotransmitters has been observed for a variety of tissues and ligands such as glucagon, insulin, TSH, LH, FSH, prostaglandins, opiates, catecholamines, carbachol, gastrin. This desensitization is produced by a number of different mechanisms including uncoupling of the receptor to the adenylate cyclase or biological responses, a decrease in the concentration of receptors (internalization, receptor degradation), progressive alteration of adenylate cyclase or phosphodiesterase activity. In gastric cells upregulation of mucosal gastrin receptors was observed in postvagotomized rats, while fasting caused a decline in receptor levels (Speir, 1982). In the human gastric cancer cell line HGT-1, chronic treatment of cultured cells with VIP produced homologous desensitization of VIP receptor activity since cAMP responses to pancreatic glucagon, and gastric inhibitory peptide remained unaffected (Gespach, 1984a). In the same model, selective disappearance of histamine H_2 receptor activity has been observed, after short-term (Gespach, 1984b and manuscript in preparation) or chronic treatment (Emami, 1985) by histamine. Figure 2 indicates that histamine H_2 receptor activity was progressively altered after short-term exposure of HGT-1 cells to histamine (half-life = 20 min). The homologous desensitization of H_2R activity by histamine or by its

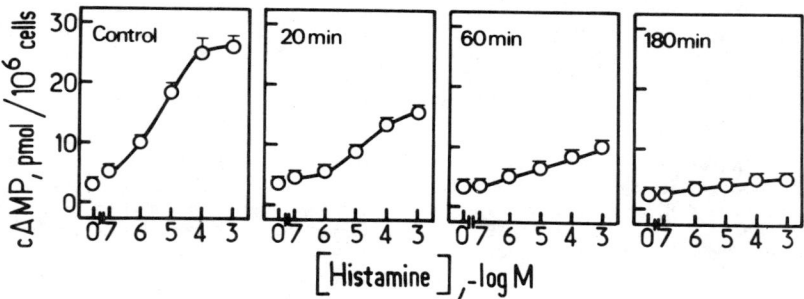

Fig. 2. Time-course of desensitization of gastric histamine H_2 receptors in HGT-1 cells. Cultured HGT-1 cells were exposed to 10^{-3} M histamine at 37°C for the indicated time, washed in culture flasks and after their collection. Isolated HGT-1 cells were then incubated in absence or in the presence of different histamine concentrations before assay of cAMP.

H_2 antagonists, such as SKF 93479, could be involved in the physiological regulation and pharmacological control of gastric cell function. Decreased histamine response has been described previously in granulocytes of asthmatic patients (H_2 receptors) and in histamine H_1 receptor-mediated glycogen hydrolysis in brain slices (Busse, 1977; Quach, 1981).

9. ONTOGENY OF GASTRIC H_2 RECEPTORS

The fetal rat stomach develops significant acidification on days 19 and 20 of gestation, spontaneously (Ducroc, 1981) or in response to histamine (Garzon, 1982). Parietal cells are demonstrable in human foetuses by 11 weeks (Salenius, 1962) and histamine H_2 receptors are functional in human (Gespach, 1981) and rat foetuses (Chérel, 1981; Gespach, 1984c), while gastrin and histamine did not stimulate acid or pepsin secretion until day 20 in the rat (Ikezaki, 1983). During the development, the general characteristics (potency and pharmacological or regulatory properties) of the histaminergic activation in rat gastric glands (fig.3) were comparable with those evidenced in adult rats (Gespach, 1984c).

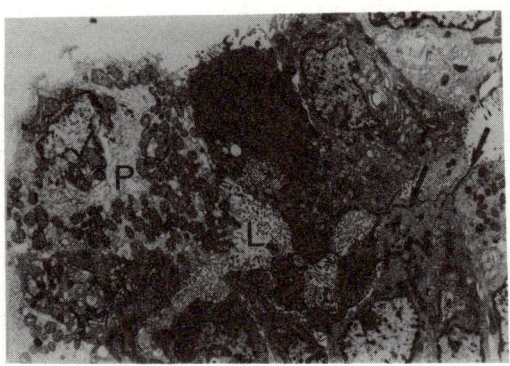

Fig. 3. Electron micrograph showing parietal cells (P) and other cell types in gastric glands isolated from the 5 day-old rat stomach. Note the good preservation of the glandular structure, including the lumen (L) and junctional complexes (at arrows). Magnification x 2000.

It is therefore likely that histamine might have a direct effect on gastric glands and may modulate their biological activities (proliferation/differentiation and function) from the neonatal period in rat. The final maturation of the H_2 receptor-dependent generating system in rat gastric glands was concomitant with dietary changes occuring after weaning at day 21 (Chérel, 1981). Similarly, maximal binding capacity of brain histamine receptors occured from 14 to 20 days post partum in the rat (Barbin, 1980; Subramanian, 1981).

CONCLUSION

Despite the intensive investigation on histamine H_2 receptors over the past 10 years, little is known about their structure and subcellular localization (Osband, 1979; Heitianu, 1982). The search of suitable agonist or antagonist reproducing all the pharmacological and biological properties of histamine stimulation or blockade would be expected for ligand binding study at physiological H_2 receptors.

REFERENCES

Ainge, G., and D. Poynter (1981). Scand. J. Gastroenterol., 16, 143-154
Albinus, M., and K. Fr. Sewing (1981). Agents and Actions, 11, 223-227
Anteunis, A., C. Gespach, A. Astésano, S. Emami, R. Robineaux, and G. Rosselin (1984). Peptides, 5, 277-283
Arrang, J.M., M. Garbarg, and J.C. Schwartz (1983). Nature, 302, 832-837
Ash, A.S.F., and H.O. Schild (1966). Br. J. Pharmacol., 27, 427-439
Ayalon, A., M.J. Sanders, L.P. Thomas, D.A. Amirian, and A.H. Soll (1982). Proc. Natl. Acad. Sci., USA, 79, 7009-7013
Barbezat, G.O., and M.I. Grossman (1971). Sciences, (N.Y.), 174, 422-424
Barbin, G., J.M. Palacios, E. Rodergas, J.C. Schwartz, and M. Garbarg (1980). Mol. Pharmacol., 18, 1-10
Barros D'sa, A.A.J., S.R. Bloom, and J.H. Barros (1975). The Lancet, 1, 886-887
Batzri, S. (1981a). Biochem. Pharmacol., 30, 3013-3016
Batzri, S. (1981b). Biochim. Biophys. Acta, 677, 521-524
Batzri, S., and J. Dyer (1981c). Biochim. Biophys. Acta, 675, 416-426
Batzri, S., J.W. Harmon, M.D. Walker, W.F. Thompson, and R. Toles (1982a). Biochim. Biophys. Acta, 720, 217-221
Batzri, S., J.W. Harmon, and M.D. Walker (1982b). Biochem. Biophys. Res. Commun., 108, 965-969
Batzri, S., J.W. Harmon, and W.F. Thompson (1982c). Mol. Pharmacol., 22, 33-40
Batzri, S., J.W. Harmon, J. Dyer, and W.F. Thompson (1982d). Mol. Pharmacol., 22, 41-47
Beaven, M.A., A.H. Soll, and K.J. Lewin (1982). Gastroenterology, 82, 254-262
Berglindh, T., and K.J. Obrink (1976a). Acta Physiol. Scand., 96, 150-159
Berglindh, T., H.F. Helander, and K.J. Obrink (1976b). Acta Physiol. Scand., 97, 401-414
Berglindh, T. (1977). Acta Physiol. Scand. 99, 75-84
Black, J.W., W.A.M. Duncan, C.J. Durant, C.R. Ganellin, and E.M. Parsons (1972). Nature, 236, 385-390
Boige, N., C. Dupont, B. Chenut, C. Gespach, and G. Rosselin (1984). Eur. J. Clin. Invest., 14, 42-48
Bunce, K.T., M. Grewal, and M.E. Parsons (1981). Br. J. Pharmacol. 73, 41-46
Busse, W.W., and J. Sosman (1977). J. Clin. Invest. 59, 1080-1087
Charbon, G.A., H.A.A. Brauwers, and A. Sala (1980). Naunyn-Schmiedeberg's Arch. Pharmacol., 312, 123-129
Chérel, Y., C. Gespach, and G. Rosselin (1981). C.R. Acad. Sci. Paris, 293, 201-206
Chew, C.S., S.J. Hersey, G. Sachs, and T. Berglindh (1980). Am. J. Physiol., 238, G312-G320
Chew, C.S. (1983). Am. J. Physiol., 245, G221-G229
Clyman, R.I., J.A. Sandler, V.C. Manganiello, and N. Vaughan (1975). J. Clin. Invest., 55, 1020-1025
Dozois, R.R., A. Wollin, R.D. Rettmann, and T.P. Dousa (1977). Am. J. Physiol., 232, E35-E38
Ducroc, R., J.F. Desjeux, B. Garzon, J.P. Onolfo, and J.P. Geloso (1981). Am. J. Physiol., 240, G206-G210
Dupont, C., C. Gespach, B. Chenut, and G. Rosselin (1980). FEBS Lett., 113, 25-28
Emami, S., C. Gespach, and G. Rosselin (1982). Gastrointestinal Hormones and Ulcer, 68th Annual Meeting of Japanese Society of Gastroenterology, Hiroshima,71
Emami, S., C. Gespach, C. Augeron, C. Laboisse, and G. Rosselin (1983a). Gut Peptides and Ulcer. In: A.Miyoshi (Ed), Biomedical Research Foundation, Tokyo, p. 64-72
Emami, S., C. Gespach, M.E. Forgue-Lafitte, Y. Broer, and G. Rosselin (1983b). Life Sci., 33, 415-423
Emami, S., C. Gespach, and H. Bodéré (1985). Agents and Actions, in the press
Fischer, D.Z., E. Meier, and D. Fitzpatrick (1981). Comp. Biochem. Physiol., 68C, 231-234
Gajtkowski, G.A., D.B. Norris, T.J. Rising, and T.P. Wood (1983). Nature, 304, 65-67

Garzon, B., R. Ducroq and J.P. Geloso (1982). J. Dev. Physiol., 4, 195-205
Gespach, C., C. Dupont, D. Bataille, and G. Rosselin (1980a). FEBS Lett., 114, 247-252
Gespach, C., D. Bataille, C. Dupont, G. Rosselin, E. Wünsch, and E. Jaeger (1980b). Biochim. Biophys. Acta, 630, 433-441
Gespach, C., C. Dupont, and G. Rosselin (1981). Experientia, 37, 866-867
Gespach, C., and J.P. Abita (1982a). Mol. Pharmacol., 21, 78-85
Gespach, C., F. Saal, H. Cost, and J.P. Abita (1982b). Mol. Pharmacol., 22, 547-553
Gespach, C., D. Bouhours, J.F. Bouhours, and G. Rosselin (1982c). FEBS Lett., 149, 85-90
Gespach, C., D. Bataille, M.C. Dutrilllaux, and G. Rosselin (1982d). Biochim. Biophys. Acta, 720, 7-16
Gespach, C., S. Emami, N. Boige, and G. Rosselin (1983a). Gut Peptides and ulcer, In: A. Miyoshi (Ed), Biomedical Research Foundation, Tokyo, p. 55-63
Gespach, C., D. Hui Bon Hoa, and G. Rosselin (1983b). Endocrinology, 112, 1597-1606
Gespach, C., I. Menez, and S. Emami (1983c). Biosci. Rep., 3, 871-878
Gespach, C., P. Mangeat, G. Marchis-Mouren and G. Rosselin (1983d). Gut Peptides and Ulcer, In: A. Miyoshi (Ed), Biomedical Research Foundation, Tokyo, p. 73-80
Gespach, C., S. Emami, and G. Rosselin (1984a). Biochem. Biophys. Res. Commun., 120, 641-649
Gespach, C., S. Emami, C. Boissard, and G. Rosselin (1984b). 7th International Congress of Endocrinology, July 1-7, Quebec, Canada, 618 (abstract)
Gespach, C., Y. Chérel, and G. Rosselin (1984c). Am. J. Physiol., 247, in the press
Grossman, M.I. (1967). Handbook of Physiology, In: C.F. Code and W. Heidel (Eds), vol. 2, Secretion, Washington, D.C., American Physiological Society, p. 835-863
Hakanson, R., B. Lilja, and Ch. Owman (1969). Histochemie, 18, 74-86
Hanssen, L.E., S. Skare, and K.F. Hanssen (1983). Hepato-Gastroenterol., 30, 73
Harvey, C.A., D.A.A. Owen, and K.D. Shaw (1980). Br. J. Pharmacol., 69, 21-27
Heltianu, C., M. Simionescu, and N. Simionescu (1982). J. Cell Biol., 93, 357-364
Hersey, S.J. (1981). Am. J. Physiol., 241, G93-G97
Hirschowitz, B.I., and G.A. Hutchison (1977). Am. J. Physiol., 233, E225-E228
Hirschowitz, B.I., J. Rentz, and E. Molina (1981). J. Pharmacol. Exp. Ther., 218 676-680
Ikezaki, M., and L.R. Johnson (1983). Am. J. Physiol., 244, G165-G170
Jacobs, D.M., and R.P. Sturtevant (1980). Cell Tissue Res., 211, 175-177
Jacobs, D.M., and R.P. Sturtevant (1982). The Anatomical Record, 203, 101-113
Kasbekar, D.K., H.A. Ridley, and J.G. Forte (1969). Am. J. Physiol., 216, 961-967
Katsumata, Y., and K. Yagi (1976). Biochem. Pharmacol., 25, 603-604
Koelz, H.R., S.J. Hersey, G. Sachs, and C.S. Chew (1982). Am. J. Physiol., 243 G218-G225
Konturek, S.J., T. Radecki, T. Demitresc,u and A. Dembinski (1974). Digestion, 10, 267-281
Koo, A. (1983). Br. J. Pharmacol., 78, 181-189
Kulkarni, P.G., F.M. Hoffman, and R.L. Shoemaker (1979). Am. J. Physiol., 236 E784-E787
Laboisse, C.L., C. Augeron, M.H. Couturier-Turpin, C. Gespach, A.M. Chéret, and F. Potet (1982). Canc. Res., 42, 1541-1548
Larsson, L.I., J. Fahrenkrug, A. Schaffalitzky de Muckadell, F. Sundler, R. Hankanson, and J.F. Rehfeld (1976). Proc. Natl. Acad. Sci. USA, 73, 3197-3200
Larsson, L.I., N. Galtermann, L. De Magistris, J.F. Rehfeld, and T.W. Schwartz (1979). Science, 205, 1393-1395
Lemmi, C.A.E. (1984). Agents and Actions, 14, 185-194
Lewin, M.J.M., F. Grelac, A.M. Chéret, E. René, and S. Bonfils (1979). Hormone Receptors in Digestion and Nutrition, In: G. Rosselin, P. Fromageot, S. Bonfils (Eds), Elsevier Biomedical Press, Amsterdam, p. 383-390
Logsdon, C.D., and T.E. Machen (1982). The Anatomical Record, 202, 73-83
Lorenz, W., A. Schauer, St Heitland, R. Calvoer, and E. Werle (1969). Naunyn-Schmiedebergs Arch. Pharmak.,265, 81-100

Major, J.J., and P. Scholes (1978). **Agents and Actions, 8**, 324-331
Mangeat, P., C. Gespach, G. Marchis-Mouren, and G. Rosselin (1982). **Regul. Peptides, 3**, 155-168
Menez, I., C. Gespach, S. Emami, and G. Rosselin (1983). **Biochem. Biophys. Res. Commun., 116**, 251-257
Nagata, H., and P.H. Guth (1983). **Am. J. Physiol., 245**, G 201-G207
Osband, M., and R. Mc Caffrey (1979). **J. Biol. Chem., 259**, 9970-9972
Perrier, C.V., and L. Laster (1970). **J. Clin. Invest., 49**, 73a
Polak, J.M., A.G.E. Pearse, L. Grimelius, S.R. Bloom, and A. Arimura (1975). **The Lancet, 1**, 1220-1222
Popielski, L. (1920). **Pfuegers Arch., 178**, 214-236
Quach, T.T., A.M. Duchemin, C. Rose, and J.C. Schwartz (1981). **Mol. Pharmacol. 20**, 331-338
Reyl, F., and M.J. Lewin (1981). **Biochim. Biophys. Acta, 675**, 297-300
Robert, A., J.E. Nezamis, and J.P. Philips (1967). **Am. J. Dig. Dis., 12**, 1073-1076
Rosa, F. (1963). **Gastroenterology, 45**, 354-363
Rosenfeld, G.C., S.J. Strada, E.J. Dial, C.F. Bearer, and W.J. Thompson (1980). **Adv. Cyclic Nucleotide Res., 12**, 255-266
Ruoff, H.J., M. Becker, B. Painz, M. Rack, K. Fr. Sewing, and H. Malchow (1979). **Eur. J. Clin. Pharmacol.,15**, 147-151
Ruoff, H.J., and W. Schepp (1984). European Histamine Research Society, Florence, 13th Meeting, 114 (abstract)
Rutten, M.J., and T.E. Machen (1981). **Gastroenterology, 80**, 928-936
Salenius, P. (1962). **Acta Anat., 50**, 1-76
Salganik, R.I., R.I. Bersimbaev, S.V. Argutinskaya, E.V. Kiseleva, N.B. Kristo-lvubova, and V.I. Deribas (1976). **Mol. Cell Biochem., 12**, 181-191
Salvati, P., and B.J.R. Whittle (1983). **Eur. J. Pharmacol., 89**, 63-68
Savany, A., and L. Cronenberger (1982). **Eur. J. Biochem., 123**, 593-599
Scholes, P., A. Cooper, D. Jones, J. Major, M. Walters, and C. Wilde (1976). **Agents and Actions, 6**, 677-682
Schultz, G., J.G. Hardman, K. Schultz, C.E. Baird, and E.W. Sutherland (1973). **Proc. Natl. Acad. Sci. USA, 70**, 3889-3893
Schusdziarra, V., D. Rouiller, V. Harris, and R.H. Unger (1981) **Regul. Peptides, 2**,353-363
Shapiro, B., K. Pienta, A. Heldsinger, and A.I. Vinik (1981). **Endocrinology, 105**, 1117-1121
Soll, A.H. (1978). **J. Clin. Invest., 61**, 381-389
Soll, A.H., and A. Wollin (1979a). **Am. J. Physiol., 237**, E444-E450
Soll, A.H., K. Lewin, and M.E. Beaven (1979b). **Gastroenterology, 77**, 1283-1290
Soll, A.H. (1980). **J. Clin. Invest., 65**, 1222-1229
Soll, A.H., K.J. Lewin, and M.A. Beaven (1981). **Gastroenterology, 80**, 717-727
Sonnenberg, A., W. Kunziker, H.R. Koelz, J.A. Fischer, and A.L. Blum (1978). **Acta Physiol. Scand., special suppl.**, 307-317
Speir, G.R., K. Takeuchi, W. Peitsch, and L.R. Johnson (1982). **Am. J. Physiol., 242**, G243-G249
Stables, R., M.J. Daly, and J.M. Humphray (1983). **Agents and Actions, 13**, 166-169
Subramanian, N., W.L. Whitmore, F.J. Seidler, and T.A. Slotkin (1981). **J. Neurochem., 36**, 1137-1141
Tepperman, B.L., E.D. Jacobson, and G.C. Rosenfeld (1979). **Life Sci., 24**, 2301-2308
Thunberg, R. (1967). **Exp. Cell Res., 47**, 108-115
Vatier, J., J.C. Robert, Ch. Poitevin, M.T. Vitré, M. Bourgeois, D. Vauché, and S. Bonfils (1982). **Gastroenterol. Clin. Biol., 6**, 617-622
Warrander, S.E., D.B., Norris, T.J. Rising, and T.P. Wood (1983). **Life Sci., 33**, 1119-1126
Wollin, A., L.D. Barnes, Y.S. Hui, and T.P. Dousa (1975). **Life Sci., 17**, 1303-1306

STIMULUS-SECRETION COUPLING IN THE PARIETAL CELL

K.-Fr. Sewing and W. Beil

Abteilung Allgemeine Pharmakologie, Medizinische
Hochschule Hannover, 3000 Hannover 61, Federal Republic
of Germany

ABSTRACT

In guinea pig isolated and enriched parietal cells in the absence of a phosphodiesterase inhibitor histamine failed to produce an accumulation of cyclic AMP and a protein kinase activation in concentrations which stimulate H^+ secretion. Only very high intracellular cyclic AMP concentrations are capable of stimulating H^+ secretion. The data suggest an alternative pathway for histamine stimulus-secretion coupling in the parietal cell. Calcium can be excluded since it inhibits K^+/H^+-ATPase in low concentrations.

KEYWORDS

Guinea pig; parietal cell; histamine; cyclic AMP; protein kinase; K^+/H^+-ATPase.

INTRODUCTION

It is well known that when the parietal cell histamine H_2-receptor gets stimulated by an adequate agonist, the K^+/H^+-ATPase in the tubulovesicular membrane starts pumping H^+ into the gastric lumen. Such a mechanism functions in the intact gastric mucosa and in isolated gastric glands or parietal cells. The conventional view how under these circumstances stimulus-secretion coupling functions and how it is usually described in review articles can be summarized as follows: exposure of a parietal cell to histamine or a histamine H_2-receptor agonist allows the affectors to bind to the histamine H_2-receptor localized at the parietal cell basolateral membrane. To the receptor an adenylate cyclase (AC) is attached which gets activated in response to reaction of the affector with the receptor. The AC in the activated state converts adenosine triphosphate (ATP) into cyclic AMP leading to an intracellular accumulation of cyclic AMP. The target for cyclic AMP is a cyclic AMP-dependent protein kinase (PK) of which - at least in other cells - one part is membrane bound and another part is soluble. In response to cyclic AMP the PK transfers phosphate from ATP to other proteins. The sequence of events which then stimulate the proton pump to secret H^+ into the gastric lumen is virtually unknown except that the pump requires a high K^+ (at least in vitro). Such a picture as complete as possible was constructed from experiments in which the whole mucosa was used or from isolated

systems in the presence of phosphodiesterase (PDE) inhibitors such as isobutyl-methylxanthine (IBMX) in order to block the enzyme which breaks down cyclic AMP to 5'-AMP. In either case the experimental design might not be quite adequate to answer the question whether or not the AC-cyclic AMP-PK system is the main pathway for histamine to stimulate H^+ secretion in the parietal cell:
1. When the whole gastric mucosa is used it cannot be decided whether any changes in cyclic AMP have to be attributed to parietal or other cells. 2. When the experiments are carried out during PDE inhibition cyclic AMP levels measured might not be representative for the processes going on under physiological conditions. Therefore a complete analysis is required which includes the complete chain of events after cellular exposure to histamine.

EXPERIMENTAL DESIGN

Guinea pig gastric mucosal cells were isolated and enriched according to Soll (1978) with the modifications used in our laboratory (Sewing et al., 1983). The cells were isolated by collagenase and pronase digestion and enriched in the Beckman elutriater system. All measurements were done on parietal cell populations (appr. 60 - 70 % pure) and on mucous cell populations (appr. 95 % pure). AC measurements were made in a cell homogenate under optimal enzyme conditions by cyclic AMP determinations in the presence of 0.1 mmol/l IBMX for PDE inhibition.
Cellular cyclic AMP in response to histamine exposure was measured in the absence and presence of 0.1 mmol/l IBMX by the Gilman assay or a radioimmunoassay.
PDE was determined by Bauer and Schwabe (1980). The procedure consists of a two-step reaction in which radioactive cyclic AMP is hydrolysed to radioactive 5'-AMP which is further broken down by a 5'-nucleotidase to radioactive adenosine (which is measured) and inorganic phosphate.
PK in response to cellular exposure to histamine was measured in a 20000 x g supernatant of a solubilized homogenate by determining the incorporation of radioactive phosphate into histone in the absence and presence of 5 µmol/l cyclic AMP. H^+ secretion of the parietal cell population (which is referred to in the discussion) was measured by Berglindh's ^{14}C-aminopyrine uptake and accumulation procedure as described by Sewing et al. (1983).

RESULTS

In both cell populations histamine stimulated adenylate cyclase activity in a concentration dependent manner. Maximal stimulation was much greater in parietal cell populations then in mucous cell populations (Fig. 1).
The difference between parietal cell and mucous cell populations was much less pronounced when the enzyme activity was related to protein instead of cell number. In spite of the marked difference in AC activity between parietal cell populations and mucous cell populations exposure of the intact cells to histamine produced a totally different effect: without PDE inhibition the maximal cyclic AMP response was greater in mucous cell populations than in parietal cell populations (Fig. 2). Taking into account the contamination of the parietal cell populations with mucous cells all increase in cyclic AMP has to be attributed to the mucous cells in the parietal cell population. In the presence of 0.1 mmol/l IBMX in both cell populations an increase in cyclic AMP concentration in response to histamine can be found.
The discrepancy between a high AC activity and the lack of an increase in cellular cyclic AMP concentration finds its explanation in PDE activities which are much higher in parietal cell populations than in mucous cell populations (Fig. 3).
In the absence of IBMX exposure of the parietal cell populations to histamine up to 10^{-3} mol/l failed to alter the PK activity ratio (activity without cyclic AMP/activity with 5 µmol/l cyclic AMP) significantly. In mucous cell populations, however, histamine stimulated the PK activitiy significantly in concentrations > 10 µmol/l. Even in the presence of 0.1 mmol/l IBMX there was only a very small histamine effect in the parietal cell populations, but the histamine effect in

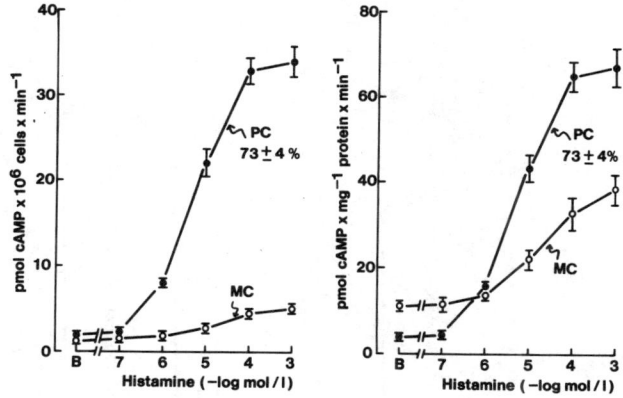

Fig. 1. Effect of histamine on guinea pig parietal cell (PC) and mucous cell (MC) adenylate cyclase. left: related to cell number, right: related to protein.

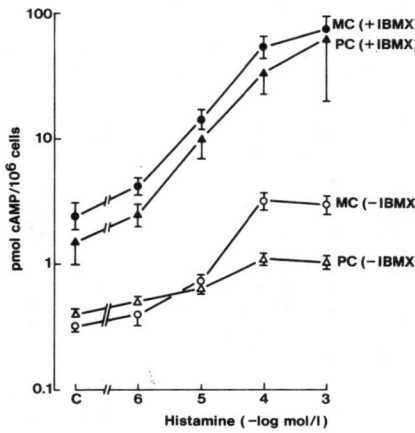

Fig. 2. Effect of histamine on parietal cell (PC) and mucous cell (MC) cyclic AMP in the absence (open symbols) and presence (filled symbols) of 0.1 mmol/l IBMX.

mucous cell populations was enhanced over the whole concentration response curve (Fig. 4).

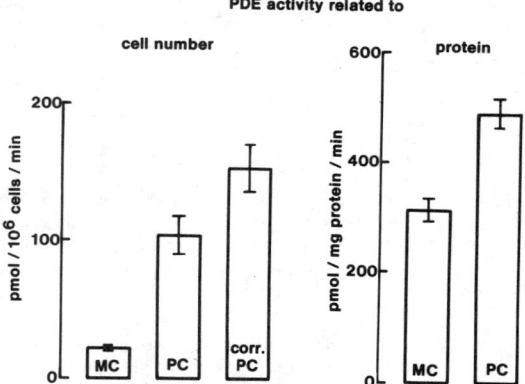

Fig. 3. PDE activity of parietal cells (PC) and mucous cells (MC), related to cell number (left) and protein (right). The columns labelled "corr." represent the parietal cell values corrected for mucous cell contamination.

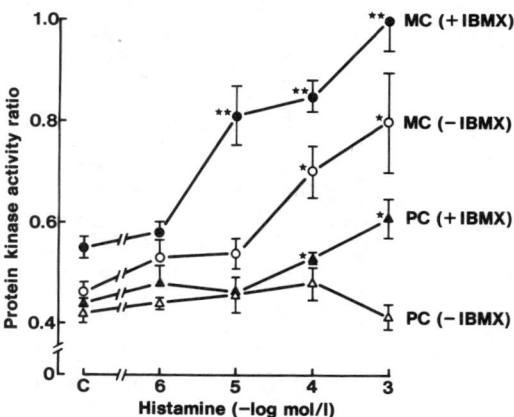

Fig. 4. Effect of histamine on PK activity ratio of guinea pig parietal cells (triangles) and mucous cells (circles) in the absence (open symbols) and presence (filled symbols) of 0.1 mmol/l IBMX. * $p < 0.05$, ** $p < 0.01$.

DISCUSSION

These data are not quite compatible with the views outlined in the introduction since the failure of histamine to increase parietal cell cyclic AMP and consequently to activate the PK points towards another mechanism of stimulus-secretion coupling at least in the guinea pig parietal cell. From studies with dibutyryl-cyclic-AMP (Sewing et al., to be published) it is known that an increase in intracellular cyclic AMP can lead to H^+ secretion but that requires threshold concentrations in the range of 50 pmol cyclic AMP per 10^6 cells. Such a concentration is hardly reached by histamine in the presence of a PDE inhibitor. A PDE inhibitor, however, was used in those studies on which the view is based, that histamine acts via cyclic AMP (Sonnenberg et al., 1978; Soll and Wollin, 1979). Studies in other species comparable to that reported here have not been done so that the question has to be left open whether this is a specific feature of guinea pigs.
It is totally unknown which alternative has to be taken into consideration. Calcium can be excluded since it has been shown to inhibit partially purified K^+/H^+-ATPase in a concentration dependent manner (Beil and Sewing, 1984). One would have to search for a mechanism that enhances the concentration of K^+ close to the proton pump for temporary stimulation or for an inhibitory mechanism that blocks the access of K^+ to the enzyme during the resting period.

ACKNOWLEDGEMENT

The studies were supported by grants from the BMFT and the Gesellschaft der Freunde der Medizinischen Hochschule Hannover.

REFERENCES

1. Bauer, A.C., and U. Schwabe (1980). Naunyn-Schmiedeberg's Arch. Pharmacol., 311, 193-198.
2. Beil, W., and K.-Fr. Sewing (1984). Br. J. Pharmacol., 82, 651-657.
3. Lowry, O.H., N.J. Rosebrough, A.L. Farr, and R.J. Randall (1951). J. biol. Chem., 193, 265-275.
4. Sewing, K.-Fr., P. Harms, G. Schulz, and H. Hannemann (1983). Gut, 24, 557-560.
5. Soll, A.H. (1978). J. clin. Invest., 61, 370-380.
6. Soll, A.H., and A. Wollin (1979). Am. J. Physiol., 237, E444-450.
7. Sonnenberg, A., W. Hunziker, H.R. Koelz, J.A. Fischer and A.L. Blum (1978). Acta physiol. scand., special suppl., 307-317.

HISTAMINE ACTION IN ISOLATED GASTRIC GLANDS AND ITS INTERACTION WITH METABOLICALLY ACTIVE SUBSTANCES

O. Nylander and K. J. Öbrink

Department of Physiology and Medical Biophysics
Biomedical Center, Uppsala University, Box 572,
S-751 23 Uppsala, Sweden

ABSTRACT

By using isolated gastric glands from rabbit it is possible to distinguish between effects on histamine release and its subsequent action on the parietal cells. Somatostatin inhibits both, but prostaglandins, especially E_1, E_2 and $16,16$-$dMeE_2$, stimulate the histamine release while they inhibit the parietal cell response. The net result from prostaglandins on an intact gastric mucosa may thus be a complicated balance between the two counteracting effects.

KEYWORDS

Histamine; Somatostatin; Prostaglandins; Isolated gastric glands; Stimulating mechanisms.

INTRODUCTION

Ever since Komarow in 1938 conclusively demonstrated that histamine and gastrin were two separate stimulants of gastric acid secretion, the physiological role of histamine has been widely discussed. The literature is wast and there are lots of reviews on the topic (e.g. Code, 1965; Wraton, 1971; Kahlson and others, 1973; Lin, 1974; Berglindh and Öbrink, 1977). Some have considered histamine as a normal physiological link in the stimulation chain whereas others have denied any such role. When it was found that the classical antihistamines did not inhibit the gastric secretion it was taken as evidence against histamine as a physiological stimulant. On the other hand when the H_2-receptor antagonists showed a potent inhibitory action it was likewise taken as a pro-histamine evidence. But still there were observations that were not in agreement with the idea of histamine as a normal physiological stimulator, (Johnsson, 1971).

HISTAMINE AS A LINK IN THE STIMULATING CHAIN

It has repeatedly been shown that histamine is present in the gastric mucosa. It appears in the gastric juice as well as in the mucosal tissue upon stimulation. But this does not prove that histamine is a mediator for secretion. It could equally well be nothing but a byproduct in the stimulation process and not itself a stimulatory link between gastrin and parietal cell secretion. Up till some years ago there was no way to differentiate between these two possibilities, the appearance of histamine in the stomach as a byproduct or as a physiological stimulator. This has been possible only with the use of isolated gastric glands.

Isolated Gastric Glands

In 1976 Berglindh and Öbrink published a report on the preparation of isolated gastric glands from the rabbit stomach. The technique, which was described in detail in their report, consists briefly of the following steps: the stomach of an anaesthetized rabbit is perfused by a retrograde injection of a warm phosphate buffer solution in the abdominal aorta at a very high pressure so as to break the capillary walls and cause a profound edema in the mucosa. This causes a mechanical separation of the gastric glands. The mucosa is removed and minced into small pieces and digested in a collagenase solution. Glands containing all the cells up to the bottom of the gastric crypts are obtained. Thus they do not contain any surface epithelial cells, nor do they contain any typical mast cells or other cells outside the gastric gland proper. Even the basilar membrane seems to be removed. They contain parietal cells, peptic cells and at least four types of endocrine cells.

Parietal cell activity in the isolated glands can only be determined indirectly in three different ways: increase in oxygen consumption; accumulation of a weak base (aminopyrine); a morphological transformation of the cells from a resting to a secreting state (Berglindh, Helander and Öbrink, 1976).

Histamine was determined according to methods descibed in the work of Bergqvist and Öbrink (1979).

Sequential Stimulation not Possible in Isolated Glands

The isolated glands are used in a suspension of Ringer's solution. In such a system a possibly normally existing sequential stimulation system can not work for the following reason: If gastrin should act on one of the endocrine cell types by liberating histamine, and if this histamine normally should act on receptors on the parietal cells, it would be necessary that the histamine reached the parietal cells in a sufficiently high concentration so as to stimulate to acid secretion. In an intact mucosa the histamine would be liberated into very narrow spaces between the glands and reach high concentrations. In a suspension of isolated glands, on the other hand, the liberated histamine would be diluted in an ocean of liquid, thus decreasing to concentrations below the threshold value for acid stimulation. This hypothesis has been thoroughly investigated (Bergqvist and Öbrink, 1976; Öbrink, 1982).

The gastric glands respond to histamine in the usual dose effect fashion (Berglindh and Öbrink, 1976). The ED-50 is around 3×10^{-6} M and the threshold value lies around 10^{-7} M. The glands do not, however, respond to pentagastrin. Analyses of histamine in the suspending medium before and after addition of different concentrations of pentagastrin showed, however, a dose-dependent liberation of histamine (Bergqvist and Öbrink, 1979), but the concentration only reached levels around 10^{-7} M. As this was the threshold region for stimulation of the parietal cells, consequently one could not expect any effect of pentagastrin on these cells due to histamine contribution. However, the sensitivity to histamine could be greatly increased, by the administration of a potent phosphodiesterase inhibitor and then this low histamine concentration was sufficient for a detectable acid response and therefore for a stimulatory effect of pentagastrin. Moreover this effect was effectively blocked by H_2-receptor antagonists. Thus it seemed quite clear that histamine did in fact act as a link between pentagastrin and acid secretion. The question whether or not gastrin also has receptors on the parietal cells is not settled. There are lots of evidence for (Soll, 1978), but in our system such receptors apparently lack the power to initiate acid secretion.

The source of the histamine in the gastric glands is not known. The usual type of mast cells seems to be absent, but as mentioned above there are at least four different types of endocrine cells that may be responsible and some are morphologically situated very close to the parietal cells and as such being candidates for the histamine liberation function (Bergqvist and others, 1980; Öbrink, 1982). The histamine content of the isolated glands is in the order of 0.4 nmoles/mg dry weight and for a maximal dose of pentagastrin roughly 5 to 15 % is released into the suspending fluid (Bergqvist and others, 1980). So far nobody has tried to exhaust the histamine content of the gastric glands and as there are small amounts of histidine decarboxylase present (Bergqvist and others, 1980) one could imagine that histamine is formed parallel to its liberation.

INTERFERENCE AT DIFFERENT STAGES IN A SEQUENTIAL STIMULATION

It now seems to be quite evident that the initiation of acid secretion is due to a stimulation chain composed of: 1) liberation of gastrin, which may take place due to vagal stimulation, chemical stimulation or distension of the antrum, followed by 2) a histamine liberation from some cells in the gastric glands and lastly 3) an effect via H_2-receptors on the parietal cells. Interfereing substances like stimulators or inhibitors of gastric acid secretion can then of course act on all these different links. We will mention a few:

Acetylcholine or carbachol has been shown to liberate histamine. The amount liberated after carbachol is similar to that after pentagastrin and can be blocked by atropin (Bergqvist and others, 1980). Acetylcholine or carbachol induces a transient increase in parietal cell activity in the rabbit gastric glands, thus indicating the presence of cholinergic receptors on the parietal cells. In the presence of low concentrations of histamine or phosphodiesterase inhibitors, the response to acetylcholine is sustained and potentiated, indicating that histamine might be involved in the stimulation of the parietal cells by acetylcholine.

Other substances interfere with the effect of histamine. For example the histamine H_2-receptor antagonists compete with the histamine itself on the parietal cells. Therefore H_2-receptor blockers have become extremely important for decreasing gastric acid secretion in ulcer patients or for eliminating the effects of histamine in the Zollinger-Ellison syndrom.

At the step beyond the histamine receptor level we have the cAMP-system. It has been shown that histamine stimulated parietal cell activity is closely associated with a marked increase in glandular cAMP (Chew, 1980). This system can be interferred with by phosphodiesterase inhibitors like isobutyl-methyl-xanthine (IMX), thus resulting in an increased effect of histamine.

Of course there are several other possibilities to interfere by metabolic inhibitors or by the specific inhibitor of the K^+/H^+-ATPase in the parietal cells (Fellenius and others, 1980).

EFFECTS OF SOMATOSTATIN AND PROSTANOIDS

When using isolated gastric glands we have the unique possibility to distinguish between: 1) actions on the histamine liberation and 2) interferences with the parietal cell activity. We will now summarize some of our findings with this model. Two groups of substances have been especially investigated in this respect namely somatostatin and prostaglandins-prostacyclin.

Effects on Histamine Liberation

We have earlier reported from this laboratory (Öbrink and others, 1984) that gastric acid inhibitors like secretin or vasopressin do not influence the histamine release elicited by pentagastrin. In a recent study (Takeuchi and others, 1982) it was reported that prostaglandins at high concentrations (more than 10^{-6} M) stimulated to acid secretion in the amphibian gastric mucosa. This stimulation was abolished by the H_2-receptor blocker methiamide or by pretreatment with 48/80. The authors suggested that high concentrations of prostaglandins (more then 10^{-6} M) might stimulate the release of endogenous histamine. We therefore undertook the investigation to see whether prostaglandins by itself could influence the histamine release. In fact we found that PGE_1 and PGE_2 both stimulate the release of histamine, Fig. 1. This happened even for low concentrations and there is no breaking point at concentrations of around 10^{-6} M. As the prostaglandins do inhibit the effect of histamine on the parietal cells, as has been previously shown (Nylander and others, 1984; Soll, 1980) and will be further documented below, we are dealing with two effects of prostaglandins opposing each other, first a concentration depending release of endogenous histamine and secondly an interference with the histamine action on the parietal cells causing a reduction in acid secretion response. It is thus quite possible that at concentrations of prostaglandins of around 10^{-6} the stimulatory effect due to histamine release will start to dominate over the inhibitory action on the parietal cell activity. In recent studies (Bergqvist and others, 1984)

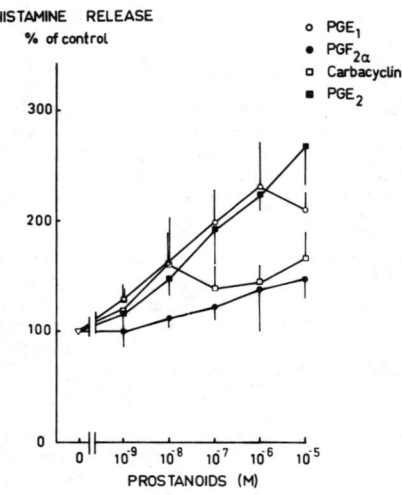

Fig. 1. The effects of prostaglandins E_1, E_2, $F_{2\alpha}$ and carbacyclin on glandular histamine release, expressed as % of control. 100 % corresponds to $0.37 \pm 0.09 \times 10^{-7}$ M histamine per 3 mg dry weight/ml. Values represent mean ± S.E.M. n = 4.

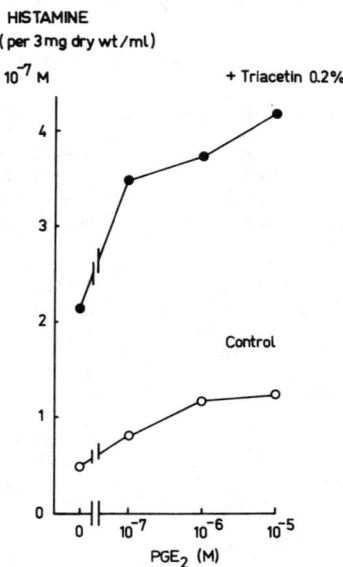

Fig. 2. Dose dependent increase of histamine release by PGE_2 alone and in combination with triacetin 0.2 %. Values are the mean of 2 experiments.

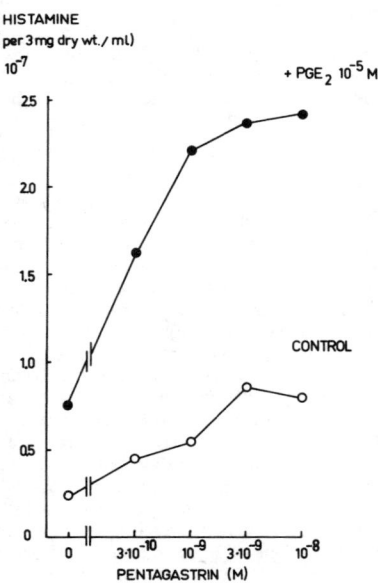

Fig. 3. A typical experiment demonstrating a dose dependent stimulation of histamine release by pentagastrin alone and in combination with PGE_2 (10^{-5} M).

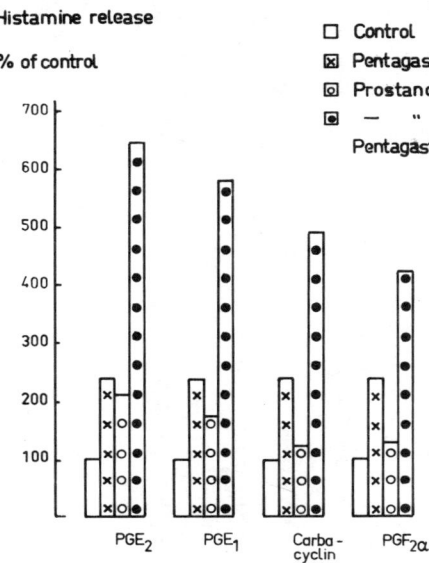

Fig. 4. Effects of pentagastrin (3×10^{-9} M), prostanoids (10^{-5} M) and their combination on histamine release expressed as % of control. Values represent the mean of 2 experiments.

we have in some detail investigated these events in our laboratory.

Prostaglandin F_2 and carbacyclin (a stabil prostacyclin analogue obtained as a kind gift from B.J.R. Whittle, Wellcome Research laboratories, UK) were also able to release histamine in the same way as PGE_1 and PGE_2 although to a somewhat lower degree (Fig. 1). 16,16-dMePGE$_2$ (a kind gift from the Upjohn Co.) exhibited the same histamine releasing property as PGE_2 (not shown in the figure) but in some preparations it was dissolved in triacetin and not in ethanol, and then the release of histamine was strongly augmented. It was then found that triacetin alone was a potent stimulant of histamine release (which 0.1 % ethanol is not). To further test this effect, triacetin at a final concentration of 0.2 % (v/v) was added to PGE_2 and the histamine release analyzed. As can be seen in Fig. 2 the PGE_2 effect was increased about 4 times. The mechanism is not clear but an additive effect of the triacetin seems to be excluded.

PGE_2 at high concentration (10^{-5} M) was added to gastric glands that were given different doses of pentagastrin, and the histamine release analyzed. Figure 3 shows a clear potentiation. Similar effects were obtained with PGE_1, $PGF_{2\alpha}$ and carbacyclin (Fig. 4).

Somatostatin was the only non cholinergic gastric acid inhibitor, that we have tried, that acted inhibitory on the histamine release. After pentagastrin stimulation an inhibition of this stimulation release up to 70-75% was obtained. See Fig. 5. This maximal inhibiton occurred at a concentraion of somatostatin of 10^{-8} M (Bergqvist and others, 1984; Öbrink and others, 1984). The effect of somatostatin on the augmented histamine release after pentagastrin-prostaglandin administration was likewise inhibited by somatostatin, Fig. 6, but it seemed more difficult to inhibit the 16,16-dimethyl PGE_2 (triacetin) induced histamine release with somatostatin.

Because of the special property of the isolated gastric glands to be rather insensitive to sequential stimulation we could not repeat the experiments of Silen and his group (Takeuchi and others, 1982) that prostaglandins at high concentrations stimulate to gastric secretion. We could only confirm their suggestions that prostaglandins do liberate histamine.

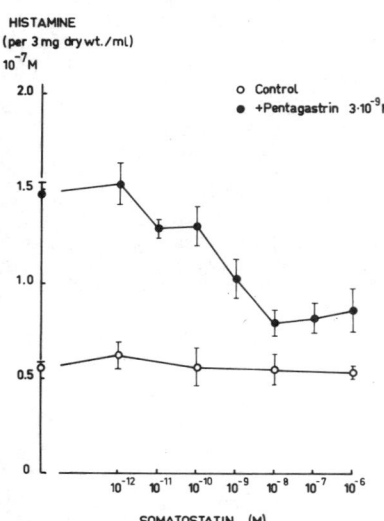

Fig. 5. Effects of somatostatin on basal and pentagastrin (3×10^{-9} M) stimulated histamine release. Values represent the mean ± S.E.M. of 3 experiments.

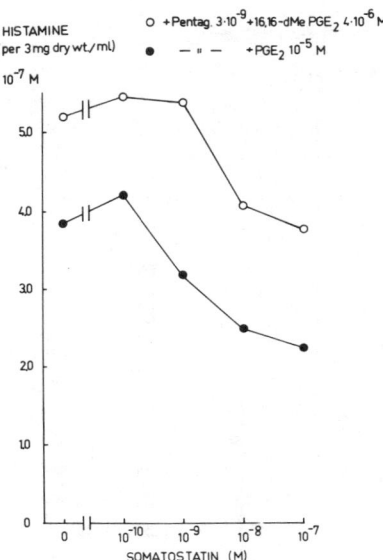

Fig. 6. Dose dependent inhibition by somatostatin of the histamine release stimulated by pentagastrin (3×10^{-9} M) and PGE_2 (10^{-5} M) or pentagastrin (3×10^{-9} M) and 16.16-dMePGE$_2$ (4×10^{-6} M). 16,16-dMePGE$_2$ contained triacetin at a concentration of 0.08 % (v/v). Values represent the mean of 2 experiments.

Effects on the Parietal Cell Activity

The second step that is possible to investigate with isolated gastric glands is the effect on the parietal cells. It has already been reported that somatostatin has a pronounced inhibitory effect on the histamine induced activity, but not on the cAMP stimulated one (Chew, 1983; Öbrink and others, 1984). Thus it was concluded that the somatostatin action took place somewhere at the adenylate cyclase level.

The effects of prostaglandins and prostacyclin have now been analyzed both on unstimulated and on histamine stimulated glands. Figure 7 shows the lack of effects of some prostanoids on the aminopyrine accumulation. Only 16,16-dMePGE$_2$ in triacetin indicates a stimulation at a concentration of 4×10^{-6} M but the effect was very poorly significant.

The effects on the histamine stimulated parietal cell activity by 16,16-dMePGE$_2$ and the cyclooxygenase inhibitor indomethacin are shown in Fig. 8, where it is clearly demonstrated that 16,16-dMePGE$_2$ inhibits and indomethacin stimulates the secretory acivity, in this case augmented by the phosphodiesterase inhibitor IMX.

It was suggested above that there could be a balance between the capacity of the prostaglandins to liberate histamine and their inhibitory action on the parietal cells. Figure 8 corroborates this view, 16,16-dMePGE$_2$ at 10^{-7} M makes a histamine concentration of more that 10^{-6} M necessary for a parietal cell response. Conversely the sensitivity of the cells will be markedly increased if the prostaglandin synthesis is inhibited.

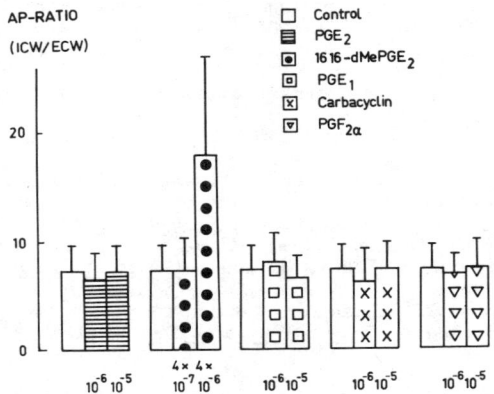

Fig. 7. The effects of different prostanoids at 2 various concentrations on basal AP-accumulation expressed as the ratio of ^{14}C-labelled aminopyrine in intracellular water to extracellular water. Mean ± S.E.M. of 3 experiments.

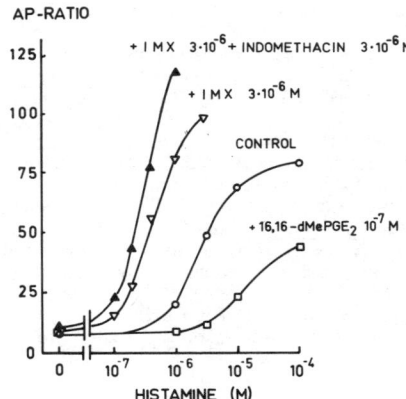

Fig. 8. Typical effects of isobutyl-methyl xanthine, IMX, (3×10^{-6} M) indomethacin (3×10^{-6} M), IMX and indomethacin combined and 16,16-dMePGE$_2$ (10^{-7} M) on histamine stimulated AP-accumulation.

CONCLUSION

The prostanoids have two opposing effects on the gastric glands: 1) They release histamine but 2) they inhibit the action of histamine on the parietal cells.

REFERENCES

Berglindh, T., H.F. Helander, and K.J. Öbrink (1976). Effects of secretagogues on oxygen consumption, aminopyrine accumulation and morphology in isolated gastric glands. Acta physiol. scand., 97, 401-414.

Berglindh, T. and K.J. Öbrink (1976). A method for preparing isolated glands from the rabbit gastric mucosa. Acta physiol. scand., 96, 150-159.

Bergqvist, E., O. Nylander, and K.J. Öbrink (1984). Dual effects of the inhibitory action of somatostatin on isolated gastric glands. (To be published).

Bergqvist, E. and K.J. Öbrink (1979). Gastrin-histamine as a normal sequence in gastric acid stimulation in the rabbit. Upsala J. Med. Sci., 84, 145-154.

Bergqvist, E., M.Waller, L. Hammar, and K.J. Öbrink (1980). Histamine as the secretory mediator in isolated gastric glands. In I. Schulz and others (Eds), Hydrogen ion transport in epithelia, Elsevier/North Holland Biomedical Press, Amsterdam. pp. 429-437

Chew, C.S.(1983). Inhibitory action of somatostatin on isolated gastric glands and parietal cells. Am. J. Physiol., 245, G221-229.

Chew, C.S., S.J. Hersey, G. Sachs, and T. Berglindh (1980). Histamine responsiveness of isolated gastric glands. Am. J. Physiol., 238, G312-320.

Code, C.F. (1965). Histamine and gastric secretion: a later look, 1955-1965. Fed. Proc., 24, 1311-1333.

Fellenius, E., T. Berglindh, A. Brändström, B. Elander, H.F. Helander, L. Olbe, G. Sachs, S.-E. Sjöstrand, and B. Wallmark (1980). The inhibitory action of sustituted benzimidazoles on isolated oxyntic glands and H^+/K^+-ATPase. In I. Schulz and others (Eds), Hydrogen ion transport in epithelia, Elsevier/North Holland Biomedical Press, Amsterdam. pp. 193-202.

Johnson, L.R. (1971). Control of gastric secretion: no room for histamine? Gastroenterology, 61, 106-118.

Kahlson, G., E. Rosengren, and S.E. Svensson (1973). Histamine and gastric secretion with special reference to the rat. In P. Holton (Ed.) Int. Encycl. Pharmacol. Ther., Sect. 39(a), Vol. 1. Pergamon Press, Oxford. pp. 41-102.

Komarov, S.A. (1938). Gastrin. Proc. Soc. Exptl. Biol. Med., 38, 514-516.

Lin, T.M. (1974). Possible relation of gastrin and histamine receptors in gastric hydrochloric acid secretion. Med. Clin. N. Am., 58, 1247-1275.

Nylander, O., E. Bergqvist, and K.J. Öbrink (1984). Endogenous prostaglandins modulate stimulation of acid formation in isolated gastric glands. In A. Allen and others (Eds), Mechanisms of mucosal protection in the upper gastrointestinal tract, Raven Press, New York. pp. 97-101.

Öbrink, K.J. (1982). Formation and liberation of histamine in isolated gastric glands and its function as a mediator to acid stimulation. In B. Uvnäs and K. Tasaka (Eds), Advances in the Biosciences, Vol. 33, "Advances in histamine research". Pergamon Press, Oxford and New York. pp. 167-176.

Öbrink, K.J., E. Bergqvist, and O. Nylander (1984). Mode of action by some acid secretion inhibitors on the stimulating mechanism in gastric epithelial cells. In J.G. Forte and F.C. Rector (Eds), Hydrogen ion transport. John Wiley & Sons, Inc. Publishers, (In press).

Soll, A.H. (1978). The interaction of histamine with gastrin and carbamylcholine on oxygen uptake by isolated mammalian parietal cells. J. Clin. Invest., 61, 381-389.

Soll, A.H. (1980). Specific inhibition by prostaglandins E_2 and I_2 of histamine-stimulated ^{14}C-aminopyrine accumulation and cyclic adenosine monophosphate generation by isolated canine parietal cells. J. Clin. Invest., 65, 1222-1229.

Takeuchi, K., K. Svanes, J. Critchlow, D. Magee, and W. Silen (1982). Prostaglandins stimulate and inhibit acid secretion in amphibian fundic mucosa. Proc. Soc. Exptl. Biol. Med., 170, 398-404.

This work was supported by the Swedish Medical Research Council (Project No 04X-151).

PROPERTIES AND FUNCTION OF MUCOSAL MAST CELLS

L. Enerbäck

Department of Pathology, University of Göteborg, Sahlgren Hospital, S 413 45 Göteborg, Sweden

ABSTRACT

Mucosal mast cells (MMC) are numerous in many species, including man, but have so far only been studied in detail in rats. MMC of the gastrointestinal tract differ in a number of ways from the connective tissue mast cells (CTMC) of other sites, including the serous coat. MMC are smaller than CTMC and contain fewer granules of more variable shape. In contrast to CTMC, they have a migratory capacity, and are often found in close relation to nerve fibers. Electron microscopy has provided evidence suggestive of a direct innervation of MMC. Histochemical and biochemical results indicate that the proteoglycan of MMC granules has a different structure from that of CTMC, the former containing an oversulphated galactosaminoglycan (chondroitin sulphate E) rather than heparin. MMC also contain a distinct serine endoprotease. They are the main repository for gut mucosal histamine, but the histamine content of the individual MMC is only one tenth of that of CTMC. Like the latter, MMC normally contain 5-hydroxytryptamine and have the capacity to store exogenous dopamine. Histamine is not released from MMC by compound 48/80 and polymyxin B, which instead induce an inverse, proliferative response. A distinctive property of MMC is their strong activation in immune responses induced by intestinal nematodes.

KEYWORDS

Mast cells; mucosal; connective tissue; basophils; rat; proteoglycan; histamine; 5-hydroxytryptamine; secretion; nematode infection.

INTRODUCTION

Until quite recently, the histamine of the gut mucosa was thought of as a non-mast cell histamine pool. The reason for this was the frequent failure to demonstrate significant numbers of mast cells in the gastrointestinal mucosa and the finding that injections of compound 48/80, a powerful histamine liberator in the rat, did not reduce the histamine content of the gut in this species. We now know that the gut mucosal histamine is stored in a specific type of mast cell which requires special fixation and staining conditions for its demonstration and is unresponsive to the degranulating action of compound 48/80. The study of the mucosal mast cells has opened new vistas in mast cell research and stimulated an interest in possible functional heterogeneities in this cell system. This paper will review some results of studies from my own and other laboratories on gastrointestinal mucosal mast cells (MMC). The properties of these cells will be compared with those of the connective tissue mast cells (CTMC) found in other locations. Although MMC are found in several species, including man, the discussion will be focused on the rat since most of what we know about MMC comes from studies of this species.

DISTRIBUTION AND STRUCTURE

After proper fixation and staining, numerous mucosal mast cells are found in the lamina propria of the entire gastrointestinal tract. The mast cell density is high compared to other tissues, higher than that of dorsal skin and about the same as in the ears. The cell numbers per unit area are somewhat higher in the ileum and jejunum than they are in the duodenum and colon (Enerbäck, 1966c). In normal rats, MMC are never found in the epithelium. They can be distinguished from CTMC by morphological criteria. MMC are smaller, of more variable shape and, as a rule, contain fewer granules of more variable size and shape (Fig. 1). The variable form of the MMC, which often show cytoplasmic processes and projections, is perhaps an expression of motility. That MMC have, in fact, a migratory capacity is shown during the "self cure" reaction of nematode infections (see below), when numerous MMC are found in the epithelium, between the individual epithelial cells. In the electron microscope the cells are found to be tightly interspersed between mesenchymal and epithelial cells, and, unlike CTMC, to have a smooth surface, lacking microvilli (Enerbäck and Lundin, 1974).

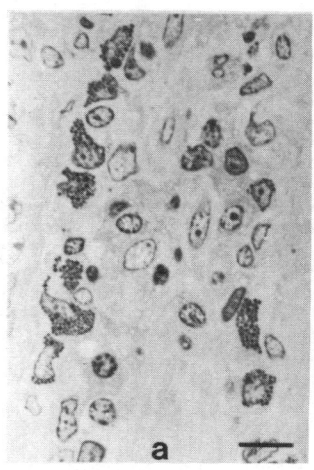 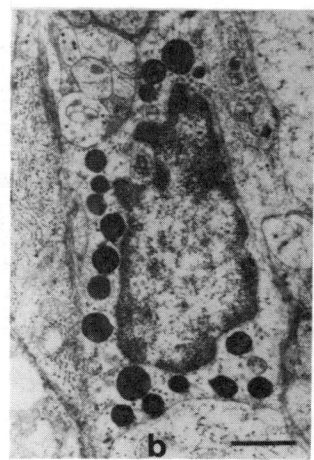

Fig. 1. Mucosal mast cells in the lamina propria of the jejunal mucosa of a normal rat.
a) Light micrograph of a toluidine blue stained Epon section. Bar 10 µm.
b) Electron micrograph. Bar 2 µm.

MMC are often found near nerve fibers of the lamina propria. In a recent study, we observed nerve terminals seemingly in direct contact with the plasma membrane of mucosal mast cells in the rat ileum (Newson and coworkers, 1983). Some of these terminals contained many clear and a few dense core vesicles (diameter 80-100 nm), while others contained mainly larger dense core vesicles (diameter around 150 nm). No attempts have been made so far to specifically identify adrenergic nerve terminals. The boutons with many clear and some larger dense core vesicles may therefore represent adrenergic and/or cholinergic nerve terminals, while the ones with predominantly larger dense core vesicles may represent peptidergic terminals. These findings strongly suggest that MMC may be directly innervated under certain conditions. More work is

Properties and function of mucosal mast cells

obviously needed before this finding can be fully evaluated. It is interesting, however, that several investigators have previously observed a close association between CTMC and nerves (for references see Newson and co-workers, 1983). Furthermore, it has been reported that both acethylcholine (Blandina and coworkers, 1980) and substance P (see Foreman and Jordan, 1983) release histamine from isolated peritoneal mast cells of the rat in vitro. It was also found that histamine was released from isolated guinea pig auricles upon vagal stimulation (Blandina and coworkers, 1983).

PROTEOGLYCAN MATRIX OF THE GRANULES

Mast cells are defined by their large cytoplasmic granules which contain a matrix of sulphated glycosaminoglycan (GAG) and protein, to which low molecular weight substances such as histamine are bound. The metachromatic staining, which is the hallmark of the mast cell, is a result of the binding of cationic dyes to anionic sites of the GAG.

Several references to mucosal mast cells can be found in the early mast cell literature (see Michels, 1938) while other, more recent papers have often denied their existence. The reason for this is that dye binding to the granules of MMC, unlike those of CTMC, is strongly dependent on the manner of fixation of the tissue. MMC were identified as a separate entity after a systematic study of the fixation and staining of rat mast cells (Enerbäck, 1966a, b). It was found that Carnoy solution and an isotonic, low concentration formaldehyde-acetic acid fixative (IFAA) preserved the staining of MMC well, while normal aldehyde fixation failed to do so. In a recent study it was found that the structural integrity of the granules of both type of mast cell is strongly dependent on ionic linkages between GAG and protein (Wingren and Enerbäck, 1983). The matrix of MMC granules was more soluble in solutions of high salt concentrations and pH than that of CTMC granules, but similar charged groups appeared to be involved in the binding. Aldehyde fixation by routine procedures was found to reversibly block the cationic dye binding of MMC granules. The dye binding groups could be unmasked by trypsination or by extreme staining times of the order of several days. On the basis of these results it was suggested that the blocking of staining by aldehydes is caused by a diffusion barrier of protein nature and that MMC and CTMC differ in terms of the spatial arrangement of GAG and protein in their granules.

In appropriately fixed tissue MMC and CTMC also differ in staining properties. In general, these differences suggest that MMC granules contain a GAG with a lower degree of sulphation than that of CTMC which is known to be heparin. Thus MMC granules stain blue with copper phthtalocyanin dyes, such as astra blue or alcian blue, in a staining sequence with safranin, while MMC granules stain red (Enerbäck, 1966b). Furthermore, the critical electrolyte concentration (Scott and Dorling, 1965) of the staining with alcian blue is substantially lower for MMC than for CTMC (Miller and Walshaw, 1972). MMC granules, unlike those of CTMC do not exhibit a fluorescent binding with the dye berberine (Wingren and Enerbäck, 1983). This fluorescent binding has a substantial degree of specificity for heparin and strongly-sulphated heparan sulphates (to be published). A staining sequence of berberine followed by toluidine blue can be used to distinguish CTMC from MMC in the same specimen.

We have recently attempted to identify the the GAG of mucosal mast cells (Enerbäck and coworkers, 1984a). For this purpose we took advantage of the fact that MMC proliferate in response to infections with the nematode N. brasiliensis, resulting in a dramatic increase in mast cell numbers and the histamine content of the mucosa (see below). Infected and control rats were injected with sodium ^{35}S sulphate, 4 times daily during a four day period, 10-13 days after infection, when the MMC of infected rats proliferate and increase greatly in number. After a further 10 days the rats were killed and tissues taken for analysis. We found a parallel increase in mast cell numbers, histamine content and ^{35}S labelled GAG (Table 1a). Analysis of the labelled polysaccharide from infected animals showed that almost 60% of this material consisted of oversulphated galactosaminoglycan, while heparin-related polysaccharides accounted for only 13% (Table 1b). The galactosaminoglycan contained 4-monosulphated and 4,6-disulphated N-acetylgalactosamine residues in approximately 5:1 molar ratio, both being linked to D-glucoronic acid residues. It is concluded that the major GAG produced by rat MMC is an oversulphated galactosaminoglycan rather than heparin. Our analytical data are in agreement with an oversulphated chondroitin sulphate of the type sometimes referred to as chondroitin sulphate E.

TABLE 1a Mucosal Mast Cells, Histamine Content and ^{35}S Labelled Glycosaminoglycans in the Jejunum of Nematode-Infected Rats

Animals[a]	Mast Cells[a,c]	Histamine[b] (ug/g tissue)	(^{35}S) Glycosaminoglycans[b] (cpm/g tissue x 10^{-3})
Infected	651±10	20.4±2.0	599±89
Controls	138±16	4.5±1.5	177±12
Infected/Controls	4.7	4.5	5.1

[a] Four rats infected with N. brasiliensis and 4 uninfected controls
[b] Mean ± S.E.
[c] Number of cells/unit mucosal length

Mast cell granules contain several proteins which have been partially characterized (Lagunoff and Pritzl, 1975). In rat mast cells there are two distinct serine proteases (Lagunoff, 1981; Woodbury and Neurath, 1980) differing in solubility, structure and antigenicity. One of these, referred to as rat mast cell protease II (RMCP II) is found in the intestinal mucosa and localized in MMC (Woodbury, Gruzensky, and Lagunoff, 1978): the other enzyme, which is the well-known mast cell chymase (Benditt and Arase, 1959), is referred to as rat mast cell protease I and mainly located in mast cells of CTMC type. Since RMCP II can be both localized microscopically and quantified by immunological methods (Woodbury and Miller, 1982) it may serve as a useful marker for MMC and their secretory activity.

TABLE 1b Composition of the ^{35}S-Labelled Glycosaminoglycan Preparations

Animals[a]	Heparin/Heparan Sulphate (%)	Galactosaminoglycans (%)	Unidentified (%)
Infected	13 (n = 3)	57 (n = 4)	30
Controls	28 (n = 2)	53 (n = 2)	19

[a] Same experiment as in Table 2a. Percent of total radioactivity; averages from 2-4 preparations, as indicated in parenthesis.

STORAGE OF BIOGENIC AMINES

Histochemical findings indicate that MMC like CTMC contain histamine (Håkansson and Owman, 1967; Miller and Walshaw, 1972). No additional storage site for histamine was found in the intestinal mucosa (Enerbäck and Wingren, 1980) in contrast to the gastric mucosa of the rat, which also contains a histamine storing enterochromaffin-like cell (Håkanson and Owman, 1967). Parallel changes in MMC numbers and histamine content during the response to N. brasiliensis infections (Befus, Johnston, and Bienenstock, 1969; Wingren and coworkers, 1983) and after repeated injections of polymyxin B (Enerbäck and coworkers, 1981) further indicate that MMC are the main repository for histamine in the intestinal mucosa. However, the histamine content of the individual MMC appears to be much lower than that of CTMC. From tissue histamine contents and mast cell densities the relative histamine content of a MMC was calculated to be only about one tenth of that of a CTMC (Enerbäck, 1981). This value agrees reasonably well with the analytical data of Befus and coworkers (1982) who measured the histamine content of isolated lymphoid cells containing about 12% MMC, and calculated the histamine content to be 1.3 pg/MMC. In contrast, about 15 pg/CTMC was found in peritoneal cell suspensions.

MMC, like CTMC, normally contain 5-hydroxytryptamine (5-HT) and take up exogenous dopamine. Both amines are stored by a reserpine sensitive mechanism (Enerbäck, 1966d; Wingren and coworkers, 1983). Again the concentration of 5-HT was found to be lower in the individual MMC than in CTMC, but increased during infections with N. brasiliensis (Wingren and coworkers, 1983). Enterochromaffin cells (ECC) are the major storage site for intestinal 5-HT. Using cytofluorometric measurements it was calculated that a MMC contains about 10% of the 5-HT content of an ECC in normal rats. Since MMC are about 3 times as frequent per unit volume of tissue, it can be estimated that up to 1/4 of the gut mucosal 5-HT may be stored in MMC.

AMINE SECRETION

A notable property of MMC is their resistance to the histamine-releasing action of polyamines, such as compound 48/80 and polymyxin B, both in vivo (Enerbäck, 1966c; Enerbäck and coworkers, 1981) and in vitro (Befus and coworkers, 1982). Repeated injections of compound 48/80 or polymyxin B for 5 days resulted in a 50 to 100 % increase in the MMC numbers and a parallel increase in mucosal histamine content. The MMC numbers then returned slowly to the control level following an exponential course. From this we calculated the half life of the newly formed mast cells to be about 40 days (Enerbäck and Löwhagen, 1979). CTMC, on the other hand, have a very long life span and do not show a significant turnover in terms of cell death and renewal.

MMC isolated from the small intestine of rats infected with N. brasiliensis responded by histamine secretion after challenge with worm specific antigen, anti IgE, concanavallin A and calcium ionophores, but were refractory to compound 48/80 and bee venom peptid 401 (Pearce and coworkers, 1982). These authors also showed that disodium cromoglycate and theophylline did not inhibit antigen induced histamine release of MMC, although effective against CTMC. These findings show that MMC differ from CTMC not only in response to secretagogues but also to modulators of secretion.

We have attempted to trace the amine secretion from MMC in vivo. An intraluminal secretion of 5-HT has been previously demonstrated both in vitro and in vivo and in several species, including the rat (Ahlman and coworkers, 1984). We therefore performed a series of intestinal perfusion experiments and measured histamine and 5-HT in the perfusates (Ahlman and coworkers, to be published). Animals in Nembutal anesthesia were ventilated on air using a rodent respirator and kept at a controlled body temperature. The proximal or distal half of the small intestine was isolated with intact vascular supply and plastic tubings inserted at each end.

The lumen was perfused with saline at a rate of 0.1 ml/min and the perfusates collected every 10 min. The amines were identified and measured with sensitive HPLC methods. Rats injected with nematode larvae and age matched controls injected with saline were perfused 14 days later, when MMC numbers and mucosal histamine content was increased 5-fold compared to controls. At this stage worms are found in the proximal segment of the intestine where many MMC have migrated into the epithelium. In the distal segment, MMC numbers and histamine content are elevated to about the same extent, but MMC are largely confined to the lamina propria and worms are absent.

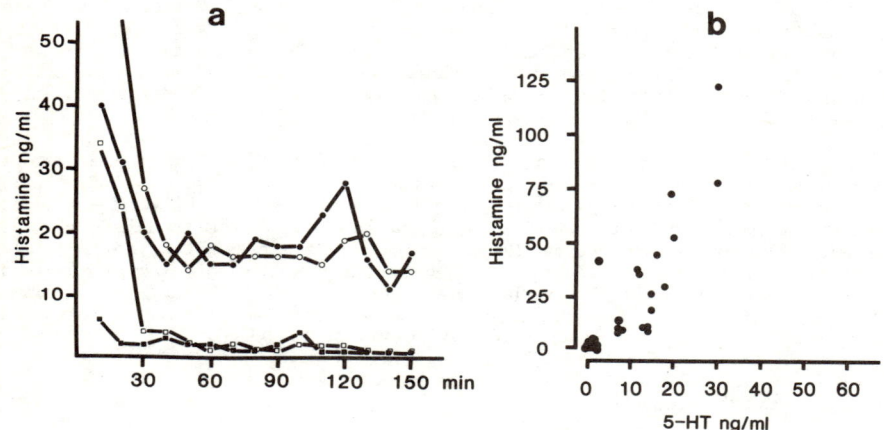

Fig. 2. Intestinal perfusion of normal and N. brasiliensis-infected rats.
a) Intraluminal histamine release from proximal (filled symbols) and distal (open symbols) intestinal segments. Each symbol represents the mean of three experiments in infected (circles) and normal (squares) animals.
b) Correlation between the concentration of histamine and 5-HT in the perfusates.

After an initial wash-out period of 30 min a steady state level of histamine secretion was obtained both in controls and in infected rats, but the histamine concentration was about 10 times higher in the latter (Fig. 2a). There was no difference in histamine secretion rate between the distal and proximal segments of the gut. In another experiment we measured histamine and 5-HT in jejunal perfusates of normal and infected rats. The concentrations of the two amines were well correlated (Fig. 2b).

These results thus suggest that histamine may be released from MMC into the gut lumen in vivo. Histamine release appears to be related to the total quantity of MMC, but does not seem to depend on the presence of intraepithelial MMC. The strong correlation between histamine and 5-HT concentration in the perfusates is of considerable interest and will be further investigated. The explanation may be that both amines are released from MMC or that amine secretion from MMC and ECC are functionally inter-related. There are no indications that the amine content of the perfusates is the result of a migration of MMC into the lumen, although this possibility cannot be wholly excluded at present. It should be noted in this context that the release of 5-HT into the gut lumen is increased by vagal stimulation (Ahlman and coworkers, 1984).

MMC PROLIFERATION IN IMMUNE RESPONSES

Intestinal helminth infections are accompanied by a massive production of IgE antibodies and a proliferation of MMC (Jarrett and Miller, 1982). The MMC response has been studied in detail in rats infected with the nematode N. brasiliensis by Miller and associates (reviewed by Miller, 1980). After skin penetration or subcutaneous injection infective larvae migrate to the intestine via the lungs, trachea, and oesophagus, moult to adult worms and start to lay eggs, which are passed in the faeces. The worms predominantly localize in the proximal part of the jejunum (MacDonald, Murray, and Ferguson, 1980). At 8 to 10 days after the infection MMC are virtually absent from the lamina propria (Miller and Jarrett, 1971). This is perhaps an effect of a non-specific mast cell degranulator produced by the worms (see Jarrett and Miller, 1982). The mast cell degranulation is followed by a proliferation of MMC reaching a maximum level of about 5 times the normal number on day 12 to 14 after the infection, when the worms are expelled from the gut by a mechanism called "self cure". During this stage MMC also migrate into the epithelium (Miller and Jarrett, 1971). Cells referred to as globule leucocytes are probably MMC which have migrated into the epithelium and partly discharged their granules (Murray, Miller, and Jarrett, 1968). The MMC proliferation is a property of the whole intestine, but the intraepithelial migration only occurs at the site of the worms (MacDonald, Murray, and Ferguson, 1980). The proliferative MMC response is immunologically mediated and dependent on the T-lymphocyte system (Mayrhofer, 1979; Befus and Bienenstock, 1979; Nawa and Miller, 1979).

The proliferative MMC response is accompanied by a parallel increase in the content of histamine and 5-HT of the gut, as discussed above. A 9-fold increase in mucosal mast cell protease content was obtained at the peak of the mast cell response (Woodbury and Miller, 1982). Concomitant immunoperoxidase studies showed that only a proportion of the MMC of the lamina propria and none of the intra-epithelial MMC contained the enzyme. A release of protease into the circulation has also been reported (Miller and coworkers, 1983).

MMC, BASOPHILS, AND BLOOD HISTAMINE

Circulating blood basophils (Ogilvie, Hesketh, and Rose, 1978) as well as elevated blood histamine levels (Roth and Levy, 1980) have been reported to occur during the N. brasiliensis infection in rats. Blood basophils are normally absent or extremely rare in rat blood, but whole blood histamine as well as free plasma histamine levels have been reported as being quite high (Almeida and coworkers, 1980). The reported values of 50 ng/ml whole blood and 17 ng/ml plasma indicate that a significant proportion of the blood histamine in normal rats is contained in the cellular fraction.

We have studied histamine levels in the gut, whole blood and plasma in relation to MMC of the gut and blood cell morphology during the course of the infection in an attempt to clarify the possible relationship between MMC and circulating blood basophils (Enerbäck and coworkers, 1984b). The results (Fig. 3) showed an increase of whole blood histamine from a control level of about 40 ng/ml to 200 ng/ml on day 12 after the infection, coinciding with the early phase of the proliferative MMC response. There was also an increase in free plasma histamine from the normal level of 15-20 ng/ml to a maximum of 80 ng/ml on day 12. Both rapidly returned towards the control level during day 16-20 while the gut histamine content remained high.

The total number of blood neutrophils increased during the early phase of the infection and there was a pronounced eosinophilia from day 10 to 16. No cells containing granules showing metachromasia or cationic dye binding at low pH levels were found in a screening which comprised 10,000 cells per specimen. During day 10 to 16 after the infection we found a number of coarsely granulated and vacuolated cells. The granules stained dark-blue with the Giemsa stain, but did not stain metachromatically with toluidine blue or with alcian blue at a low pH. We interpret this change as being equivalent to the so-called toxic granulation occurring in human neutrophils during certain infections. It may have been mistaken for a specific basophilic granulation by previous investigators. Apparently, mature granulated basophils are absent from or extremely rare in rat blood. The cellular repository for the blood histamine in normal as well as nematode infected rats remains unclear. We have suggested, as a working hypothesis, that the histamine is contained in a circulating progenitor cell for MMC which may have the ability to synthesize the amine and store it in a loosely bound state, but has not yet acquired the ability to assemble the specific cytoplasmic granules. The absence of such granules would make the histamine highly susceptible to leakage into the plasma which would in turn explain the unexpectedly high plasma histamine levels that are obtained in the rat. An alternate explanation of the high blood histamine levels during the nematode infection could be that it is a result of a release from MMC. The time course of the changes in blood histamine, as well as the absence of evidence of histamine uptake by leucocytes tend to make this alternative the less likely of the two.

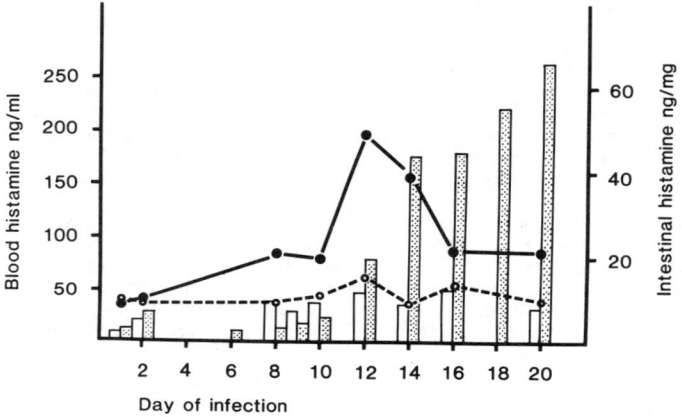

Fig. 3. Concentration of histamine in whole blood (circles) and intestine (bars) during the course of an infection with N. brasiliensis. Each symbol represents the mean of three infected (filled symbols) or control rats (open symbols, broken line).

DERIVATION OF MMC

The origin of mast cells has been the subject of controversy for a long time. However, recent studies by Kitamura and associates on mutant mice genotypes have shown that there are two hierarchial classes of mast cell precursor (Kitamura, Sonoda, and Yokoyama, 1983). The primary progenitor is a circulating, bone marrow derived precursor originating from the multipotential haemopoietic stem cell (CFU-S). This primary progenitor may be regulated by long-range, differentiating factors and, in turn, gives rise to a localized, tissue-bound mast cell precursor whose differentiation may be locally regulated. Kitamura's work concerns CTMC, and MMC were not specifically studied. However, the results neatly explain the existence of specific mast cell phenotypes such as MMC in special tissue sites.

Another important recent development is the demonstration by several groups of the growth of mast cells from haemopoietic tissues of mice in vitro (reviewed by Jarrett and Haig, 1984). These mast cells proliferate in the presence of a lymphokine promoting the cycling of multipotential stem cells, called IL3 (Ihle, Rebar, and Keller, 1982). The cultured cells appear to have the MMC rather than the CTMC phenotype and at least one such cell line produces chondroitin sulphate E instead of heparin (Razin and coworkers, 1982). Moreover, Jarrett and associates have cultured mast cells from normal rat bone marrow, stimulated by factors released from lymphocytes by N. brasiliensis antigen, or by concanavallin A. These mast cells were identified as MMC on the basis of their histochemical, and biochemical properties, including the content of a chondroitin sulphate-like proteoglycan and the MMC specific serine endoprotease RMCP II (Jarrett and Haigh, 1984).

CONCLUSION

The findings summarized in this paper identify MMC as a specific cell line within the mast cell system, phenotypically different from the connective tissue mast cells of other sites. It is obvious that the specific properties of MMC must be considered when the role of these cells in physiological and pathological reactions is considered. The distribution of the MMC phenotype in species other than the rat and in other tissues are important issues for future studies. It is also essential that the degree of heterogeneity of the mast cell system is further explored.

ACKNOWLEDGEMENTS

Part of the work reported in this paper was carried out at the authors laboratory with support from the Swedish Medical Research Council (Project 2235).

I wish to thank Gun Augustsson, Anita Olofsson, and Marie Svensson for skilful technical assistance and Annika Dahlqvist for expert secretarial aid.

REFERENCES

Ahlman, H., K. Grönstad, O. Nilsson, and A. Dahlström (1984). Biogenic Amines, 1, 63-73.
Almeida, A. P., W. Flye, D. Deveraux, Z. Horakova, and M. A. Beaven (1980). Comp. Biochem. Physiol., 67C, 187-190.
Befus, A. D., and J. Bienenstock (1979). Immunology, 38, 95-101.
Befus, A. D., N., Johnston, and J. Bienenstock (1979). Exp. Parasitol., 48, 1-8.
Befus, A. D., F. L. Pearce, J. Gauldie, P. Horsewood, and J. Bienenstock (1982). J. Immunol., 128, 2475-2480.
Benditt, E. P., and M. Arase (1959). J. Exp. Med., 110, 451-460.
Blandina, P., R. Fantozzi, P. F. Mannaioni, and E. Masini (1980). J. Physiol., 301, 281-293.
Blandina, P., M. Barattini, R. Fantozzi, E. Masini, and P. F. Mannaioni (1983). Agents and Actions, 13, 179-182.
Enerbäck, L. (1966a). Acta Path. Microbiol. scand., 66, 289-302.
Enerbäck, L. (1966b). Acta Path. Microbiol. scand., 66, 303-312.
Enerbäck, L. (1966c). Acta Pathol. Microbiol., 66, 313-322.
Enerbäck, L. (1966d). Acta Pathol. Microbiol. Scand., 67, 365-369.
Enerbäck, L. (1981). Monographs in Allergy, 17, 222-232.
Enerbäck, L., S. O. Kolset, M. Kusche, A. Hjerpe, and U. Lindahl (1984a). Submitted for publication.
Enerbäck, L., G. Lindenger, T. van Loo, and G. Granerus (1984b). Submitted for publication.
Enerbäck, L., and P. M. Lundin (1974). Cell Tissue Res., 150, 95-105.
Enerbäck, L., and G.-B. Löwhagen (1979). Cell Tissue Res., 198, 209-215.
Enerbäck, L., G.-B. Löwhagen, O. Löwhagen, and U. Wingren (1981). Cell Tissue Res., 214, 239-246.
Enerbäck, L., and U. Wingren (1980). Histochemistry, 66, 113-124.
Foreman, J., and C. Jordan (1983). Agents and Actions, 13, 105-116.
Håkansson, R., and C. Owman (1967). Life Sci, 6, 759-766.
Ihle, J. N., L. Rebar, and J. Keller (1982). Immunol. Rev., 63, 5-32.
Jarrett, E. E. E., and H. R. P. Miller (1982). Prog. Allergy, 31, 178-233.
Jarrett, E. E. E., and D. M. Haig (1984). Immunology Today, 5, 115-119.
Lagunoff, D., and P. Pritzl (1975). Arch. Biochem. Biophys., 173, 554-563.

Lagunoff, D. (1981). Neutral proteases of mast cells. In E. L. Becker, A. S. Simon, K. F. Austen (Eds.), Biochemistry of Acute Allergic Reactions, Vol. 14. Kroc Foundation Ser. New York: Liss. 350 pp.
Kitamura, Y., T. Sonoda, and M. Yokoyama (1983). Differentiation of tissue mast cells. In S.-A. Killmann, E. P Cronkite, and C. N. Müller-Berat (Eds.), Haemopoietic Stem Cells, Munksgaard, Copenhagen, pp 350-361.
MacDonald, T. T., M. Murray, and A. Ferguson (1980). Exp. Parasitol., 49, 9-14.
Mayrhofer, G. (1979). Immunology, 47, 312-322.
Michels, N. A. (1938). The mast cells. In Downey's Handbook of Haematology, 1:232-372. Republished in Mast cells and basophils. Padawer. J Ed (1963) Ann N. Y. Acad. Sci. 103, Appendix.
Miller, H. R. P., and W. F. H. Jarrett (1971). Immunology, 20, 277-288.
Miller, H. R. P., and R. Walshaw (1972). Am. J. Path., 69, 195-208.
Miller, H. R. P. (1980). Biologie Cell, 39, 229-232.
Miller, H. R. P., R. G. Woodbury, J. F. Huntley, and G. Newlands (1983). Immunology, 49, 471-479.
Murray, M., H. R. P. Miller, and W. F. H. Jarrett (1968). Lab. Invest., 19, 222-234.
Nawa, Y., and H. R. P. Miller (1979). Cell Immunol., 42, 225-239.
Newson, B., A. Dahlström, L. Enerbäck, and H. Ahlman (1983). Neuroscience, 10, 565-570.
Ogilvie, B. M., P. M. Hesketh, and M. E. Rose (1978). Exp. Parasitol., 46, 20-30.
Pearce, F. L., A. D. Befus, J. Gauldie, and J. Bienenstock (1982). J. Immunol., 128, 2481-2486.
Razin, E., R. L. Stevens, F. Akiyama, K. Schmid, and K. F. Austen (1982). J. Biol. Chem., 257, 7229-7236.
Roth, R. L., and D. A. Levy (1980). Exp. Parasitol., 50, 331-341.
Scott, J. E. and J. Dorling (1965). Histochemie, 5, 221-233.
Wingren, U., and L. Enerbäck (1983). Histochem. J., 15, 571-582.
Wingren, U., L. Enerbäck, H. Ahlman, S. Allenmark, and A. Dahlström (1983). Histochemistry, 77, 145-158.
Wingren, U., Å. Wastesson, and L. Enerbäck (1983). Int. Archs. Allergy appl. Immun., 70, 193-199.
Woodbury, R. G., G. M. Gruzenski, and D. Lagunoff (1978). Proc. Natl. Acad. Sci. USA, 75, 2785-2789.
Woodbury, R. G., and H. R. P. Miller (1982). Immunology, 46, 487-495.
Woodbury, R. G., and H. Neurath (1980). FEBS Lett., 114, 189-206.

Actions and Role of Histamine in the Cardiovascular System

PHYSIOLOGY AND PHARMACOLOGY OF CARDIAC HISTAMINE, REVISITED

P. F. Mannaioni

Department of Pharmacology, Florence University, School of Medicine, Viale Morgagni 65, 50134 Florence, Italy

ABSTRACT
The state of the art on the physiology and pharmacology of cardiac histamine is revisited, aiming to identify the unsettled aspects of the histaminergic regulations of myocardial functions.

KEYWORDS
Histamine; histamine release; cardiac functions.

In 1961 ERSPAMER wrote on histamine in the central nervous system: "Histamine has been ignored for a long time by several investigators as a second - class amine. But this amine, however annoying the fact may be, has the same citizenship right as catecholamines or 5-hydroxytryptamine" (Erspamer, 1961). At the present, after the breakthrough achieved by Black and co-workers (1972) with the invention of H_2-receptor antagonists and the accompanying taxonomy of H_1 and H_2 receptors in the heart and peripheral vessels, there are no questions that histamine belongs to the realm of cardiovascular physiology and pharmacology. Indeed, a variety of exhaustive reviews has appeared on this issue in recent years (Mannaioni, 1972; Levi, Owen and Trzeciakowski, 1982) rendering the task of revisiting the physiological aspects and the pharmacological implications of histamine in the cardiovascular system apparently ripetitive.
At first sight, it might be said that histamine has already met the criteria which have been used historically to define acetylcholine and noradrenaline as the basic modulators of myocardial functions, these criteria being the synthesis from physiologically occuring compounds, the storage into definite cellular sites, the uptake, release and metabolism, the receptor populations subserving the effects of exogenous and endogenous histamine, which can be mimicked or antagonized by specific compounds. However, the task of revisiting cardiovascular histamine may be revived by looking more insight into the variegate aspects of the histaminergic physiology and pharmacology in the heart and peripheral vessels.
In spite of its presence in the mammalian heart in concentrations far exceeding those of noradrenaline and acetylcholine, the origin of cardiac histamine

has not been conclusively demonstrated; either histamine is formed in situ, or the heart takes up histamine from the blood. How much of the histamine formed in situ contributes to the steady-state level of histamine in the heart is not clear: formation of histamine has been shown in the guinea-pig and rat heart, but only at a very negligible extent. A first issue to be revisited in detail is therefore represented by the very presence of histamine in the heart, to be accounted for either by the local decarboxylation of histidine (within mast-cell or non-mast cell storage sites) or by an active uptake from the circulation.

The heart takes up histamine in all the animal species examined. However, the bulk of histamine taken up is quickly catabolized into acid metabolites and Nτ-methyl-histamine, making unlikely that the uptake of the preformed amine contributes entirely to building up cardiac histamine stores, unless the minute amounts of unchanged amine escaping metabolism slowly accumulates into the storage sites.

The capacity for effecting the uptake of histamine is greatly reduced in guinea-pig hearts which have been depleted of mast cells by combining (+) tubocurarine with antigen, thus indicating mast cells as the main repository of cardiac histamine. However, mast cells cannot account for the uptake of histamine in the rat heart, since compound 48/80 reduces the endogenous histamine stores without measurably affecting ^{3}H-histamine decline in the heart. A second debatable issue lays therefore into the identification of the cell(s) which store histamine in the heart, and into the distinction between mast cell and non-mast cell histamine kinetics. The concept of non-mast cell histamine has been recently strengthened by the discovery of the W-W^1 inbred mice, genetically deprived of mast cells but still containing histamine in their tissues.

A fluorishing information is now available on the release of histamine by the mammalian heart, starting from the pioneering work of Cesaris-Demel (1910). The stimuli leading to liberation of cardiac histamine can be classified as immunological (as in cardiac anaphylaxis), chemical (compound 48/80; calcium ionophore A23187) and pharmacological (+-tubocurarine; tolazoline and burimamide; corticotrophin and synthetic analogs; morphine; the anthracycline antibiotics).

A settled argument is represented by the actions exerted by endogenously released or by the exogenously administered histamine on the main parameters of cardiac functions. The pattern of cardiac reaction to an effective dose of histamine entails an increase in the rate and amplitude of contraction, a delay in atrio-ventricular conduction, abnormalities of origin and spread of excitation in the ventricles, and a marked reduction of coronary outflow, the effects being species-dependent.

The taxonomy of the receptors subserving the cardiac effects of histamine has been analyzed in detail, by using as specific pharmacological tools the histamine H_1 and H_2-receptors agonists and antagonists. A variety of careful studies has mapped these receptors as predominant H_2, mediating the increase in sinus rate, ventricular contractility and the increase in atrial and ventricular automaticity; while the increase of atrial contractility, of atrio-ventricular conduction time and the decrease of coronary flow would be mediated by H_1-receptors. However, an overview of the histamine action on the heart leads to the idea of a dishomogenous distribution of H_1 and H_2 receptors, which may be influenced by the animal species, the experimental setting, the temperature of incubation, without any significant correlation between binding studies (^{3}H-mepyramine) and the pharmacodynamic effects. Some of the cardiovascular effects induced by histamine in the experimental animals can be extrapolated to man, in vivo.

A great deal of experimental evidences have been provided in the recent years on the biochemical and electrophysiological basis of cardiac histamine actions. Among them, the demonstration that the positive inotropic effect of histamine is mediated by 3'-5'-cyclic-AMP through the activation of an adenyl-cyclase system separate from that of catecholamines (an H_2-response), and by an H_2-receptor mediated increase in calcium transmembrane influx. Electrophysiological studies have shown that histamine increases the slope of pace-maker potentials in the sinoatrial node cells of rabbit and guinea-pig heart and in human right atrial fibre, while it decreases the duration of action potential in papillary muscles and ventricular strips of guinea-pig heart. These effects are blocked by burimamide and by cimetidine and mimicked by H_2-agonists. On the other hand, H_1-receptor agonists ('2-pyridyl-ethylamine) increase the duration of the action potential in the guinea-pig left atrium in a way similar to that described by De Mello (1976) in right ventricular strips of the guinea-pig heart and by Eckel and co-workers (1982) in human papillary muscles. Moreover, histamine induces automaticity in silent preparations, restores the excitability of heart preparations blocked by tetrodotoxin or by high potassium concentration and induces oscillatory activity in sheep Purkinje fibers depolarized by low-potassium medium (Mugelli and co-workers, 1980).

Notwithstanding, the most controversial question throughout the whole history of cardiac histamine has been the physiological functions, as opposed to its role in cardiac pathology. This second issue has been clarified by the repeated demonstration of the arrhythmogenic actions of histamine in humans (Levi and co-workers, 1981) and in the experimental animals, relevant in the pathogenesis of cardiac disorders in drug-induced anaphylaxis, and by the implication of histamine in inducing a variant angina pectoris. The pharmacology of cardiac histamine is on its way (see Giotti and Zilletti, 1976, for a review) especially focused on the protection afforded by cimetidine after experimental infarction in the guinea-pig, and the alleged benefits of a therapy with H_2-receptor agonists in patients with catecholamine-refractory heart failure.

However, little is known on the physiological stimuli capable of releasing cardiac histamine. From this standpoint, two recent pieces of evidence are worth mentioning: a) the demonstration that histamine is released together with noradrenaline from the isolated guinea-pig heart upon stimulation of sympathetic nerves (Levi and Roby, 1981); b) the demonstration that histamine is released together with acetylcholine in the isolated, vagally innerved, guinea-pig auricles upon vagal stimulation, and that the release of histamine is paralleled to a significant diminution in mast cell count (Blandina and co-workers, 1983). If the parasympathetic and sympathetic innervation of cardiac mast cells would turn to be true, the cardiac histaminergic system might represent an additional control of cardiovascular homeostasis, according to the concept of "the other receptor system", envisaged by Bristow, Ginsburg and Harrison (1982).

REFERENCES

Black, J. W., W. M. Duncan, C. J. Durant, G. R. Ganellin, and M. E. Parsons (1972). Definition and antagonism of histamine H_2-receptors. Nature, 236, 385-390.
Blandina, P., M. Barattini, R. Fantozzi, E. Masini, and P. F. Mannaioni (1983). Histamine release by vagal stimulation. Agents and Actions, 13, 179-182.
Bristow, M. R., R. Ginsburg, and D. C. Harrison (1982). Histamine and the

human heart: the other receptor system. Amer. J. Cardiol., 49, 249-251.
Cesaris-Demel, A. (1910). Recherches sur l'anaphylaxie: sur le mode de se comporter du coeur isolé d'animaux sensibilisés. Arch. It. Biol., 54, 141-152.
De Mello, W. C. (1976). On the mechanism of histamine action in cardiac muscle Eur. J. Pharmacol., 35, 315-324.
Eckel, L., R. W. Gristwood, H. Nawrath, D. A. A. Owen, and P. Satter (1982). Inotropic and electrophysiological effects of histamine on human ventricular heart muscle. J. Physiol., 330, 111-123.
Erspamer, V. (1961). Pharmacologically active substances of mammalian origin. Ann. Rev. Pharmacol., 1, 175-218.
Giotti, A., and L. Zilletti (1976). Antiarrhythmic actions of anti-histamines. In L. Szekeres (Ed.), Pharmac. Ther. B, Vol. 2, Pergamon Press, pp. 863-900.
Levi, R., J. R. Malm, F. O. Bowman, and M. R. Rosen (1981). The arrhythmogenic actions of histamine on human atrial fibers. Circulation Res., 49, 545-550.
Levi, R., D. A. A. Owen, and J. Trzeciakowski (1982). In C. R. Ganellin, and M. E. Parsons (Ed.), Pharmacology of histamine receptors, Wright-PSG, Bristol, London, Boston, Chap. 6, pp. 236-297.
Levi, R., and A. Roby (1981). Histamine, adrenergic transmission and cardiac function. Eight International Congress of pharmacology, abstracts, 1602.
Mannaioni, P. F. (1972). Physiology and pharmacology of cardiac histamine. Arch. Int. Pharmacodyn., 196, 64-78.
Mugelli, A., L. Mantelli, S. Manzini, and F. Ledda (1980). Induction by histamine of oscillatory activity in sheep purkinje fibers and suppression by verapamil or lidocaine. J. Cardiovasc. Pharmac., 2, 9-15.

IgE-MEDIATED HYPERSENSITIVITY AND ISCHEMIA AS CAUSES OF ENDOGENOUS CARDIAC HISTAMINE RELEASE[1]

R. Levi, A. Wolff, D. A. Robertson and L. Michael Graver

Department of Pharmacology, Cornell University Medical College, 1300 York Avenue, New York, NY 10021, USA

ABSTRACT

Our previous studies in the guinea pig have implicated histamine in the pathogenesis of cardiac dysfunctions associated with immediate hypersensitivity. We have now studied histamine release, and associated functional changes, in human heart tissue immunologically challenged in vitro. Pectinate muscles were isolated from human atrial appendages, removed routinely during corrective cardiac surgery, and allowed to beat spontaneously in a tissue bath. Challenge with human IgE-specific antibodies caused a marked increase in spontaneous rate and contractility which was antagonized by cimetidine. Thus, IgE-mediated hypersensitivity can result in functionally significant histamine release from human myocardium.

Release of cardiac histamine by various stimuli is known to provoke ventricular arrhythmias. Since ventricular arrhythmias are common in the course of myocardial ischemia and infarction, we determined whether cardiac histamine is released by coronary artery occlusion, and - if so - whether histamine release is associated with ventricular arrhythmias. The left anterior descending coronary artery was occluded in anesthetized dogs. Coronary sinus histamine concentration increased about 10-fold (as contrasted with a 21% decrease in coronary sinus flow). Cardiac histamine efflux directly correlated with the number of ventricular premature beats during the first 30 minutes of occlusion. The mean peak coronary sinus histamine concentration was significantly greater in dogs that suffered ventricular fibrillation than in those that did not. Cardiac histamine efflux correlated directly with infarct size. Thus, cardiac histamine is released as an acute response to coronary artery occlusion and may mediate ischemic ventricular arrhythmias.

KEYWORDS

Human Cardiac Anaphylaxis; Myocardial Ischemia; Histamine Release; Cardiac Arrhythmias; Cimetidine

---

[1]Supported by grants from the National Institutes of Health (GM 20091 and HL 18828), by the Veterans Administration (V.A. general research funds), by a Predoctoral Fellowship in Pharmacology from the Pharmaceutical Manufacturers Association Foundation, and by an Arietta S. Livanos Research Fellowship in Surgery and Pharmacology.

IgE-MEDIATED HISTAMINE RELEASE FROM HUMAN HEART TISSUE

Studies from several laboratories, including ours, have implicated a number of pharmacologic mediators, such as histamine, prostaglandins, leukotrienes and platelet-activating factor, in the pathogenesis of cardiac dysfunctions associated with immediate hypersensitivity (Feigen and Prager, 1969; Levi et al, 1982a; Levi et al, 1984). These investigations have utilized various animal models, especially the guinea pig, for its proverbial sensitivity to histamine. The results of these studies clearly designate the heart as a major target organ in systemic acute allergic reactions (Capurro and Levi, 1975; Zavecz and Levi, 1977) and offer an explanation of cardiovascular dysfunctions reported to occur in humans during systemic anaphylaxis (Bernreiter, 1959; Booth and Patterson, 1970; Criep and Woehler, 1971; Sullivan, 1982). Indeed, the human heart is rich in histamine, which can be readily released in vitro by therapeutic concentrations of drugs such as morphine (Levi et al, 1982b); furthermore, histamine has potent arrhythmogenic effects on the human heart in vitro (Levi et al, 1981).
Recently, we have provided the direct demonstration of histamine release, and associated functional changes, in human heart tissue immunologically challenged in vitro (Graver et al, 1983).
Specimens of human atrial tissue were removed from the atriotomy site during the cardio-pulmonary bypass procedure in corrective cardiac surgery. Institutional and Federal regulations for the protection of human subjects were observed. Pectinate muscles were excised from the surgical specimen and allowed to beat spontaneously in an isolated organ bath containing oxygenated Tyrode's solution at 37°C; isometric contractile force was measured with a force-displacement transducer (Guo et al, 1983). The remaining portion of the surgical specimen was chopped into small fragments and added to the bath, so as to provide a greater source of mediators. After a period of equilibration, the tissue was challenged immunologically either with goat serum containing antibodies specifically directed against human IgE or with control sera. Two control sera were used, one was the specific goat serum from which anti-human IgE's had been removed by affinity chromatography, the other was non-specific goat serum. Samples of the bath fluid were taken before and at various intervals after specific or control immunologic challenge, and were assayed for histamine by the radioenzymatic microassay of Beaven et al (1982).
Pectinate muscles responded to specific immunologic challenge with a progressive increase in the rate and force of spontaneous contractions which reached a maximum within 5 minutes of the challenge; this response was accompanied by histamine release. Neither functional changes nor histamine release occurred upon re-challenge with specific serum. Minimal changes occurred when tissues were incubated with either of the control sera specified above. When atrial tissues were immunologically challenged in the presence of cimetidine, histamine release was not significantly modified, whereas the positive inotropic and chronotropic effects were markedly attenuated. A quantitative description of our findings is offered in Table 1.

TABLE 1 Responses of Human Right Atrial Tissue to Immunologic Challenge In Vitro and their Modification by Cimetidine

	Control*	Specific Immunologic Challenge**	
		Untreated	Cimetidine (3uM)
Contraction (% increase)	0.8±1.9***	43±7	9±9
Rate (increase in beats/min)	0	8±1	2±1
Histamine Release (ng/100mg)	0.23±0.1	1.1±0.1	0.7±2.9

*Incubated with goat antiserum directed against horseradish peroxidase.
**Challenged with goat antiserum directed against human IgE.
***All values are means (±S.E.M.); n=3-7.

Our data indicate that IgE-mediated hypersensitivity can result in functionally-significant histamine release from human myocardium and that changes in rate and contractility are probably mediated by H_2-receptors. Our findings further suggest that the human heart may participate as a target organ in systemic acute allergic reactions.

MYOCARDIAL ISCHEMIA AS A CAUSE OF HISTAMINE RELEASE FROM THE CANINE HEART

Although histamine release from the hypoxemic heart was recognized half a century ago (Anrep et al, 1936) and later suspected to be arrhythmogenic (Harris, 1950), only recently has our laboratory documented that cardiac histamine is released as an acute response to coronary artery occlusion and that histamine release correlates with ventricular arrhythmias (Wolff et al, 1984).
We occluded the left anterior descending (LAD) coronary artery in pentobarbital-anesthetized, open-chest dogs for periods ranging from 30 minutes to 22 hours. Samples of coronary sinus blood were assayed for histamine by the radioenzymatic micromethod of Beaven et al (1982). Coronary sinus histamine concentration rose from baseline levels of 0.06±0.03 to 0.61±0.11 ng/ml (n=14; p<0.001) within 14.8±2 minutes of occlusion. In contrast with this 10-fold increase in histamine concentration, the coronary sinus flow is known to decrease by only 21%, following the acute occlusion of the left anterior descending coronary artery (Lombardi et al, 1983). This excludes that the increase in histamine concentration may simply reflect the decline in coronary sinus flow. Most interestingly, cardiac histamine efflux directly correlated with the number of ventricular premature beats (VPBs) occurring within the first 30 minutes of occlusion, in those dogs not suffering ventricular fibrillation (10/14). Thus, for cumulative (i.e. 30-min) coronary sinus histamine concentrations ranging between 0 and 5 ng/ml there was a mean of 68 VPBs (N=7), whereas in the 5-10 and 10-15 ng/ml range, mean VPBs increased to 255 (N=2) and 514 (N=1), respectively. In the other 4 dogs, ventricular fibrillation occurred: peak coronary sinus histamine concentration averaged 0.86 ng/ml, as compared with 0.37 ng/ml in the 10 dogs which had VPBs but did not fibrillate (p=0.05). Thus, the frequency of VPBs appears to correlate with the amounts of histamine continuously released from the heart, whereas the incidence of ventricular fibrillation appears to coincide with large bursts of cardiac histamine release. We also measured infarct size by the nitro-blue tetrazolium method (Nachlas and Shnitka, 1963) in 6 dogs with LAD coronary artery occlusion. We found that cardiac histamine efflux correlated with infarct size: with mean infarct sizes of 3.7, 7.8 and 15.5 g (N=2 for each group), mean cumulative (i.e. 30-min) coronary sinus histamine concentrations increased from 1.50 to 4.69 and 10.97 ng/ml, respectively.
Our findings are the first documentation of cardiac histamine release as an acute response to coronary artery occlusion. Since histamine efflux appears to correlate directly with the incidence and the severity of ventricular arrhythmias, our data further suggest that cardiac histamine release may at least in part mediate ischemic ventricular dysrhythmias.

ACKNOWLEDGEMENTS

Dr. A.A. Wolff was also associated with the Division of Cardiology, Dept. of Medicine, New York Veterans Administration Medical Center, New York University School of Medicine, New York, N.Y. 10010.
We wish to acknowledge the invaluable technical assistance of Dr. Aida A. Chenouda and Mr. Pedro Dedos, the kind cooperation of the Divisions of Thoracic Surgery and Surgical Pathology of the New York Hospital-Cornell Medical Center, and the excellent secretarial assistance of Ms. Claudia B. Gross.

REFERENCES

Anrep, G.V., G.S. Barsoum, and M. Talaat (1936). J. Physiol., 86, 431-451.
Beaven, M.A., A. Robinson-White, N.B. Roderick, and G.L. Kauffman (1982). Klin. Wochenschr., 60, 873-881.
Bernreiter, M. (1959). J.A.M.A., 170, 1628-1630.
Booth, B.H., and R. Patterson (1970). J.A.M.A., 211, 627-631.
Capurro, N., and R. Levi (1975). Circulation Res., 36, 520-528.
Criep, L.H., and T.R. Woehler (1971). Ann. Allergy, 29, 399-409.
Feigen, G.A., and D.J. Prager (1969). Amer. J. Cardiol., 24, 474-491.
Graver, L.M., R. Levi, A.A. Chenouda, C.G. Becker, and W.A. Gay, Jr. (1983). Circulation, 68 III, 332.
Guo, Z.G., R. Levi, L.M. Aaronson, and W.A. Gay, Jr. (1983). J. Pharmacol. Methods, 9, 127-135.
Harris, A.S. (1950). Circulation, 1, 1318-1328.
Levi, R., J.A. Burke, and E.J. Corey (1982a). In B. Samuelsson and R. Paoletti (Eds.), Adv. Prost. Thrombox. Leukotr. Res., Vol. 9, Raven Press, New York. pp. 215-222.
Levi, R., J.A. Burke, Z.-G. Guo, Y. Hattori, C.M. Hoppens, L.M. McManus, D.J. Hanahan, and R.N. Pinckard (1984). Circ. Res., 54, 117-124.
Levi, R., A.A. Chenouda, J. Trzeciakowski, Z.-G. Guo, L.M. Aaronson, R.D. Luskind, C.-H. Lee, W.A. Gay, V.A. Subramanian, J.C. McCabe, and J.C. Alexander (1982b). Klin. Wochenschr., 60, 965-971.
Levi, R., J.R. Malm, F.O. Bowman, and M.R. Rosen (1981). Circulation Res., 49, 545-550.
Lombardi, F., R.L. Verrier, and B. Lown (1983). Am. Heart J., 105, 958-965.
Nachlas, M.M., and T.K. Shnitka (1963). Am. J. Path., 42, 379-406.
Sullivan, T.J. (1982). J.A.M.A., 248, 2161-2162.
Wolff, A.A., R. Levi, V.J. Fisher, and A.A. Chenouda (1984). Fed. Proc., 43, 458.
Zavecz, J.H., and R. Levi (1977). Circulation Res., 40, 15-19.

HISTAMINE AND MYOCARDIAL DYSFUNCTION

R. W. Gristwood, D. A. A. Owen, P. Romanec and K. A. Sampford

Smith Kline and French Research Limited, The Frythe, Welwyn, Hertfordshire, UK

ABSTRACT

The mammalian heart contains large quantities of histamine which may be released, leading to functional changes, during treatments which cause mast cell degranulation (including anaphylaxis). We have measured histamine release from the heart in further models of experimental cardiac injury in guinea-pigs and rats.

In the perfused isolated rat heart the "calcium paradox" procedure led to severe cardiac damage. Large quantities of both creatine kinase and histamine were detected in the coronary effluent. In guinea-pigs the calcium paradox procedure led to the release of creatine kinase, but histamine release was only detected in 2 out of 6 hearts.

Ischaemia-induced injury in rat hearts, (5% of normal flow for 30 mins), led to the release of creatine kinase and histamine. In guinea-pig hearts, this ischaemia led to more variable damage. In damaged hearts histamine release was detected only in trace quantities. Histamine release could be consistently detected in the coronary effluent from guinea-pig hearts exposed to a more severe ischaemia.

These studies extend the conditions of experimental cardiac damage in which histamine is released and also emphasise that this potentially important feature of cardiac injury shows quantitative differences between species.

KEYWORDS

Histamine release; Calcium paradox; Myocardium; Ischaemia; Reperfusion; Creatine kinase

INTRODUCTION

The aetiology of injury related myocardial dysfunction is not fully understood. It is known that endogenous cardioactive mediators such as prostaglandins E_2 and $F_{2\alpha}$ (Block, Poole and Vane, 1974; Wennmalm, Chanh and Junstad, 1974) and noradrenaline (Wollenberger and Shahab, 1965) may be released in association with myocardial injury and may contribute to the resultant myocardial dysfunction.

Histamine is present, in large quantities, in the heart of most species including man (Mannaioni, 1972). It is possible that histamine may also be released during myocardial injury. This could be of clinical importance since histamine has been found to elicit major changes in cardiac function in various species (McNeill, 1982) including man (Gristwood, Lincoln and Owen, 1980). The concept of histamine release from tissues following injury is well established (Horokova and Beaven, 1974; Markley and colleagues, 1975). However, to date the possibility of injury induced release of myocardial histamine has not been investigated in detail, but restricted to studies with procedures known to degranulate mast cells e.g. anaphylaxis, compound 48/80 (Levi and Guo, 1982).

In this study we have investigated whether endogenous myocardial histamine is released during myocardial injury. For these experiments we have chosen two experimental models of myocardial injury (calcium paradox and ischaemia/ reperfusion) and two species (rat and guinea-pig). The calcium paradox causes severe myocardial damage (as assessed by creatine kinase release) whereas the ischaemia/reperfusion method caused a less severe myocardial damage. Both of these methods of inducing myocardial damage have been well characterised in the rat (Apstein and colleagues, 1977; Hearse, Humphrey and Bullock, 1978).

MATERIALS AND METHODS

Animals and Preparation

Male rats, Wistar strain, were in the weight range 230-280 g. Male guinea-pigs, Dunkin-Hartley strain, were in the weight range 500-600 g. All animals were treated with heparin (5000 IU/kg i.p.). 20 minutes later, animals were killed by either cranial impact (rats) or cervical dislocation (guinea-pigs). The heart was quickly excised and placed in ice-cold perfusion medium until beating ceased. The heart was then set up as a Langendorff preparation.

The Perfusion Medium

The constituents of the perfusion medium were (in mmol/l):- NaCl, 124, KCl, 4.7; $MgCl_2$, 1.0; $NaHCO_3$, 2.4; NaH_2PO_4, 0.5; Glucose, 11.0; $CaCl_2$, 2.4. The medium was gassed with 95:5 O_2/CO_2 gas mixture at 37.5°C. In the calcium-free perfusion medium, the 2.4 mM $CaCl_2$ was omitted. Care was taken to avoid calcium contamination of the calcium-free medium, by inclusion of 0.1 mmol/l of the disodium salt of ethylene diamino tetra-acetic acid (EDTA) in the medium. 0.1 mmol/l EDTA was also included in the calcium containing perfusion medium but this had been prechelated with equimolar quantities of $CaCl_2$ before inclusion.

Protocol

Calcium Paradox

The hearts from rat or guinea-pig were perfused at a temperature of 37.5°C and at a constant pressure of 75 cm H_2O. All hearts were initially perfused for a stabilisation period of 30 minutes, afterwhich the hearts were exposed to 20 minutes calcium-free perfusion and then reperfused with their original perfusion medium for 10 minutes.

Ischaemia/Reperfusion

Rats

In this series of experiments the rat hearts were perfused using a constant flow system. The flow during the 30 minute equilibration period was maintained at 8.0 ml/min with a Watson-Marlow peristaltic pump. During the ischaemic period the flow was reduced to 5% (0.4 ml/min) maintained by a second pump (Pharmacia P1 peristaltic pump). The 5% low flow was continued for 30 minutes. Finally on reperfusion the flow was restored to 8.0 ml/min for 10 minutes.

Guinea-pigs

Two series of experiments have been completed. In the first, an ischaemic period of 30 minutes at 5% flow (i.e. normal flow 14 ml/min, ischaemia flow 0.7 ml/min) followed by 10 minutes reperfusion at 14 ml/min. In order to elicit more consistent injury to guinea-pigs hearts, it was necessary to use a more severe procedure. The guinea-pig hearts were initially perfused at a rate of 14.0 ml/min. During the ischaemic period, flow was halted completely for 1 hour. The hearts were then reperfused at 14.0 ml/min for 30 minutes.

Parameters Measured

In all experiments isometric tension was recorded via a Statham UC3 strain gauge attached by cotton to the apex of the left ventricle, the signal was recorded on an MX2 Lectromed recorder. The resting tension was set at 1 gram. Coronary flow was measured by collection and later analysed for its creatine kinase activity and its histamine content.

Creatine kinase was measured on an Abbot VP bichromatic autoanalyser, using SK&F Spinchem diagnostic reagents. This assay is based upon an enzymatically coupled assay (Oliver, 1955). Creatine Kinase (CK) is a cytosolic enzyme and its presence in the coronary perfusate is used in these experiments as an indication of the severity of damage the heart has undergone.

The histamine content of the coronary perfusate for the calcium paradox experiments was measured using a double-isotope radio-enzymatic assay (Gristwood, Lincoln, Owen and Smith, 1981). In brief, histamine was methylated to N-tele-methylhistamine in the presence of N-histamine methyl transferase, using S-adenosyl-6-[methyl-^{3}H]-methionine as the methyl donor. [U-^{14}C]-histamine was used to correct for efficiency of methylation and extraction. A modification of this assay, using the method of N-tele-methylhistamine extraction from the chloroform phase described by Keeling, Smith and Tipton (1984), was required to analyse the lower histamine content of the coronary perfusate of the ischaemia/reperfusion experiments.

RESULTS

Calcium Paradox

The procedure of calcium paradox led to severe cardiac damage in both rats and guinea-pigs. The release of creatine kinase into the coronary effluent was similar in both species; a cumulative release of approximately 2000 units/g dry weight of heart occurring within 10 minutes of reperfusion (Fig. 1).

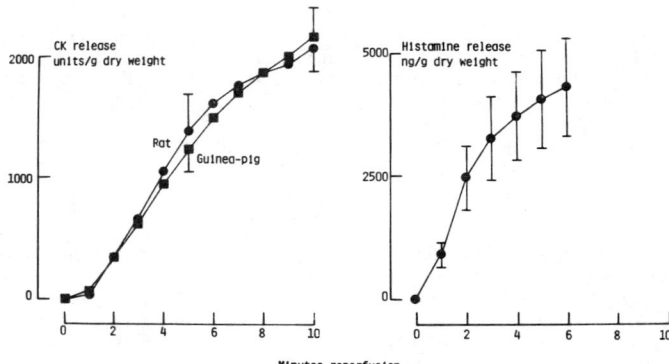

Fig. 1. Left: The cumulative release of creatine kinase (CK), during reperfusion with normal perfusion medium after a period of calcium-free perfusion (the calcium paradox), from rat (●) and guinea-pig (■) Langendorff heart preparations (n=3 and 6 respectively). Right: The cumulative release of histamine from rat hearts in response to the calcium paradox (n=4). Release of histamine from guinea-pig hearts in response to the calcium paradox (not shown) could only be detected in 2 out of 6 preparations. Means ± s.e.m. are indicated.

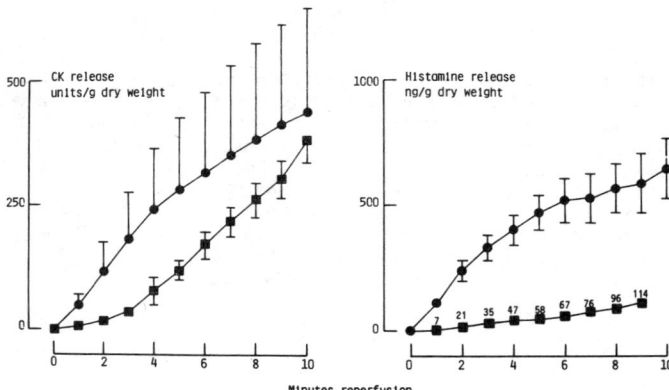

Fig. 2. Left: The cumulative release of CK, during reperfusion after a 30 min period ischaemia (5% flow), from rat (●) and guinea-pig (■) Langendorff heart preparations (n=6 and 3 respectively). Right: The cumulative release of histamine from rat (●) and guinea-pig (■) hearts on reperfusion, after the ischaemia described above (n=6 and 3 respectively); release of histamine from guinea-pig hearts was at the limits of detection of the histamine assay. Means ± s.e.m. are indicated.

In rat hearts, the calcium paradox injury led to consistent release of histamine into coronary effluent cumulative release approximately 5 µg/g dry weight of heart (Fig. 1). In guinea-pig hearts, consistent evidence of histamine release could be obtained in one preparation only with sporadic evidence of histamine detected in a further heart. In 4 of the 6 preparations, no histamine could be detected in the coronary effluent at any time after reperfusion with calcium.

Ischaemia/reperfusion

A period of ischaemia, 5% flow for 30 minutes, elicited moderate cardiac injury, as assessed by release of creatine kinase into the coronary effluent, in both rats and guinea-pigs (Fig. 2). In rat hearts, this injury was associated with release of histamine into the coronary effluent, total cumulative release approximately 500 ng/g dry weight (Fig. 2). In guinea-pig hearts, trace quantities of histamine could be detected in all coronary samples on reperfusion, although the concentrations measured were very close to the limits of detection and should be judged as semi-quantitative measurements.

In guinea-pig hearts, a more severe procedure was additionally employed (no flow for 60 minutes followed by reperfusion). This procedure caused consistent release of histamine into the coronary effluent on reperfusion after the no flow procedure.

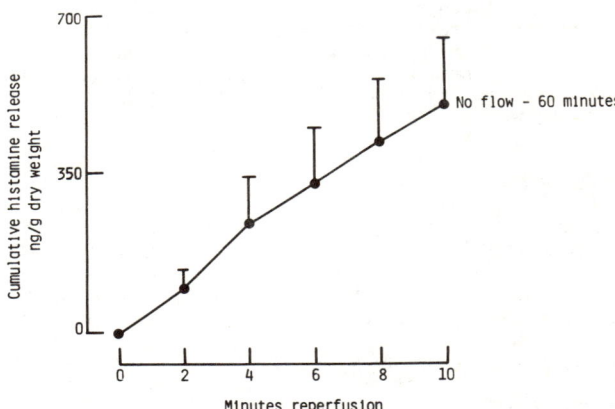

Fig. 3. The cumulative release of histamine into the coronary effluent during reperfusion after a 60 minute period of no-flow in the guinea-pig Langendorff heart preparation (n=3). Mean ± s.e.m. are indicated.

DISCUSSION

Cardiac damage is known to release a range of cardio-active agents e.g. arachidonic acid metabolites (Block, Poole and Vane, 1974; Wennmalm, Chanh and Junstad, 1974; Sakai, Ito and Ogawa, 1982) catecholamines (Wollenberger and Shahab, 1965; Rochette and colleagues, 1980). The present studies provide evidence that cardiac damage additionally causes release of myocardial histamine although there are clear quantitative differences in the coronary histamine content following cardiac injury in rats and guinea-pigs. Previous studies had shown release of myocardial histamine by known mast cell degrangulation procedures e.g. anaphylaxis (Levi and Guo, 1982).

The procedures of calcium paradox and ischaemia followed by reperfusion have been used to assess the potential benefits of agents in the treatment of cardiac dysfunction (Nayler, 1980; Ashraf and colleagues, 1982; Jolly, Menahan and Gross, 1981) and are considered to be useful experimental model of myocardial injury. The demonstration that these procedures release myocardial histamine, implies that this cardioactive amine must also be considered as a factor which might influence myocardial function following injury.

The clear difference in histamine release measured as coronary sinus histamine content may reflect differences in the release of histamine by injury in these species. An alternative explanation may be suggested by the observation that the guinea-pig heart and its microvasculature has a very high histamine metabolising capacity which substantially exceeds that of the rat heart (Robinson-White and Beaven, 1982). It may be that release of histamine by cardiac injury is similar in both species but that the guinea-pig heart is able to metabolise this histamine prior to appearance in the coronary effluent whereas the lesser metabolic capacity of the rat heart allows ready detection of coronary histamine content.

Histamine produces major changes in cardiac function in man (Eckel and colleagues, 1982; Gristwood, Lincoln and Owen, 1980). The evidence that myocardial injury causes release of histamine implies that this amine should be considered as one of the endogenous cardioactive mediators released and which may influence cardiac function following myocardial injury. Studies are currently in progress to try to establish the role of histamine in the functioning of the injured heart.

REFERENCES

Ashraf, M., M. Onda, Y. Hirohata, and A. Schwartz (1982). Therapeutic effect of diltiazem on myocardial cell injury during the calcium paradox. J. Mol. Cell. Cardiol., 14, 323-327.
Apstein, C. S., L. Deckelbaum, M. Mueller, L. Hogopian, and W. B. Hood (1977). Graded global ischaemia and reperfusion: Cardiac function and metabolism. Circulation, 55, 864-872.
Block, A. J., S. Poole, and J. R. Vane (1974). Modification of basal release of prostaglandins from rabbit isolated hearts. Prostaglandins, 7, 473-486.
Eckel, L., R. W. Gristwood, H. Nawrath, D. A. A. Owen, and P. Satter (1982). Inotropic and electrophysiological effects of histamine on human ventricular heart muscle. J. Physiol., 330, 111-123.
Gristwood, R. W., J. C. R. Lincoln, and D. A. A. Owen (1980). Effects of histamine on human isolated heart muscle: Comparison of effects with noradrenaline. J. Pharm. Pharmacol., 32, 145-146.
Gristwood, R. W., J. C. R. Lincoln, D. A. A. Owen, and I. R. Smith (1981). Histamine release from human right atrium. Br. J. Pharmacol., 74, 7-8.
Hearse, D. J., S. M. Humphrey and G. R. Bullock (1978). The oxygen paradox and the paradox: Two facets of the same problem. J. Mol. Cell. Cardiol., 10, 641-668.
Horakova, Z., and M. A. Beaven (1974). Time course of histamine release and oedema formation in the rat paw after thermal injury. Eur. J. Pharmacol., 27, 305-312.
Jolly, S. R., L. A. Menahan, and G. J. Gross (1981). Diltiazem in myocardial recovery from global ischaemia and reperfusion. J. Mol. Cell. Cardiol., 13, 359-372.

Keeling, D. J., I. R. Smith, and K. F. Tipton (1984). A coupled assay for histidine decarboxylase: in vivo turnover of this enzyme in mouse brain. Naunyn-Schmiedeberg's Arch. Pharmacol., 326, 215-221.

Levi, R., and Z. Guo (1982). Roles of histamine and cardiac dysfunction. In: B. Uvnas and K. Tasaka (Eds). Advances in histamine research. (Advances in Biosciences vol. 33), 213-322, Pergamon Press.

Mannaioni, P. F. (1972). Physiology and pharmacology of cardiac histamine. Arch. Int. Pharmacodyn. Ther., 196, Supplement, 64-78.

Markley, K., Z. Horakova, E. T. Smallman, and M. A. Beaven (1975). The role of histamine in burn, tourniquet and endotoxin shock in mice. Eur. J. Pharmacol., 33, 255-265.

McNeill, J. H. (1982). Cardiac histamine receptors: Species and regional differences. In: B. Uvnas and K. Tasaka (Eds). Advances in histamine research. (Advances in Biosciences, vol. 33), 233-242, Pergamon Press.

Nayler, W. G. (1980). The pharmacological protection of the ischaemic heart: The use of calcium and beta-adrenoceptor antagonists. Eur. Heart J., 1, (supplement B), 5-13.

Oliver, I. (1955). A spectrophotometric method for the determination of creatine phosphokinase and myokinase. Biochem. J., 61, 116-122.

Robinson-White, A., M. A. Beaven (1982). Presence of histamine and histamine metabolising enzymes in rat and guinea-pig microvascular endothelial cells. J. Pharmacol. Exp. Ther., 223, 440-445.

Rochette, L., J. P. Didier, D. Moreau, and J. Bralet (1980). Effect of substrate on release of myocardial norepinephrine and ventricular arrhythmias following reperfusion of the ischemic isolated working rat heart. J. Cardiovasc. Pharmacol., 2, 267-279.

Sakai, K., J. Ito, and K. Ogawa (1982). Role of endogenous prostacyclin and thromboxane A_2 in the ischemic canine heart. J. Cardiovasc. Pharmacol., 4, 129-135.

Wennmalm, A., P. H. Chanh, and M. Junstad (1974). Hypoxia causes prostaglandin release from perfused rabbit hearts. Acta Physiol. Scand., 91, 133-135.

Wollenberger, A., and L. Shahab (1965). Anoxia-induced release of noradrenaline from the isolated perfused heart. Nature, 207, 88-89.

HISTAMINE MODULATION OF CARDIAC SYMPATHETIC RESPONSES

S. S. Gross and R. Levi

Department of Pharmacology, Cornell University Medical College, 1300 York Avenue, New York, NY 10021, USA

ABSTRACT

We have found that histamine attenuates the increases in contractility, heart rate and coronary resistance evoked by stellate ganglion stimulation in the isolated guinea pig heart. This modulatory effect occurs with low concentrations of histamine ($< 3 \times 10^{-7}$M) relative to that necessary to elicit direct cardiac actions. Two lines of evidence indicate that the modulatory effect of histamine involves a postjunctional action: 1) histamine is equipotent in its attenuation of responses elicited by either sympathetic nerve stimulation or intracardiac administration of norepinephrine, and 2) histamine does not depress the sympathetic nerve stimulation-evoked release of norepinephrine from the heart. Pharmacological analysis suggests that the sympathetic modulatory action of histamine is mediated by an H_2-receptor. The physiological relevance of these findings is suggested by our observation that significant quantities of histamine are released following sympathetic nerve stimulation. The magnitude of nerve stimulation-evoked histamine release is frequency-dependent and may be subject to autoinhibition since the H_2-blocker tiotidine enhances histamine overflow 3-fold. We have also found that cardiac responses to sympathetic stimulation are potentiated and/or prolonged in the presence of tiotidine. Our findings suggest that histamine may play a physiological role in the modulation of cardiac sympathetic responses.

KEYWORDS

Histamine Release; Sympathetic Modulation; Cardiac Histamine; Cardiac Function; Histamine: Cardiac Effects; Tiotidine

INTRODUCTION

An intimate anatomical relationship between mast cells and sympathetic nerves has been observed in vascular tissue (Dzielak et al, 1983). In the heart, the distribution of histamine parallels that of norepinephrine (Giotti et al, 1966). Furthermore, cardiac sympathetic nerves contain histamine in very high concentrations (von Euler, 1966; Ryan and Brody, 1970, and 1972). Recognition of the association between histamine and sympathetic nerves has prompted several investigators to assess whether histamine may modulate noradrenergic responses in cardiovascular tissues. Accordingly, histamine has been found to reduce the field stimulation-induced efflux of radioactivity from (^{3}H)-norepinephrine preloaded guinea pig atrial tissue (Rand et al, 1982), dog saphenous vein and tibial artery (McGrath and Shepherd, 1976). These studies suggest that histamine attenuates responses to sympathetic nerve stimulation by a pre-junctional mechanism of action whereby norepinephrine release is reduced. This effect appears to be mediated by H_2-receptors. Consistent with an action on norepinephrine release, histamine inhibits the positive chronotropic response to right cardiac sympathetic nerve stimulation in the dog, but not the tachycardia obtained with intravenous norepinephrine administration (Lockhandwala, 1978; Kimura and Satoh, 1983). Similarly, histamine inhibits the vasoconstrictor response to sympathetic stimulation in the isolated gracilis muscle of the dog, but not the response elicited by the administration of norepinephrine (Powell, 1979). Although all of these observations indicate that histamine may modulate sympathetic activity by a pre-junctional mechanism, histamine also inhibits responses elicited by exogenously administered norepinephrine in the dog hindpaw (Powell, 1979). Therefore, in addition to a pre-junctional action, a post-junctional action has been implicated for histamine's attenuation of sympathetic responses. Whether any of these effects of histamine occur under physiological conditions remains to be established.

A major interest of our laboratory has been to elucidate cardiovascular dysfunctions caused by histamine in a variety of pathophysiological conditions (Levi and Allan, 1980; Levi et al,1982a and 1982b). Our recent finding that significant quantities of histamine are co-released with norepinephrine following cardiac sympathetic nerve stimulation (Guo et al., 1983; Gross et al., 1984a and 1984b) has led us to consider the intriguing possibility that histamine may also participate in the normal physiological control of the heart. To test this hypothesis, we have used as a model the spontaneously beating guinea pig heart (Langendorff preparation), isolated with its sympathetic innervation intact. This preparation allows one to measure physiological responses elicited by direct nerve stimulation, concomitant with the release of endogenous transmitter.

ATTENUATION OF CARDIAC SYMPATHETIC RESPONSES BY HISTAMINE

Cardiac sympathetic nerve stimulation causes frequency-dependent increases in left ventricular contractile force (LVCF), heart rate (HR) and coronary resistance (perfusion pressure, PP). Intracardiac histamine administration causes increases in contractility and rate and a decrease in coronary resistance. Thus, the responses of the heart to histamine are in the same direction as (LVCF and HR), or in opposition (PP) to, the responses elicited by sympathetic nerve stimulation. However, cardiac perfusion with 3×10^{-7}M histamine, a dose which has little effect on the heart, greatly attenuates the responses elicited by sympathetic nerve stimulation (fig. 1). This attenuation of sympathetic responses is rapidly reversed following histamine washout. The time course of responses elicited by stimulation of cardiac sympathetic nerves, in the absence or presence of 3×10^{-7}M histamine, is shown in fig. 2. Although histamine causes a significant depression of the 3 sympathetic responses monitored (i.e., LVCF, HR and PP), it does not significantly alter the release of norepinephrine into the coronary effluent (norepinephrine overflow, NEO). This is surprising because other laboratories have reported that histamine attenuates adrenergic responses by an inhibition of norepinephrine release, i.e., by a pre-junctional mechanism. We questioned whether our inability to detect a decrease in stimulation-evoked norepinephrine release in the presence of histamine may have resulted from norepinephrine losses by reuptake (uptake$_1$ and uptake$_2$) and catabolism. However, even when stimulation-evoked norepinephrine overflow was increased 9-fold by blockade of reuptake (uptake$_1$ with desmethylimipramine 10^{-7} M and uptake$_2$ with 10^{-5} M hydrocortisone), and by antagonism of the auto-inhibition of norepinephrine release (with 10^{-7} M yohimbine), histamine potently depressed the response of the heart to sympathetic stimulation, yet, it did not reduce NEO (Gross et al., 1984a).

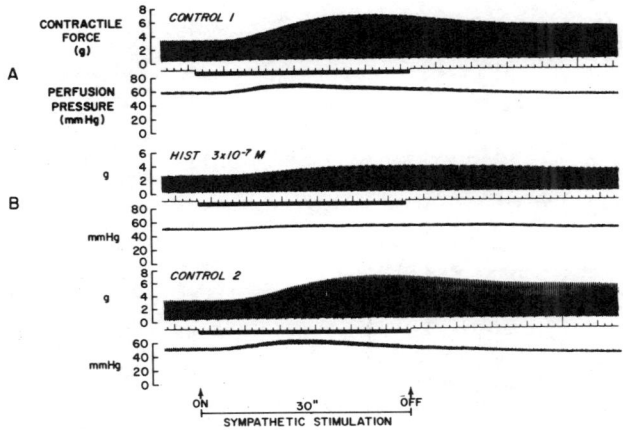

Fig. 1. Effect of histamine on responses of the isolated guinea pig heart to sympathetic nerve stimulation.
A typical recording is displayed which shows the changes in left ventricular contractile force and perfusion pressure in response to sympathetic stimulation at 8 Hz for 30 seconds: (panel A) control stimulation; (panel B) stimulation in the presence of histamine; (panel C) control stimulation following histamine washout. Fifteen-minute intervals were provided for recovery between successive stimulation periods.

Since auto-inhibition of norepinephrine release occurs preferentially at low frequencies of nerve stimulation (Yamaguchi et al., 1977), we investigated whether the same might be true for histamine (Gross et al., 1984a). We found that histamine is a potent inhibitor of cardiac sympathetic responses also at lower frequencies of stimulation (i.e. 2 and 4 Hz). Nonetheless, histamine did not significantly reduce NEO at any stimulation frequency tested.
Our inability to attribute the attenuation of cardiac sympathetic responses by histamine to a pre-junctional action, as we had originally expected, led us to test the alternate possibility, i.e., that histamine acts post-junctionally. We found that, in analogy to its action on nerve stimulation-evoked responses, histamine also attenuated the increases in LVCF, HR and PP when elicited by the intracardiac administration of norepinephrine. Indeed, the dose-response relationships for histamine-induced modulation of cardiac responses, either to sympathetic nerve stimulation or to administered norepinephrine, are virtually identical (fig. 3). We conclude, therefore, that histamine modulates cardiac sympathetic responses by a post-junctional action, i.e., an action on the heart and not on the nerve.

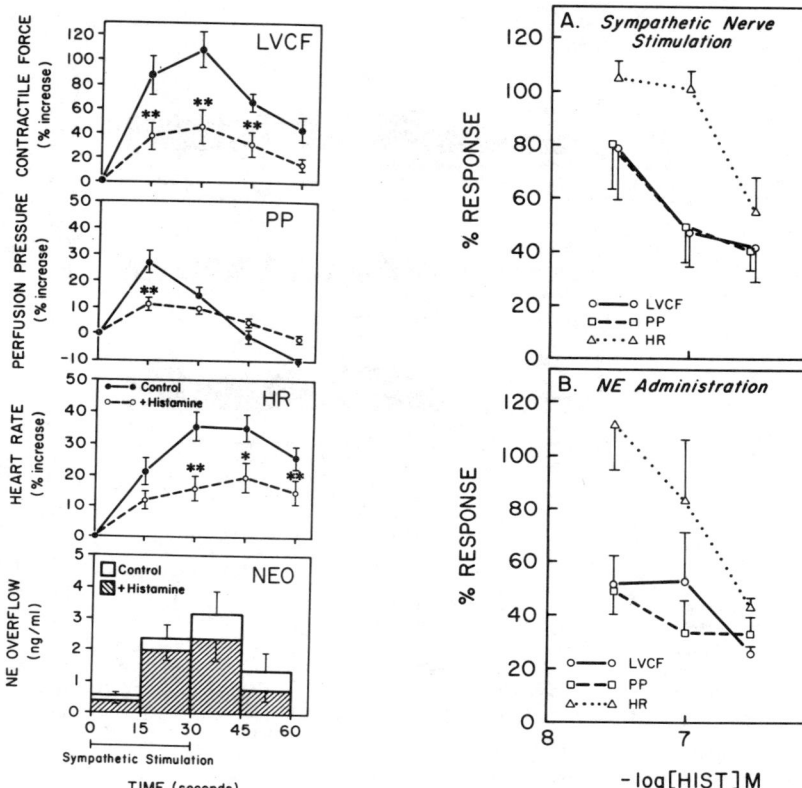

Fig. 2. Time course of stimulation-induced responses and norepinephrine overflow in isolated guinea pig hearts in the absence or presence of histamine. Maximum increases in left ventricular contractile force (LVCF), coronary perfusion pressure (PP), heart rate (HR), and norepinephrine overflow (NEO) were recorded during four consecutive 15-second intervals commencing with nerve stimulation (8 Hz; 30 sec), in control preparations (closed circles) or in the presence of 3×10^{-7} M histamine (open circles). Before stimulation, LVCF, HR, and PP were 3.3 ± 0.3 g, 209 ± 6 beats/min, and 52.6 ± 4.4 mm Hg, respectively. Points and bars represent means ($\pm$SEM) of 4-6 experiments.*,** = significant depression of responses by histamine at the 0.05 and 0.01 level, respectively, as determined by paired t-test.

Fig. 3. Dose-response relationship for histamine-induced attenuation of adrenergic responses. Adrenergic responses

were elicited by sympathetic nerve stimulation at 8 Hz for
30 seconds (panel A) and by direct cardiac administration
of 160 ng NE (panel B). Maximum increases in LVCF
(circles), PP (squares), and HR (triangles) in the absence
of histamine are taken as control (=100%).
Changes elicited by 3×10^{-7} M histamine prior to
stimulation were +26.4±12.6%, -23.5±5.3%, and +12.5±5.1%
for LVCF, PP, And HR, respectively (mean ± SEM). Points
are the mean changes (± SEM, n = 6) from control induced by
histamine at the indicated concentrations.

That histamine-induced modulation of sympathetic responses is mediated by an
H_2-receptor is suggested by the observation that dimaprit, a selective
H_2-agonist mimics the action of histamine while the selective H_2-antagonist
tiotidine inhibits it (Gross et al., 1984a and 1984b). Furthermore, the
H_1-antagonist mepyramine has little effect on histamine's sympathetic modulatory
effect (Gross and Levi, unpublished data).

RELEASE OF CARDIAC HISTAMINE BY SYMPATHETIC NERVE STIMULATION

A physiological relevance for the modulatory action of histamine is suggested by
our finding that significant quantities of histamine, are released from the heart
following sympathetic nerve stimulation. Thus, a stimulation frequency of 8 Hz
results in an approximate 4-fold increase over the basal level of histamine in the
coronary effluent. Whereas the concentration of norepinephrine in the coronary
effluent increases significantly during a 30-second period of nerve stimulation,
histamine does not increase until the 30-second period following cessation of
stimulation. Thus, the overflow of norepinephrine from the
sympathetically-stimulated heart occurs prior to that of histamine. This
observation suggests the possibility that norepinephrine may serve as the trigger
for histamine release. Indeed, like sympathetic stimulation, the administration
of a bolus injection of norepinephrine to the heart (160 ng) elicits the release
of endogenous cardiac histamine (fig. 5). Thus, we hypothesize that
neurally-released norepinephrine may trigger the release of histamine, which may
then attenuate norepinephrine-mediated cardiac responses.

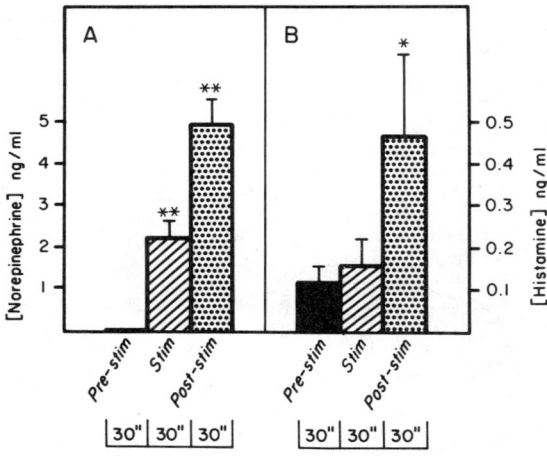

Fig. 4. Sympathetic nerve stimulation-induced overflow of

NE and histamine into the coronary perfusate of isolated guinea pig hearts. Endogenous NE (panel A) and histamine (panel B) were assayed in the perfusate before, during, and after a 30-second period of nerve stimulation at a frequency of 8 Hz. Values represent the mean concentration obtained (± SEM) with n = 6 for NE and n = 9 for histamine. *P<0.05 and **P<0.01 indicate a significant increase in concentration with respect to prestimulation levels.

The release of cardiac histamine increases with increasing frequencies of sympathetic nerve stimulation (fig. 6). Most interesting is our finding that H_2-receptor blockade may further enhance histamine release evoked by sympathetic stimulation. Whereas 100 nM tiotidine has no effect on norepinephrine overflow, it causes a 3-fold increase in histamine release by 2 Hz nerve stimulation (fig 6). This suggests that histamine release may be subject to auto-regulation, perhaps by a mechanism analogous to that described for norepinephrine (Starke, 1977; Westfall, 1977). The site from which histamine is released and verification of an auto-regulatory mechanism awaits further investigation.

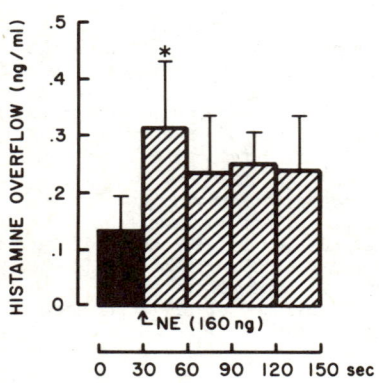
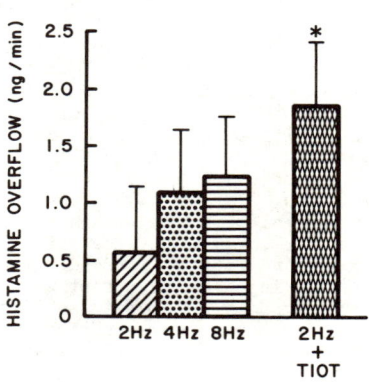

Fig. 5. Norepinephrine-induced release of endogenous cardiac histamine. Langendorff guinea pig hearts were perfused with Krebs solution at constant flow (4 ml/min). At the indicated time, a bolus dose of 160 ng norepinephrine was administered intraaortically. Bars represent the mean histamine concentration ± SEM (n = 10), present in the cardiac effluent during a given 30-second interval. *Indicates a significant increase in histamine release at the 0.05 level.

Fig. 6. Effect of sympathetic nerve stimulation frequency and tiotidine on cardiac histamine release. Sympathetic nerves were stimulated at the indicated frequency for a period of 30 seconds in the absence or presence of 100 nM tiotidine. Bars represent the mean concentration of histamine ± SEM present in the coronary effluent (n = 6-10), collected during a 60-second interval commencing with nerve stimulation. *Indicates a significant increase in histamine release with tiotidine when compared to nerve stimulation in its absence.

Although histamine is released following cardiac sympathetic nerve stimulation, to substantiate a physiological role for histamine it is necessary to demonstrate that its concentration at the receptor site is sufficient to attenuate the responses to neurally released norepinephrine. In an attempt to address this issue, we have studied the time course of cardiac responses to sympathetic stimulation in the presence of concentrations of an H_2-receptor antagonist which eliminate histamine's attenuation of cardiac responses (Gross et al, 1984a). If nerve stimulation releases enough histamine to attenuate cardiac sympathetic responses, the response of the heart to sympathetic stimulation should be potentiated and/or prolonged in the presence of the antihistamine. Indeed, we found that tiotidine prolongs the increases in LVCF and PP, as well as prolongs and potentiates the increase in HR (Gross et al, 1984a). These findings provide evidence that nerve stimulation may release sufficient quantities of histamine to attenuate sympathetic responses.

CONCLUSIONS

Our results demonstrate that histamine: a) is released upon cardiac sympathetic nerve stimulation, b) attenuates cardiac sympathetic responses via a post-junctional mechanism and c) may modulate its own release. Moreover, evidence has been provided that these phenomena occur under normal physiological conditions. Thus, our findings suggest that histamine may play a role in the normal regulation of cardiac responses to sympathetic nerve stimulation.

ACKNOWLEDGEMENTS

Figures 1-4 of this communication were reproduced from Gross et al. (1984a) by permission of the American Heart Association, Inc. This research was supported by NIH grants GM 20091 and HL 18828, and by a fellowship from the New York Association. We also wish to acknowledge the invaluable technical assistance of Dr. A.A. Chenouda and the excellent secretarial skills of Ms. Claudia B. Gross.

REFERENCES

Dzielak, D.J., A. Thureson-Klein, and R.L. Klein (1983). Blood Vessels, 20, 122-134.
von Euler, U.S. (1966). In M. Rocha e Silva (Ed.), Histamine and Anti-Histamines, Springer-Verlag, New York. pp. 318-333.
Giotti, A., A. Guidotti, P.F. Mannaioni, and L. Zilletti (1966). J. Physiol., 184, 924-941.
Gross, S.S., Z.-G. Guo, R. Levi, W.H. Bailey, and A.A. Chenouda (1984). Circ. Res., 54, 516-526.
Gross, S.S., R. Levi, W.H. Bailey, and A.A. Chenouda (1984). Fed. Proc., 43, 458.
Guo, Z.-G., S.S. Gross, R. Levi, and W.H. Bailey (1983). Fed. Proc., 42, 907.
Kimura, T., and S. Satoh (1983). Br. J. Pharmacol, 78, 733-738.
Levi, R., And G. Allan (1980). In M. Bristow (Ed.), Drug-Induced Heart Disease, Elsevier-North Holland Biomedical Press, Amsterdam, pp. 377-395.
Levi, R., J.A. Burke, and E.J. Corey (1982). In B. Samuelsson and R. Paoletti (Eds.), Adv. Prostagl. Thrombox. Leukotr. Res., Vol. 9, Raven Press, New York. pp. 215-222.
Levi, R., A.A. Chenouda, J. Trzeciakowski, Z.-G. Guo, L.M. Aaronson, R.D. Luskind, C.-H. Lee, W.A. Gay, V.A. Subramanian, J.C. McCabe, and J.C. Alexander (1982). Klin. Wochenschr., 60, 965-971.
Lokhandwala, M.F. (1978). J. Pharmacol. Exp. Ther., 206, 115-122.

McGrath, M.A., and J.T. Shepherd (1976). *Circ. Res.*, 39, 566-573.
Powell, J.R. (1979). *J. Pharmacol. Exp. Ther.*, 208, 360-365.
Rand, M.J., D.F. Storey, and H.K. Wong-Dusting (1982). *Br. J. Pharmacol.*, 75, 57-64.
Ryan, M.J., and M.J. Brody (1970). *J. Pharmacol. Exp. Ther.*, 174, 123-132.
Ryan, M.J., and M.J. Brody (1972). *J. Pharmacol. Exp. Ther.*, 181, 83-91.
Starke, K. (1977). *Rev. Physiol. Biochem. Pharmac.*, 77, 1-124.
Westfall, P.C. (1977). *Physiol. Rev.*, 57, 659-728.

A NEW THERAPEUTIC APPROACH IN CONGESTIVE HEART FAILURE: COMBINED PHOSPHODIESTERASE-INHIBITION WITH SIMULTANEOUS H_2-RECEPTOR STIMULATION

G. Baumann, D. Mercader, B. Permanetter,
U. Busch, K. Ningel, A. Wirtzfeld and H. Blömer

1st Department of Medicine, Klinikum rechts der Isar,
Technical University of Munich,
Federal Republic of Germany

ABSTRACT

The highly selective H_2-receptor agonist impromidine (IMP) proved to be a marked positive-inotropic compound for treatment of catecholamine-insensitive heart failure. ARL-115 BS, in contrast, is generally accepted as a potent phosphodiesterase inhibitor. The aim of the present study was to clarify whether the positive-inotropic effect of IMP and dobutamine (DOB) could be potentiated by ARL-115 BS. Results: In the isolated guinea pig heart the dose-response curve for IMP on LV_{dP}/dt starts at 5×10^{-11} moles reaching its peak response at 2×10^{-9} moles. In the presence of ARL-115 BS in a concentration which per se lead to an average increase of cardiac contractile parameters by 50%, the dose-response curve for IMP was significantly shifted to the left by more than one order of magnitude. A similar effect was observed for selective ß-receptor stimulation by DOB in normal hearts. - In 8 patients with congestive cardiomyopathy DOB increased cardiac output by 25% with no significant effect on pulmonary artery pressure, wedge pressure as well as right and left heart filling pressures. In the presence of ARL-115 BS there was a significant improvement of all contractile parameters. IMP induced a 200-300% increase in cardiac output and normalisation of all pressures at a dose of 40µg/kg/h. In the presence of ARL-115 BS comparable improvement of all above parameters was achieved at only 5-10µg/kg/h. After a 5 days period of treatment with either IMP or ARL-115 BS + IMP there was a marked increase (+65%) in ß-receptor-mediated contractile response of the heart to dobutamine indicating a partial recovery of the ß-adrenoceptor stimulation mechanism.- These results suggest that combined therapy with ARL-115 BS and IMP or DOB may be a new therapeutic approach in congestive heart failure especially in view of a long-term treatment to prevent development of "down-regulation" of cardiac H_2- and $ß_1$-receptors induced by IMP and DOB.

KEYWORDS

Congestive cardiomyopathy; H_2-receptor; $ß_1$-receptors; adenylate cyclase; phosphodiesterase; theophylline; ARL-115 BS; tachyphyllaxis; receptor down regulation; catecholamines.

INTRODUCTION

Myocardial contractility is under the regulatory control of the adrenergic nervous system. Meanwhile there is striking evidence suggesting that remarkable changes in cardiac contractility and myocardial metabolism occur in diverse heart diseases causally involving a considerable impairment of the ß-adrenergic stimulation mechanism (Baumann et al., 1980, 1981a,b,c, 1982, 1983a; Bristow et al.,1982; Colucci et al., 1981; Lehmann et al., 1981; Thomas and Marks, 1978). Recent reports from our department (Baumann et al., 1980, 1981a,b,c, 1982, 1983a,b) indicate that in the non-ischemic surviving myocardium a pronounced specific impairment of the ß-adrenergic stimulation mechanism concerning sympathetic stimulation of cardiac contractility and adenylate cyclase activity occurrs in the whole surviving myocardium after coronary occlusion. These effects have been shown to be most likely the result of a decreased number of sarcolemmal ß-receptors induced by increased levels of circulating catecholamines following acute myocardial infarction. In contrast to this, the response to histamine which is known to act via specific H_2-receptors was found to be essentially unaltered in the same hearts. The development of specific histaminergic agonists which selectively activate H_2-receptors devoid of the well-known disadvantageous side effects of histamine (presumably H_1-receptor-mediated side effects) led us to investigate the positive-inotropic effects in the catecholamine-insensitive surviving myocardium after coronary occlusion (Baumann et al., 1981c, 1982, 1983b). In these studies the H_2-receptor agonist IMP turn out to be an effective potent stimulator of cardiac contractile force in hearts which were refractory to indirect and direct sympathetic stimulation with tyramine and isoprenaline, respectively.

The present contribution aimed to characterize the functional status of the ß-adrenoceptor stimulation mechanism in patients with class IV congestive cardiomyopathy. In addition the hemodynamic effects of the H_2-receptor agonist IMP were evaluated in the same patients and compared to the DOB-mediated positive-inotropic action. Furthermore, we intended to elucidate whether a simultaneous phosphodiesterase inhibition by ARL-115 BS or theophylline is capable to potentiate the inotropic action of IMP and DOB.

METHODS

Patients

Twenty one consecutive patients (age 24-70 years) fulfilling the entry criteria were studied in the coronary care unit. In these patients the existence of coronary artery disease and valve disorders was excluded by clinical examination and heart catheterisation including coronary angiography prior to IMP treatment. The cardiac serum enzymes, serum electrolytes, blood coagulation status and urea as well as serum creatinine were determined every 12 hours. On admission to the study all patients were in regular sinus rhythm and without severe hypotension. All of them were on diuretic treatment (furosemide or etacrynic acid). On admission, 17 of them received digitalis, none of them had received catecholamines or opiates within 24 hours prior to the study. A written consent was obtained from each patient or his nearest relatives and the study was agreed by the Ethic Committee of the Technical University of Munich. For further details see Baumann et al., 1984.

RESULTS

Hemodynamic effects of impromidine and dobutamine in 21 patients with class IV congestive cardiomyopathy

In order to characterize the in vivo effects of an H_2-receptor stimulation in man a clinical trial with IMP was undertaken in patients with catecholamine-insensitive heart failure due to stage IV congestive cardiomyopathy. IMP was applied in different concentrations (infusion rates 20-60µg/kg/hr) and the hemodynamic effects compared to those of a maximal dose of the ß-adrenoceptor agonist DOB (up to 900 µg/kg/hr). As can be seen from Fig. 1, dobutamine only weekly increased cardiac output in 5 patients and was without any significant effect in the others. A similar lack of effect could be established for pulmonary capillary wedge pressure which decreased in only 4 patients whereas it remained unchanged in the others. In contrast to this however, IMP induced a considerable increase in cardiac output and a drastic decrease in pulmonary artery wedge pressure (Fig. 2), though the degree of the IMP-induced hemodynamic changes varied considerably at the different concentrations. Concommittant with these findings there was a decrease in right atrial pressure, pulmonary systolic, diastolic and mean pressure and a decrease in

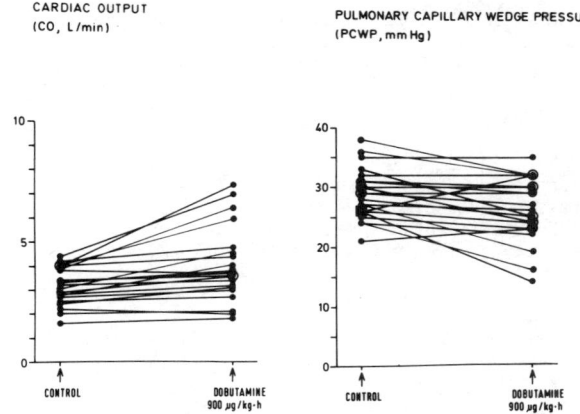

Fig. 1. Hemodynamic effects of dobutamine in 21 patients with congestive cardiomyopathy.

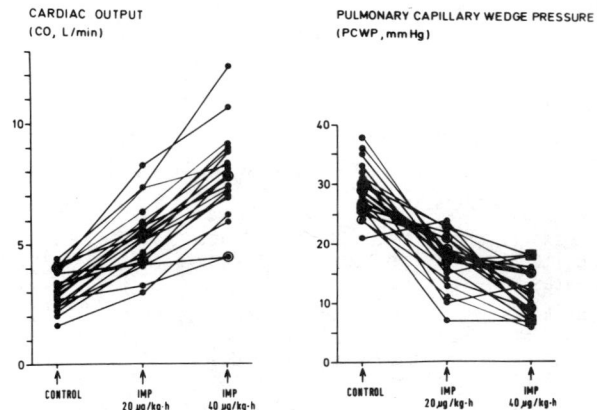

Fig. 2. Hemodynamic effects of impromidine in the same patients.

systemic arterial blood pressure as well as systemic vascular resistance, whereas heart rate remained unchanged (Table 1). The latter results suggest that the hemodynamic in vivo effects of IMP are of a more complex nature and not only based upon the direct positive-inotropic effect of this compound.

Effect of long-term stimulation with impromidine on myocardial responsiveness to H_2-receptor stimulation

Of course the question arises for how long such an H_2-receptor stimulation remains effective. Up to date the longest stimulation period with IMP in patients was 5 days and we noticed a loss of sensitivity by nearly 20% thereafter. Therefore we checked the efficacy of such an H_2-receptor stimulation in the guinea pig for periods of up to 14 days with 4 different infusion rates.

It is obvious from Fig. 3 that application of IMP at a dose of 10 µg/kg/hr (upper curve) did not alter sensitivity of the heart even after 14 days. In contrast, there was a considerable loss of sensitivity to H_2-receptor stimulation if IMP was ad-

TABLE 1 Hemodynamic effects of IMP in 21 patients with congestive cardiomyopathy
         (For details see text)

	Control	IMP
RA (mm Hg)	13.8 ± 3.2	5.5 ± 1.8 *
PA syst./diast. (mm Hg)	55.1 ± 8.3/27.5 ± 3.4	23.6 ± 7.2/14.9 ± 3.2 **
PCWP (mm Hg)	29.4 ± 5.1	14.4 ± 4.8 **
MABP (mm Hg)	85 ± 7	70 ± 4 *
CI (L/min/m^2)	1.8 ± 0.9	4.5 ± 2.3 **
TPAR (dyne s cm^{-5}/m^2)	3625 ± 375	1178 ± 428 **

Statistically different from controls: *p< 0.05, **p< 0.01. Mean values ± SD.
RA=right atrial pressure, PA=pulmonary artery pressure, PCWP=pulmonary capillary wedge pressure, MABP=arterial blood pressure, CI=cardiac index, TPAR=total peripheral arterial resistance. IMP=impromidine (40 μg/kg/h).

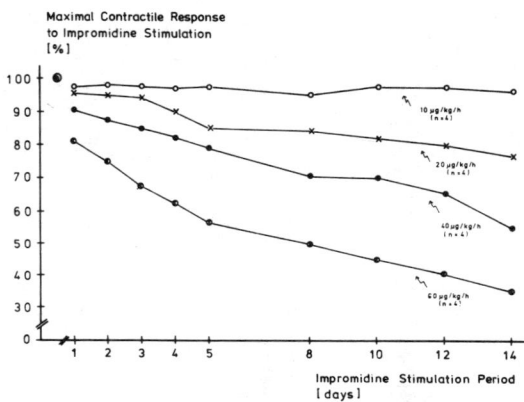

Fig. 3. Loss of cardiac response to IMP after continuous H_2-receptor stimulation for periods up to 14 days and 4 different infusion rates.

ministered at 20 and 40 with a maximal loss of response by nearly 70% after 2 weeks, if 60 μg/kg/hr IMP were continuously applied. This clearly indicates that continuous infusion of IMP definitely leads to a dose- and time-dependent specific damage or desensitization of cardiac H_2-receptors.

Effect of the phosphodiesterase inhibitor ARL-115 BS on position and sloap of dose-response curves for IMP and DOB on contractile parameter of the isolated perfused guinea pig heart.

In view of the rapid desensitization of cardiac H_2-receptors by continuous infusion of IMP it seems of interest to investigate whether the cyclic-AMP-mediated positive-inotropic effect of IMP could be further enhanced by simultaneous application of ARL-115 BS, a potent phosphodiesterase inhibitor, thereby preventing degradation of cyclic-AMP. In order to examine this hypothesis the hemodynamic effect of IMP and isoprenaline in the presence and absence of ARL-115 BS were evaluated in the isolated perfused guinea pig heart. As can be seen from Fig. 4 the dose response curve for IMP in the presence of ARL-115 BS is shifted to the left. Stimulation of left ventricular dp/dt begins at 4×10^{-11} and reaches a maximum at 4×10^{-9} moles. In the presence of ARL-115 BS the dose response curve on left ventricular dp/dt begins at 4×10^{-11} and plateaus at 4×10^{-10} moles. Comparing the EC_{50} values this means, that the dose response curve for IMP is shifted to the left by nearly one order of magnitude. This implies that the concentration of IMP can be reduced to 1/10th in the presence of ARL-115 BS though providing the same degree of cardiac stimulation. In contrast, there was no significant difference in the presence of

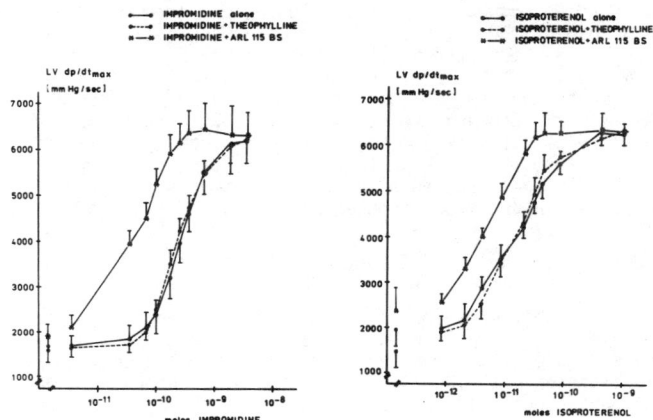

Fig. 4. Effect of simultaneous phosphodiesterase inhibition by ARL-115 BS on position of the dose-response curves of IMP (left) and isoproterenol (right) in the isolated guinea pig heart.

theophylline which is confined to the extracellular space - even if applied in a relatively high dose of 10^{-4} moles.
Similar results as shown here for IMP were although obtained for ß-adrenergic stimulation with isoproterenol in the normal guinea pig heart. As can be seen from Fig. 4 theophylline did not change position or sloap of the curves significantly whereas ARL-115 BS markedly shifted the dose-response curve to the left to a similar degree as pointed out for IMP.

Effect of combined administration of ARL-115 BS and IMP in 8 patients with congestive cardiomyopathy.

Since both compounds IMP and ARL-115 BS were under clinical investigation in our intensive care unit last year it seemed of interest to check whether results of these experimental studies could be also verified under in vivo conditions in patients with congestive cardiomyopathy where IMP already proved to be beneficial under certain conditions. In the 8 patients studied average basal cardiac output was 3.5 l/min (Fig. 5). IMP 5 and 10 µg/kg/hr did not increase cardiac output in these

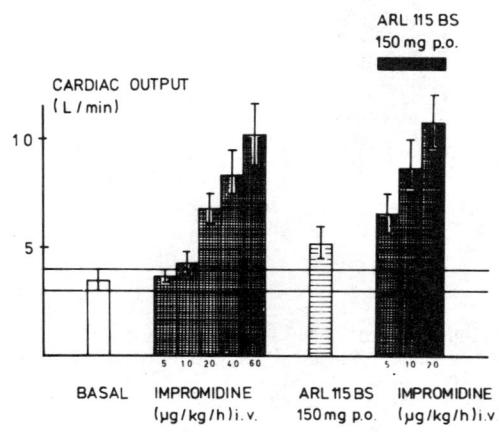

Fig. 5.
Effect of ARL-115 BS on IMP stimulation of cardiac output in 8 patients with congestive cardiomyopathy.
(For details see text)

rather low concentrations. There was a marked increase at 20, 40 and 60µg/kg/hr with a maximal cardiac output of 10 l/min. In the presence of ARL-115 BS administered orally in a dose of 150 mg, which per se only marginally increased cardiac output there was now a marked supra-additive response at 5 and 10 µg IMP indicating a shift of the IMP curve to the left. This means that identical cardiac output levels were obtained though the IMP dose could be reduced to $1/4^{th}$ or $1/5^{th}$ in the presence of ARL-115 BS. Comparative studies with DOB in the presence and absence of ARL-115 BS (results not shown) also revealed a tendency for a leftward shift in the presence of ARL-115 BS, though values were not statistically different. The poor effect of DOB in these patients may reflect the previously mentioned specific damage of sarcolemmal ß-receptors induced by excessive levels of circulating endogenous catecholamines.

Effect of continuous treatment with ARL-115 BS and IMP on ß-adrenoceptor mediated contractile effects.

In order to clearify whether stimulation by ARL 115 BS and/or IMP could eventually improve responsiveness of the ß-adrenergic stimulation mechanism cardiac effects of DOB were re-evaluated after a 5 days period of stimulation with either ARL 115 alone or in combination with IMP. The dose of both compounds were adjusted to give a cardiac output of about 5 l/min. As can be seen from Fig. 6 DOB only marginally increased cardiac output in response to 2.5, 5.0, 7.5 and 10.0 µg/kg/min before beginning of alternative stimulation. The evaluation of hemodynamic potencies of DOB after a 5 days treatment period with ARL-115 BS or the combination ARL-115 BS + IMP clearly demonstrated a statistically significant increase in the DOB-mediated positive-inotropic action of cardiac contractile parameters. DOB now induced a 2-fold increase in cardiac output at 5.0 and 7.5 µg/kg/min. A similar beneficial effect could also be established for pulmonary capillary wedge pressure which decreased now in all patients as a result of an improved left ventricular performance in the presence of DOB. These results suggest that periodical cardiac stimulation distinct from ß-receptors definitely improves the stimulation potency of the ß-adrenergic system leading - at least in part - to a restoration of the ß-adrenoceptor-adenylate cyclase system.

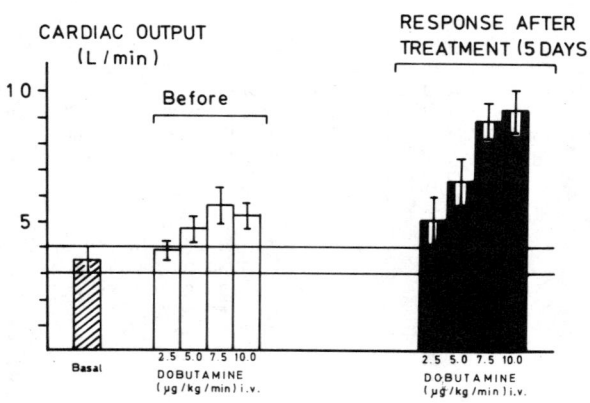

Fig. 6.

Improvement of ß-adrenoceptor-mediated cardiac contractility following a 5 days treatment with ARL-115 BS and IMP. (For details see text)

DISCUSSION

Sarcolemmal alterations of the failing myocardium have been the subject of several studies from our laboratory during the past few years. A recent report from our laboratory exhibited essential alterations in the non-ischemic surviving myocardium of the same hearts that have been subjected to myocardium infarction. It could be shown that the dose-response curve for isoproterenol on the right ventricular dp/dt$_{max}$ was significantly shifted to the right in hearts in which strictly left ventricular myocardial infarctions had been produced by coronary ligation. In contrast to this, the positive-inotropic response to histamine was not altered. Stimulation rates of adenylate cyclase activity by isoproterenol in right ventricular membrane preparations of the same hearts were reduced by 70% three days postinfarction whereas histamine and NaF revealed stimulation rates equivalent to controls. ß-receptor binding studies indicated a 74% loss of ß-receptors and a lowered affinity of the remaining stereospecific receptors. It seems of importance that all these changes could be effectively prevented by pretreating the animals with reserpine prior to the operation or by treatment with metoprolol during the whole postinfarction period. These observations clearly demonstrate the detrimental effects in terms of specific damage of sarcolemmal ß-receptors by increased levels of circulating catecholamines in the postinfarction period. In summary, we interpreted our results as a pathophysiologic mechanism according to which the whole surviving myocardium progressively looses its physiological ability to adapt to stress situations or to increased requirements of the body by means of an enhanced cardiac output mediated by catecholamines (Baumann et al., 1981).

In another recent study two new histaminergic H$_2$-receptor agonistic compounds were characterized in the guinea pig and human myocardium (Baumann et al., 1982). Both substances, IMP and dimaprit, exerted pronounced inotropic effects, most likely due to the activation of the membrane bound adenylate cyclase by increasing myocardial cyclic-AMP levels as well as by directly stimulating the enzyme in a particulate membrane preparation. These effects could not be abolished by the ß-blocking agent metoprolol but on the other hand were completely antagonized by the selective H$_2$-antagonist cimetidine.

Previous findings and the result of the present studies strongly suggest that a causality exists between the observed decrease in inotropic action of ß-receptor agonists, the diminished ß-adrenergic response of myocardial adenylate cyclase and the loss in number of sarcolemmal ß-receptors, leading to a specific impairment of the ß-adrenoceptor system, presumably caused by prolonged exposure of the heart to increased levels of endogenous catecholamines. Such a mechanism could also recently be confirmed for congestive heart failure due to mitral- and aortic valve disorders (Baumann et al., 1983). Compared to a collective of patients with pure mitral valve stenosis the response of cardiac adenylate cyclase activity to isoproterenol showed a marked decrease (-90%) in patients with severe combined mitral and aortic valve disease. Similar changes were observed in direct receptor binding studies with ^{3}H-dihydroalprenolol, in which the reduction of ß-receptor density was in the same order of magnitude. In contrast, however, stimulation rates of the enzyme by IMP and binding capacity of ^{3}H-tiotidine to cardiac H$_2$-receptors were found unaltered in the same membrane preparations of all patients. Furthermore, there was no significant difference in maximal NaF-induced stimulation of cardiac adenylate cyclase and no significant difference in maximal binding capacity and affinity of ^{3}H-QNB to cholinergic muscarinic receptors. These findings emphasize the specifity of the process and strongly suggest that this mechanism is triggered directly by endogenous catecholamines and exclusively involves cardiac ß-receptors resulting in a decrease in their number according to the severity of left ventricular dysfunction.

The results of the present pilot study demonstrate that under in vivo conditions in humans the H$_2$-receptor system is not affected and consequently not involved in the pathophysiologic process as demonstrated for the ß-adrenoceptor mechanism. IMP showed a marked positive-inotropic effect when given in doses between 20 and 60 µg/kg/hr as continuous infusion for up to 48 hours. There was a constant increase in cardiac output (2-3 fold the baseline values) a pronounced decrease in pulmonary wedge pressure by 70% as well as decrease in pulmonary artery pressure by 45% and right ventricular filling pressure. In the presence of the phosphodiesterase inhibitor ARL-115 BS quantitatively comparable effects were achieved at much lower concentrations of IMP (5 and 10 µg/kg/hr). This means that the dose-response curve for IMP is shifted to the left under in vivo conditions as well.

IMP not only turned out to be a potent positive-inotropic agent but also considerably lowered pre- and afterload values. In order to differentiate between these effects, comparative studies with nitroglycerin, nitroprusside and prazosine were performed in some patients. Nitroprusside and prazosine, by arteriolar dilation

could be expected to exert their major influence on the failing ventricle by reduction of its afterload. In contrast nitroglycerin, by predominant venous dilation and increase in venous capacitance, could be expected to exert its major hemodynamic influence on the heart by reduction in its preload. The resulting effects on the function curve of the failing left ventricle in all patients was only moderate. At roughly similar levels of right heart filling pressure and dilation of the arteriolar resistance vessels by these compounds there was a far greater increase in cardiac output under IMP than that induced by dilation of venous capacitance vessels (nitroglycerin) or pure reduction of afterload (nitroprusside, prazosine).
This indicates that in the patients studied IMP primarily increased cardiac output as the result of its direct positive-inotropic effect rather than by decreasing pre- and afterload.

In conclusion, present results with IMP so far support our previous suggestion (Baumann et al., 1980, 1981a,b,c,1982, 1983a,b) that the combined vasodilator and inotropic actions of IMP may be of value in the treatment of severe cardiac failure at least in some patients. Administration of IMP allows discontinuation of orally effective drugs, e.g. nitrates and alpha-blockers thus preventing tolerance to this class of compounds. Furthermore treatment with IMP to stimulate the H_2-receptor system offers the additional chance of a simultaneous treatment with ß-blocking agents (Swedberg et al., 1979). This would allow the physiologic ß-adrenergic system to recover without the risk of inducing myocardial failure. As far as a combined therapy with phosphodiesterase inhibitors is concerned our results so far suggest that combined therapy with ARL-115 BS and IMP may be usefull, especially in view of a long-term treatment to prevent a specific damage of cardiac H_2- and $ß_1$-receptors induced by IMP or DOB, respectively.

In this latter respect it seems, that balanced manipulation of the circulation in myocardial failure is now feasible and worthy of further studies in these high risk patients. However we wish to emphasize that - however attractive these pharmacodynamic arguments are - it is still quite unknown or at least uncertain which of these particular hemodynamic manipulations offer the patients the most benefit either in the short term or in the long one. In case that such an H_2-receptor stimulation turns out to be of future importance we should be aware of the fact that IMP is not expected to be the optimal H_2-receptor agonist for several reasons:

(1) The synthesis of IMP is too complicated and therefore very expensive,
(2) the effects of IMP - though a short acting agent - are difficult to control and its administration absolutely requires invasive techniques for continuous assessment of hemodynamic parameters, and
(3) the unpredictable effects of IMP on cardiac afterload in a normal collective of patients.

All these facts make it necessary to develop H_2-agonistic compounds which selectively discriminate H_2-receptors, for example cardioselective compounds devoid of effects on the pheripheral vascular smooth muscle.

ACKNOWLEDGEMENT

Supported by the Deutsche Forschungsgemeinschaft (DFG) by Grant Ba 666/1, 666/2-2 and 666/2-3.

REFERENCES

REFERENCES

Baumann, G., G. Rieß, W.D. Erhardt, S.B. Felix, and H. Blömer (1980). Z. Kardiol., 69, 209.
Baumann, G., J. Schrader, and E. Gerlach (1981a). Circulation Res., 48, 259-266.
Baumann, G., G. Rieß, W. Erhardt, et al. (1981b). Am. Heart J., 101, 569-581.
Baumann, G., S.B. Felix, J. Schrader, et al. (1981c). Res. exp. Med. (Berl.), 179, 81-98.
Baumann, G., S.B. Felix, G. Rieß, U. Loher, L. Ludwig, and H. Blömer (1982). J. cardiovasc. Pharmac., 4, 542-553.
Baumann, G., D. Mercader, S.B. Felix, U. Loher, L. Ludwig, H. Sebening, S. Hagl, F. Sebening, and H. Blömer (1983a). J. cardiovasc. Pharmac., 5, 618-625.
Baumann, G., S.B. Felix, G. Rieß, U. Loher, L. Ludwig, and H. Blömer (1983b). Ag. Actions (in press)
Baumann, G., B. Permanetter, and A. Wirtzfeld (1984). Pharmac. Ther., 24, 165-177.
Bristow, M.R., R. Ginsburg, W.B.S. Minobe, et al. (1982). N. Engl. J. Med., 307, 205-211.
Colucci, W.S., R.W. Alexander, G.D. Williams, et al. (1981). N. Engl. J. Med., 305, 185-190.
Lehmann, M., J. Keul, H. Löllgen, and H. Just (1981). Z. Kardiol., 70, 238-244.
Owen, D.A.A., C.A. Harvey, and R.W. Gristwood (1979). J. Pharm. Pharmac.,31, 577-582.
Thomas, I.A. and M.G. Marks (1978). Am. J. Cardiol., 41, 233-243.

POSSIBLE INVOLVEMENT OF BRAIN HISTAMINE IN THE REGULATION OF BLOOD PRESSURE

A. Philippu

Department of Pharmacodynamics and Toxicology, University of Innsbruck, A-6020 Innsbruck, Austria

ABSTRACT

To investigate the possible involvement of histamine in the central regulation of the arterial blood pressure, the posterior hypothalamus was superfused with CSF through a push-pull cannula and the release of endogenous histamine was determined in the superfusate.

In anaesthetized cats, experimentally induced blood pressure changes enhanced the rate of release of histamine in the posterior hypothalamus.

In the hypothalamus of unanaesthetized, spontaneously hypertensive rats the rate of release of histamine was higher than that in the hypothalamus of normotensive (Wistar Kyoto strain) animals.

Superfusion of the cat hypothalamus with histamine increased the rates of release of endogenous dopamine, noradrenaline and adrenaline. Superfusion with 2-(2-aminoethyl)thiazole (H_1-agonist) enhanced, while superfusion with mepyramine (H_1-antagonist) decreased the rates of release of noradrenaline and adrenaline. Superfusion with dimaprit (H_2-agonist) enhanced the rates of release of all three catecholamines. Thus, catecholaminergic neurons of the hypothalamus seem to possess histamine receptors which may modulate the release of catecholamines.

KEYWORDS

Hypothalamus; histamine; hypertension; push-pull cannula; catecholamines; SHR; dimaprit; 2-(2-aminoethyl)thiazole; mepyramine.

INTRODUCTION

In recent years several neurotransmitters of the brain have been implicated in the central regulation of the arterial blood pressure. The following main criteria should be fulfilled to postulate the involvement of a transmitter in blood pressure homeostasis.

1. The presence of the neurotransmitter in neurons of those brain areas which are involved in blood pressure regulation.

2. The ability of the substance, when centrally applied, to alter the arterial blood pressure and/or to influence blood pressure changes elicited by electrical stimulation of various brain areas.

3. Inhibition by central application of specific antagonists of the blood pressure changes induced by the exogenously applied neurotransmitter.

4. Alteration by an experimentally induced change in blood pressure of the rate of release of the neurotransmitter from its nerve terminals to counteract the blood pressure change.

Central application of histamine leads to a rise in the arterial blood pressure (Trendelenburg, 1957) and enhances the pressor response to electrical stimulation of the hypothalamus as well (Philippu and Wiedemann, 1981). Rise in blood pressure and enhancement of the pressor response by histamine are inhibited by histamine antagonists (Sinha and co-workers, 1969; Philippu and Wiedemann, 1981). Recently, histaminergic nerve endings and cell bodies were described in the posterior hypothalamus (Wilcox and Seybold, 1982; Watanabe and co-workers, 1983). On the other hand, electrical stimulation of this hypothalamic area elicits a rise in blood pressure. These findings seem to support the hypothesis that histaminergic neurons of the brain are involved in the regulation of the arterial blood pressure.

In the following results will be presented showing that experimentally induced blood pressure changes alter the release of endogenous histamine in the hypothalamus.

RESULTS AND DISCUSSION

Changes in Blood Pressure Increase the Rate of Release of Endogenous Histamine in the Posterior Hypothalamus

The experiments were carried out in anaesthetized cats. The posterior hypothalamus was superfused with artificial CSF through a push-pull cannula (Philippu, Przuntek and Roensberg, 1973) and the release of endogenous histamine was determined in the superfusate by the radioenzymatic assay of Enna and Snyder (1976) as modified by Philippu and co-workers (1982). To experimentally increase the arterial blood pressure, noradrenaline or tramazoline were injected intravenously. To elicit a fall of blood pressure, controlled bleeding was carried out, or nitroprusside was injected intravenously. A long-lasting fall of blood pressure was induced by intravenous injection of chlorisondamine. Finally, a biphasic change in blood pressure was elicited by transection of the spinal cord at C1/C2.

Experimentally induced increases and decreases in the arterial blood pressure enhanced the rate of release of endogenous histamine. However, the enhanced rate of release of the amine seemed to last shorter than the change in the arterial blood pressure (Philippu and co-workers, 1983).

Enhanced Release of Endogenous Histamine in the Posterior Hypothalamus of Hypertensive Rats

Determination of the histamine concentrations in the brains of spontaneously hypertensive rats (SHR) led to conflicting results. Chalmers and co-workers (1979) found the histamine levels of SHR to be unchanged, while Spector, Tarver and Berkowitz (1972) and Correa and Saavedra (1981) reported increased levels of histamine in various hypothalamic nuclei of SHR.

Both findings may be associated with unchanged, increased or decreased rates of release of histamine. In an attempt to directly determine the rate of release of histamine in the rat hypothalamus, a guide cannula was stereotaxically inserted into the posterior hypothalamus of 60-day old normotensive (WKy) and spontaneously hypertensive rats. Some days after operation a push-pull cannula was inserted into the guide cannula and the hypothalamus of conscious, freely moving rats was superfused with CSF.

The rate of release of histamine in SHR was found to be significantly higher than the rate of release in normotensive rats (SHR: 470 $\pm$ 27 fmol/min, normotensive rats: 328 $\pm$ 20 fmol/min; mean values of 7-9 experiments $\pm$ S.E.M.) (Tuomisto and co-workers, 1983).

Since experimentally induced blood pressure changes elicit a short-lasting increase in the release of histamine in the cat hypothalamus (see above), it is not certain whether the increased release of histamine in SHR is due to the high blood pressure. Alternatively, the enhanced rate of release of histamine might indicate that this amine is involved in the development and/or maintenance of hypertension in SHR. Irrespective of their interpretation, the results indicate that in conscious SHR the rise in blood pressure is also associated with an enhanced release of histamine in the hypothalamus.

Histamine Agonists and Antagonists Influence the Release of Endogenous Catecholamines in the Cat Hypothalamus

Histamine enhances the release of noradrenaline from peripheral tissues after preloading them with the tritiated catecholamine (Flacke and co-workers, 1967; Enero and Langer, 1975; Starke and Weitzell, 1978; Marco and co-workers, 1980). Histamine also increases the release of radioactive noradrenaline from brain slices (Subramanian and Mulder, 1977) and synaptosomes (Tuomisto and Tuomisto, 1980). We investigated the effects of histamine agonists and antagonists on the release of endogenous catecholamines in the hypothalamus of the anaesthetized cat. For this purpose the posterior hypothalamus was superfused with CSF that contained various histamine agonists and/or antagonists and the release of dopamine, noradrenaline and adrenaline was determined in the superfusate by a radioenzymatic assay after separation by thin layer chromatography (Philippu, Dietl and Sinha, 1979).

Hypothalamic superfusion with histamine greatly enhanced the release of dopamine, noradrenaline and adrenaline in the posterior hypothalamus. The effect of histamine was calcium-dependent, since superfusion with calcium-free CSF abolished the release of noradrenaline and adrenaline and greatly diminished that of dopamine. The H_1-agonist 2-(2-aminoethyl)thiazole increased the rates of release of noradrenaline and adrenaline without affecting the release of dopamine, while superfusion with the H_1-antagonist mepyramine inhibited the release of noradrenaline and adrenaline, but not that of dopamine. On the other hand, the H_2-agonist dimaprit enhanced the rates of release of all three catecholamines. The releasing effect of dimaprit was abolished when the hypothalamus was superfused with the agonist in the presence of the H_2-antagonist ranitidine. These results suggest that H_1- and H_2-receptors are involved in the release of noradrenaline and adrenaline by histamine. The findings also indicate that H_2-receptors are implicated in the release of dopamine. However, it should be mentioned that the releasing effect of histamine on all three catecholamines was inhibited by mepyramine (Philippu and co-workers, 1984). Thus, the involvement of H_1-receptors in the release of dopamine by histamine cannot be excluded with certainty. Hence, histamine receptors located on catecholaminergic neurons of the hypothalamus seem to influence the release of catecholamines.

As mentioned above, histamine-containing cell bodies and nerve endings have been identified in the hypothalamus (Wilcox and Seybold, 1982; Watanabe and co-workers, 1983). Moreover, histaminergic interneurons seem to be present in this brain region (Prast, Saxer and Philippu, in preparation). The location of histamine receptors on catecholaminergic neurons and the release by histamine of catecholamines indicate that in vivo endogenous histamine might modulate the release of catecholamines. Since catecholaminergic neurons of the hypothalamus are involved in the regulation of blood pressure (Sinha, Dietl and Philippu, 1980; Dietl and co-workers, 1981; Philippu, 1984), it cannot be excluded that the effect of histamine on blood pressure is partly due to modulation of the release of catecholamines.

REFERENCES

Chalmers, J. P., P. C. Howe, J. C. Provis,and M. J. West (1979). Cardiac and central histamine in spontaneously hypertensive and stroke-prone rats. In P. Meyer, H. Schmitt (Eds.), Nervous System and Hypertension, John Wiley, Chichester. pp. 244-252.

Correa, F. M. A., and J. M. Saavedra (1981). Increase in histamine concentrations in discrete hypothalamic nuclei of spontaneously hypertensive rats. Brain Res., 205, 445-451.

Dietl, H., A. Eisert, A. Kraus, and A. Philippu (1981). The release of endogenous catecholamines in the cat hypothalamus is affected by spinal transection and drugs which change the arterial blood pressure. J. Auton. Pharmac., 1, 279-286.

Enero, M. N., and S. Z. Langer (1975). Pharmacological effects of histamine on the isolated nictitating membrane. Brit. J. Pharmacol., 53, 431-432.

Enna, S. J., and S. H. Snyder (1976). A simple, sensitive and specific radioreceptor assay for endogenous GABA in brain tissue. J. Neurochem., 26, 221-224.

Flacke, W., D. Atanackovic, R. A. Gillis, and M. H. Alper (1967). The action of histamine on the mammalian heart. J. Pharmacol. Exp. Ther., 155, 271-278.

Marco, E. J., G. Balfagón, J. Martín, B. Gómez, and S. Lluch (1980). Indirect adrenergic effect of histamine in cat cerebral arteries. Naunyn-Schmiedeberg's Arch. Pharmacol., 312, 239-243.

Philippu, A., H. Przuntek, and W. Roensberg (1973). Superfusion of the hypothalamus with gamma-aminobutyric acid: Effect on release of noradrenaline and blood pressure. Naunyn-Schmiedeberg's Arch. Pharmacol., 276, 103-118.

Philippu, A., H. Dietl, and J. N. Sinha (1979). In vivo release of endogenous catecholamines in the hypothalamus. Naunyn-Schmiedeberg's Arch. Pharmacol., 308, 137-142.

Philippu, A., and K. Wiedemann (1981). Hypothalamic superfusion with histamine agonists and antagonists modifies the pressor response to hypothalamic stimulation. J. Auton. Pharmac., 1, 111-117.

Philippu, A., U. Hanesch, R. Hagen, and R. L. Robinson (1982). Release of endogenous histamine in the hypothalamus of anaesthetized cats and conscious, freely moving rabbits. Naunyn Schmiedeberg's Arch. Pharmacol., 321, 282-286.

Philippu, A., R. Hagen, U. Hanesch, and U. Waldmann (1983). Changes in the arterial blood pressure increase the release of endogenous histamine in the hypothalamus of anaesthetized cats. Naunyn-Schmiedeberg's Arch. Pharmacol., 323, 162-167.

Philippu, A., M. Bald, A. Kraus, and H. Dietl . In vivo release by histamine agonists and antagonists of endogenous catecholamines in the cat hypothalamus. Naunyn-Schmiedeberg's Arch. Pharmacol., (in press).

Sinha, J. N., M. L. Gupta, and K. P. Bhargava (1969). Effect of histamine and antihistaminics on central vasomotor loci. Eur. J. Pharmacol., 5, 235-238.

Sinha, J. N., H. Dietl, and A. Philippu (1980). Effect of a fall of blood pressure on the release of catecholamines in the hypothalamus. Life Sci., 26, 1751-1760.

Spector, S., J. Tarver, and B. Berkowitz (1972). Catecholamine biosynthesis and metabolism in the vasculature of normotensive and hypertensive rats. In K. Okamoto (Ed.), Spontaneous Hypertension, Springer Verlag, Berlin. pp. 41.

Starke, K., and R. Weitzell (1978). Is histamine involved in the sympathomimetic effect of nicotine? Naunyn-Schmiedeberg's Arch. Pharmacol., 304, 237-248.

Subramanian N., and A. H. Mulder (1977). Modulation by histamine of the efflux of radiolabeled catecholamines from rat brain slices. Eur. J. Pharmacol., 43, 143-

152.
Trendelenburg, U. (1957). Stimulation of sympathetic centres by histamine. Circul. Res., 5, 105-110.
Tuomisto, J., and L. Tuomisto (1980). Effects of histamine and histamine antagonists on the uptake and release of catecholamines and 5-HT in brain synaptosomes. Med. Biol., 58, 33-37.
Tuomisto, L., A. Yamatodani, H. Dietl, U. Waldmann, and A. Philippu (1983). In vivo release of endogenous catecholamines, histamine and GABA in the hypothalamus of Wistar Kyoto and spontaneously hypertensive rats. Naunyn-Schmiedeberg's Arch. Pharmacol., 323, 183-187.
Watanabe, T., Y. Taguchi, H. Hayashi, J. Tanaka, S. Shiosaka, M. Tohyama, H. Kubota, Y. Terano, and H. Wada (1983). Evidence for the presence of a histaminergic neuron system in the rat brain. An immunohistochemical analysis. Neurosci. Lett., 39, 249-254.
Wilcox, B. J., and V. S. Seybold (1982). Localization of neuronal histamine in the rat brain. Neurosci. Lett., 29, 105-110.

MULTIPLE ACTIONS OF HISTAMINE ON CEREBRAL BLOOD VESSELS

P. M. Gross

Departments of Neurological Surgery and Neurobiology and Behavior, State University of New York, Stony Brook, New York, USA

Abstract

Responses of cerebral arteries, arterioles, capillaries and veins to histamine and its pharmacological agonists are examined. The studies indicate that cerebral arterial smooth muscle responds to histamine with relaxation, capillaries become more permeable to circulating solutes, and cerebral veins are unresponsive.

Keywords

pial arteries and veins; cerebral vascular resistance; cerebral blood flow; capillary permeability; blood-brain barrier; sympathetic nerves

INTRODUCTION AND LITERATURE REVIEW

There has been interest for several decades about how histamine affects blood vessels in the brain. Until recently, the techniques for studying cerebral vascular physiology were limited and yielded unsatisfying information. Four general categories of studies concerning histamine in the cerebral circulation can be classified from the literature over the past 60 years. They can be grouped according to: 1) pial arteries and veins, 2) cerebral blood flow, 3) interaction with other mediators of cerebrovascular control, and 4) the capillary system ("blood-brain barrier"). Before updating our understanding of histamine's roles in the cerebral circulation, I will briefly review older studies, which although providing only limited details, were important in establishing critical directions for the advances of the last few years.

Pial Circulation

In 1929, Forbes and his colleagues reported that systemically administered histamine dilated the brain's arterial system, a concept that was poorly understood for decades thereafter (Sokoloff, 1959). The results from Forbes' studies are not easily interpreted because histamine produced decreases in arterial blood pressure and increases in vascular caliber. If one is observing the pial arterial system as Forbes did, these results would lead to assertions that dilatation of the vessels must have occurred from histamine's direct action on arterial smooth muscle. It was not understood then that histamine does not penetrate the blood-brain barrier from systemic administration (Snyder, Axelrod and Bauer, 1964; Oldendorf, 1971). Its apparent effects on the brain arterial supply are probably indirect, being the result of autoregulatory dilatation to the systemic hypotension, a vasomotor mechanism quite different (Lassen, 1974) from active relaxation of cerebrovascular smooth muscle that was implied from the studies of Forbes and coworkers (1929).

Differences in the manner in which histamine has been introduced to the pial vasculature have produced conflicting results. In studies involving superfusion of histamine over the entire cortical field, Raper and colleagues (1972) found increases in arteriolar caliber in cats, and Rosenblum (1976) reported no effect on pial arteries in mice. When histamine is discretely administered by perivascular microinjection, however, pial arteries and arterioles always respond with concentration-dependent dilatation (Wahl and Kuschinsky, 1979).

The response of cerebral venules and veins in vivo is an important determinant to capillary blood flow, pressure and filtration, as has been discussed for several non-neural organs (Haddy, 1960; Diana and Kaiser, 1970; Owen, 1977). Studies in peripheral vascular beds of vasoactive agents, including histamine, indicate that the precapillary resistance vessels are generally more responsive to these stimuli than capacitance vessels (Sharpey-Shafer and Ginsberg, 1962). Consecutive vascular segments may even have opposite responses to the same stimulus. In skeletal muscle and skin preparations, histamine dilates arteries and constricts veins (Powell and Brody, 1976). Such factors as vascular wall structure, wall tension, and receptor density and distribution within smooth muscle layers may be important to segmental differences in response to histamine between arteries and veins. These factors have not been systematically evaluated in the cerebral venous system.

Cerebral Blood Flow

Even in the last few years, there have been reports of increased cerebral blood flow resulting from intravascular histamine administration. Critical appraisal of these studies reveals the following difficulties: 1) flow measurements were obtained from large extracranial arteries supplying the brain (Tindall and Greenfield, 1973; Saxena, 1975; Spira and coworkers, 1978). It is unlikely that such determinations accurately reflect cerebral perfusion. Blood flow estimates from large cranial vessels in dogs and cats are especially difficult to interpret because the extracerebral vascular anatomy in these species is complex and may involve shunting of blood between muscular and cerebral vessels during intravascular stimuli (Heistad and coworkers, 1980; Gross, Harper and Teasdale, 1981a); 2) studies using perfused brain (Muravchick and Bergofsky, 1976) or venous outflow (Carpi, Cartoni and Giardini, 1972) techniques require deep anesthesia and extensive surgery. They are unlikely to provide reliable data.

Until recently, there were no studies of regional heterogeneity in the brain during histamine administration, of receptor types that may be involved, or of potential influences exerted by histamine on tissue metabolism, a factor that has important consequences on establishing vascular resistance in the nervous system.

Interaction With Other Vasomotor Mediators

Histamine is synthesized and/or stored in peripheral autonomic nerves (Ryan and Brody, 1970). The amine is richly concentrated in post-ganglionic sympathetic nerves (Ryan and Brody, 1970), and is avidly sequestered by sympathetic axons in the rabbit iris (Ehinger, 1974). Although not yet demonstrated histochemically, histamine may be present in cerebrovascular sympathetic nerves, and may have a role in modulating nervous activity at the sympathetic neurovascular junction. Bevan, Duckles and Lee (1975) showed that histamine could modify basilar arterial responses to transmural nerve stimulation and exogenous norepinephrine in vitro. Similar responses have been found in dog saphenous vein

(McGrath and Shepherd, 1976), rabbit ear artery (Foldes and Hall, 1979), and rabbit ganglia (Brimble and Wallis, 1973). In each of these studies conducted in vitro, a potentiating effect of histamine on noradrenergic responses was found to be linked to H_1 histamine receptors. The organization and function of histamine receptors at noradrenergic nerve endings must be complex, however, because sympathetic effects in myocardium, skeletal muscle arteries, and ganglia are inhibited, rather than potentiated, by stimulation of H_2 receptors (Brimble and Wallis, 1973; McGrath and Shepherd, 1976; Lokhandwala, 1978; Powell, 1979). Given that histamine has this diversity of influence on neural factors in peripheral organs, it was important to understand its influence on the sympathetic control of cerebrovascular resistance and capacitance.

Capillaries

In qualitative studies published some 30 years ago, it was established that blood-borne histamine could increase the passage into brain of the protein-bound dye, neutral red, and antibiotics such as penicillin and streptomycin (Hurst and Davies, 1950; Foldes and Kelentei, 1954). Studies since than have failed to confirm histamine-induced increases in the permeability of cerebral capillaries (Gabbiani, Badonnel and Majno, 1970; Rapoport, 1976; Bradbury, 1979). There are several factors that may account for these inconsistencies. Included are the route, concentration and duration of the histamine administered, physical characteristics of the tracer used for study, and possible differences in response between species. In that histamine is a constituent of cerebral perivascular mast cells (Head and coworkers, 1980), its receptors are present in microvessel fractions (Peroutka and coworkers, 1980), and a histamine-sensitive adenylate cyclase is located in cortical capillaries (Karnushina and coworkers, 1980), it is likely that histamine is involved in regulation of endothelial function in the nervous system. Only until recently, however, were studies performed to demonstrate where and to what extent in the CNS histamine has effects and over what receptor system(s) its influence is mediated.

The summary above presents a brief historical perspective of studies searching for histamine roles in the cerebral circulation. It is clear that a considerable base of information has been established from experiments both in the brain and, to an even greater extent, in peripheral organ blood vessels. Collectively, these efforts have cultivated further investigations from which the following analyses and concepts emerged.

RECENT ADVANCES

The influence by histamine on cerebral arterial and venous smooth muscle has been evaluated by studies of vessels in vitro and in situ and by measurements of cerebral blood flow. Histamine likely has interactions with other vasomotor mediators such as the norepinephrine released from stimulation of sympathetic nerves. Effects of histamine on the cerebral capillary system have been tested with dyes, drugs, and radiolabeled tracer solutes. The interpretations from these various approaches are discussed below and in a recent review (Gross, 1982). They are summarized in Fig. 1.

Pial Circulation

Three types of studies published in the 1970's and 80's were important to fulfilling questions about histamine action on pial arteries and veins.

First, in vitro experiments with cat middle cerebral arteries established that histamine H_1 and H_2 receptors were present in smooth muscle layers of this vessel (Edvinsson and Owman, 1975). This finding was subsequently confirmed by additional studies using the same preparation but with selective

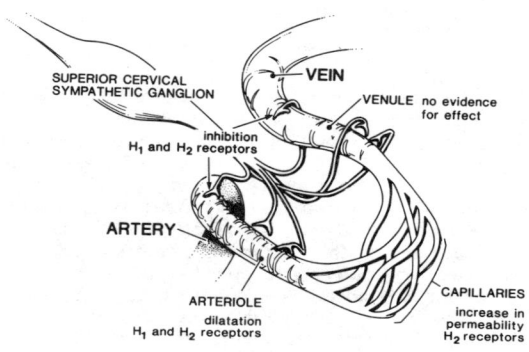

Fig. 1. Multiple actions of histamine on cerebral blood vessels.

agonists of H_1 and H_2 receptors, 2,2-pyridylethylamine (PEA) and impromidine, respectively (Edvinsson, Gross and Mohamed, 1983). H_2 receptors mediate considerable relaxation of precontracted artery segments in vitro. The response is dependent on the amount of tone the vessel has before stimulation by the bath agent. Selective stimulation of arterial H_1 receptors by PEA produces only small dilatatory responses in vitro.

Second, concentration-response curves for histamine were systematically produced for pial arteries in situ by Wahl and Kuschinsky (1979). With the perivascular microinjection technique, these investigators demonstrated 1) a maximal effect of histamine at about 10 uM (33% increase in arteriolar diameter from control), 2) a pronounced rightward shift of the curve in the presence of cimetidine (H_2 receptor antagonist), and 3) no significant effect of mepyramine (H_1 receptor antagonist) on the histamine concentration-response curve. Dilatatory responses to histamine were not further reduced by combined treatment with the two antagonists. These studies were critically important to understanding histamine effects on cerebral arterial smooth muscle because perivascular microinjection mimics the route of histamine stimulation from mast cells or from histaminergic fibers innervating the vasculature.

Third, the description and availability of selective agonists and antagonists for histamine provided opportunities for further evaluation of the significance of histamine receptors in this vascular bed in situ. The syntheses by Durant and coworkers (1975; 1978) of PEA (H_1) and impromidine (H_2) were essential in establishing these new pharmacological opportunities.

Wahl and Kuschinsky (1979) did not include an evaluation of histamine effects on cerebral veins, and, therefore, a comparison of relative responses between consecutive vascular segments was not possible. Furthermore, they did not examine responses to selective stimulation by agonists. For these two reasons, new experiments were undertaken using the same preparation and method as Wahl and Kuschinsky. Studies were done with PEA, impromidine and histamine in both arterioles and in veins (Gross, Harper and Teasdale, 1981b). Both groups of vessels had resting diameters of from 50 to 150 microns. In arterioles, a hierarchy of responses was discerned for the histamine agents. The order and magnitude (maximal response, respective concentration) of arteriolar dilatation was impromidine (+43%, 1 uM) > histamine (+28%, 100 uM) > PEA (+17%, 100 uM). The dilatations from impromidine and PEA were effectively reduced by prior microapplication of 10 uM doses of their respective antagonists, metiamide and mepyramine (Edvinsson, Gross and Mohamed, 1983).

Pial veins and venules were unresponsive to any of the histamine agents (Gross, Harper and Teasdale, 1981b). The studies were conducted with concentrations of histamine and its agonists at doses that produced the most marked arterial responses. The absence of histaminergic effects on pial veins compared to arterioles during abluminal stimulation may be explained by relatively thinner layers of venous smooth muscle, lower prestimulation tone in the veins, or a lower density of smooth muscle receptors for histamine in veins.

Cerebral Blood Flow

The previous studies on histaminergic regulation of blood flow in the brain did not establish clearly the relevance of cerebral endothelial cells (the "blood-brain barrier") in determining whether the amine directly or indirectly affects cerebrovascular resistance. A technique for transiently disrupting the barrier function of brain capillaries and arterioles was used to "expose" cerebral arterial smooth muscle to intravascularly administered histamine and its agonists (Gross, Harper and Teasdale, 1981a). The method involves injecting a hypertonic solution into the carotid arterial supply over a brief period short enough so that carotid hemodynamics are not seriously disturbed but long enough so that an osmotic effect is imparted to the endothelial cells. The result establishes in rats a condition of about 30 minutes wherein the blood-brain barrier is about 4-times more permeable than normal (Hardebo, 1980; Gross, Harper and Teasdale, 1981a).

By comparing the effects of carotid arterial infusion of histamine on cerebral blood flow in rats without and with blood-brain barrier disruption, two important concepts were established: 1) histamine does not affect cerebral blood flow when it is given by arterial infusion in rats with an intact blood-brain barrier. This concept also applies to humans (Olesen, 1982); and 2) histamine has concentration-related effects on cerebrovascular resistance. The largest changes in blood flow (+31%) were found in structures perfused primarily by carotid arterial and middle cerebral arterial blood. The effects could be mimicked both by H_1 and H_2 receptor agonists (PEA and dimaprit), and they could be attenuated during histamine infusion by prior treatment with either mepyramine or metiamide. Furthermore, the influence by histamine appears to be purely vascular because there were no effects on tissue glucose utilization in the same structures that had such pronounced increases in blood flow (Gross, Harper and Teasdale, 1981a).

Interaction With Other Vasomotor Mediators

The contiguous relationship in the vicinity of cerebral vessels of neurotransmitter substances, their nerves, and storage compartments suggests that a functional interaction probably exists to modulate vascular resistance from moment to moment during neural and humoral stimuli. Histamine is stored in cerebral perivascular mast cells (Head and coworkers, 1980) and in a nonmast cell pool within vessel walls (El-Ackad and Brody, 1974). Furthermore, it may be situated in neural storage granules at sympathetic endings within vascular smooth muscle (Ryan and Brody, 1972) or within vascular processes of its own putative cell bodies. These points suggest studies to examine possible overlaps of control between vasomotor mediators located near cerebral vessels.

One such step was taken to test the interaction between sympathetic vasoconstrictory and histaminergic vasodilatatory influences in cerebral arteries and veins (Gross, Harper and Teasdale, 1983). Electrical stimulation of sympathetic nerves in anesthetized cats causes constriction of pial arteries and veins (about 8% decrease in vessel diameter). In arteries, simultaneous perivascular microapplication of concentrations of histamine, PEA or impromidine, in doses that produced about the same amount of dilatation, prevented constriction during nerve stimulation. With higher concentrations of the histamine agents, the arterial response was always dilatation rather than constriction. Veins constrict as much as arteries during nerve stimulation, but do not dilate in response to histamine. There was no constriction of veins during nerve stimulation when histamine, PEA or impromidine was microinjected next to the vessel. These findings suggest that, if histamine is released simultaneously with norepinephrine during sympathetic nerve activity in cerebral vessels, the constriction normally resulting from sympathetic stimulation alone is opposed.

There are numerous other candidate transmitter substances that may affect cerebral vascular regulation. An important field of future research will be to expand our understanding of how these agents are influential independently and simultaneously with other liberated mediators. Such substances that have already been evaluated with respect to their interaction with histamine are arachidonic acid derivatives (Juan and Sametz, 1980; Baenziger and coworkers, 1981; Dux and coworkers, 1982) and peptides (Fjellner and Hagermark, 1981; Skofitsch and coworkers, 1983).

Capillaries

The findings of increased cerebral capillary permeability to histamine, published more than thirty years ago by Hurst and Davies (1950) and Foldes and Kelentei (1954), have been confirmed recently by independent investigations in two laboratories. Carotid arterial infusion of histamine in pharmacological concentrations produced in anesthetized rats increases in transcapillary influx of sucrose, alpha-aminoisobutyric acid, horseradish peroxidase, and albumin. An increase in water content in the ipsilateral hemisphere was accompanied by ultrastructural signs of glial edema (Dux and Joó, 1982; Gross and coworkers, 1982). In both studies, an increase in the number of pinocytotic vesicles was found from electron microscopic examination of the endothelial cells in parietal cortex, a particularly provocative result that may be linked to the presence of histamine-sensitive adenylate cyclase within endothelial membranes or cytoplasm (Karnushina and coworkers, 1980). This process is specifically related to stimulation of histamine H_2 receptors (Karnushina and coworkers, 1980; Dux and Joó, 1982; Gross and coworkers, 1982).

Two additional noteworthy concepts were revealed from the studies of histamine and its effect on blood-brain transfer of small solutes such as sucrose (Gross and coworkers, 1982). First, the increase in permeability was regionally nonuniform. Higher rates of transfer were found in cortex than in hippocampus. This result may indicate a heterogeneous density of histamine receptors in brain microvessels. Second, the effect of histamine on capillary permeability was time-dependent. Increases in transfer were as large 30 minutes after the histamine infusion as they were during infusion. Two hours after termination of the infusion, there were no changes in permeability. It is possible that a time-dependent activation process of histamine receptors by enzymes such as adenylate cyclase (Joó, 1979) is reflected by this finding.

Acknowledgments

I thank Beverly Gabriel for producing the typescript and Kathy Gebhart for drawing the figure.

References

Baenziger, N. L., F. J. Fogerty, L. F. Mertz and L. F. Chernuta (1981). Regulation of histamine-mediated prostacyclin synthesis in cultured human vascular endothelial cells. Cell 24:915-923.

Bevan, J. A., S. P. Duckles and T. J. F. Lee (1975). Histamine potentiation of nerve and drug induced responses of a rabbit cerebral artery. Circ. Res. 36:647-653.

Bradbury, M. W. B. (1979). The Concept of a Blood-Brain Barrier. Chichester, Wiley.

Brimble, M. J. and D. I. Wallis (1973). Histamine H_1 and H_2 receptors at a ganglionic synapse. Nature 246:156-158.

Carpi, A., C. Cartoni and V. Giardini (1972). Segmental effects of histamine, acetylcholine and bradykinin on cerebral vessels. Arch. Int. Pharm. 196:111-112.

Diana, J. N. and R. S. Kaiser (1970). Pre- and post-capillary resistance during histamine infusion in isolated dog hindlimb. Am. J. Physiol. 218:132-142.

Durant, G. J., C. R. Ganellin and M.E. Parsons (1975). Chemical differentiation of histamine H_1- and H_2-receptor agonists. J. Med. Chem. 18:905-909.

Durant, G. J., W. A. M. Duncan, C. R. Ganellin, M. E. Parsons, R. C. Blakemore and A. C. Rasmussen (1978). Impromidine (SK&F 92676) is a very potent and specific agonist for histamine H_2-receptors. Nature 276:403-405.

Dux, E. and F. Joó (1982). Effects of histamine on brain capillaries. Exp. Brain Res. 47:252-258.

Dux, E., F. Joó, A. Gecse, Z. S. Mezei, L. Dux, J. Hideg and G. Telegdy (1982). Histamine-stimulated prostaglandin synthesis in rat brain microvessels. Agents Actions 12:146-148.

Edvinsson, L. and Ch. Owman (1975). A pharmacological comparison of histamine receptors in isolated extracranial and intracranial arteries in vitro. Neurology 25:271-276.

Edvinsson, L., P. M. Gross and A. Mohamed (1983). Characterization of histamine receptors in cat cerebral arteries in vitro and in situ. J. Pharmacol. Exp. Ther. 225:168-175.

Ehinger, B. (1974). Uptake of histamine or histamine metabolites into sympathetic nonadrenergic axons. Acta Physiol. Scand. 90:218-225.

El-Ackad, T. M. and M. J. Brody (1974). Fluorescence histochemical localization of nonmast cell histamine. In Neuropsychopharmacology Series, 359, Excerpta Medica, Amsterdam, pp. 551-559.

Fjellner, B. and O. Hägermark (1981). Studies on pruritogenic and histamine-releasing effects of some putative peptide neurotransmitters. Acta derm.-vener. Stockh. 61:245-250.

Foldes, A. and R. C. Hall (1979). The effects of histamine on responses of the rabbit ear artery to electrical stimulation and to exogenous noradrenaline. Brit. J. Pharmacol. 67:329-335.

Földes, I. and B. Kelentei (1954). Studies on the haemato-encephalic barrier II. The effects of histamine with special reference to the passage of antibiotics. Acta Physiol. Acad. Sci. Hung. 5:149-161.

Forbes, H. S., H. G. Wolff and S. Cobb (1929). The cerebral circulation X. The action of histamine. Am. J. Physiol. 89:266-272.

Gabbiani, G., M. C. Badonnel and G. Majno (1970). Intra-arterial injections of histamine, serotonin and bradykinin: a topographic study of vascular leakage. Proc. Soc. Exp. Biol. Med. 135:447-452.

Gross, P. M., A. M. Harper and G. M. Teasdale (1981a). Cerebral circulation and histamine. I. Participation of vascular H_1- and H_2-receptors in vasodilatatory responses to carotid arterial infusion. J. Cereb. Blood Flow Metab. 1:97-108.

Gross, P.M., A. M. Harper and G. M. Teasdale (1981b). Cerebral circulation and histamine. 2. Responses of pial veins and arterioles to receptor agonists. J. Cereb. Blood Flow Metab. 1:219-225.

Gross, P. M. (1982). Cerebral histamine: indications for neuronal and vascular regulation. J. Cereb. Blood Flow Metab. 2:3-23.

Gross, P. M., G. M. Teasdale, D. I. Graham, W. J. Angerson and A. M. Harper (1982). Intra-arterial histamine increases blood-brain transport in rats. Am. J. Physiol. 243:H307-H317.

Gross, P. M., A. M. Harper and G. M. Teasdale (1983). Interaction of histamine with noradrenergic constrictory mechanisms in cat cerebral arteries and veins. Can. J. Physiol. Pharmacol. 6l:756-763.

Haddy, F. J. (1960). Effect of histamine on small and large vessel pressures in the dog foreleg. Am. J. Physiol. 198:161-168.

Hardebo, J. E. (1980). A time study in rat on the opening and reclosure of the blood-brain barrier after hypertensive or hypertonic insult. Exp. Neurol. 70:155-160.

Head, R. J., J. T. Hjelle, B. Jarrott, B. Berkowitz, G. Cardinale and S. Spector (1980). Isolated brain microvessels: preparation, morphology, histamine and catecholamine contents. Blood Vessels 17:173-186.

Heistad, D. D., M. L. Marcus, S. I. Said and P. M. Gross (1980). Effect of acetylcholine and vasoactive intestinal peptide on cerebral blood flow. Am. J. Physiol. 239:H73-H80.

Hurst, E. W. and O. L. Davies (1950). Studies on the blood-brain barrier II. Attempts to influence the passage of substances into the brain. Brit. J. Pharmacol. 5:147-163.

Joó, F. (1979). Significance of adenylate cyclase in the regulation of the permeability of brain capillaries. In B.B. Mrsulja, M. Rakie, I. Klatzo and M. Spatz (Eds.), Pathophysiology of Cerebral Energy Metabolism, Plenum, New York, pp. 211-237.

Juan, H. and W. Sametz (1980). Histamine-induced release of arachidonic acid and of prostaglandins in the peripheral vascular bed: mode of action. Arch. Pharmacol. 314:183-190.

Karnushina, I. L., J. M. Palacios, G. Barbin, E. Dux, F. Joó and J. C. Schwartz (1980). Studies on a capillary-rich fraction isolated from brain: histaminic components and characterization of the histamine receptors linked to adenylate cyclase. J. Neurochem. 34:1201-1208.

Lassen, N.A. (1974). Control of cerebral circulation in health and disease. Circ. Res. 34:749-760.

Lokhandwala, M. F. (1978). Inhibition of sympathetic nervous system by histamine: studies with H_1- and H_2-receptor antagonists. J. Pharmacol. Exp. Ther. 206:115-122.

McGrath, M. A. and J. T. Shepherd (1976). Inhibition of adrenergic neurotransmission in canine vascular smooth muscle by histamine: mediation by H_2-receptors. Circ. Res. 39:566-573.

Muravchick, S. and E. H. Bergofsky (1976). Adrenergic receptors and vascular resistance in cerebral circulation of the cat. J. Appl. Physiol. 40:797-804.

Oldendorf, W. H. (1971). Brain uptake of radiolabeled amino acids, amines, and hexoses after arterial injection. Am. J. Physiol. 221:1629-1639.

Olesen, J. (1982). Effects of circulating monoamines and related substances on rCBF in man; in Heistad, Marcus, Cerebral blood flow: effects of nerves and neurotransmitters. Elsevier/North-Holland, New York, pp. 183-188.

Owen, D. A. A. (1977). Histamine receptors in the cardiovascular system. Gen. Pharmacol. 8:141-156.

Peroutka, S. J., M. A. Moskowitz, J. F. Reinhard, Jr. and S. H. Snyder (1980). Neurotransmitter receptor binding in bovine cerebral microvessels. Science 208:610-612.

Powell, J. R. and M. J. Brody (1976). Identification and specific blockade of two receptors for histamine in the cardiovascular system. J. Pharmacol. Exp. Ther. 196:1-14.

Powell, J.R. (1979). Effects of histamine on vascular sympathetic neuroeffector transmission. J. Pharmacol. Exp. Ther. 208:360-365.

Raper, A. J., H. A. Kontos, E. P. Wei and J. L. Patterson, Jr. (1972). Unresponsiveness of pial pre-capillary vessels to catecholamines and sympathetic nerve stimulation. Circ. Res. 31:257-266.

Rapoport, S. I. (1976). Blood-Brain Barrier in Physiology and Medicine, Raven, New York.

Rosenblum, W. I. (1976). Pial arteriolar responses in the mouse brain revisited. Stroke 7:283-287.

Ryan, M. J. and M. J. Brody (1970). Distribution of histamine in the canine autonomic nervous system. J. Pharmacol. Exp. Ther. 174:123-132.

Ryan, M. J. and M. J. Brody (1972). Neurogenic and vascular stores of histamine in the dog. J. Pharmacol. Exp. Ther. 181:83-91.

Saxena, P. R. (1975). The significance of histamine H_1 and H_2 receptors on the carotid vascular bed in the dog. Neurology 25:681-687.

Sharpey-Schafer, E. P. and J. Ginsberg (1962). Humoral agents and venous tone: effects of catecholamines, 5-hydroxytryptamine, histamine, and nitrites. Lancet December 29: 1337-1340.

Skofitsch, G., J. Donnerer, S. Petronijevic, A. Saria and F. Lembeck (1983). Release of histamine by neuropeptides from the perfused rat hindquarter. Arch. Pharmacol. 322:153-157.

Snyder, S. H., J. Axelrod and H. Bauer (1964). The fate of ^{14}C-histamine in animal tissues. J. Pharmacol. Exp. Ther. 144:373-379.

Sokoloff, L. (1959). The action of drugs on the cerebral circulation. Pharmacol. Rev. 11:1-85.

Spira, P. J., E. J. Mylecharane, J. Misbach, J. W. Duckworth and J. W. Lance. (1978). Internal and external carotid vascular responses to vasoactive agents in the monkey. Neurology 28:162-173.

Tindall, G. T. and J. C. Greenfield (1973). The effects of intra-arterial histamine on blood flow in the internal and external carotid artery of man. Stroke 4:46-49.

Wahl, M. and W. Kuschinsky (1979). The dilating effect of histamine on pial arteries of cats and its mediation by H_2 receptors. Circ. Res. 44:161-165.

Role of Histamine in Immune Responses

LYMPHOCYTES AND HISTAMINE, A NEW ENTRY TO IMMUNOREGULATION

J.-F. Bach, L. Chatenoud and M. Dy

INSERM U25, Hôpital Necker, 161 rue de Sèvres,
75015 Paris, France

INTRODUCTION

Histamine has been known for a long time to be one of the main end-products of immediate hypersensitivity reactions. Its role in IgE-mediated anaphylaxis and atopy is well established, even if other mediators also intervene in a major fashion. Recently, other properties of histamine related to the immune system have been revealed, which suggest that it could play an important role in the regulation of immune responses.

IMMUNOPHARMACOLOGICAL EFFECTS OF HISTAMINE

Histamine modulates the function of most cells involved in immune responses (Plaut and Lichtenstein, 1982). The suppressive effect on lymphocyte proliferative responses was one of the first to be recognized. Histamine exerts its inhibitory activity only at high concentrations (10^{-4}M) when optimal concentrations of mitogens are used (e.g., concanavalin A) (Plaut, Nordin and Thomas, 1980; Wang and Zweiman, 1978). However, the inhibition of lymphocyte proliferation is induced by lower histamine concentrations ($10^{-6} - 10^{-7}$M) for mixed lymphocyte reactions and mitogens used at suboptimal concentrations. Effects of cell mediated immunity are also suppressed by histamine (10^{-6}M) and its two major aspects : T-cell mediated cytotoxicity (Plaut, Nordin and Thomas, 1980; Yellin 'and others', 1979) and lymphokine production (Rocklin, 1976). All these effects are opposed by H2 antihistamine drugs, indicating that they are mediated by H2 receptors. Regulatory T cells are also affected by histamine, particularly suppressor T cells. It was initially shown that histamine inhibited the induction of suppressor cells at high concentrations, an effect surprisingly blocked by H1 antagonists (Askenase, Gundeson and Graziano, 1980). More recently, Rocklin (1977) has shown that histamine was in fact capable of activating suppressor cells generated following concanavalin A-induced polyclonal activation. This effect, which is mediated by a T-cell produced soluble factor (histamine suppressor factor), probably explains some of the histamine properties mentioned above (Rocklin, 1977). Histamine may also suppress antibody formation in vitro and NK cell cytotoxicity. This wide range of activities presents the problem of a putative common mode of action. The first and main question relates to the existence of histamine receptors on lymphocytes and their involvement in the histamine immunopharmacological effects. Several approaches argue in favor of the presence of histamine receptors on certain lymphoid cell populations. Lymphocytes form rosettes with histamine coated cells (Saxon, Morledge and Bonavida, 1977) and are retained on histamine coated columns (Ballet and Merler, 1976). Preliminary studies have been performed with radiolabeled ligands with H1 or H2 receptor specificity (Osband and Mc Caffrey, 1979). It is only fair to say that if all these studies have revealed the indubitable presence of histamine binding sites on lymphoid cells, no sufficient evidence has yet been collected to assess the existence of true histamine receptors on lymphocytes. The possibility of non specific binding has not yet been totally excluded, even if the various lymphoid subsets do not bind histamine equally : in particular, the suppressor T cell subpopulation, one of the potential targets of histamine has been reported to be selectively retained on histamine-coated columns, but the specificity of this retention has been questioned because of the low avidity of histamine binding to lymphocytes. Most data pertinent to the receptor problem are based upon pharmacological studies using histamine antagonists. At variance with anaphylactic effects, which are essentially mediated by H1 receptors, it is apparent that the immunoregulatory effects of histamine are generally blocked by H2 rather than H1 antagonists. This is not, however, a general rule, and again high antagonist concentrations must be used. In some cases neither H1 nor H2 antagonists significantly blocks the histamine effects. In addition, inhibitors, particularly cimetidine, have been shown to have significant effects in vitro in the absence of histamine, which may be interpreted either as a direct effect of the compound, or an inhibition of the histamine produced during the in vitro reaction, for example by phagocytic cells.

Another important problem is that of the cellular mode of action of histamine. It is interesting that histamine induces a rise in cyclic AMP levels and that its immunoregulatory effects parallel, in several regards, those of another agent known to increase lymphocyte cyclic AMP levels, prostaglandin E2. The precise level of action of histamine (or cyclic AMP) is not known. It may act upon cellular proliferation, cell metabolic activity or directly upon the cell membrane as suggested by direct short term effects on lymphocyte membranes : histamine inhibits E rosette formation by T cells mixed with sheep red blood cells and, as we shall see below, cimetidine or histamine agonists (Birch and Polmar, 1981) alters the phenotypic expression of differentiation antigens defined by monoclonal antibodies.

IN VIVO RELEVANCE OF HISTAMINE IMMUNOREGULATORY PROPERTIES. THE EFFECT OF CIMETIDINE TREATMENT.

All data mentioned above are derived from in vitro experiments whose artificial nature is well appreciated. Experiments with H2 antagonists have provided some indication that histamine could have a true immunoregulatory function in vivo. Indeed, cimetidine has been shown to enhance delayed type hypersensitivity reactions in patients with normal (Avella 'and others', 1978) or depressed (Jorizzo 'and others", 1980) cell-mediated immunity. In vivo treatment with cimetidine has also been shown to augment mitogen responsiveness and tumor rejection (Osband 'and others', 1981) and skin grafts (Golberg 'and others', 1979). These effects are in keeping with the numerous reports of heightened in vitro immune responses induced by the addition of relatively potent cimetidine concentrations (Gifford, Hatfield and Schmidtke, 1980).

The mechanism of action of cimetidine in vivo on immunological parameters is not clear. Recent data obtained in our laboratory (Chatenoud 'and others', 1982) indicate that several targets may be involved. We initially observed that cimetidine given orally, at doses of 400-600 mg/day, to hemodialyzed patients altered T cell phenotypes with an increase in the percentage of $OKT8^+$ cells (which include suppressor T cells), a rather unexpected finding, since the working hypothesis was that cimetidine enhanced immunity by inhibiting suppressor T cell function. In fact, further investigation showed that the increased number of $OKT8^+$ cells was the consequence of an augmented $OKT4^+$ $OKT8^+$ pool; i.e., cells that express both the T4 and T8 markers. This overlap is usually not found in peripheral blood and is only seen on immature T cells, such as those found in the thymus. It is unlikely that cimetidine acted in these patients by promoting the release of thymocytes from the thymus, since doubly labeled cells could also be induced in vitro using normal peripheral blood lymphocy   and, more informatively, using purified OKT4+ cells separated by panning from OKT8+ cells. In any case, if it is assumed that cimetidine acts in vivo by blocking the physiological effects of histamine (rather than showing a direct pharmacological effect), these results suggest that histamine could contribute to the control of lymphocyte membrane activity. Its action on the T cell differentiation antigen T8 could have counterparts in other membrane receptors involved in the various lymphocyte functions. It is interesting, in this regard, to note that the T8 molecule itself has recently been shown to participate in antigen recognition by the suppressor/cytotoxic T cell subset.

Our studies with cimetidine-treated patients have also revealed an increased production of interleukin 2 (IL-2) lymphokine known to enhance the differentiation of cytotoxic T cells and to promote T cell growth in vitro. This cimetidine effect could be related to the suppressive effect of histamine on lymphocyte proliferation discussed above, which is dependent upon the presence of interleukin 2. It is reminiscent of the effect of monocyte-produced PGE2 which suppresses IL-2 production by activating suppressor T-cells. It is possible, although not proven, that histamine and PGE2 interact by modulating IL-2 production. Indeed, Rocklin has suggested that histamine could induce the production of histamine suppressor factor (HSF) which would itself stimulate monocyte synthesis of immunosuppressive PGE2. (this volume).

HISTAMINE PRODUCTION DURING NON IgE-MEDIATED IMMUNE RESPONSES.

Most of the immunoregulatory effects of histamine discussed so far involve cell-mediated immunity which develops at the antigen site. In order to assess the physiological role of histamine in the regulation of these immune responses it is essential to know whether all participants in the histamine-induced immunoregulation are present at the site of T-cell-mediated immune reactions. Recent studies performed in our laboratory indicate that histamine could indeed be produced in allografts undergoing rejection (Dy 'and others', 1981) and possibly during other T-cell mediated immunological responses. High histamine levels are found in the supernatants from secondary mixed lymphocyte reactions performed by mixing lymphocytes from a skin allograft recipient with allogeneic lymphocytes from the skin donor strain. Studies showing the incorporation of labeled histidine into histamine and increased levels of histidine decarboxydase demonstrated that histamine is indeed synthesized during the reaction. This histamine synthesis is secondary to the action of a lymphokine (non antigen specific T cell product) called HCSF (histamine producing cell stimulating factor). This lymphokine is also fabricated by concanavalin A stimulated T cells, which suggests its possible intervention in the generation of the T cell mediated suppression discussed above. HCSF has been purified and shown to be a glycoprotein with a mol.wt of approximately 30.000   KD. HCSF stimulates histamine synthesis in bone marrow cells and to a slighter degree in other lymphoid organs. Another lymphokine, called interleukin 3 (IL-3), has also been shown to stimulate histamine synthesis and to promote histamine production and cell differentiation. HCSF and IL-3 are closely related chemically and could represent variants of the same molecule (Ihle ' and others', 1983). Alternatively, HCSF and IL-3 could be two totally separate molecules with overlapping activities. Recent data obtained in our laboratory indicate that chemical differences exist between the two molecules, thus leaving the question open. HCSF could intervene in vivo by increasing histamine synthesis in immune reactions involving T cell activation. Thus, HCSF and histamine synthesis are dramatically increased at the time of worm rejection in Nippostrongylus brasiliensis infested rats (Abbud Filho 'and others', 1983). It remains to be determined, however, whether HCSF target cells are present at the same of the immunological reaction. HCSF is most active on bone marrow cells where it probably interacts with a subset of mast-cell like cells. It will be important to better characterize this cell type and search for its presence in allograft or delayed type reactions which has already been proven in certain settings (i.e., in the basophil associated delayed type Jones-Motes reaction) but remains to be established on a larger scale.

CONCLUSIONS

Immunoregulation involves a complex series of events in which several cellular populations interact either directly or via the intermediary of humoral mediators. Some of these cellular interactions, either positive (helper) or inhibitory (suppressive), are antigen specific. Others are not antigen specific and generally operate through soluble mediators such as monokines, (interleukin 1), lymphokines (interleukin 2), suppressor factors and prostaglandins. The entirety of the data reviewed in this article suggests that histamine could be one of these mediators. If this were to be confirmed, it would be interesting that whereas its primary significance in anaphylaxis and atopy would be lost, histamine would now be considered in the context of several other potent mediators, such as serotonin, or SRS-A, and could acquire a new and important role in immunity, as an important intermediate in immunoregulation, notably in the generation of non antigen specific suppressor mechanisms.

REFERENCES

Abbud Filho, M., M. Dy, B. Lebel, G. Luffau, and J. Hamburger (1983). Eur. J. Immunol., 13, 841-847.
Askenase, P.W., L. Gundeson, and F. Graziano (1980). Late cutaneous reactions mediated by serum rich in guinea-pig IgE antibody. Abstract 13.3.01. Abstracts of the 4th International Congress of Immunology, Paris.
Avella, J., H.J. Binder, J.E. Madsen, and P.W. Askenase (1978). Lancet., 1, 624.
Ballet, J.J., and E. Merker (1976). Cell. Immunol., 24, 250-269.
Birch, R.E., and S.H. Polmar (1981). Cell. Immunol., 57, 455-467.
Chatenoud, L., S. Berrih, M.C. Bene, H. Kreis, and J.F. Bach (1982). J. Clin. Immunol., 3, 61-66.
Dy, M., B. Lebel, P. Kamoun, and J. Hamburger (1981). J. Exp. Med., 153, 293-309.
Gifford, R.R.M., S.M. Hatfield, and J.R. Schmidtke (1980). Transplantation, 29, 143-148.
Golberg, E.H., J.S. Goodwin, S.E. Arrit, and R.C. Williams (1979). Transplantation, 28, 432-433.
Ihle, J.N., J. Keller, S. Orozlan, L.E. Henderson, T.D. Copeland, F. Fitch, M.B. Prystowsky, E. Goldwasser, J.W. Schrader, E. Palszynski, M. Dy, and B. Lebel, (1983). J. Immunol. 131, 282-287.
Jorizzo, J.L., W.M. Sams, B.V. Jegasothy, and A.J. Olansky (1980). Annals Intern. Med., 92, 192-195.
Osband, M., and R. Mc Caffrey (1979). J. Biol. Chem., 254, 9970-9972.
Osband, M., Y.J. Shen M. Shlesinger, A. Brown, D. Hamilton, E. Cohen, P. Lavin, and R. Mc Caffrey (1981). Lancet, 1, 636-638.
Plaut, M., and L.M. Lichtenstein (1982). Histamine and immune response. Pharmacology of Histamine Receptors, Wright-PSG, Bristol.
Plaut, M., L. Nordin, and L.L. Thomas (1980). Fed. Proc., 39, 445. (abstr.)
Rocklin, R.E. (1976). J. Clin. Invest., 57, 1051-1058.
Rocklin, R.E. (1977). J. Immunol., 118, 1734-1738.
Saxon, A., V.D. Morledge, and B. Bonavida (1977). Clin. Exp. Immunol., 28, 394-399.
Wang, S.R., and B. Zweiman (1978). Cell. Immunol., 36, 28-36.
Yellin, T.O., S.H. Buck, D.J. Gilman (1979). Pharmacologist, 21, 266 (abstr.)

HISTAMINE-INDUCED SUPPRESSOR CELL RESPONSES IN NORMAL AND ATOPIC SUBJECTS

R. E. Rocklin

Tufts University Medical School, Boston, MA, USA

ABSTRACT

Histamine-induced suppressor T cell function is mediated in part through the production of a suppressor lymphokine termed HSF. The latter is produced by stimulating a subpopulation of H_2 receptor-bearing T lymphocytes with histamine. HSF in turn augments the production of prostaglandin by monocytes. These latter compounds are thought to be intimately involved in the effector stage of this reaction and may directly suppress lymphocyte proliferation or lymphokine production or further activate suppressor T cells. In addition, indomethacin, a cyclo-oxygenase pathway inhibitor, can reverse histamine-induced suppression. In addition to its role in the effector stage, the monocyte is also known to be required in the activation of histamine-induced suppressor cell. A monokine, IL-1, has been shown to augment lymphocyte activation in response to histamine.

Atopic subjects have recently been documented to have reduced histamine-induced (but not Con A-induced) suppressor T cell function and to have decreased phenotypic expression of T cell H_2 receptors but not of T cell H_1 receptors, when compared to nonatopic controls. Since proper functioning of the above suppressor system involves obligatory interactions between lymphocytes and monocytes, it is possible that a defect in lymphocyte and/or monocyte function or a defect in the response to, or production of, monokines, such as IL-1 and prostaglandins, could explain the abnormal histamine-suppressor response seen in atopic subjects. However, recent studies show that lymphocytes from atopic patients fail to produce normal amounts of a suppressor factor lymphokine (HSF) when stimulated by histamine. This response cannot be corrected by the exogenous addition of IL-1. If HSF is exogenously provided to cultures of atopic monocytes, their production of PGE_2 is reduced as compared to the amount produced from monocytes of normal subjects. These data suggest that there may be an underlying defect in the immunoregulatory system of the mononuclear cells of atopic patients.

KEYWORDS

Histamine; suppressor cells; lymphocytes; atopic disease; suppressor lymphokine; prostaglandins; interleukin I.

INTRODUCTION

Regulation of the immune response is similar to other complex biologic processes in that it is modulated by a series of positive and negative factors. A major negative regulatory influence is provided by suppressor T cells (Cantor and Gershon, 1979). Suppressor lymphocytes can be activated *in vitro* by various stimuli including specific antigens, mitogens, antigen-antibody complexes and histamine. This activation process involves the participation of macrophages, inducer T lymphocytes and suppressor cell precursors. Mature suppressor T cells are a lineage distinct from helper, lymphokine producing and cytotoxic T lymphocytes and are themselves a heterogeneous population. Signals from cell to cell in immunoregulatory systems may be mediated by soluble suppressor factors. Indeed, the addition of soluble suppressor factors to some *in vitro* systems such as antibody formation and allogeneic lymphocyte reactions may substitute for the presence of intact suppressor cells.

Recent studies have demonstrated that histamine activates human suppressor cells *in vitro* (Beer et al, 1982a, 1982b; Rocklin et al, 1980; Thomas et al, 1981). Highly purified populations of human T cells, but not of B cells, produced a histamine-induced suppressor factor (HSF) in response to varying concentrations of histamine (10^{-9} - 10^{-4}M). The histamine dose response curves for the generation of HSF were variable from one individual to another. In some instances, high concentrations of histamine (10^{-5} - 10^{-4} M) were required to produce HSF whereas in other instances, low concentrations (10^{-8} - 10^{-6} M) generated peak HSF responses. Ongoing DNA metabolism was not required for the release of HSF as evidenced by the finding that mitomycin-C treatment did not diminish its production. The T cells that synthesized HSF expressed an H_2-receptor, were retained on columns containing insolubilized histamine, were found within the OKT8-positive population, and comprised 50 percent of the population of T cells that possess Fc receptors for IgG (T_γ) (Damle and Gupta, 1981; Lima and Rocklin, 1981).

Human HSF has been characterized by enzyme treatment, sensitivity to reduction and alkylation, by molecular sieve chromatography and polyacrylamide gel electrophoresis (Rocklin et al, 1983). HSF was found to have a wide pH stability (pH 3-10), sensitivity to temperatures greater than 80°C, and found to have the properties of a glycoprotein by virtue of its sensitivity to chymotrypsin, sodium periodate and neuraminidase. HSF did not appear to have serine groups in its active site since its biologic activity remained intact following treatment with irreversible serine esterase inhibitors. HSF did not appear to have inter- or intra-molecular disulfide bridges because treatment with denaturing and/or reducing agents followed by alkylation did not significantly alter its suppressor activity. Molecular sieve chromatography employing Sephadex G-100 revealed an apparent molecular weight for HSF of 25,000-40,000. Electrophoresis of HSF in polyacrylamide gels under nonreducing conditions revealed two regions of activity, one region migrating with albumin and the other anodal to albumin.

The metabolic requirements for the generation of histamine-induced suppressor cells has recently been investigated (Rocklin and Haberek-Davidson, 1984). The generation of histamine-induced suppressor cells was shown to require active cellular metabolism since inhibitors of transcription, translation, oxidative phosphorylation and glycolysis significantly reduced their activity. Furthermore, inhibitors of cytoskeletal function such as colchicine and cytochalasin B also markedly reduced suppressor activity. There was no apparent requirement for DNA synthesis in the generation of suppressor cells. These agents may interfere with critical lymphocyte-macrophage interactions (described below) that are required for intact suppressor responses.

The requirement for the presence of monocytes in the activation and expression of histamine-induced suppressor activity has recently been explored. Histamine activation of human suppressor T cells was shown to require the presence of monocytes (Beer et al, 1982a, 1982b). T lymphocyte populations containing less than two percent monocytes were unable to be activated by histamine to exert a suppressor influence. If, during the generation phase, the T cell population was reconstituted by the readdition of 5-10 percent autologous monocytes, subsequent exposure to histamine resulted in suppressor activity. The requirement for intact monocytes in the activation process could be bypassed by suspending the T lymphocytes in culture fluids derived from activated monocytes. This supernatant factor was subsequently identified as being interleukin I (Beer et al, 1982b). Interleukin I by itself did not activate suppressor T cells non-specifically, but instead behaved as an accessory factor that was required for the generation of histamine-induced suppressor T cells.

Further investigation has also revealed a requirement for monocytes in the effector stage of histamine-induced suppressor activity (Beer et al, 1982a; Rocklin et al, 1983). The removal of monocytes from both the suppressor and target cell populations resulted in a marked reduction of histamine-induced suppressor activity despite the addition of human interleukin I to the assay. Thus, unlike the generation phase of suppressor cell activation where a monocyte-derived factor could partially replace or augment the function of intact monocytes, the effector phase appeared to require the presence of monocytes or a factor not present in the dialyzed, partially purified monocyte culture fluids for full expression of histamine-induced suppressor activity. Furthermore, the addition of indomethacin (a prostaglandin synthesis inhibitor) during the effector phase abrogated histamine-induced suppression when monocytes were present. In contrast, indomethacin had no effect on the generation of suppressor cells. These latter observations led to the demonstration that supernatants from histamine stimulated mononuclear cells induced monocytes, but not lymphocytes, to increase their production of prostaglandins and thromboxane B_2. Collectively, these data suggest that HSF mediated inhibition of lymphocyte proliferation may occur in part through the augmented production of prostaglandins and/or thromboxane B_2 by human monocytes. Figure 1 presents a model illustrating the cellular interactions between lymphocytes and monocytes involved in the activation of suppressor cells and the expression of their activity.

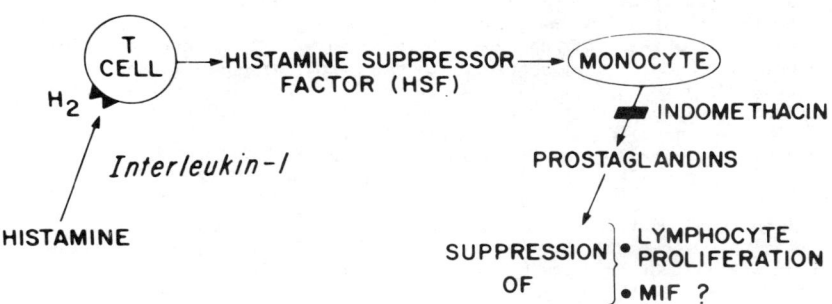

Fig. 1. Proposed model of *in vitro* monocyte-lymphocyte interactions required for generation and expression of histamine-induced suppression.

An evaluation of non-specific suppressor cell function in patients with atopic disorders (rhino-conjunctivitis and/or asthma) has revealed a subtle defect. Mononuclear cells from allergic patients have generated less histamine-induced suppressor activity compared to non-atopic control subjects (Beer et al, 1982c). This defect in suppressor cell response was not "global" and appeared to be specific for histamine because their response to another suppressor signal, concanavalin A, was normal. In the process of investigating the mechanism related to this diminished response to histamine, it was found that the number of H_2-receptor bearing T lymphocytes (but not H_1-receptor bearing T cells) was decreased in these atopic patients. One explanation for the reduced functional suppressor response to histamine as well as the reduced phenotypic expression of H_2-receptors in the atopic population is that they represent secondary changes resulting from chronic *in vivo* exposure of their lymphocytes to circulating histamine, rather than primary abnormalities inherent to the atopic diathesis. This question was addressed when non-atopic patients with systemic mastocytosis (a disease characterized by elevated levels of circulating histamine) had their histamine responsive suppressor cells evaluated (Beer et al, 1982c). In this latter group of patients, the suppressor cell response to histamine was normal, as was the expression of H_1- and H_2-receptors on their T lymphocytes. This observation mitigates against the observed abnormalities in atopics as representing secondary changes from *in vivo* "desensitization" or receptor "down regulation". Rather, the suppressor cell abnormalities observed in allergic subjects may reflect a primary defect inherent to the atopic diathesis.

Since proper functioning of the above histamine activatable suppressor system involves obligatory interactions between lymphocytes and monocytes, it is possible that a defect in lymphocyte and/or monocyte function, or a defect in the response to, or production of monokines, such as interleukin 1 and prostaglandins, could explain the abnormal histamine suppressor response observed in atopic subjects. An analysis was carried out of the *in vitro* components of histamine activated mononuclear cells from atopic patients with regard to their production of the suppressor lymphokine (HSF) and a monocyte function, namely HSF-augmented production of prostaglandin E_2 (PGE) (Matloff et al, 1983). Blood mononuclear cells from atopic patients and non-atopic controls were preactivated with histamine or Con-A and their ability to suppress lectin-stimulated lymphocyte proliferation was measured. While cells from some atopics had normal amounts of inhibition, the mean percent suppression by histamine stimulated atopic mononuclear cells was significantly reduced compared to the mean suppression exerted by mononuclear cells from normal subjects (Fig. 2). The addition of interleukin 1 to either mononuclear cells or nylon wool purified T cells did not restore the histamine suppressor response of atopics to the normal range (Matloff et al, 1983).

Cells from atopic patients and controls were stimulated in the presence or absence of histamine to generate HSF (Matloff et al, 1983). The results of these experiments indicated that HSF production by atopic mononuclear cells was significantly reduced compared to that of normal mononuclear cells (Fig. 3). The exogenous addition of interleukin 1 to the atopic cultures did not significantly increase HSF activity to normal levels. Since atopic mononuclear cells did not produce a suppressor signal in response to histamine, it was important to determine whether this signal, if provided exogenously, would stimulate atopic monocytes to produce prostaglandin. The results of these experiments demonstrated that monocytes from atopic patients synthesized approximately tenfold less PGE_2 compared to monocytes from control subjects (Matloff et al, 1983). Differences in the baseline levels of PGE_2 synthesized by monocytes from atopic and control subjects did not account for the reduction observed in the atopic group (Fig. 4).

In view of the T cell dependence for the regulation of IgE antibody production, overproduction of specific IgE observed in allergic disease might be a consequence of altered regulatory function. In humans, it has been demonstrated that atopic individuals have reduced proportions of T cells with surface membrane receptors for the Fc portion of IgG and that after successful immunotherapy, the proportions of these cells reaches normal levels (Canonica et al, 1979). Cells within the

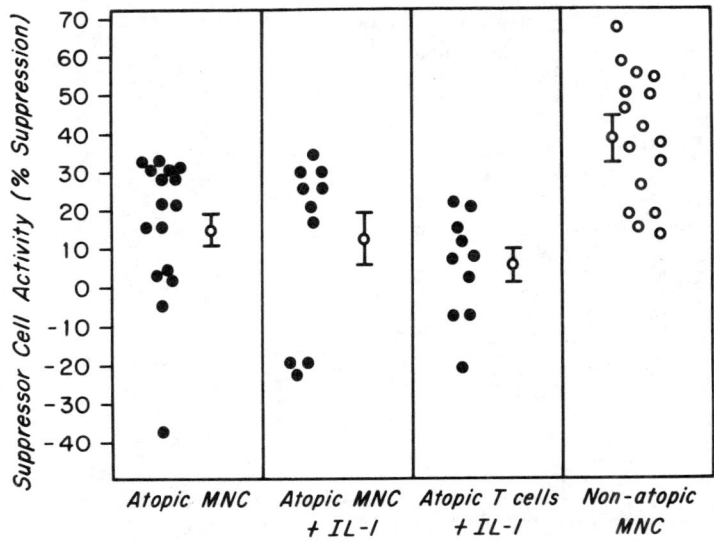

Fig. 2. Histamine-induced suppression by atopic mononuclear or T cells cultured in the absence or presence of IL-1 employing the co-culture technique. The suppressor-cell response by atopic cells was significantly reduced ($p<0.01$) compared to cells from control subjects. The addition of IL-1 did not substantially increase the suppressor activity.

latter subpopulation are known to regulate immunoglobulin synthesis by suppressing T-dependent B cell differentiation. Furthermore, it has been described above that T lymphocytes bearing H_2-receptors and expressing suppressor activity following stimulation with histamine also possess Fc receptors for IgG. It is possible then that the observed abnormalities in atopic subjects reflects an *in vivo* deficiency in antigen non-specific and/or antigen-specific suppressor cell activity, either or both of which may be necessary for the dampening of IgE antibody production. Evidence for this hypothesis is indirectly provided by a study in which it was demonstrated that ragweed antigen-specific suppressor T lymphocytes could be detected in ragweed allergic individuals during 6 and 12 months of immunotherapy, but not prior to therapy (Rocklin et al, 1980). When lymphocytes were taken from treated patients and passed over columns containing insolubilized histamine, antigen-specific suppressor cells that could be activated by ragweed antigen were deleted. These results suggested that antigen-specific suppressor T cells belonging to the subpopulation of lymphocytes bearing histamine receptors were generated during antigen desensitization, and failure to detect these cells in untreated patients may be a reflection of the underlying defect leading to the atopic diathesis.

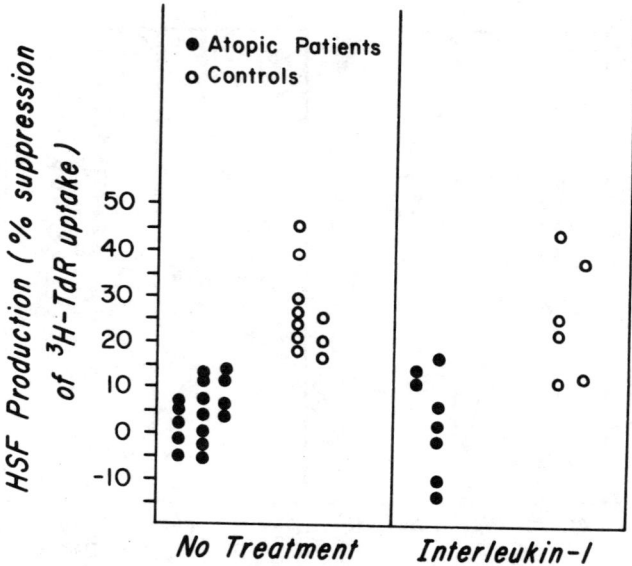

Fig. 3. HSF production by mononuclear cells from atopic patients and control subjects.

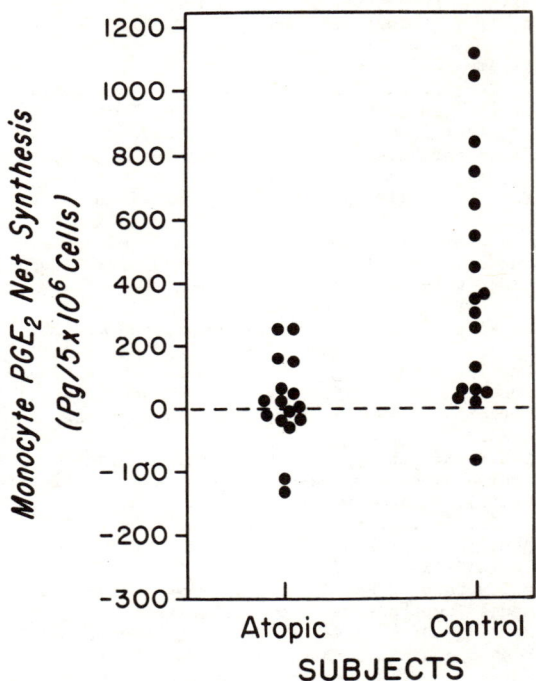

Fig. 4. PGE$_2$ production by HSF-stimulated monocytes obtained from atopic patients and normal subjects.

REFERENCES

Beer, D., C. Dinarello, L. Rosenwasser, and R. E. Rocklin (1982a). Cellular interactions in the generation and expression of histamine and concanavalin A-induced suppressor activity. *Cell. Immunol.*, 69, 101-112.

Beer, D., L. Rosenwasser, C. Dinarello, and R. E. Rocklin (1982b). Supernatants containing human leukocyte pyrogen replace the adherent cell requirement in human suppressor cell systems. *J. Clin. Invest.*, 70, 393-400.

Beer, D. J., M. E. Osband, R. P. McCaffrey, and R. E. Rocklin (1982c). Nonspecific suppressor cell function in atopic individuals. *N. Engl. J. Med.*, 306, 454-458.

Canonica, G. W., M. C. Mingan, G. Melioli, and L. Morretta (1979). Imbalances of T cell subpopulations in patients with atopic diseases and effect of specific immunotherapy. *J. Immunol.*, 123, 2669-2674.

Cantor, H., and R. K. Gershon (1979). Immunological circuits: cellular composition. *Fed. Proc.*, 38, 2058-2077.

Damle, N. K., and S. Gupta (1981). Autologous mixed lymphocyte reaction in man. II. Histamine-induced suppression of the autologus mixed lymphocyte reaction by T cell subsets defined with monoclonal antibodies. *J. Clin. Immunol.*, 1, 241-247.

Lima, M., and R. E. Rocklin (1981). Histamine modulates *in vitro* IgG production by human mononuclear cells. *Cell. Immunol.*, 64, 324-336.

Matloff, S. M., I. Kiselis, and R. E. Rocklin (1983). Reduced production of histamine-induced suppressor factor (HSF) by atopic mononuclear cells and decreased prostaglandin E_2 output by HSF-stimulated atopic monocytes. *J. Allergy Clin. Immunol.*, 72, 359-364.

Rocklin, R. E., J. Beard, S. Gupta, R. A. Good, and K. S. Melmon (1980). Characterization of the human blood lymphocytes that produce a histamine-induced suppressor factor (HSF). *Cell. Immunol.*, 51, 226-233.

Rocklin, R. E., A. L. Sheffer, D. R. Greineder, and K. S. Melmon (1980). Generation of antigen-specific suppressor cells during allergy desensitization. *N. Engl. J. Med.*, 302, 1213-1219.

Rocklin, R. E., A. Blidy, and M. Kamal (1983). Physicochemical characterization of human histamine-induced suppressor factor. *Cell. Immunol.*, 76, 243-252.

Rocklin, R. E., I. Kiselis, D. J. Beer, P. Rossi, F. Maggi, and J. Bellanti (1983). Augmentation of prostaglandin and thromboxane production *in vitro* by monocytes exposed to histamine-induced suppressor factor (HSF). *Cell. Immunol.*, 77, 92-98.

Rocklin, R. E., and A. Habarek-Davidson (1984). Pharmacologic modulation *in vitro* of human histamine-induced suppressor cell activity. *Int. J. Immunopharmacol.*, (In Press).

Thomas, Y., R. Huchet, and D. Grandjon (1981). Histamine-induced suppression of lymphocyte mitogenic responses. *Cell. Immunol.*, 59, 268-276.

HISTAMINE INDUCED INHIBITION OF INTERLEUKIN-2 SYNTHESIS AND ACTIVITY IN MAN

R. Huchet

INSERM U267, 14-16 avenue Paul-Vaillant-Couturier, 94804
Villejuif Cedex, France

ABSTRACT

In these experiments the mechanisms underlying the inhibitory activity of histamine on human lymphocyte response to PHA were investigated by the analysis of its interference with interleukin 2 (IL-2) synthesis and activity. Histamine inhibits IL-2 synthesis by the whole lymphocyte population and by the T4 and T8 lymphocytes. In addition histamine interaction with T lymphocytes leads to the release of a factor which inhibits the activity of IL-2 on its target cells.

KEYWORDS

Histamine inhibitory activity. IL-2 synthesis. Normal human lymphocytes. Inhibitory factor with anti IL-2 activity.

INTRODUCTION

Histamine is found endowed of the ability to inhibit mainly cell-mediated immunity as shown by numerous studies in guinea pigs (Rocklin, 1976, 1977, Rocklin and co-workers, 1978), in mice (Plaut and co-workers, 1973, 1975, Suzuki and Huchet, 1981, 1982) and in man (Ballet and Merler, 1976, Strannegard, 1976, Wang and Zweiman, 1978, Thomas, Huchet and Grandjon, 1981). The main feature of these inhibitory activities is the specificity of the interaction of histamine with H_2 receptor bore by T lymphocytes. This inhibition occurs either as a consequence of the functional inactivation of lymphocytes related to an increase in c.AMP (Bourne and co-workers, 1974), or as an induction of suppressor cells (Thomas, Huchet and Grandjon, 1981) leading to the release of inhibitory factors which in man inhibit the lymphocyte response to mitogens, and the functions of helper T cells (Rocklin and co-workers, 1980, Garovoy, Reddish, Rocklin, 1983).

The inhibitory activity of histamine and of the suppressor factor it induces, in the lymphocyte response to mitogens like PHA, raises the question of the interference of these activities with the mechanisms underlying T cell activation, namely IL-2 synthesis and activity. The experiments reported here were undertaken in order to analyse this question.

METHODOLOGY

Assay for IL-2 Synthesis by Normal Human Lymphocytes.

Mononuclear cells were prepared by density gradient centrifugation of heparinized blood over Ficoll-Paque (Pharmacia). The mononuclear cell suspension at 10^6 cells/ml, and irradiated (5000 r) Daudi cell line at the concentration of 2×10^5 cells/ml, were cultured in RPMI 1640 supplemented with L glutamine, gentalline and 1% AB serum. The cell suspension was first incubated for 4 hours at 37°C in a 5% CO_2 atmosphere with PHA (Difco) at a dilution of the mitogen giving an optimal stimulation of lymphocytes, and with TPA (20 ng/ml). At the end of this period the cells were washed 3 times and resuspended in RPMI supplemented as indicated above and cultured for 36 hours in 5% CO_2 atmosphere. Finally the cell suspension was centrifuged and the supernatant was dialysed against PBS for 24 hours and against RPMI for 6 hours. The supernatants were then sterilized by millipore filtration and stored frozen at -20°C.

The same assay for IL-2 production was performed after various treatments of the mononuclear cell population : a) with anti T4 or anti T8 monoclonal antibodies (Ortho) + complement in order to deplete selectively a given T lymphocyte subclass from the whole mononuclear cell population, (the remaining cells are referred respectively T8 and T4 lymphocytes, and include monocytes) ; b) with histamine : the cells were incubated for 3 hours at various molar concentrations in RPMI without AB serum ; c) both.

Assay for IL-2 Activity.

The IL-2 activity of the supernatants obtained was tested on the T cell blasts obtained after a 3 day culture period of lymphocytes with PHA. At the end of this period blast cells were isolated after centrifugation on Ficoll metrizoate (d = 1065) and resuspended in RPMI 1640 supplemented with human AB serum, glutamine and gentalline, at the concentration of 10^5 cells/ml. This cell suspension was distributed in 0.1 ml fraction in microtiter well (in Falcon microtissue culture plate (3042) with 0.1 ml of the supernatants of IL-2 activity to be determined for a three day culture period at 37°C in an humidified atmosphere of air (95%) and CO_2 (5%). For the evaluation of blast multiplication reflecting IL-2 activity, 0.2 u Ci of tritiated thymidine was added for the last six hours of culture. Cultures were harvested after pulsing a Mash II harvester on glass wool filters and were counted in a liquid scintillation counter. Each sample of IL-2 at a given dilution was studied in quadruplicate. Results are expressed by the arithmetic mean $\pm$ S.D.

RESULTS

Study of the Inhibitory Activity of Histamine on IL-2 Synthesis.

Lymphocytes were incubated with histamine at various molar concentrations for 3 hours at 37°C in RPMI without AB serum and after 3 washes assayed for IL-2 synthesis. Results in Table I show that a 3-fold reduction of the IL-2 synthesis is observed at 10^{-5} and 10^{-6}M and a noticeable reduction is observed in some experiments (like in experiment n° 2) at 10^{-8} M.

TABLE 1 Inhibitory Activity of various Molar Concentrations of Histamine on IL-2 Synthesis

Molar concentration of histamine	IL-2 activity	
	Exp. 1	Exp. 2
-	23 900 + 2 300	65 600 + 5 200
$10^{-5}M$	8 450 + 2 100	21 200 + 700
$10^{-6}M$	14 400 + 1 400	9 200 + 2 200
$10^{-7}M$	17 800 + 2 500	20 200 + 1 300
$10^{-8}M$	21 200 + 700	38 600 + 4 300

Inhibitory Activity of Histamine on IL-2 Synthesis by Lymphocyte Subpopulations

The inhibitory activity of histamine on IL-2 production by whole lymphocyte population T4 and T8 lymphocytes is reported in Table 2. At $10^{-5}M$, histamine inhibits IL-2 synthesis by each of these populations, at the different dilutions tested, albeit at different extent for each population.

TABLE 2 Study of the IL-2 Activity of the Supernatant of Lymphocytes Preincubated with Histamine (10^{-5} M) and cultured for IL-2 Production.

Source of supernatant		IL-2 activity of the supernatant at different dilutions		
Lymphocyte population	Histamine 10^{-5} M	1/2	1/4	1/8
Whole mono-nuclear cell population	-	27 275 + 4 000	15 780 + 5 000	6 020 + 1 100
	+	1 840 + 430	730 + 160	300 + 70
T4	-	23 080 + 3 300	9 100 + 1 100	5 680 + 1 250
	+	6 200 + 1 350	2 665 + 770	1 320 + 220
T8	-	7 180 + 950	2 620 + 150	1 200 + 150
	+	1 120 + 200	630 + 90	460 + 80

Study of the Anti IL-2 Activity of the Supernatant obtained Histamine Induced Inhibition of IL-2 Synthesis.

The supernatants of lymphocytes preincubated with histamine, exhibiting a severe reduction of IL-2 synthesis, were tested for their ability to interfere with the activity of a standard batch of IL-2. For this purpose 50 µl of undiluted supernatant of various cellular sources, with reduced IL-2 activity, or 50 µl of RPMI (control) were mixed with 50 µl of a standard batch of IL-2, at different dilutions, and added to 0.1 ml of T cell blasts. The IL-2 activity was measured 3 days later.

Results in Table 3 indicate that the supernatant of whole lymphocyte populations and of T8 lymphocytes, preincubated with histamine interferes with the activity of the standard batch of IL-2 leading to a 3-fold reduction of the latter, whereas the T4 supernatant exhibits only a marginal interference with IL-2 activity. This inhibition of IL-2 is quite similar to that described previously in mice by Hardt and co-workers (1980). These results indicate that histamine can act at the efferent arm of the triggering event related to IL-2, by inhibiting IL-2. However, this inhibitory factor was not found present in all the supernatants of lymphocytes preincubated with histamine and exhibiting a severe reduction of IL-2 activity. This led us to investigate whether IL-2 could not act directly on lymphocytes synthesizing IL-2.

TABLE 3 IL-2 Inhibitory Activity of the Supernatant of Lymphocytes Preincubated with Histamine (10^{-5} M) and with PHA and Daudi Cell Line Thereafter.

Experimental groups		Activity of the standard batch of IL-2 at the following dilutions in 50 ul		
		1/2	1/4	1/8
IL-2 + RPMI	50 µl 50 µl	27 200 ± 5 900	19 700 ± 300	9 500 ± 2 400
IL-2 + whole lymphocyte population supernatant	50 µl 50 µl	22 250 ± 3 300	5 900 ± 800	3 700 ± 200
IL-2 + T4 supernatant	50 µl 50 µl	22 300 ± 2 400	13 600 ± 3 300	7 500 ± 400
IL-2 + T8 supernatant	50 µl 50 µl	19 500 ± 1 800	6 200 ± 1 000	3 500 ± 500

Effect of Irradiation on the Histamine Induced Inhibition of IL-2 Synthesis.

The aim of this experiment was to get insight into the mechanism of histamine induced inhibition of IL-2 synthesis since it was shown on the one hand that histamine induced suppressor cells are radio-sensitive (Thomas, Huchet, Grandjon, 1981) and on the other hand that IL-2 synthesis is not altered after irradiation (Ruscetti and Gallo, 1981). For this purpose lymphocytes after preincubation with histamine 10^{-6} M, were irradiated (1200 r) or not, and assayed for IL-2 synthesis. The results of this experiment in Table 4 indicate that histamine induced inhibition of IL-2 synthesis is not altered after irradiation : lymphocytes preincubated with histamine exhibit the same suppression of IL-2 synthesis whether irradiated or not.

These results indicate therefore that the inhibitory activity of histamine can be observed in conditions where the activity histamine induced suppressor cells is destroyed. These results suggest that histamine could act directly on lymphocytes synthesising IL-2.

TABLE 4 Effect of Preincubation of Normal Human Lymphocytes with Histamine on their ability to synthetise IL-2.

Experimental groups :	IL-2 activity of the supernatant at the following dilutions		
	1/2	1/4	1/8
1. Preincubation with histamine 10^{-6} M	8 100 $\pm$ 300	4 000 $\pm$ 500	2 300 $\pm$ 600
2. No treatment	85 700 $\pm$ 7 200	49 100 $\pm$ 13 000	17 600 $\pm$ 3 200
3. Preincubation with histamine 10^{-6} and irradiation 1200 r thereafter	5 900 $\pm$ 800	3 500 $\pm$ 200	1 800 $\pm$ 200
4. Irradiation 1200 r	86 200 $\pm$ 1 800	41 500 $\pm$ 7 400	17 500 $\pm$ 2 000

CONCLUSION

Histamine induced inhibition of lymphocyte response to PHA is related to a reduction of IL-2 synthesis and in some cases to the production of a factor which inhibits the activity of IL-2 at the level of its target cell.

ACKNOWLEDGMENTS

This work was supported by grant n° 819 from UER Kremlin Bicêtre and grant n° 3070 from Association pour la Recherche sur le Cancer (Villejuif).

REFERENCES

Ballet, J.J., E. Merlet (1976). Cell Imm. 24, 250-269.
Bourne, H.R., L.M. Lichtenstein, K.L. Melmon, C.S. Henney, and Y. Weinstein. (1974). Science, 184, 19-28.
Garovoy, M.R., M.A. Reddish, and R.E. Rocklin. (1983). J. Imm. 130, 357-361.
Hardt, C., M. Rollinghoff, K. Pfizenmaier, H. Mosmann, and H. Wagner. (1981). J. Exp. Med., 154, 262-274.
Plaut, M., L.M. Lichtenstein, E. Gillepsie, and C.S. Henney. (1973). J. Imm. 111, 389-394.
Plaut, M., L.M. Lichtenstein, and C.S. Henney. (1975). J. Clin. Invest., 55, 856-874.
Rocklin, R.E. (1976). J. Clin. Invest., 57, 1051-1058.
Rocklin, R.E. (1977). J. Imm., 118, 1734-1738.
Rocklin, R.E.,D. Entredemer, B.M. Littman, K.L. Melmon. (1978). Cell. Imm., 37, 162-173.
Rocklin, R.E., J. Bréard, S. Gupta, R.A. Good, and K.L. Melmon. (1980). Cell. Imm., 51, 226-237.
Ruscetti, F.W., and R.C. Gallo. (1981). Blood, 57, 379-394.
Strannegard, I.L., and O. Strannegard. (1977). Scand. J. Imm., 6, 1225-1231.
Suzuki, S., and R. Huchet. (1981). Cell. Imm., 62, 396-405.
Suzuki, S., and R. Huchet. (1982). Cell. Imm., 68, 349-358.
Thomas, Y., R. Huchet, and D. Grandjon. (1981). Cell. Imm., 59, 268-275.
Wang, R.S., and B. Zweiman. (1978). Cell. Imm., 36, 28-36.

HISTAMINE-INDUCED HUMAN LYMPHOKINES AFFECTING T-LYMPHOCYTE MOTILITY

D. J. Beer, W. W. Cruikshank, J. S. Berman and D. M. Center

Pulmonary Center, Evans Memorial Department of Clinical Research, Boston University School of Medicine, Boston, MA 02118, USA

ABSTRACT

Although functional histamine receptors have generally been restricted to those human T lymphocytes expressing suppressor cell functions, more recent evidence suggests that histamine receptor-bearing human T lymphocytes are functionally heterogeneous and capable of other immunomodulatory activities. Lymphocyte chemoattractant factor (LCF) is a cationic sialoprotein with an apparent MW of 56,000, whose production is limited to histamine-type 2 (H_2) receptor-bearing human T cells. LCF is selectively chemokinetic for T lymphocytes, and presumably contributes to the recruitment of effector lymphocytes at inflammatory sites. In addition to LCF, Sephadex G-100 gel filtration of histamine-induced lymphocyte supernatants revealed two regions of migration inhibitory activity for T-cells. These regions corresponded to MWs of 70-80,000 ($LyMIF_{75K}$) and 30-40,000 ($LyMIF_{35K}$). $LyMIF_{75K}$ had a single pI of 7.5-8.0 and its biologic activity was sensitive to trypsin but not to neuraminidase and heat. $LyMIF_{35K}$ had a single pI of 8.5 and its biologic activity was sensitive to neuraminidase and heat but not to trypsin. Lymphocytes incubated with histamine and diphenhydramine produced LCF but neither LyMIF, whereas cells incubated with histamine in the presence of cimetidine produced both LyMIFs but not LCF. These data suggest that a subset of lymphocytes defined by the presence of histamine-type 1 (H_1) receptors are capable of producing two distinct species of lymphocyte migration inhibitory activity. These cells may contribute to the immobilization of effector T lymphocytes chemokinetically attracted to certain inflammatory sites.

KEY WORDS

Histamine, lymphokines, histamine-type 1 receptors, lymphocyte migration inhibitory factors, inflammation.

INTRODUCTION

The human T lymphocyte subset is heterogeneous, both on the basis of phenotypic membrane macromolecules and functional capabilities. Among the former, some T cells bear receptors for vasoactive amines (Melmon, Rocklin, and Rosenkranz, 1981). Experiments in a number of species have suggested that vasoactive amines may play an important role in regulating immune responses both _in vivo_ and _in vitro_ (reviewed in Rocklin and Beer, 1983; Beer, Matloff, and Rocklin, 1984). Although histamine receptors generally have been restricted to human OKT8+ suppressor cells (Damle and Gupta, 1981), this report will demonstrate that T cells bearing histamine receptors are themselves phenotypically and functionally heterogeneous. Employing an *in vitro* microchemotaxis assay to assess lymphocyte migration, we have recently identified and characterized a histamine-induced lymphokine, lymphocyte chemoattractant factor (LCF) which is selectively chemokinetic for T cells. LCF is a cationic (pI 9.0) sialoprotein with a molecular weight (MW) of 56,000 daltons, that is produced only by H_2 receptor-bearing lymphocytes (Center, Cruikshank, Berman, and Beer, 1983). LCF presumably contributes to the recruitment of effector T lymphocytes to lymphocyte-mediated inflammatory reactions. In the course of experiments designed to purify the lymphotactic lymphokine (LCF) from histamine-stimulated T cell supernatants, Sephadex G-100 molecular sieve chromatography demonstrated two simultaneously generated non-cytotoxic inhibitors of T lymphocyte migration (lymphocyte migration inhibitory factors, LyMIFs) which had not been characterized previously. In this communication, we will detail our investigations concerning these histamine-induced lymphocyte migration inhibitory factors which are products of H_1 receptor-bearing cells and then discuss the relationship of *in vitro* observations to *in vivo* cell-mediated immune events.

METHODS

Generation of Supernatants

Normal human peripheral blood mononuclear cells (PBMC) were employed as the source of lymphocyte migration inhibitory lymphokines. Mononuclear cell populations were cultured at a concentration of 2×10^6 cells/ml in the presence or absence of histamine dihydrochloride (10^{-9} to 10^{-3}M) for 24 hours at 37°C in a 5% CO_2 humidified atmosphere. In some experiments, cimetidine or diphenhydramine were added to the cell cultures. The cell free supernatants were harvested, dialyzed, and, in certain experiments, concentrated by lyophilization to 1/15 – 1/30 of the original volume.

Cell Migration

Lymphocyte migration inhibitory activity was assessed employing a modification of a Boyden chamber technique (Center, Cruikshank, Berman, and Beer, 1983), utilizing human blood or rat splenic T lymphocytes as the responding cell pool. To determine the effect on lymphocyte migration of an experimental sample, 50 ul of a lymphocyte suspension containing 10×10^6 cells/ml in tissue culture medium enriched with 0.4% bovine serum albumin (BSA) were placed in the upper compartment of 48-well micro-chemotaxis chambers separated by 8 um nitrocellulose micropore filters from 30 ul of M199-HPS alone (control) or experimental samples. Lymphocyte migration experiments were carried out for 3 hours at 37°C in a 5% CO_2 moist atmosphere. The filters were fixed, stained, dehydrated and quantified by counting the total number of cells migrating beyond a fixed distance, using 10 um increments, in five high power fields (hpf) in duplicate micropore filters. Counting depth was adjusted to give control numbers of 10-25 cells. Results were calculated as mean cells/hpf ± SD. Meaned data from similar experiments underwent analysis of variance to determine statistical signficance. In all figures, experimental data will be expressed as mean percent of migration under control conditions ± SD.

Characterization of Lymphokines

Concentrated supernatants of histamine-stimulated PBMC were dialyzed against PBS and applied to a Sephadex G-100 column. Fractions with lymphocyte migration inhibitory activity as assessed in a micro-chemotaxis assay were dialyzed against distilled water, concentrated 10-fold, and subjected to isoelectric focusing in sucrose with ampholytes in the 7-10 pH range. Fractions eluted with a peristaltic pump were assessed for pH, dialyzed against PBS, and assayed for migration inhibitory activity.

RESULTS

While low doses of concentrated crude histamine-induced lymphocyte supernatants enhanced lymphocyte migration, higher doses inhibited lymphocyte migration (Table 1).

Table 1 Lymphocyte Migratory Responses To Increasing Concentrations of Crude Supernatant Dilutions

	0[a]	1:10	1:3	1:1	3:2	Neat[b]
Crude[c]	100±10	118±18	235±28*	252±12*	102±12	72±6*

[a] "0" refers to migration under control conditions.
[b] Neat refers to undiluted material (30 ul).
[c] Crude histamine-induced lymphocyte supernatants, concentrated fifteen-fold and tested for ability to alter T lymphocyte migration in various doses (mean ± SEM, n = 3-6) where control was 14.8 ± 1.6 cells.
* $p < 0.01$.

This observation is explained by the findings of Sephadex G-100 molecular sieve chromatography of concentrated histamine-stimulated mononuclear cell supernatants which revealed three regions of interest (Fig. 1). A region of human blood and rat splenic T lymphocyte migration enhancement, previously characterized (Center, Cruikshank, Berman, and Beer, 1983) and corresponding to a MW of 56,000 daltons was flanked by two areas of inhibition of T lymphocyte migration. These activities were found in the supernatants of histamine stimulated cells but not in column fractions from control supernatants, whether assayed with human T cells (Fig. 1A) or rat splenic T lymphocytes (Fig. 1B). One region of migration inhibitory activity eluted just prior to bovine serum albumin and corresponded to a MW of 70-80,000 daltons ($LyMIF_{75K}$). The second region of migration inhibitory activity eluted just after ovalbumin and corresponded to a MW of 30-40,000 daltons ($LyMIF_{35K}$). The generation of these lymphokines was maximal in the presence $10^{-4}M$ histamine, but was observed over a wide range of concentrations from $10^{-7}M$ to $10^{-3}M$. Viability of lymphocytes incubated for 3 hours in $LyMIF_{75K}$ or $LyMIF_{35K}$ was > 95% as assessed by exclusion of Trypan blue dye. There were no differences noted between the migratory responses to either LyMIF of human blood T lymphocytes or rat splenic T lymphocytes. The data for all further experiments are expressed as the rat splenic T lymphocyte migratory response.

To determine the cell of origin of the LyMIFs, supernatants were generated utilizing PBMC stimulated for 24 h with histamine alone, or in combination with the H_2 antagonist cimetidine ($10^{-5}M$) or the H_1 antagonist diphenhydramine ($10^{-5}M$). These supernatants were lyophilized and subjected to Sephadex G-100 gel filtration as described above, and column fractions assessed for their effect on lymphocyte migration (Fig. 2). Histamine stimulation of T lymphocytes resulted in the production of LCF and both LyMIFs. Incubation of T lymphocytes with histamine plus cimetidine resulted in selective production of $LyMIF_{35K}$ and $LyMIF_{75K}$; no LCF was produced. In contrast, supernatants generated by T cells incubated with histamine and diphenhydramine produced LCF, while no $LyMIF_{35K}$ or $LyMIF_{75K}$ were detected. Gel filtration of lyophilized supernatants from T cells incubated with either cimetidine or diphenhydramine alone or with a combination of histamine, cimetidine and diphenhydramine revealed no fractions with significant LCF or LyMIF activity.

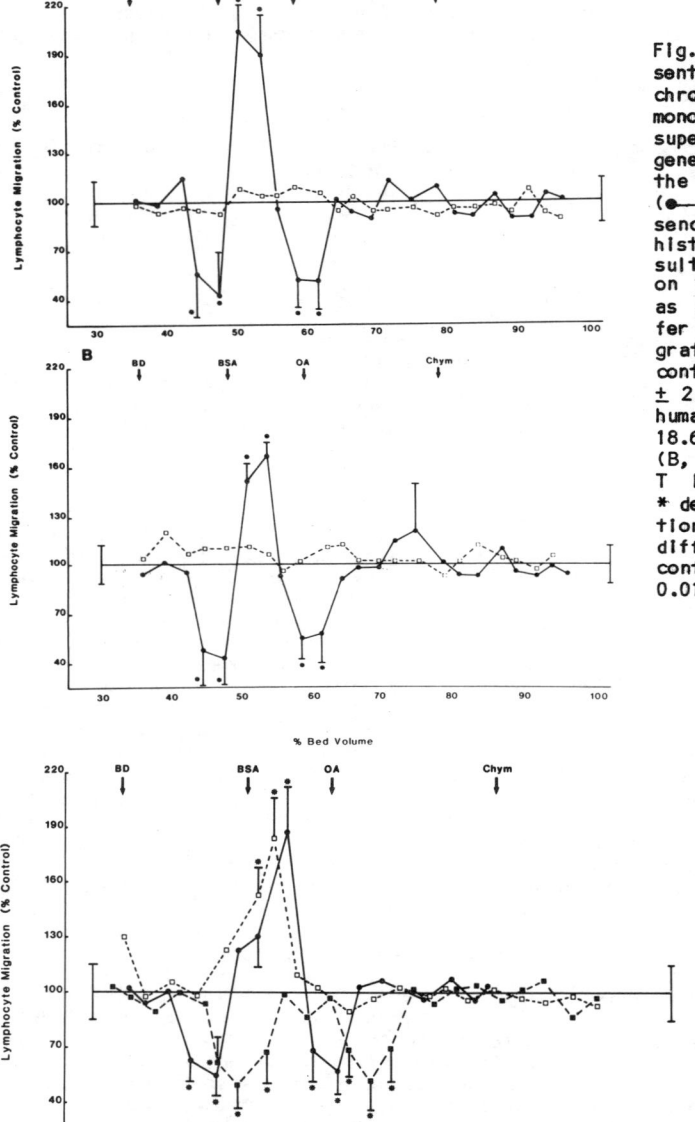

Fig. 1. Representative G-100 chromatograms of mononuclear cell supernatants generated in the presence (●—●) or absence (□—□) of histamine. Results expressed on the ordinate as percent buffer control migration, where controls were 15 ± 2.2 cells (A, human T) and 18.6 ± 1.9 cells (B, rat splenic T lymphocytes). * denotes migration that was different from control (p < 0.01).

Fig. 2. Sephadex G-100 chromatograms of concentrated mononuclear cell supernatants, incubated in the presence of histamine (●—●), histamine plus cimetidine (■—■), or histamine plus diphenhydramine (□—□). Lymphocyte migration is expressed on the ordinate as percent of buffer control, where control migration was 15.3 ± 1.6 cells. * denotes migration that was different from control (p < 0.01).

To further characterize the LyMIFs, pooled material from molecular sieve chromatography was subjected to isoelectric focusing in sucrose (Fig. 3). $LyMIF_{75K}$ had a single isoelectric point of 7.5-8.0. Focusing of $LyMIF_{35K}$ revealed a single area of inhibitory activity with an isoelectric point of 8.5-8.8. Wide range focusing using ampholytes with a pH range of 3-10 did not reveal any other species possessing LyMIF activity.

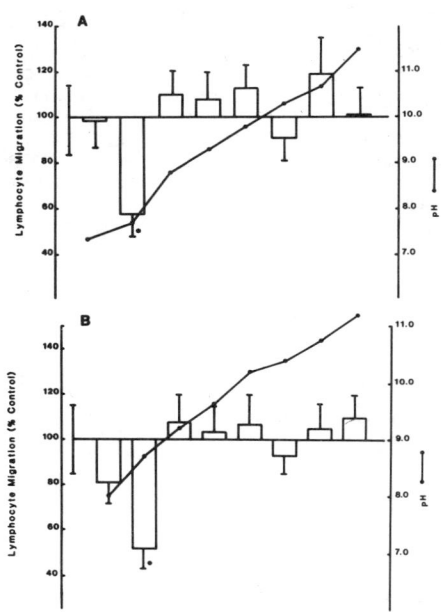

Fig. 3. Isoelectric focusing of active fractions from Sephadex G-100 chromatography of (A) $LyMIF_{75K}$ and (B) $LyMIF_{35K}$. Lymphocyte migratory responses are expressed on the ordinate as percent of migration in buffer control alone, where controls were 14.4 ± 2.0 (A) and 17.9 ± 2.5 (B) cells. Expressed on the opposite ordinates are the pH measurements of the individual fractions (•—•). * denotes migration that was different from control ($p < 0.01$).

Separately pooled G-100 $LyMIF_{75K}$ and $LyMIF_{35K}$ were subjected to enzymatic degradation with trypsin or neuraminidase and to heat treatment (56°C for 30 min). The lymphokines were exposed to trypsin at concentrations of $10^{-7}M$ or $10^{-5}M$ for 20 minutes; the trypsin was subsequently inactivated by the addition of an excess of soybean trypsin inhibitor (SBTI) and these mixtures of lymphokine, trypsin and SBTI assessed for its effect on lymphocyte motility (Table 2). Trypsin inactivated by SBTI had no effect on lymphocyte migration. The biologic activity of $LyMIF_{75K}$ but not that of $LyMIF_{35K}$ was sensitive to treatment with trypsin. The biologic activity of $LyMIF_{75K}$ was unaffected by pretreatment with neuraminidase, even at concentrations as high as 10^{-5} M (Table 2). In contrast, the biologic activity of $LyMIF_{35K}$ was sensitive to pretreatment with neuraminidase. Neuraminidase alone did not significantly alter lymphocyte migration. The biologic activity of $LyMIF_{75K}$ was heat stable while that of $LyMIF_{35K}$ was heat labile (Table 2).

DISCUSSION

These experiments provide evidence for the existence of two distinct, non-cytotoxic inhibitors of lymphocyte migration produced by H_1 receptor-bearing human blood T lymphocytes stimulated with histamine. These lymphocyte migration inhibitory lymphokines appear to be distinct from human lymphokines with migration inhibitory activity for cell types other than lymphocytes (Table 2) and, in addition, different from the two previously described histamine-induced lymphokines, histamine-induced suppressor factor (HSF) and LCF. HSF has been physicochemically characterized and shown to be two species of acidic glycoproteins with MWs between 25-40,000 daltons (Rocklin, Blidy, and Kamal, 1983), thus clearly differentiating this factor from $LyMIF_{35K}$ and $LyMIF_{75K}$. The other lymphokine that is elaborated in response to histamine, LCF, has a MW of 56,000, and an isoelectric point of 9.0-9.4. Of particular interest is the observation that these lymphocyte migration inhibitory factors are produced by histamine's interaction with an H_1 receptor on human lymphocytes, in contrast to HSF and LCF, which are produced by histamine interacting with H_2 receptors.

Table 2 Physicochemical Characteristics of Human Migration Inhibitory Lymphokines

	Molecular Weight	pI	Heat	Trypsin	Neuraminidase
Lymphocyte Migration Inhibitory Factor ($LyMIF_{75K}$)	70-80,000	7.5-8.0	Stable	Sensitive	Stable
Lymphocyte Migration Inhibitory Factor ($LyMIF_{35K}$)	30-40,000	8.5-8.8	Sensitive	Stable	Sensitive
Macrophage Migration Inhibitory Factors (MIF)					
First Day pH 5	23,000	4.3-5.2	N.D.	Sensitive	Stable
Second Day pH 3	65,000	2.4-3.3	Stable	Stable	Sensitive
Second Day pH 5	23-42,000	4.3-5.6	N.D.	Stable	Sensitive
Leukocyte Migration Inhibitory Factor (LIF)	68,000	5.0-5.5 8.0-8.5	Stable	N.D.	Stable
Tumor Migration Inhibitory Factor (TMIF)	5-10,000	N.D.	Stable	Sensitive	N.D.

Because other lymphokine activities have not been found as products of histamine-stimulated lymphocytes, histamine has been considered a ligand capable of induction of selective protein elaboration. Interestingly, all lymphokines found to be induced by histamine alter lymphocyte functions. HSF is a soluble suppressor factor which inhibits lymphocyte blastogenesis, lymphokine production, and generation of helper cell activity (Beer, Matloff, and Rocklin, 1984). LCF is selectively chemokinetic for T lymphocytes (Center, Cruikshank, Berman, and Beer, 1983), and $LyMIF_{75K}$ and $LyMIF_{35K}$ are inhibitors of T lymphocyte migration. Histamine may act as a limited regulatory stimulus to T lymphocyte subsets which act to modify the functions of other lymphocytes.

The finding of simultaneous generation of chemoattractant and immobilizing lymphokines is consistent with the pattern and proposed mechanism of accumulation of other leukocytes to sites of activated lymphocytes (Altman, 1978), particularly when the chemoattractant is predominantly chemokinetic in nature. Thus monocytes (Ward, Remold, and David, 1969) and polymorphonuclear leukocytes (Ward and Volkman, 1975) are attracted by chemoattractant lymphokines and are immobilized by macrophage migration inhibitory factor (MIF) (Bloom and Bennett, 1966) and leukocyte inhibitory factor (LIF) (Rocklin, 1974), respectively. Along these lines, checkerboard analyses of purified LCF demonstrated this T cell chemoattractant to be chemokinetic in nature (Center, Cruikshank, Berman, and Beer, 1983). High-dose inhibition of migration is not a characteristic of LCF and thus is not an adequate explanation of lymphocyte immobilization at sites of inflammation. However crude supernatants from histamine-activated lymphocytes induce stimulation of migration at low concentrations and inhibition of lymphocyte migration at high concentrations (Table 1). This phenomenon is explained by the generation of a lymphocyte chemokinetic factor (i.e., LCF) whose effect is demonstrable at lower concentrations than a simultaneously generated inhibitor of lymphocyte migration (i.e., LyMIFs). The stimulation of migration with low concentrations of crude lymphokine supernatant and inhibition at high concentrations is consistent with the postulated mechanism in vivo where distant cells must necessarily first sense low levels of lymphokines. When these leukocytes migrate closer to sites of lymphocyte activation, thereby experiencing higher concentrations of lymphokines, immobilization of the cells would occur.

Prior investigations have demonstrated the presence of basophils and mast cells at sites of lymphocyte-mediated inflammatory responses (Askenase, 1979; Epstein, Fukuyama, Danno, and Kwan-Wong, 1979). In addition, multiple IgE-independent triggers for release of intracellular histamine have been described (Thueson, Speck, Lett-Brown, and Grant 1979; Dy and Lebel, 1983). Although histamine traditionally has been considered as an effector molecule of immediate hypersensitivity, the above observations coupled with our recent findings of histamine induction of lymphocyte chemoattractant factors places histamine into the broader category of an autacoid capable of functioning as a physiological modulator of cellular immune responses.

REFERENCES

Altman, L.C. (1978). Leukocyte Chemotaxis: Methods, Physiology, and Clinical Implications, Raven Press, New York. pp. 267-287.
Askenase, P.W. (1979). J. Allergy Clin. Immunol. 64, 79-89.
Beer, D.J., S.M. Matloff, and R.E. Rocklin (1984). Advances in Immunology, vol. 35, Academic Press, Orlando. pp. 209-268.
Center, D.M., W.W. Cruikshank, J.S. Beran, and D.J. Beer (1983). J. Immunol., 131, 1854-1859.
Damle, N.K. and S. Gupta (1981). J. Clin. Immunol., 1, 241-249.
Dy, M. and B. Lebel (1983). J. Immunol., 130, 2343-2347.
Epstein, W.L., K. Fukuyama, K. Danno, and E. Kwan-Wong (1979). J. Pathol., 127, 207-215.
Melmon, K.L., R.E. Rocklin, and R.P. Rosenkranz (1981). Am. J. Med., 71, 100-106.
Bloom, B.R. and B. Bennett (1966). Science, 153, 80-82.
Rocklin, R.E. (1974). J. Immunol., 112, 1461-1466.
Rocklin, R.E. and D.J. Beer (1983). Advances in Internal Medicine, Vol. 28, Year Book Medical Publishers, Chicago. pp. 225-251.
Rocklin, R.E., A. Bildy, and M. Kamal (1983). Cell. Immunol., 76, 243-252.
Thueson, D.O., L.S. Speck, M.A. Lett-Brown, and J.A. Grant (1979). J. Immunol., 123, 626-632.
Ward, P.A., H.G. Remold, and J.R. David (1969). Science, 163, 1079-1081.
Ward, P.A. and A. Volkman (1975). J. Immunol., 115, 1394-1398.

MODULATION OF CYTOTOXIC T LYMPHOCYTE RESPONSES BY HISTAMINE

M. Plaut, A. Kagey-Sobotka and A. R. Jacques

Division of Clinical Immunology, Department of Medicine, Johns Hopkins University School of Medicine at The Good Samaritan Hospital, Baltimore, MD 21239, USA

Supported by Grant AI 12810 of the National Institutes of Health.

Publication #568 of the O'Neill Research Laboratories of The Good Samaritan Hospital.

ABSTRACT

The activity of cytotoxic T lymphocytes (CTL) is inhibited by histamine. Because of controversy in the recent literature, we have re-evaluated the receptor specificity of histamine-lymphocyte interactions. Histamine acts via a specific histamine-type 2 (H_2) receptor, since its inhibition is paralleled by low concentrations of dimaprit, and the inhibition by both histamine and dimaprit is reversed by H_2 antagonists, with dissociation constants of antagonist-receptor complexes identical to those of H_2 receptors on other tissue types. High concentrations of dimaprit and nor-dimaprit inhibit CTL activity, but these effects are not reversed by H_2 antagonists. Histamine and its agonists mediate similar effects on mitogen-induced proliferation of human peripheral T lymphocytes.

We have carried out experiments to evaluate situations which might influence histamine-mediated control of CTL activity--both the level of production of histamine and the level of sensitivity of responder cells to histamine. In vitro CTL generation was inhibited by histamine. To determine whether histamine was generated endogenously, we measured its production in mixed leukocyte cultures (MLC). Within 48 hours, histamine was secreted in such MLC, and greater amounts were produced by culturing spleen cells from 10-17 day immune mice than from non-immune mice. The histamine was newly synthesized, as its production was ablated by alpha-fluoromethyl-histidine, an inhibitor of histidine decarboxylase.

Our studies of the histamine sensitivity of responder cells were prompted by our observation that following in vivo immunization, the CTL activity of spleen cells was inhibited much more by histamine (> 40%) and other cAMP agonists than was the activity of peritoneal cells (10% inhibition by histamine). To determine responsiveness of CTL to cAMP agonists, CTL populations were transferred either intraperitoneally or intravenously into non-immune syngeneic recipients, and the responsiveness of CTL that were in recipient spleen, peritoneum or lung was tested. CTL were found to change their cAMP responsiveness within 24-48 hours after transfer. Regardless of whether the donor CTL populations had high or low responsiveness to cAMP, the activity of CTL in recipient spleen was inhibited 25%, 45% and 75% by 10^{-5}M histamine, 10^{-6}M PGE_2 and 10^{-3}M dibutyryl cAMP, and the activity of CTL in recipient peritoneum was inhibited 10-21%, 11-20% and 38-65% by the same three cAMP agonists. Thus, the local environment is the major determinant of the cAMP responsiveness of CTL.

These results establish mechanisms whereby histamine production, and environmentally determined histamine sensitivity of effector populations, interact to determine the level of control of immune responses by histamine.

KEYWORDS

T lymphocytes, cytotoxicity, histamine, histamine synthesis, local environment.

ABBREVIATIONS

CTL:	Cytotoxic T lymphocytes
αFMH:	Alpha-fluoromethylhistidine
H1:	Histamine - Type 1
H2:	Histamine - Type 2
K_B value:	antagonist-receptor dissociation constant
PBMC:	Peripheral blood mononuclear cells

INTRODUCTION

Our research has focused on the mechanisms by which endogenous mediators, especially histamine, regulate the function of T lymphocytes. Much of our work has examined control of mouse cytotoxic T lymphocytes (CTL), but we have also demonstrated that histamine modulates the function of human peripheral blood T lymphocytes.

We have been interested in histamine because we believe that it is a physiologic regulator of both immediate hypersensitivity reactions (basophil secretion) and cell mediated reactions (effector function of both CTL and delayed hypersensitivity T cells) (Plaut, 1982; Lichtenstein, 1975; Plaut, 1975; Rocklin, 1976). These inhibitory actions of histamine are mediated by specific H2 receptors. Perhaps the most interesting concept is that the inhibitory action of histamine is targeted to only a subset of immune and inflammatory cells, since some cell populations bear functional H2 receptors and others do not. For example, splenic CTL obtained after in vivo immunization are inhibited by histamine, but CTL obtained after in vitro immunization are not inhibited (Plaut, 1979). Suppressor T cells appear to be preferentially activated by histamine (Beer, 1984; Suzuki, 1982; Birch, 1982). This concept of specific targeting by histamine apparently applies not only to T lymphocyte subsets, but to differences between individuals in lymphocyte subsets (Beer, 1984; Staszak, 1980). Atopic individuals appear to have normal levels of circulating suppressor T cells (at least in terms of effectiveness of con A in activating them) but have a deficit of functional H2 receptors on circulating suppressor T cells (Beer, 1984).

The present paper deals with three aspects of histamine-T cell interaction. First, it re-evaluates the H2 receptor specificity of the action of histamine agonists on lymphocytes. Then, it discusses two levels of control of histamine-T cell interaction—control of the concentration of free histamine and control of the display of functional H2 receptors. Both increased production of histamine, and increased display of H2 receptors, occur late in the immune response, suggesting that histamine acts selectively to inhibit events in the late immune response.

METHODS

Reagents: Histamine was obtained from Sigma Chemical Company, St. Louis, MO. The following were kindly supplied: dimaprit, nor-dimaprit, burimamide, metiamide and cimetidine by Dr. Michael Parsons, Smith, Kline, French Laboratories; tiotidine by ICI Laboratories; ranitidine by Glaxo Laboratories; alpha-fluoromethylhistidine (αFMH) by Drs. Alan Rosenthal and Hans Zweerink, Merck and Company.

Mice and Immunization: C57 BL/6 ($H-2^b$) mice were immunized intraperitoneally with 10^7 cells of the P815 ($H-2^d$) cell line. P815 cells were used as target cells after labelling with ^{51}Cr (Plaut, 1979).

Mixed Lymphocyte Culture to Generate Histamine: Spleen cells (1×10^7) were incubated with 2×10^5 mitomycin C-treated P815 cells, in phenol red-free, serum-free RPMI 1640, with or without L-histidine (10^{-4}M), in 2 ml in wells of Costar plates, for up to 72 hours. At the end of that time, the cells were centrifuged, and the cell-free supernatant was assayed for histamine by the automated fluorometric technique of Siraganian (1975).

Cell Transfer: C57 BL/6 immune spleen cells (1×10^8) were injected either intraperitoneally or intravenously (in 1 ml RPMI 1640 medium) into syngeneic mice. After 48 hours, the recipient mice were killed, and single cell suspensions were prepared from the spleens and peritonea. Data from each recipient were calculated separately (Plaut, 1984).

Cytolytic Assay: Spleen cells (usually 1×10^7) or peritoneal cells (usually 1×10^6) were incubated with 2×10^5 or 2×10^4 ^{51}Cr-P815 cells, respectively, with or without histamine agonists and antagonists, in RPMI 1640 + 5% FCS, in 0.2 ml in wells of V-bottom microtiter plates, for up to 4 hours. At the end of incubation, an aliquot of the cell-free supernatant was assessed for ^{51}Cr content, and % ^{51}Cr release was calculated. Percent inhibition by histamine agonists was calculated relative to % ^{51}Cr release in drug-free wells (Plaut, 1975; Plaut, 1979).

Human Peripheral Blood Mononuclear Cell Proliferation Assay: Human peripheral blood mononuclear cells (PBMC) were obtained from normal laboratory personnel, using Hypaque-Ficoll separation of venous blood. PBMC (2×10^5) were incubated in 0.2 ml in round-bottom wells of microtiter plates, with suboptimal doses of concanavalin A (3 μg/ml), with or without histamine agonists and antagonists, for 72 hours, with a terminal 6 hour pulse of ^{3}H-thymidine (2 mCi/mM, 0.1 μCi/plate). The plates were harvested, washed and assayed by liquid scintillation spectroscopy. Percent inhibition by histamine agonists was calculated relative to ^{3}H-thymidine uptake (and incorporation into DNA) in drug-free wells.

RESULTS AND DISCUSSION

A. Histamine Receptor Specificity

We have previously demonstrated that the effector activity of mouse CTL is inhibited by histamine and that this histamine effect is mediated through H2 receptors. Histamine also induces an increase in the cAMP levels of spleen cells, suggesting that H2 receptors activate adenylate cyclase (Plaut, 1975; Plaut, 1973). The specificity of the H2 receptor was confirmed by Schild plots (Fig. 1) for inhibition of CTL activity by histamine, alone and in the presence of increasing concentrations of the H2 antagonist, burimamide. Burimamide shifted the histamine dose-response curve in parallel to the right. Such plots yielded the expected K_B value of 10^{-5}M for burimamide (Plaut, 1975).

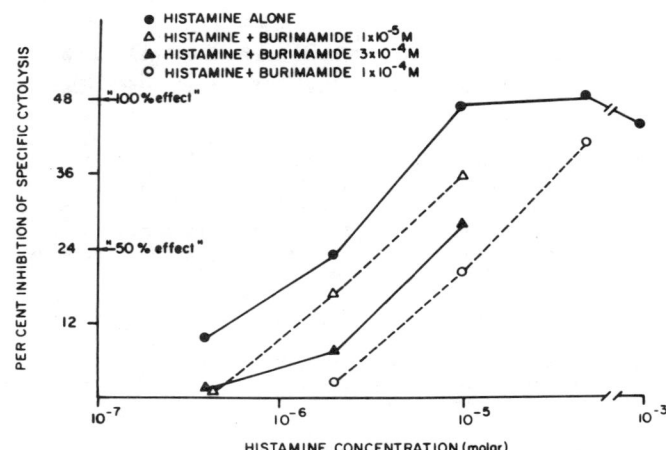

Fig. 1   Inhibition of CTL activity by histamine, alone or in the presence of burimamide. From Plaut, 1975; reproduced from The Journal of Clinical Investigation, by copyright permission of The American Society for Clinical Investigation.

The specificity of the H2 receptor has been demonstrated on another inflammatory cell, the basophil, where histamine inhibits antigen-induced release of histamine, and H2 antagonists reverse the inhibition, with K_B values identical to those in other tissues (Plaut, 1982; Lichtenstein, 1975). Moreover, H2 antagonists alone augment histamine release with a potency that parallels their H2 blocking activity, apparently because the antagonists block the negative feedback effect of histamine (released from some basophils, and then inhibiting release from other basophils) (Tung, 1982). Recently, the H2 specificity of histamine on lymphocytes and neutrophils has been questioned, principally because nor-dimaprit, an inactive congener of the H2 agonist dimaprit, inhibits the effector function of these cells (Gordon, 1981; Vickers, 1982). Hence, we have re-examined the specificity of action of histamine and its agonists on the activity of in vivo-generated splenic CTL. Histamine, dimaprit and 4-methylhistamine inhibited CTL activity. Maximal inhibition by histamine occurred at 10^{-5}M concentrations, and comparable levels of inhibition occurred at about $3-5 \times 10^{-5}$M for the other agonists. However, 2-methylhistamine and 2-pyridylethylamine, which are H1 agonists but weak H2 agonists, inhibited CTL activity only at high concentrations (10^{-3}M). These agonists had parallel dose-response curves for inhibiting CTL activity and for inducing increases in cAMP in spleen cell populations. The only exception was dimaprit, which at 10^{-3}M inhibited CTL activity more than histamine, but induced a relatively small cAMP increase.

The H2 specificity of the inhibitory action of histamine on CTL activity was established by Schild plots, which yielded estimated K_B values for H2 antagonists (10^{-5}M for burimamide, 10^{-6}M for metiamide and cimetidine, 10^{-7}M for ranitidine, slightly less than 10^{-7}M for tiotidine) that were similar to those for H2 receptors on other tissues. The dose-response inhibition curves for low concentrations of dimaprit ($\leq 10^{-4}$M) were shifted to the right by H2 antagonists, as expected for an H2 agonist. However, while dimaprit at high concentrations ($>10^{-4}$M), and nor-dimaprit (3×10^{-5}M -10^{-3}M) inhibited CTL activity, their inhibition was not reversed by H2 agonists. Thus, nor-dimaprit and high concentrations of dimaprit inhibited by non-H2-mediated mechanisms.

We have also found that histamine and H2 agonists inhibited the con A-induced proliferation of human PBMC cells, and that this inhibition was reversed by H2 antagonists. As shown in Fig. 2, dimaprit had a biphasic dose-response curve on inhibiting proliferation of human PBMC. Inhibition by low concentrations was reversed by cimetidine. High concentrations of dimaprit inhibited 100%, and this inhibition was not reversed by cimetidine. Also, nor-dimaprit

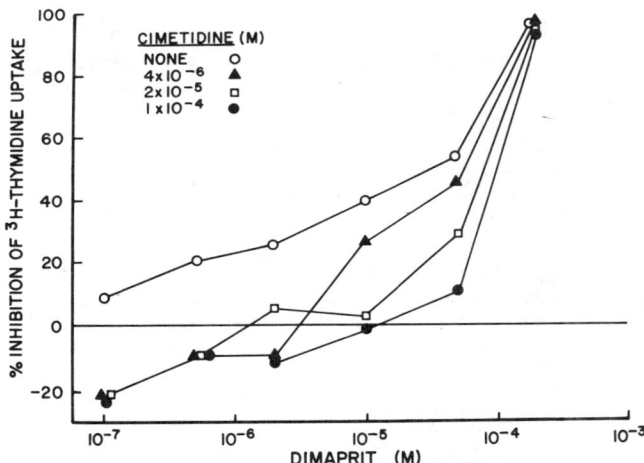

Fig. 2 Inhibition of con A-induced proliferation of human peripheral blood mononuclear cells by dimaprit, alone and in the presence of various concentrations of cimetidine.

inhibited, but the inhibitory effect was not reversed by H2 antagonists. Thus, the inhibitory effects of histamine agonists on con A-induced proliferation of human PBMC were similar to their effects on mouse CTL activity.

B. Regulation of Histamine Synthesis

Dy and co-workers (1981) have shown that mixed lymphocyte cultures induce histidine decarboxylase activity and the appearance of free histamine in culture supernatants. We have extended their work. As shown in Table I, at time 0 we found little cell associated or free histamine in culture, because there were few mast cells in these spleen cell preparations. After 48 hours, there was 12.6 ng histamine in the supernatant. Little histamine was stored

TABLE I Histamine synthesis following culture of 10^7 immune spleen cells with mitomycin C-treated allogeneic cells: Effect of αFMH

Time (Hrs.)	Histamine (Total ng)			
	Histidine-free medium		Histidine-containing medium	
	Cells	Supt	Cells	Supt
0	0.3	0.4	0.3	1.8
48 (No Drug)	0.1	0.8	0.5	12.6
48 (αFMH,10^{-5}M)	0.1	1.0	0.1	0.8

intracellularly. This level of histamine represented new synthesis, since it was blocked by culture in the presence of the histidine decarboxylase inhibitor, αFMH, as well as by culture in histidine-free medium.

Dy (1981) also previously reported that allograft-immunized spleen cells produce more histamine during a mixed lymphocyte reaction than non-immune. We have confirmed this result with our spleen cells from alloimmunized mice. While non-immune spleen cells generated 6 ng/ml histamine, 10-17 day-immune CTL generated 14-16 ng/ml. This increased histamine generation by immune cells may reflect changes both in numbers of histamine synthesizing cells, and in the level of production of a lymphokine (IL-3-like) that stimulates histamine synthesis (Dy, 1981; Ihle, 1983; Guy-Grand, 1984). The increase in histamine production occurs at the same time that functional histamine H2 receptors on CTL are increased (see below), so that the newly produced histamine can interact with H2 receptors.

C. Regulation of H2 Receptor Display on CTL

We have observed that different CTL populations differ in their capacity to be inhibited. Thus, the activity of splenic CTL obtained following in vivo immunization is inhibited by cAMP agonists, but splenic CTL after short-term culture are minimally inhibited by these agonists (Plaut, 1979, 1983). Furthermore, during the primary immune response, there are marked changes in both CTL activity, and the level of inhibition by cAMP agonists (Plaut, 1975, 1981, 1984). Thus, splenic CTL activity peaked on day 10, then fell. The inhibition by cAMP agonists of splenic CTL activity increased during the immune response. The most dramatic increase in inhibition is that by histamine. Maximal inhibition by histamine (i.e., inhibition by 10^{-5}M or 10^{-4}M histamine) increased progressively, from < 10% on day 8 to > 40% on day 14-18. Furthermore, in contrast to inhibition of day 14-18 splenic CTL, day 14-18 peritoneal CTL were inhibited only 10% by histamine (Plaut, 1984). Such differences in inhibition could be intrinsic properties of the CTL, but also could be accounted for by differences in the local environment of spleen vs. peritoneum. To test the role of the environment, we transferred immune splenic populations either intraperitoneally or intravenously into non-immune syngeneic mice, then tested CTL activity in recipient spleen and peritoneum. In parallel experiments, we transferred 8 day-immune vs. 14-15 day-immune CTL intraperitoneally (Plaut, 1984). The frequency of peritoneal-homing CTL was approximately 10-fold higher than that of spleen, but the level of CTL activity in both organs was sufficiently high to measure inhibition of activity accurately. As shown in Table II, the percent inhibition by cAMP agonists of the activity of 8 day CTL was much lower than that of 15 day CTL. Following transfer, inhibition of "spleen-homing" was greater than that of the starting

TABLE II Effect of Transferring 8 day immune vs. 15 day immune spleen cells into syngeneic recipients, on inhibition of CTL activity in recipient spleen and peritoneum[a]

	Percent inhibition by	
	Hist	PGE_2
8 Day Cells	$10^{-5}M$	$10^{-6}M$
Donor Cells	3	10
Recipient Peritoneum	5 ± 2	11 ± 2
Recipient Spleen	22 ± 6	39 ± 4
15 Day Cells		
Donor Cells	23	23
Recipient Peritoneum	16 ± 2	18 ± 1
Recipient Spleen	27 ± 10	40 ± 8

[a]Results of a single experiment, with transfer of each donor population into 2 mice, are shown. Results are mean $\pm$ S.E.M. Detailed statistical analysis of multiple experiments with 8 vs. 14-15 day immune mice is presented elsewhere (Plaut, 1984).

population. From the data in Table II, and other experiments, inhibition by each agonist of spleen-homing CTL was the same (i.e., histamine = 25% inhibition, PGE_2 = 45%, dibutyryl cAMP = 75%) regardless of whether the CTL were derived from 8 vs. 14-15 day immune cells, even though inhibition of the two donor CTL populations was very different.

Inhibition by cAMP agonists of spleen-homing CTL was found to be much greater than that of peritoneal-homing CTL. The recipient local environments are the major variables in these cell transfer experiments. Therefore, the local environment of spleen vs. peritoneum is the major determinant of the responsiveness of CTL to cAMP agonists. However, the level of inhibition by cAMP agonists of peritoneal-homing CTL derived from 8 day donor cells was significantly lower than that derived from 14-15 day donor cells, so the responsiveness to cAMP agonists of the starting population plays some role in determining the responsiveness of peritoneal-homing cells.

If immune spleen populations were cultured for 24 hours with P815 cells and IL-2-containing supernatants, the inhibition by cAMP agonists became very low (Plaut, 1984). When such cells were transferred intraperitoneally, the levels of inhibition by cAMP agonists of both peritoneal-homing and spleen-homing CTL were similar to those shown in Table II (Plaut, 1984). When immune spleen populations were transferred intravenously, the inhibition by cAMP agonists of spleen-homing CTL was similar to that in Table II. Peritoneal-homing cells had much lower activity after intravenous than intraperitoneal transfer, but the inhibition by cAMP agonists of peritoneal CTL was similar to that shown in Table II (Plaut, 1984).

Thus, the susceptibility of CTL to the inhibitory effects of histamine and
other cAMP agonists is not affected by the route of cell transfer, and is not
an intrinsic property of CTL populations, but is determined by the local
environment.

The identity of cellular or secreted local factors that regulate cAMP agonist
responsiveness is unknown (cf. Lipschultz, 1981). Local, external factors may
regulate not only the histamine responsiveness of different subpopulations of
CTL, but also that of CTL early vs. late in the immune response. Perhaps local
factors also regulate the differences in display of H2 receptors on
inflammatory cell subsets in man, and even may explain differences in H2
receptor display on suppressor T cells between non-atopic and atopic
individuals.

CONCLUDING REMARKS

Newly synthesized histamine is probably a major source of endogenous histamine
for regulation of T lymphocyte function. However, human mononuclear
cell-derived factors, including a potent macrophage-derived factor that we have
recently identified, induce rapid release of histamine from human basophils
(Schulman, 1984). Since basophil infiltrates do occur in cell-mediated
reactions including allograft rejection (Askenase, 1979), such basophils may be
another endogenous source of regulatory histamine. The relative importance of
these sources of histamine is not known.

Histamine production, and histamine sensitivity of effector populations, are
two mechanisms for control of histamine-T cell interactions. Further work is
necessary to understand fully these interactions.

REFERENCES

Askenase, P.W. (1979). Mechanisms of hypersensitivity: cellular interactions.
Basophil arrival and function in tissue hypersensitivity reactions. J.
Allergy Clin. Immunol., 64, 79-89.

Beer, D.J., and R.E. Rocklin. (1984). Histamine-induced suppressor cell
activity. J. Allergy Clin. Immunol., 73, 439-452.

Birch, R.E., A.K. Rosenthal, and S.H. Polmar. (1982). Pharmacological
modification of immunoregulatory lymphocytes. II. Modulation of T lymphocyte
cell surface characteristics. Clin. Exp. Immunol., 48, 231-238.

Dy, M., B. Lebel, P. Kamoun, and J. Hamburger. (1981). Histamine production
during the anti-allograft response. Demonstration of a new lymphokine
enhancing histamine synthesis. J. Exp. Med., 153, 293-309.

Gordon, D., G.P. Lewis and A. Nouri. (1981). Inhibition of lymphocyte
proliferation by histamine and related compounds not mediated via H1- or H2-
receptors. Br. J. Pharmacol., 74, 137-141.

Guy-Grand, D., M. Dy, G. Luffau, and P. Vassali. (1984). Gut mucosal mast
cells: Origin, traffic, and differentiation. J. Exp. Med., 160, 12-28.

Ihle, J.N., J. Keller, S. Oroszlan, L.E. Henderson, T.D. Copeland, F. Fitch, M.B. Prystowsky, E. Goldwasser, J.W. Schrader, E. Palaszynski, M. Dy, and B. Lebel. (1983). Biologic properties of homogenous interleukin 3. I. Demonstration of Wehi-3 growth factor activity, mast cell growth factor activity, P cell-stimulating factor activity, colony-stimulating factor activity, and histamine-producing cell-stimulating factor activity. J. Immunol., 131, 282-287.

Lichtenstein, L.M., and E. Gillespie (1975). The effects of H1 and H2 antihistamines on allergic histamine release and its inhibition by histamine. J. Pharmacol. Exp. Ther., 192, 441-450.

Lipshultz, S., J. Shanfeld, and S. Chacko. (1981). Emergence of β-adrenergic sensitivity in the developing chicken heart. Proc. Natl. Acad. Sci. USA, 78, 288-292.

Plaut, M., L.M. Lichtenstein, E. Gillespie, and C.S. Henney. (1973). Studies on the mechanism of lymphocyte-mediated cytolysis. IV. Specificity of the histamine receptor on effector T cells. J. Immunol., 111, 389-394.

Plaut, M., L.M. Lichtenstein, and C.S. Henney (1975). Properties of a subpopulation of T cells bearing histamine receptors. J. Clin. Invest., 55, 856-874.

Plaut, M. (1979). The role of cyclic AMP in modulating cytotoxic T lymphocytes I. In vivo-generated cytotoxic lymphocytes, but not in vitro-generated cytotoxic lymphocytes, are inhibited by cyclic AMP-active agents. J. Immunol., 123, 692-701.

Plaut, M. (1981). Increased responsiveness to cyclic AMP-active agents during the immune response in vivo. Immunopharmacol., 3, 107-116.

Plaut, M., and L.M. Lichtenstein (1982). Histamine and immune responses. In Pharmacology of Histamine Receptors, C.R. Ganellin and M.E. Parsons (Eds.) John Wright and Sons Ltd., Bristol, U.K., pp. 392-435.

Plaut, M., G. Marone, and E. Gillespie. (1983). The role of cyclic AMP in modulating cytotoxic T lymphocytes. II. Sequential changes during culture in responsiveness of cytotoxic T lymphocytes to cAMP-active agents. J. Immunol., 131, 2945-2952.

Plaut, M., L. Nordin, M.C. Liu, and A.R. Jacques. (1984). The role of cAMP in modulating cytotoxic T lymphocytes (CTL). III. The local in vivo environment determines the cAMP responsiveness of CTL. J. Immunol., in press.

Rocklin R.E. (1976). Modulation of cellular immune responses in vivo and in vitro by histamine receptor-bearing lymphocytes. J. Clin. Invest., 52, 1051-1058.

Schulman, E.S., D. Proud, M.C. Liu, D.W. MacGlashan, Jr., L.M. Lichtenstein, and M. Plaut. (1984). Human lung macrophages induce histamine release from basophils and mast cells. Amer. Rev. Resp. Dis., submitted.

Siraganian, R.P. (1975). Refinements in the automated fluorometric histamine analysis system. J. Immunol. Methods, 7, 283-290.

Staszak, C., J.S. Goodwin, G.M. Troup, D.R. Pathak, and R.C. Williams, Jr. (1980). Decreased sensitivity of prostaglandin and histamine in lymphocytes from normal HLA-B12 individuals: A possible role in autoimmunity. J. Immunol., 125, 181-185.

Suzuki, S., and R. Huchet. (1982). Properties of histamine-induced suppressor factor in the regulation of lymphocyte responses to PHA in mice. Cell. Immunol., 68, 349-358.

Tung, R., A. Kagey-Sobotka, M. Plaut, and L.M. Lichtenstein. (1982). H2 antihistamines augment antigen-induced histamine release from human basophils in vitro. J. Immunol., 129, 2113-2115.

Vickers, M.R., K. Milliner, D. Martin, and C.R. Ganellin. (1982). Histamine-induced inhibition of lymphocyte proliferation and lysosomal enzyme release from polymorphs may not be mediated via H1- or H2-receptors. Agents and Actions, 5, 630-634.

ALTERATIONS IN IMMUNOREGULATORY T-LYMPHOCYTE PHENOTYPE AND FUNCTION: ACTION OF H_1 AND H_2 HISTAMINE AGONISTS

R. E. Birch and S. H. Polmar

Department of Pediatrics, Washington University School of Medicine, St. Louis, Missouri 63178, USA

ABSTRACT

Brief incubation of peripheral blood T-lymphocytes with the H_2-Histamine agonist, Impromidine (1-100μM, 45 min., 37° C) results in increased RFcγ expression and OKT8 reactivity accompanied by a decline in OKT4 reactivity. These alterations in phenotype are subsequently accompanied by induction of immunosuppressive activity for PWM driven B-cell differentiation within a fraction of T-lymphocytes previously observed to phenotypically and functionally T-helper cells. Moreover, the Impromidine induced alterations in T-cell phenotype and function are preceded by activation of adenylate cyclase and methyl transferase. Conversely, incubation of T-lymphocytes with the H_1-histamine agonist 2-pyridylethylamine results in loss of RFcγ expression and OKT8 reactivity within the suppressor T-cell subset but causes no change on OKT4 reactivity. These changes in phenotype are indicative of loss of suppressor cell activity within the suppressor T-cell subset. Histamine receptor specific alterations in immunoregulatory phenotype and function provide a model for analysis of the pharmacologic basis of immunoregulatory events.

KEYWORDS

H_1-Histamine receptor; H_2-Histamine receptor; Immunoregulation; Induced Immunoregulation; Induced Immunosuppression.

INTRODUCTION

The inducible suppressor cell in the human has been examined by a number of researchers (Rola-Plezczynski, 1982; Thomas, 1982; Birch, 1980; Birch, 1982c and d; Rocklin, 1980). It is interesting that no two of these inducible suppressor cells are identical. They may very in terms of specificity, radiosensitivity or mode of induction as well as in aspects of surface phenotypic characteristics. Nonetheless, it is clear that there are cells within the OKT4 reactive T-cell subset capable of being induced to act as suppressor cells themselves or of inducing the development of suppressor cells. Our laboratory has examined two modes of induction of immunosuppression and the biochemical mechanisms required for the generation of immunosuppressive activity. We have observed that both adenosine and the H_2-histamine agonist, Impromidine, can trigger a subset of T-helper cells (T_H cells) to undergo alterations of cell surface phenotype with the ultimate induction of immunosuppressive activity (Birch, 1980; Birch 1982c; Birch 1982d). In the adenosine system we observed that the interaction of adenosine with its T-cell surface receptor results in a step-wise series of biochemical events which include activation of adenylate cyclase, phospholipid methylation, activation of phospholipase, as well as arachidonic acid release and metabolism via either the lipoxygenase or cyclooxygenase pathways (Birch 1982a; Mandler 1982). In the present studies, we have extended this analysis of induction of immunosuppression to the H_1-and H_2-histamine receptor specific compounds, 2-pyridylethylamine (2PE) and Impromidine.

METHODS

Preparation of peripheral blood lymphocytes, B-cells, T-cells and T-cell subsets have been reported previously (Birch, 1980 and 1982c). Analysis of surface markers and lymphocyte surface receptors have been described in detail elsewhere (Birch, 1980; Birch, 1982d). Pokeweed mitogen driven B-cell differentiation was determined by the detection of either cytoplasmic immunoglobulin containing plasma cells as measured by cytoplasmic immunofluoresence or secreted IgG as measured by ELISA (Birch, 1982c; Voller, 1979).

In the analysis of biochemical processes initiated by histamine receptor specific agents, the following assays were utilized: Cellular cyclic AMP was measured by modification of the method of Brown and co-workers (1971) employing bovine heart protein kinase as the binding protein.

Phospholipid methylation and arachidonic release was determined by methods previously described by Hirata and co-workers (1978) and Parker and co-workers (1979).

All histamine receptor agonists employed in the studies were kindly provided by B.N. Dracott (SmithKline and French Research Ltd., Wellwyn, England).

RESULTS AND DISCUSSION

THE EFFECT OF IMPROMIDINE UPON T-LYMPHOCYTE PHENOTYPE

In previous studies (Birch, 1980; 1982c; 1982d) we reported that brief exposure of T_H-cells to Impromidine (1-100μM, 45 mins., 37°C) resulted in an approximately two-fold increase in the expression of receptors for the Fc portion of IgG (RFcγ). This increase in RFcγ was accompanied by a decreased OKT4 reactivity and increased OKT8 reactivity. In time course studies it was observed that a 45 minute incubation with Impromidine (1μM) at 37°C followed by removal of the drug from the lymphocyte suspension resulted in a non-reversible change from helper to suppressor phenotype.

In the present studies, we have confirmed these findings and have demonstrated that Impromidine incubation can induce changes in the T-lymphocyte surface markers at concentrations as low as 0.1μM with maximal changes at 1-100μM (Figure 1). Reactivity with OKT4 decreased from 51-37% at concentrations of Impromidine of 1μM or more. Increases in OKT8 reactivity are observed at all concentrations examined. Increases in RFcγ expression appear to be maximal at 1-100μM.

As shown in Table 1 the action of Impromidine is selective in effecting primarily cells within the T-helper/inducer cell population (T_H), enriched for H_2 receptor positive cells and the OKT4 antigen. In studies on cell suspensions depleted of OKT8 reactive cells, it was observed that Impromidine induced an eighteen-fold increase in OKT8 reactivity (from 1.2 to 19.2%).

In panning experiments separating H_2-receptor positive cells from H_2-receptor negative cells the receptor positive population displayed similar surface marker changes subsequent to Impromidine exposure. In the H_2-receptor positive fraction, RFcγ expression was increased to 26.6% and OKT8 reactivity to 37% from untreated levels of 15.7% and 15.8%, respectively. Moreover, OKT4 reactivity decreased to less than 50% of the untreated level. Conversely, the H_2-receptor negative lymphocyte suspensions showed no alterations in surface marker expression except for small decreases in RFcγ and OKT8 reactivity after incubation with Impromidine.

Selection of T_H and T suppressor (T_S) cells by theophylline sensitivity also resulted in the T_H subset demonstrating phenotypic and functional changes after Impromidine incubation. The theophylline resistant sheep erythrocyte rosetting T_H fraction displayed both increased RFcγ expression and OKT8 reactivity accompanied by a decline in OKT4. The theophylline sensitive T_S-subset showed no increase in RFcγ.

THE EFFECT OF IMPROMIDINE UPON T_H-CELL FUNCTION

The ability of T_H-cells to facilitate B-cell differentiation was measured in seven day cultures stimulated with pokeweed mitogen (PWM). Peripheral blood lymphocyte suspensions were separated into T and B cell subpopulations by sheep erythrocyte rosetting and Ficoll-Hypaque density gradient centrifugation. The non-rosetting, non-T-cells were employed as the B-cell source in the B-cell differentiation assays. The rosetting T-cells were either used in unfractionated suspension or were further separated to T_H and T_S cell subsets. In studies examining the effect of Impromidine (1μM) upon T_H-cell function, it was observed that the helper cell subset lost its ability to facilitate PWM-driven B-cell differentiation to immunoglobulin containing plasma cells after exposure to Impromidine (Figure 2). That this loss of helper cell activity was in fact induction of immunosuppressive activity within the T_H-cell subset was shown by the finding that the addition of Impromidine treated T_H-cells to a suspension of 5×10^4 B-cells plus 5×10^4 untreated T_H-cells resulted in a marked decrease in plasma cells.

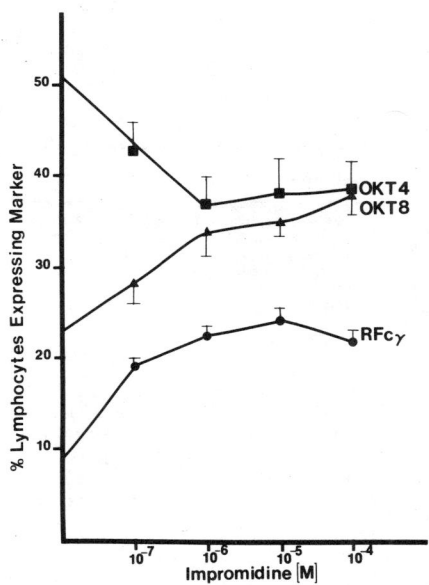

Fig. 1. The effect of Impromidine concentration upon T-lymphocyte surface marker expression. T-lymphocytes (2×10^6 cells/ml) were incubated with Impromidine (10^{-7} to 10^{-4}M) for 45 minutes at 37°C. After incubation the cell suspensions were washed to removed the Impromidine and assayed for RFcγ (●——●) expression as well as OKT4 (■——■) and OKT8 (▲——▲) reactivity.

TABLE 1: THE EFFECT OF H_2 AGONIST, IMPROMIDINE, UPON T-LYMPHOCYTE SUBSET PHENOTYPE

Subset	Impromidine[a]	% Lymphocytes ± SEM[b]		
		RFcγ	OKT4	OKT8
Unfractionated T cells	−	9.4±1.3	59.5±3.8	17.9±2.3
	+	18±2.5	47±3.2	28±3.5
OKT8 depleted[c]	−	7.5	57.5	1.2
	+	11.1	43.01	19.2
H_2-Histamine Receptor+[c]	−	15.8±4.1	66±5.3	15.7±4.7
	+	26.6±1.6	31.3±3.5	37.0±4.0
H_2-Histamine Receptor−	−	18.0±4.6	37.6±3.7	48.6±6.7
	+	12.1±2.2	40.2±4.6	33.6±3.3
Theophylline Resistant[d] (Helper)	−	7.2±1.3	66.3±3.0	19.9±2.4
	+	16.9±1.2	52.9±3.5	39.3±8.3
Theophylline Sensitive (Suppressor)	−	35.9±3.0	27.6±3.4	44.5±2.5
	+	37.9±2.6	ND	ND

[a] Cells were incubated with Impromidine (10^{-5}M) for 45 minutes prior to assay.
[b] The percentage of 200 viable cells expressing each surface marker ± SEM.
[c] T-lymphocyte suspensions were depleted of OKT8 or H_2-histamine receptor bearing cells by panning techniques.
[d] Theophylline sensitive and resistant T-cells were selected by the ability to rosette with sheep erythrocytes after incubation with theophylline (1mM, 60 min., 37°C)

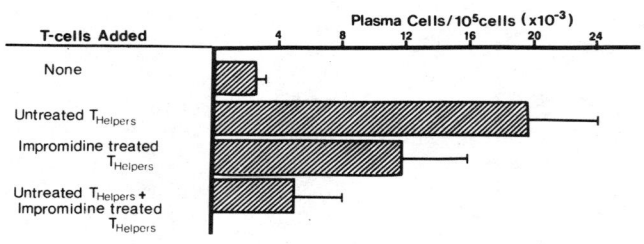

Figure 2. The effect of Impromidine upon T-cell function. Suspensions of T_H-cells were incubated with Impromidine (10^{-5}M) for 60 minutes, followed by washing to remove the drug. The treated T-cells (5×10^4 cells/well) were then added to suspensions of 5×10^4 B-cells alone or 5×10^4 B-cells plus 5×10^4 T_H-cells and incubated in the presence of PWM for 6 days. B-cell differentiation to cytoplasmic immunoglobulin containing plasma cells was assayed by staining with fluorescein labelled antiglobulin reagents.

In studies examining PWM driven B-cell differentiation into immunoglobulin secreting cells, Impromidine (10μ M) treatment was also observed to inhibit T-cell ability to facilitate differentiation (Figure 3). In culture suspensions in which increasing numbers of T-cells were added to 5×10^4 B-cells, the Impromidine treated preparations elicited approximately one-half the level of secreted IgG observed in suspensions utilizing untreated T-cells. This loss of helper activity has been shown to in fact be induction of suppression and not merely loss of helper cell function or number (Birch 1980; 1982c and d).

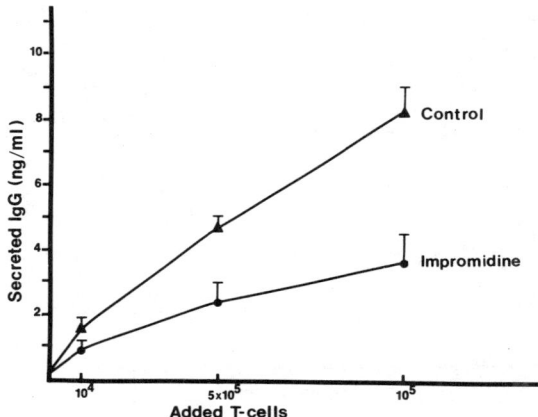

Fig. 3. Impromidine inhibits the ability of T-lymphocytes to facilitate PWM driven B-cell differentiation to IgG secreting plasma cells. Suspensions of 5×10^4 B-cells plus increasing numbers of treated (●—●) and untreated (▲—▲) T-cells were incubated for 7 days at $37°C$ in 5% CO_2 in the presence of PWM. At 7 days the culture supernatants were harvested and secreted IgG assayed by ELISA.

BIOCHEMICAL EVENTS ASSOCIATED WITH IMPROMIDINE INDUCED IMMUNOSUPPRESSION

It has been reported that the interaction of adenosine with its cell surface receptor results in activation of adenylate cyclase and synthesis of cyclic AMP (Marone, 1978; Mandler, 1982; Schwartz, 1978). Moreover, we subsequently observed that adenosine induced immunosuppression required a sequence of biochemical steps which began with adenylate cyclase activation but also included phospholipid methylation and metabolism as well as the products of subsequent cell associated fatty acid metabolism (Birch, 1982a and b).

In the present study, incubation of T-lymphocytes with (1µM) Impromidine resulted in synthesis of cyclic AMP that reached a level of 12 pmoles/10^6 cells within 1 minute (Figure 4). By 10 minutes the level of cyclic AMP reached its peak of 14 pmoles/10^6 cells and subsequently began to decline so that measurable cyclic AMP returned to background levels at 30 minutes of incubation. This pattern of cyclic AMP synthesis is similar to that observed with adenosine incubation, although the peak is broader and takes longer to return to control levels (Mandler, 1982).

Methylation of phospholipids is an event associated with membrane perturbation and alterations in cell surface. The studies illustrated in Figure 5 indicate a progressive increase in methyl group incorporation into membrane phospholipid that is increased as late as 180 minutes after Impromidine exposure. Impromidine induced [^3H] -CH_3 incorporation remains at control levels until approximately 30 minutes into the incubation period but begins to rise and continues to increase to as much as 0.3 pmoles/10^6 cells, whereas the untreated control remains at a relatively constant level of 0.15 pmoles/10^6 cells throughout the incubation period.

It has been suggested that the products of fatty acid metabolism and particularly arachidonic acid metabolites produced via the cyclooxygenase pathway or the lipoxygenase pathway play an important role in the generation of immunosuppressive

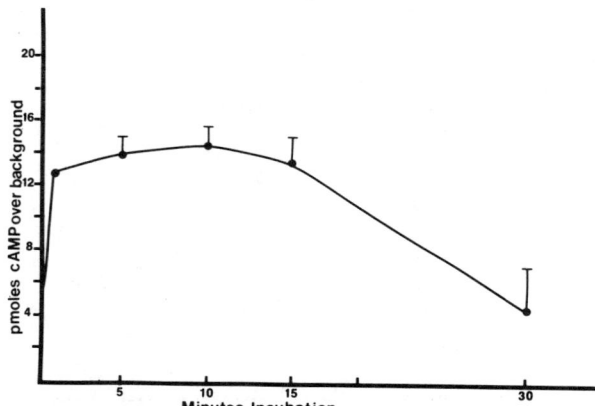

Fig. 4. Impromidine induces activation of adenylate cyclase and synthesis of cAMP in T-cells. T-lymphocytes were incubated with Impromidine (10^{-5}M) for up to 30 minutes. Aliquots of 10^6 cells were taken at each time point, boiled to kill phosphodiesterase activity and assayed for cAMP by the method of Brown (1971).

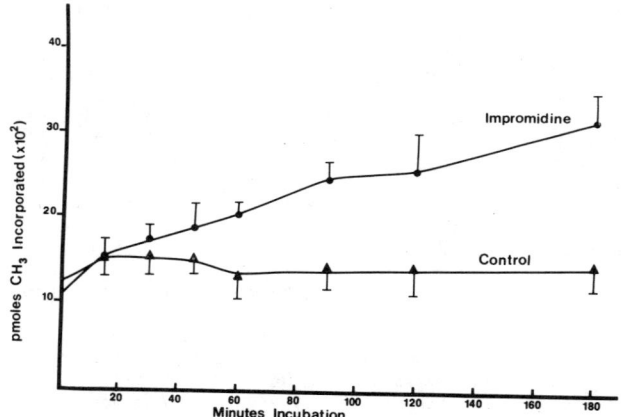

Figure 5. Incubation with Impromidine induces T-lymphocytes to undergo methylation of membrane phospholipids. T-lymphocyte suspensions (2×10^6 cells/ml) were incubated with (●——●) and without (▲——▲) Impromidine (10^{-6}M) for up to 180 mins. At each time point the reaction was stopped by the addition of cold TCA. The precipitate was pelletted and phospholipid extracted by the method of Hirata (1979).

activity (Goodwin, 1980; Rola-Plezczynski, 1983). Indeed we have found in adenosine induced immunosuppression that arachidonic acid is released from adenosine treated T-lymphocytes after 30-60 minutes of incubation. In contrast, T-lymphocytes incubated with Impromidine failed to demonstrate increased arachidonic acid release. Specifically, although Impromidine elicits persistent phospholipid methylation, released [^{14}C]-arachidonic acid does not increase above control levels during the incubation period studied (Figure 6). That is not to say that the event

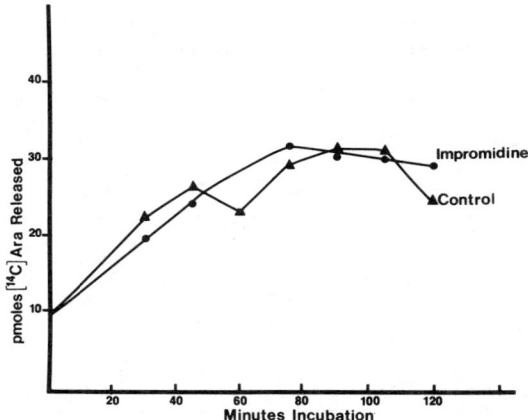

Fig. 6. Incubation with Impromidine (10^{-6}M) does not elicit release of arachidonic acid by T-lymphocytes. Arachidonic acid (^{14}C) prelabelled suspensions of T-lymphocytes (2×10^6 cells/ml) were incubated with Impromidine for up to 120 min. At each time point the cells were pelletted and the supernatant assayed for released ^{14}C-arachidonic acid by the method described by Parker (1979).

does not occur at some later point. It may be that Impromidine elicits a much slower chain of biochemical events than those associated with adenosine induced immunosuppression, which are nearly complete within 45 minutes of adenosine exposure (Birch 1982a and b). Alternatively, while adenosine causes arachidonate release from T-lymphocytes, the H_2-agonist may be incapable of inducing T-lymphocyte arachidonic acid release. It is also possible that arachidonic acid release and metabolism occur in this system but take place in another cell such as the macrophage. Wadee and Rabson (1983) have demonstrated phospholipid metabolites such as phosphatidyl inositol and phosphatidylethanolamine may function as intercellular signals in the development of immunosuppressive activity involving arachidonic acid.

THE EFFECT OF THE H_1-HISTAMINE AGONIST, 2-PYRIDYLETHYLAMINE UPON T-LYMPHOCYTE PHENOTYPE AND FUNCTION

Unlike the H_2-histamine agonists, the H_1-receptor specific agent 2-pyridylethylamine (2PE) does not act upon the T_H cell subset nor does incubation with 2PE result in the enhanced immunosuppression or biochemical events observed after incubation with the H_2-agonists. Incubation of T-lymphocytes with 2PE(10^{-4}M) for 60 minutes resulted in decreased RFcγ expression and OKT8 reactivity but no significant change in OKT4 (Table 2). Moreover, the action of 2PE appears to be specific for T-cell subsets displaying a suppressor cell phenotype. This is indicated by the observation that only the H_2-receptor negative and theophylline sensitive suppressor T-cell subsets display changes in cell surface phenotype after incubation with 2PE. That the loss of suppressor cell phenotype reflects altered suppressor cell phenotype reflects altered suppressor cell activity is indicated by the observation that 2PE treated theophylline sensitive T_S-cells lose the ability to suppress pokeweed mitogen driven B-cell differentiation to cytoplasmic immunoglobulin containing plasma cells (Figure 7). Previous studies have indicated that this loss of suppression is not the result of suppressor cell death or loss but rather alterations in cell activity (Polmar 1980). It should also be noted that in direct contrast to Impromidine, 2PE did not activate adenylate cyclase and subsequent synthesis of cyclic AMP (data not shown).

TABLE 1: THE EFFECT OF H_1-HISTAMINE AGAINST 2-PYRIDYLETHYLAMINE UPON T-LYMPHOCYTE SUBSETS

Subset	2PE[a]	% Lymphocytes ± S.E.M.[b]		
		RFcγ	OKT4	OKT8
Unfractionated T-cells	−	9.4±1.3	59.5±6.2	17.9±2.3
	+	6.3±1.9	48.5±2.5	6.6±2.5
H_2-Histamine Receptor[+][c]	−	15.8±4.1	66±3.3	37±4.0
	+	16±2.1	56±3.5	20±6.0
H_2-Histamine Receptor[−]	−	18.0±4.6	37.6±3.7	48.6±6.7
	+	10.5±1.5	34.6±0.6	8.2±3.6
Theophylline Resistant[d]	−	8.6±1.9	66.3±3.0	18.9±2.4
(Helper)	+	10.5±0.5	ND	ND
Theophylline Sensitive	−	42.3±5.0	27.6±3.4	44.5±2.5
(Suppressor)	+	13.9±1.5	ND	ND

[a] Cell suspensions were incubated with 2-pyridylethylamine (10^{-4}M) for 60 minutes at 37°C prior to assay.

[b] The percentage of 200 viable cells expressing RFcγ or reacting with the OKT4 or OKT8 antibodies.

[c] H_2-Histamine receptor[+] cells were selected by panning on Seragen H_2-Cell Ect plates

[d] Theophylline resistant and sensitive T-cells were selected by the ability of the T-cells to rosette with sheep erythrocytes after incubation with theophylline (1mM, 60 min., 37°C).

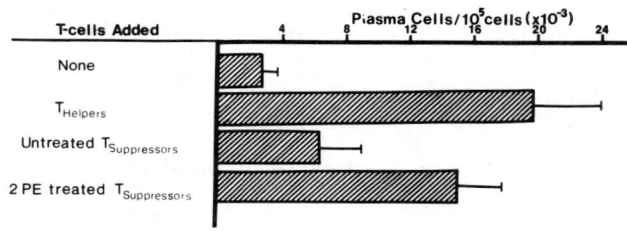

Fig. 7. Incubation with 2-pyridylethylamine results in a loss of suppressor T-cell activity. T_S-lymphocytes were incubated with or without 2PE (10^{-4}M) for 60 min. and the drug removed by washing. To assay PWM driven B-cell differentiation 5X10^4 B-cells were mixed with 5X10^4 treated or untreated T-cells and incubated at 37°C in 5% CO_2 for 6 days. B-cell differentiation was assessed by intracytoplasmic immunoglobulin detected with fluorescein conjugated antiglobulin reagents.

In summary, receptor specific histamine analogs have dramatic effects upon T-lymphocyte immunoregulatory activity as well as the expression of surface antigens. H_1 and H_2 histamine agonists act on different T-cell populations and have precisely opposite actions. 2PE, an H_1-histamine agonist, inhibits suppressor activity and expression of suppressor associated surface antigens while Impromidine, an H_2 agonist, enhances suppression and suppressor associated antigens. While the biochemical mechanisms observed in H_2-receptor associated suppression are similar to those observed in adenosine induced immunosuppression, significant differences also exist including slower kinetics and the absence of demonstrable T-lymphocyte arachidonic acid release with Impromidine. Important questions requiring study include: (1) the surface phenotype of the histamine responsive cells, (2) the relationship of H_2-induced immunosuppression to the adenosine-induced immunosuppression system, (3) the identity of the phospholipid metabolites important in H_2-induced immunosuppression, and (4) the possible relationships to other H_2-induced suppression systems in which glycoprotein lymphokines (e.g. HSF) have been identified.

ACKNOWLEDGEMENTS

These studies were supported by NIH grants AI20086 and AI17570.

REFERENCES

Bessler, H., M. Djaldetti and C. Moroz (1982). Cell Immunol., 73, 216-229.
Birch, R.E., R. Mandler, S.E. Rudolph and S.H. Polmar (1982a). Int. J. Immunopharm., 4, 294.
Birch, R.E., R. Mandler, S.A. Rudolph and S.H. Polmar (1982b). Fed. Proc.,41,799.
Birch, R.E. and S.H. Polmar (1981). Cell. Immunol., 57, 455-67.
Birch, R.E. and S.H. Polmar (1982c). Clin. Exp. Immunol., 48, 218-230.
Birch, R.E., A.K. Rosenthal and S.H. Polmar (1982d). Clin. Exp.Immunol.,48, 231-38.
Brown, B.L., J.D.M. Albano, B. Ekins and A.M. Sgherzi (1971). Biochem. J. 121, 561-2.
Goodwin, J.S. and D.R. Webb (1980). Clin. Immunol. and Immunopathol., 15, 106-22.
Hirata, F., O.H. Viveros, E.J. Diliberto and J. Axelrod (1978). Proc. Nat'l Acad. Sci. - USA, 75, 1781-21.
Mandler, R., R.E. Birch, S.H. Polmar, G.M. Kammer and S.A. Rudolph (1982). Proc. Nat'l. Acad.Sci.-USA, 79, 4542-46.
Marone, G. , M. Plaut and L.M. Lichtenstein (1978). J. Immunol., 11, 2153-9.
Parker, C.W., J.P. Kelly, S.F. Falkenheim and M.G. Huber (1979). J. Exp. Med., 149, 1487-1503.
Polmar, S.H. and R.E. Birch (1980). In R.S. Krakauer and M.K. Cathcart (eds), Autoimmunity and Immunoregulation, Elsevier, North Holland,Amsterdam pp. 11-19.
Rocklin, R., J. Breard, S. Gupta, R.A. Good and K.L. Melmon (1980). Cell.Immunol., 51, 226-37.
Rola-Plezczynski, M., P. Borgeat and P. Sirois (1982). Biochem. Biophys. Res. Commun., 198, 1531-7.
Rola-Plezczynski, M., and M. Sirois (1983). In P.J. Piper (ed.). Leukotrienes and Other Lipoxygenase Products, Wiley and Sons, London, p. 234-40.
Schwartz, A., R.C. Stern and S.H. Polmar (1978). Clin. Exp. Immunol. Immunopathol., 9, 499-505.
Thomas, Y., L. Rogozinski, O.H. Grigoyen, H.H. Shen, M.A. Talle, G. Goldstein and L. Chess (1982)., J. Immunol., 128, 1386-90.
Voller, A., D.E. Bidwell and A. Bartlett (1979). The Enzyme Linked Immunosorbent Assay (ELISA). Dynatech Laboratories, Inc., Alexandria VA.
Wadee, A.A. and A.R. Rabson (1983). J. Immunol., 130, 2271-6.

Mechanisms of Histamine Release

MOLECULAR AND BIOCHEMICAL MECHANISMS OF IgE-MEDIATED HISTAMINE RELEASE FROM MAST CELLS

T. Ishizaka

Subdepartment of Immunology, The Johns Hopkins University School of Medicine at the Good Samaritan Hospital, 5601 Loch Raven Blvd., Baltimore, MD 21239, USA

ABSTRACT

Bridging of IgE receptors on rat mast cells results in the activation of membrane associated putative proteolytic enzyme followed by activation of both methyltransferases and adenylate cyclase. The receptor bridging also induces mobilization of cytoplasmic calcium influx, as demonstrated by using Quin-2 fluorescence. Inhibitors of methyltransferases inhibit not only phospholipid methylation but also all biochemical events induced by receptor bridging. The results indicate that the activation of methyltransferases is involved in IgE-mediated calcium influx and mediator release. Our results also suggest that the activation of the putative proteolytic enzyme(s) and methyltransferase I, induced by the bridging of IgE-receptors, results in the enhancement of PI turnover in rat mast cells. Mast cells release histamine upon exposure to nonspecific stimuli, such as compound 48/80, Ca-ionophore C3a, and C5a. Biochemical events leading to histamine release by the secretagogues are reviewed in comparisons with IgE-mediated histamine release.

KEY WORDS

IgE receptor, proteolytic enzyme, methyltransferases, Quin-2, ^{45}Ca influx, histamine and arachidonate release, PI turnover, 1, 2-diacylglycerol formation.

INTRODUCTION

Mast cells and basophilic granulocytes bear specific receptors for IgE, which bind IgE molecules with high affinity, and the reactions of cell-bound IgE antibodies with multivalent antigen initiate the release of a variety of preformed and newly generated mediators, such as histamine and leukotrienes (Ishizaka and Ishizaka, 1975).

In the past several years, we analyzed IgE-mediated triggering mechanisms of mediator release in purified rat peritoneal mast cells. This presentation is to review biochemical cascade involved in triggering mast cells for mediator release.

TIRGGERING SIGNALS OF IgE-DEPENDENT MEDIATOR RELEASE

In order to analyze immunological mechanisms involved in initial triggering events in mast cells for IgE-mediated histamine release, we prepared rabbit antibodies against IgE receptors on rat mast cells. Divalent anti-receptor antibodies induced histamine release from rat mast cells, without participation of IgE. The results indicated that bridging of IgE receptors is responsible for triggering mast cells for mediator release (Ishizaka and Ishizaka, 1978). In the IgE-mediated reactions, IgE-receptors serves as an anchor for specific IgE antibody molecule. Once IgE antibody binds to the receptor with high affinity, cell-bound IgE molecules permit antigen to bridge adjacent receptor molecules which in turn initiates process of histamine release. Since no immunoglobulin other than IgE will bind to IgE-receptors with high affinity, triggering of histamine release through IgE receptors will be mediated only by IgE antibodies.

STIMULATION OF METHYLTRANSFERASES AND ADENYLATE CYCLASE BY BRIDGING OF IgE RECEPTORS

Bridging of IgE receptors on rat mast cells induced a marked increase in ^{45}Ca influx followed by histamine release. Since Ca^{2+} is essential for mast cell activation, we examined possible participation of membrane-associated enzymes in Ca^{2+} influx induced by receptor bridging. Our results revealed that challenge of purified normal rat mast cells with $F(ab')_2$ fragments of anti-receptor antibody or anti-IgE resulted in a marked increase in incorporation of ^3H-methyl group into phospholipids and a monophasic rise in intracellular cAMP. Both responses reached maximum at 15 sec after the challenge. The phospholipid methylation is followed by an increase in ^{45}Ca uptake and release of both histamine and arachidonates. ^{45}Ca uptake reached plateau at 2 min and the maximum release of histamine and arachidonates were observed within 3 min (Fig. 1). In contrast, Fab' monomer of anti-receptor antibody or anti-IgE failed to induce these responses (Ishizaka and co-workers, 1981).

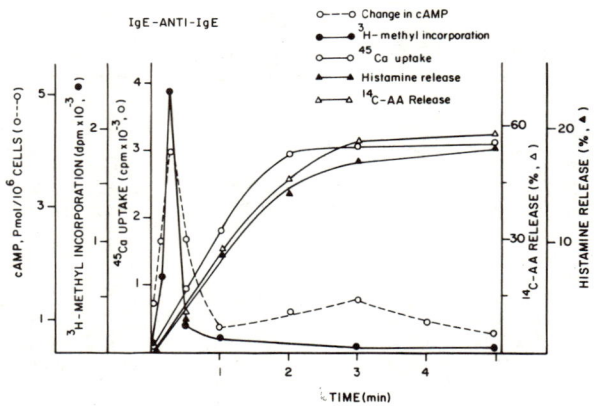

Fig.1. Kinetics of ^3H-methyl incorporation into phospholipids (●), ^{45}Ca uptake (o), change in cAMP level (●), and the release of both histamine (▲) and ^{14}C-AA (Δ) in rat mast cells induced by divalent anti-IgE. The same purified rat mast cells sensitized with IgE were used for all measurements.

It was also found that preincubation of purified mast cells with inhibitors of phospholipid methylation, such as 3-deaza adenosine (ADO) together with L-homocysteine thiolactone, or 5'-deoxy-5'-(isobutylthio)-3-deaza adenosine (3-deaza SIBA), resulted in not only inhibition of phospholipid methylation, but also all of biochemical events induced by receptor bridging i.e., cAMP rise, ^{45}Ca influx and release of both histamine and arachidonates, in a similar dose response fashion (Fig. 2). These results suggest that phospholipid methylation induced by receptor bridging is intimately involved in IgE-mediated Ca^{2+} influx and mediator release.

Recently, we determined changes in cytoplasmic Ca^{2+} in rat mast cells following receptor bridging using the fluorescent probe Quin-2 in collaboration with Drs. J. R. White and R. Sha'afi (White and co-workers, 1984). A marked increase in Quin-2 fluorescence was observed when sensitized mast cells loaded with Quin-2 were exposed to specific antigen. The Quin-2 signal reached maximum within 20 sec after the challenge and then gradually declined. Even in the presence of EGTA (Ca^{2+} concentration equivalent to $6 \times 10^{-7}M$), a substantial increase in Quin-2 fluorescence was observed, indicating that bridging of cell-bound IgE molecules by multivalent antigen induced not only Ca^{2+} influx but also mobilization of cytoplasmic Ca^{2+} (Fig. 3). It was also found that pretreatment of mast cells with inhibitors of methyltransferases resulted in the inhibition of both antigen-induced increase in Quin-2 fluorescence and histamine release.

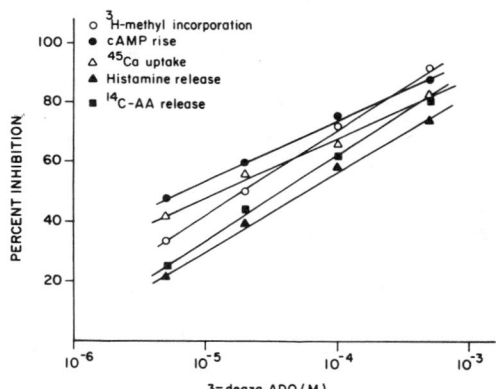

Fig. 2. Inhibition of anti-IgE-induced ^{3}H-methyl incorporation (o), ^{45}Ca uptake (Δ), cAMP rise (●), histamine release (▲) and ^{14}C-arachidonic acid release (■) by 3-deaza adenosine. Purified rat mast cells sensitized with IgE were preincubated with various concentrations of 3-deaza adenosine together with 100 μM of L-homocysteine thiolactone at 37°C for 1 hr. The cells were then challenged with an optimal concentration of anti-IgE.

Subsequently, a supporting evidence for an essential role of methyltransferases in IgE-mediated histamine release was provided by McGivney and co-workers (1981), using variants of histamine releasing subline of rat basophilic leukemia (RBL) cells. It was found that variants of RBL cells deficient in one of methyltransferases were incapable of releasing histamine by IgE and anti-IgE. When these cells were hybridized, however, some of hybrids, which restored two methyltransferases, gave IgE-mediated histamine release. The results support the concept that methyltransferases are involved in the transduction of IgE-mediated triggering signals to the process of mediator release.

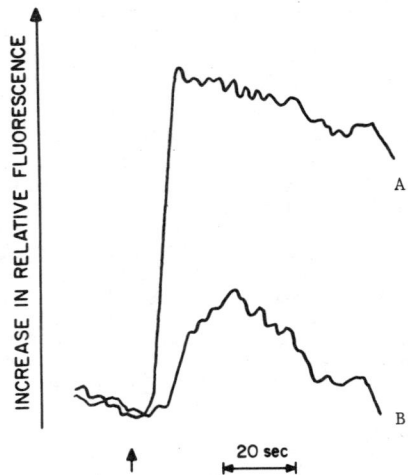

Fig. 3. The increase in cell-associated Quin-2 fluorescence in the presence and absence of extracellular Ca^{2+}. Purified mast cells sensitized with anti-DNP IgE antibody and loaded with Quin-2 were suspended in HEPES buffer containing 1.6 mM Ca^{2+} and 1 mM Mg^{2+} and challenged with an optimal concentration of $DNP_{13}HSA$ (A). EGTA (3 mM) was added to the cells 1 min before antigen challenge (B).

POSSIBLE PARTICIPATION OF MEMBRANE ASSOCIATED PROTEOLYTIC ENZYMES IN INITIAL MAST CELL ACTIVATION

A question to be asked is whether methyltransferases are the first enzyme activated by receptor bridging, or some other enzymes are activated prior to methyltransferases. Earlier studies by Austen and Brocklehurst (1960) and others strongly suggested involvement of a membrane associated proteolytic enzyme in the early stage of antigen-induced histamine release from mast cells. Our results confirmed their observations that potent inhibitor of serine esterases, such as diisopropylfluorophosphate (DFP) and p-nitrophenyl pentylphosphonate inhibited both phospholipid methylation and an initial rise in cAMP induced by receptor bridging. In contrast, non-phosphorylating analogues of the phosphonates had much less inhibitory effects. Furthermore, substrate and inhibitors of chymotrypsin, trypsin and chymase inhibited both phospholipid methylation and an initial rise in cAMP with comparable concentration. The inhibition by these inhibitors are reversible: when mast cells were preincubated with these inhibitors, washed and then challenged with anti-receptor antibody or anti-IgE in the absence of the inhibitor, neither phospholipid methylation nor cAMP rise was inhibited. These results were confirmed using isolated plasma membranes of rat mast cells (Ishizaka and Ishizaka, 1984). It appears that a membrane associated proteolytic enzyme is activated by receptor bridging, and a cleavage product by this enzyme may be involved in the activation of methyltransferases and adenylate cyclase. The putative proteolytic enzyme may be a key enzyme in the induction of initial triggering signals for mediator release.

POSSIBLE ROLE OF PHOSPHOLIPID METHYLATION IN THE ACTIVATION OF PHOSPHOLIPID-DIACYLGLYCEROL CYCLE

Bridging of IgE-receptors on mast cells also induces alterations in phospholipid and diacylglycerol metabolism. Kennerly and co-workers (1979) observed that anti-IgE induced a selective ^{32}P incorporation into phosphatidic acid (PA), phosphatidylinositol (PI) and phosphatidylcholine (PC) in early stages of mast cell activation. Further studies by Sullivan (1981) demonstrated that the activation of rat mast cells resulted in accumulation of 1, 2-diacylglycerol (DAG) followed by the formation of monoacylglycerol (MAG) and free fatty acids. A marked loss of radiolabeled phosphatidylinositol (PI) and a concurrent accumulation of DAG in rat mast cells following antigen stimulation were also demonstrated by Ishizuka and Nozawa (1983).

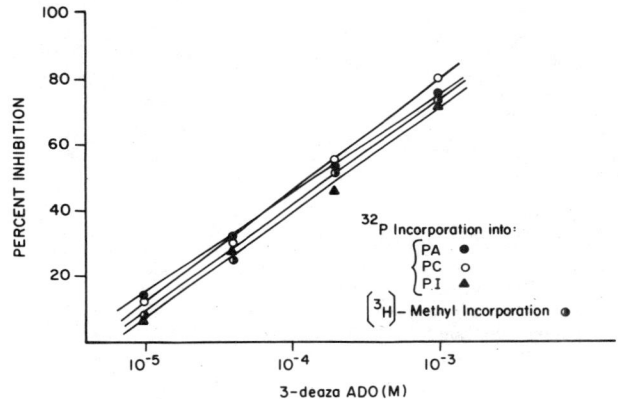

Fig. 4. Inhibition of anti-IgE induced ^3H-methyl incorporation into phospholipids and ^{32}P incorporation by 3-deaza adenosine (ADO). Purified rat mast cells sensitized with IgE were preincubated with various concentrations of 3-deaza-ADO together with 100 μM L-homocysteine thiolactone at 37°C, for 1 hr, and then challenged with anti-IgE. ^{32}P incorporation into PA, PI, PC was analyzed after 10 min incubation, while ^3H-methyl incorporation into phospholipids was determined at 15 sec after the challenge.

In order to analyze possible interrelationship between phospholipid methylation and PI turnover, we studied effect of inhibitors of phospholipid methylation on ^{32}P incorporation into PA, PI and PC. As shown in Fig. 4, preincubation of rat mast cells with 3-deaza ADO together with homocysteine thiolactone resulted in inhibition of both the incorporation of ^3H methyl group into phospholipids and the selective incorporation of ^{32}P into PA, PI and PC in an identical dose response fashion. Another inhibitor of phospholipid methylation, i.e., 3-deaza SIBA, gave identical results. Furthermore, addition of methyl donor, S-adenosyl-L-methionine (SAM) in the reaction system reversed the inhibition of ^{32}P incorporation by 3-deaza ADO or 3-deaza SIBA, suggesting that accumulation of S-adenosyl-L-homocysteine or its analogues was responsible for the inhibition of ^{32}P incorporation. More recent experiments carried out in collaboration with Dr. T. Sullivan have shown that inhibitors of phospholipid methylation, such as 3-deaza-ADO or 3-deaza-SIBA inhibited the formation of DAG and that the inhibition of DAG formation by the methyltransferase inhibitors was reversed by the addition of S-adenosyl-L-methionine (Table 1).

TABLE 1. EFFECTS OF INHIBITORS OF PHOSPHOLIPID METHYLATION ON DAG FORMATION AND HISTAMINE RELEASE

PREINCUBATION WITH	CHALLENGE ANTIGEN	SAM	[^{3}H]-METHYL IN PHOSPHOLIPIDS	DAG	HISTAMINE RELEASE
			DPM/10^6 CELLS	PMOLE/10^6 CELLS	%
NONE	DNP-HSA	−	3544	167	40
		+	3551	174	39
3-DEAZA SIBA	DNP-HSA	−	644	35	11
		+	2521	196	36
3-DEAZA ADO + HCY	DNP-HSA	−	620	45	13
		+	3188	163	38
NONE	NONE	−	618	26	4
		+	607	48	3

Mast cells sensitized with anti-DNP IgE antibody were pre-incubated with 3-deaza SIBA (0.4 mM) or 3-deaza ADO (0.5 mM) together with Hcy (0.1 mM) for 1 hr, at 37°C, then challenged with DNP$_{13}$ HSA in the presence or absence of SAM (5 mM). ^{3}H methyl incorporation, 1, 2-diacylglycerol (DAG) formation and histamine release were determined at 15 sec, 10 min and 5 min, after the challenge, respectively.

Hirata and Axelrod (1978) demonstrated that the first methyltransferase methylates phosphatidylethanolamine (PE) to form phosphatidyl-N-monomethyl ethanolamine (PME) and the second methyltransferase adds two methyl groups successively to form phosphatidylcholine (PC). Thus, we determined as to whether the activation of both methyltransferases was required for stimulation of PI turnover. Since the first enzyme is Mg^{2+}-dependent, purified rat mast cells were challenged in the presence of Mg^{2+} and EGTA, or in the presence of Ca^{2+} and Mg^{2+}, and incorporation of both ^{3}H-methyl groups and ^{32}P into phospholipids were analyzed by thin layer chromatography. The results showed that in the presence of both Ca^{2+} and Mg^{2+}, the two methyltransferases were activated to form PME, phosphatidyl-N, N-dimethyl ethanolamine (PDE) and PC. In the presence of Mg^{2+} and EGTA, formation of PME was predominant, indicating that only the first methyltransferase was fully activated under this condition. However, ^{32}P incorporation in PA, PI and PC was comparable in the two conditions. The results suggest the activation of the first methyltransferase is sufficient for the activation of enzymes involved in PI turnover. Since accumulation of PME in the plasma membrane is known to reduce membrane viscosity and affects many membrane events, one may speculate that such changes in the plasma membrane may be responsible for the stimulation of phospholipid diacylglycerol cycle. Further studies indicated that inhibitors and substrates of proteolytic enzymes, which prevented phospholipid methylation, also inhibited ^{32}P incorporation into PA, PC and PI, and formation of DAG. The concentrations of the inhibitors required for 50% inhibition of the ^{32}P incorporation and DAG formation were comparable to that required for 50% inhibition of phospholipid methylation. These results indicate that the activation of a proteolytic enzyme and methyltransferase I are involved in the activation of phospholipid diacylglycerol cycle.

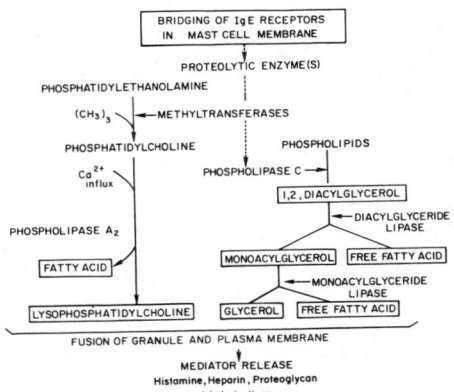

Fig. 5. Biochemical cascade for IgE-dependent mediator release from rat mouse mast cells.

Biochemical cascades involved in IgE-mediated activation of rat mast cells for mediator release are summarized in Fig. 5. Bridging of IgE receptors activates membrane-associated putative proteolytic enzyme followed by activation of both methyltransferases and adenylate cyclase. Accumulation of monomethylated phospholipids in the plasma membrane by activation of methyltransferase I appears to be sufficient for stimulation of PI turnover. Once mast cells are activated through the biochemical pathways, lysophospholipid would be generated by the action of phospholipase A_2, and both DAG and MAG will be generated by action of phospholipase C and diacylglyceride lipase. Since these substances are powerful membrane fusogens, they may facilitate granule membrane fusion and mediator release. At the same time, free arachidonic acid released through the two pathways will be metabolized to generate many biologically active lipid mediators, such as prostaglandins and leukotrienes.

Biological significance of an initial rise in cAMP is not clear. As demonstrated by Lewis and his co-workers (1979) on rat mast cells, 10 μM indomethacin, which completely inhibits prostaglandin synthesis, failed to inhibit an initial rise in cAMP in both purified human lung mast cells and cultured human basophils. The results indicated that an initial rise in cAMP is not due to prostaglandin synthesis. Furthermore, evidence was obtained that β-adrenergic receptors are not involved in the activation of adenylate cyclase induced by bridging of IgE receptors (Ishizaka and co-workers, 1981). Holgate and his co-workers (1980) demonstrated that bridging of IgE molecules on rat mast cells resulted in the activation of adenylate cyclase, activation of cAMP-dependent protein kinase and granule secretion, and speculated that an initial rise in cAMP may be an essential step in histamine releasing process. However, it is also possible that cAMP rise could provide "off" signal after the histamine releasing cascade was initiated by an elevation of phospholipid methylation.

BIOCHEMICAL EVENTS INVOLVED IN MEDIATOR RELEASE FROM MAST CELLS BY NON-SPECIFIC STIMULI

Mediator release from mast cells is induced not only by specific ligand-receptor interaction, but also by various nonspecific stimuli. Among them, important ligands from the biological viewpoints are complement-derived peptides, C5a and C3a which are generated during inflammation. Biochemical cascades activated by complement-derived peptides, C5a and C3a, are similar to IgE-mediated activation in rat mast cells. Challenge of rat mast cells with anaphylatoxin C5a resulted in stimulation of phospholipid methylation, and an increase in ^{45}Ca uptake which are followed by the release of histamine and arachidonate. As demonstrated in IgE-mediated activation, inhibitors of phospholipid methylation inhibited these biochemical events induced by the peptides, suggesting that phospholipid methylation is involved in transduction of C5a-, C3a- induced triggering signals for mediator release. An interesting finding was that C5a-, C3a- induced cAMP rise was much slower than that induced by bridging of IgE receptors. Furthermore, the cAMP rise by C5a and C3a was completely inhibited by the presence of 10 µM indomethacin, indicating that the increase is the result of prostaglandin synthesis. Since indomethacin does not inhibit C5a induced histamine release from rat mast cells, it appears that the increase in cAMP is not involved in C5a-induced histamine release.

Compound 48/80 and Ca-ionophore A23187 also induce histamine release from rat mast cells. Different from IgE-mediated or anaphylatoxin-mediated histamine release, however, both compound 48/80 and Ca-ionophore failed to induce phospholipid methylation. These compounds directly induce mobilization of intracellular Ca^{2+} and Ca^{2+} influx which were followed by mediator release. Our recent studies using Quin-2 fluorescence demonstrated that phorbol 12-myristate 13-acetate induces histamine release from rat mast cells without increasing intracellular Ca^{2+} (White and co-workers, 1984). These results reflect complexity of activation processes for mediator release from mast cells.

In summary, bridging of IgE-receptors on rat mast cells induces phospholipid methylation, a monophasic rise in intracellular cAMP, mobilization of intracellular Ca^{2+} and an increase in Ca^{2+} influx. These responses are followed by the release of both histamine and arachidonate. Inhibitors of methyltransferases inhibit not only phospholipid methylation but also an increase in intracellular Ca^{2+} and mediator release, suggesting that the activation of methyltransferase, induced by receptor-bridging, is intimately involved in the increase in Ca^{2+} uptake and mediator release. Bridging of IgE-receptors also induces a selective incorporation of ^{32}PO into phosphatidic acid (PA), phosphatidylcholine (PC) and phosphatidylinositol (PI), and the formation of diacylglycerol (DAG). Preincubation of rat mast cells with inhibitors of methyltransferases inhibited both phospholipid methylation and ^{32}PO incorporation into PA, PI and PC and formation of DAG in a similar dose response fashion. Our results suggest that the activation of methyltransferase I, which catalyzes the formation of phosphatidyl-N-monomethylethanolamine from phosphatidylethanolamine, is involved in the stimulation of PI turnover. It was also found that inhibitors of serine protease inhibited all of biochemical events induced by receptor bridging i.e., phospholipid methylation, cAMP rise, Ca^{2+} influx, the release of both histamine and arachidonate, and PI turnover. It appears that membrane-associated proteolytic enzyme is activated by receptor-bridging, and this enzyme may play a crucial role in the induction of IgE-mediated triggering signals for mediator release.

Biochemical events induced by nonspecific ligands differ depending on ligand. Anaphylatoxin C5a and C3a induces phospholipid methylation and ^{45}Ca uptake followed by histamine and arachidonate release. Compound 48/80 and Ca-ionophore A23187 induce the mobilization of intracellular Ca^{2+} and Ca^{2+} influx but failed to induce phospholipid methylation. Phorbol 12-myristate 13-acetate induces histamine release from rat mast cells without increasing intracellular Ca^{2+}. The findings reflect complexity of activation process for mediator release.

ACKNOWLEDGEMENT

I would like to express my gratitude for the collaboration with the following investigators; Dr. K. Ishizaka, D. H. Conrad, E. S. Schulman, J. R. White, Mr.

A. R. Sterk and Mrs. C. G. L. Ko, The Johns Hopkins University, Baltimore, MD. Dr. R. I. Sha'afi, University of Connecticut Health Center, Farmington, CT., and Dr. T. J. Sullivan, University of Texas Health Science Center at Dallas, TX. Their excellent collaboration and assistance made it possible for me to carry on this series of studies. My special appreciation goes to Dr. T. E. Hugli, Scripps Clinic, La Jolla, CA. and Dr. P. M. Henson, National Jewish Hospital, Denver, CO., for preparations of purified C5a and C3a, and Dr. J. C. Powers, Georgia Institute of Technology, Atlanta, GA. for synthesized substrates and inhibitors of chymase and tryptase. These materials were invaluable in my studies.

This work was supported by research grant AI-10060 from USPHS and a grant from the Lillia Babbit Hyde Foundation. This is publication No. 567 from the O'Neill Laboratories at the Good Samaritan Hospital, Baltimore, MD.

REFERENCES

Austen, K. F. and W. W. Brocklehurst (1978). J. Exp. Med., 113: 521-539.
Hirata, F. and J. A. Axelrod (1978). Proc. Natl. Acad. Sci. (USA) 76: 2348-2352.
Holgate, S. T., R. A. Lewis and K. F. Austen (1980). Proc. Natl. Acad. Sci. (USA) 77: 6800-6804.
Ishizaka, T. and K. Ishizaka (1975). Progress in Allergy 19: 60-121.
Ishizaka, T. and K. Ishizaka (1978). J. Immunol., 120: 800-805.
Ishizaka, T., F. Hirata, A. R. Sterk, K. Ishizaka and J. A. Axelrod (1981). Proc. Natl. Acad. Sci. (USA) 79: 6812-6816.
Ishizaka, T. and K. Ishizaka (1984). Proc. Allergy 34: 188-235.
Ishizuka, Y. and Y. Nozawa (1983). Biochem. Biophys. Res. Commun. 117: 710-717.
Kennerly, D. A., T. J. Sullivan and C. W. Parker (1979). J. Immunol., 122: 152-159.
Lewis, R. A., S. T. Holgate, L. J. Roberts, II., J. F. Maguire, J. A. Oates and K. F. Austen (1979). J. Immunol., 123: 1633-1638.
McGivney, A., F. T. Crew, F. Hirata, J. A. Axelrod and R. P. Siraganian (1981). Proc. Natl. Acad. Sci. (USA) 78: 6176-6180.
Sullivan, T. J. (1981). In: Biochemistry of the Acute Allergic Reactions, E. L. Becker, A. S. Simon and K. F. Austen, p. 229-238, Alan R. Liss Co., New York.
White, J. R., T. Ishizaka, K. Ishizaka and R. I. Sha'afi (1984). Proc. Natl. Acad. Sci. (USA) 81: 3978-3982.

MAST CELL HETEROGENEITY DIFFERENTIAL RESPONSIVITY TO HISTAMINE LIBERATORS AND ANTI-ALLERGIC DRUGS

F. L. Pearce*, H. Ali*, K. E. Barrett*,
A. D. Befus**, J. Bienenstock**, J. Brostoff***,
M. Ennis*, K. C. Flint***, N. McI. Johnson***,
K. B. P. Leung* and P. T. Peachell*

*The Department of Chemistry, University College London,
London, UK
**The Department of Pathology, McMaster University,
Hamilton, Ontario, Canada
***The Medical Unit and Department of Immunology,
Middlesex Hospital Medical School, London, UK

ABSTRACT

Examples are provided of the functional heterogeneity of mast cells from different locations. Mast cells from various species and even from given tissues within a particular animal are shown to differ in their responses to histamine liberators and anti-allergic drugs. The pharmacological and clinical significance of these findings are discussed.

KEYWORDS

Allergy; anti-allergic drugs; histamine; histamine-liberators; mast cells; mast cell heterogeneity.

INTRODUCTION

Mast cells are widely distributed throughout the human body but are found predominantly in those areas which come into most frequent contact with foreign substances, namely in the loose connective tissue of the bronchi, conjunctiva, gut, ear, nose, throat and skin. Activation of these cells leads to the release of a variety of newly synthesised and preformed inflammatory mediators exemplified by the autacoid histamine. These mediators then act on distinct effector cells to produce the symptoms of allergy and anaphylaxis.

The pathophysiological stimulus for the release of histamine from the mast cell is provided by the combination of specific antigen with reaginic antibody fixed to the cell surface. In addition, secretion may be induced by a variety of pharmacological agents which act independently of the immunological mechanism. Given the widespread distribution of the mast cell, it is fundamental to our understanding of the aetiology and prophylaxis of allergic conditions to appreciate that mastocytes from different locations may show marked variations in their functional properties. In particular, they may differ in their responses both to histamine liberators and to anti-allergic drugs. The former effect is of clear importance in view of the fact that a number of compounds in clinical use may act as histamine liberators in appropriate experimental situations. The latter effect is of obvious relevance in the development of new compounds directed against specific inflammatory conditions.

In order to characterize an agent as a histamine liberator two basic approaches are possible. Firstly, parenteral administration of the compound should lead to a degranulation of mast cells *in situ* and a corresponding depletion of histamine in affected tissues *in vivo*. These effects will lead to an elevation in the plasma level of the amine and produce characteristic, systemic anaphylactoid responses. Secondly, the compound should induce a release of histamine from isolated tissues or free mast cells *in vitro*. Large numbers of mast cells occur in the serosal cavities of some rodents, particularly the rat, and may be isolated from these sources by simple lavage. Significant numbers of mast cells may also be isolated from the airways of man by bronchoalveolar lavage (Flint and others, 1984). Unfortunately, free serosal cells do not occur in significant quantities in other animals and for this reason, and in order to make further comparative studies, methods have been developed for the enzymic dissociation of intact tissues into their component cells. The preparations thus obtained are morphologically intact, biochemically unimpaired and provide ideal models for the study of functional heterogeneity. The present article will compare the responsivity of these cells to defined histamine liberators and anti-anaphylactic drugs. In total, several hundred agents have been found to release histamine from mast cells. For this reason, the current work will concentrate on a small number of examples which are of particular interest either because of their wide usage, their high degree of selectivity, or their clinical importance.

DIFFERENTIAL EFFECTS OF HISTAMINE LIBERATORS

Compound 48/80

Compound 48/80 is a synthetic polyamine produced by the acid-catalysed condensation of p-methoxy-N-methylphenethylamine and formaldehyde. The compound is one of the most widely used and best studied histamine liberators and is often described as a "classical mast cell degranulating agent". In fact, the compound shows a very high degree of selectivity in its action. Parenteral administration produces a severe or fatal anaphylactoid reaction in the rat, cat and dog but has a limited or negligible effect in the rabbit, mouse, guinea pig, hamster, man and monkey (for references see Pearce, 1982a). The systemic responses in the former species are accompanied by a marked degranulation of mast cells and a depletion of histamine in a variety of connective tissues. However, mast cells in the mucosa of the gastrointestinal tract are completely unresponsive to compound 48/80. In fact, the latter cells provide a particularly striking example of heterogeneity within a single species (for a review see Enerbäck, 1981). The distribution of mast cells in the small bowel of the rat has been investigated by ultrastructural and histochemical techniques. Small numbers of mast cells occur in the outer serosal layers and resemble the connective tissue cells found in various organs. In contrast, the mast cells in the mucosal layers differ dramatically in their ultrastructural, cytochemical, biochemical and functional properties. These cells, originally referred to as "atypical mast cells", are smaller than the connective tissue cells, have a lower histamine content, a negligible content of serotonin, and possess fewer granules. The latter consist of a relatively soluble matrix containing an unidentified, poorly sulphated glycosaminoglycan which is distinct from heparin. These properties require that special conditions of fixation and staining be used to demonstrate characteristic metachromasia in this cell type. The mucosal cells have a short life-span and proliferate in thymus dependent fashion in response to certain parasitic infections. They also contain an antigenically distinct serine protease which has been used as a marker in ontogenic studies. Differential fixation and staining also indicates a similar heterogeneity of mast cells in the gastrointestinal tract of man (Strobel and others, 1981).

The specificity of compound 48/80 *in vivo* is mirrored by studies on isolated cells and tissues *in vitro*. Rat peritoneal and pleural cells respond strongly to the amine. Mesenteric, pulmonary and cutaneous cells show significant reactivity, while cardiac and intestinal cells are totally unresponsive (Fig. 1a). Pulmonary or mesenteric mast cells of the guinea pig and man are also unreactive (Barrett, Ennis and Pearce, 1983; Ennis, 1982; Ennis and Pearce, 1980), as are human basophil leucocytes (Foreman and Lichtenstein, 1980) and mastocytes obtained by human bronchoalveolar lavage (unpublished work). Additional examples of the variation in response to compound 48/80 have recently been summarized (Pearce 1982a, 1983).

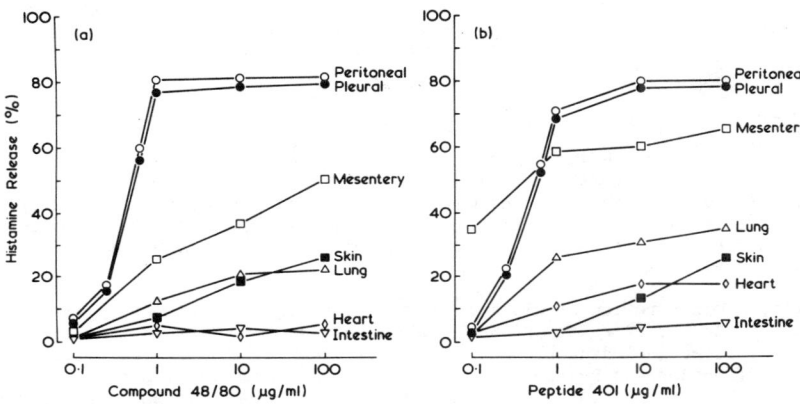

Fig. 1. Histamine release from isolated rat mast cells treated with (a) compound 48/80 and (b) peptide 401.

Peptide 401

Peptide 401, the mast cell degranulating (MCD) peptide from bee venom, is a basic molecule composed of twenty-two amino acid residues. Comparative studies have shown that the molecule strongly resembles compound 48/80 in its specificity and mode of action. Parenteral administration produces an acute, systemic reaction in the rat but is virtually without effect in the mouse, guinea pig or rabbit (Breithaupt and Habermann, 1968). The peptide is a potent liberator of histamine from rat peritoneal and pleural mast cells *in vitro*, being rather more active than compound 48/80 on a molar basis (Barrett and Pearce, 1982). Pulmonary and particularly mesenteric cells of the rat are also reactive but cutaneous and cardiac cells are rather resistant. Rat intestinal mast cells are again totally unresponsive to the peptide. These data are summarized in Fig. 1b. Studies with fluorescently labelled peptide 401 have shown that the mucosal cells, unlike those in the connective tissues, do not bind the peptide and may thus lack the appropriate receptors for the molecule (Befus and others, 1982). Peritoneal mast cells from the mouse and hamster are less responsive than those of the rat (Barrett and Pearce, 1983; Leung and Pearce, 1984) whereas human basophil leucocytes (Assem and Atkinson, 1973), human lung mast cells obtained by enzymic dispersion (Ennis, 1982) or bronchoalveolar lavage (unpublished work), and guinea pig mast cells from the heart, lung and mesentery (Ali and Pearce, 1985; Barrett, Ennis and Pearce, 1983; Ennis and Pearce, 1980) are all totally unreactive.

Polylysine and Polymyxin

Polylysine and the peptide antibiotic polymyxin both produce systemic reactions in the rat (Bushby and Green, 1955; Rothschild, 1966). Polylysine is also an effective histamine liberator in the cat and dog (Rothschild, 1966) but polymyxin is much less reactive in these species (Bushby and Green, 1955). Both agents are potent releasers of histamine from isolated rat peritoneal mast cells (Ennis, Pearce and Weston, 1980; Peachell and Pearce, 1984) and resemble compound 48/80 and peptide 401 in being much less active against guinea pig and human mast cells. However, polylysine appears to have a broader spectrum of activity than the latter polycations. It is an effective releaser of histamine from peritoneal mast cells of the mouse and hamster (Barrett and Pearce, 1982; Leung and Pearce, 1984) and from human basophil leucocytes (Foreman and Lichtenstein, 1980) but is inactive against human bronchoalveolar lavage cells (unpublished work). Polymyxin is weakly active against peritoneal cells of the mouse but moderately effective against those of the hamster (Peachell and Pearce, 1984).

Dextran

Dextran is a branched chain homopolymer of α-D-glucopyranosyl residues. The native material is extremely polydisperse but by means of controlled hydrolysis and careful fractionation, samples may be prepared of defined molecular weight range. These substances are used clinically as plasma substitutes and blood volume expanders. Dextran also provides one of the best examples of a highly specific histamine liberator.

Parenteral administration of clinical dextran produces an acute anaphylactoid reaction in the rat (Parratt and West, 1957) but is completely without effect in any other species including the mouse, hamster, rabbit, guinea pig, pigeon and dog (for references see Pearce, 1982a). The systemic reaction in the rat is accompanied by a striking elevation in the level of plasma histamine and a marked degranulation of mast cells in those areas in which the inflammatory response is most marked, namely in the dorsal skin and pads of the feet and in the ears and muzzle (Parratt and West, 1957). Mast cells in the ventral abdominal skin are, however, relatively unaffected. Dextran also provides an interesting example of the genetic control of mast cell reactivity. By selective breeding, Harris, Kalmus and West (1963) have produced a pure strain of Wistar rat that is refractory to the systemic effects of clinical dextran. This hereditary trait is carried by an autosomal, recessive gene. The origin of the effect is discussed further below.

The specific action of dextran is also manifest *in vitro*. The polysaccharide is an effective releaser of histamine from peritoneal and pleural mast cells of the rat and has some effect on isolated connective tissue but not mucosal mast cells of this animal (Barrett, Ali and Pearce, 1984; Barrett and Pearce, 1982; Barrett and Pearce, 1983; Befus and others, 1982; Ennis and Pearce, 1980). However, it is completely inactive against pulmonary or mesenteric mast cells of the guinea pig and man and against peritoneal cells of the hamster and mouse (Barrett and Pearce, 1983; Barrett, Ennis and Pearce, 1983; Ennis, 1982; Ennis and Pearce, 1980; Leung and Pearce, 1984). Dextran appears to produce its effects on responsive mast cells by interaction with specific glucoreceptors on the plasma membrane (Moodley, Mongar and Foreman, 1982). Isolated peritoneal cells from rats bred for their resistance to the parenteral administration of clinical dextran (see above) do not respond to the polysaccharide *in vitro* but react normally to other immunological and pharmacological stimuli. Ludowyke and coworkers (1982) have shown that the plasma membranes of these cells contain a specific polypeptide which is deficient in the mast cells of normal, dextran-sensitive animals. They suggested that this protein may down-regulate or uncouple the dextran receptor in non-responsive rats, rendering the cells insensitive to the polysaccharide. A similar mechanism, or complete absence of the receptor, could operate in the other examples cited.

Phosphatidylserine (PS)

While PS does not itself release histamine in the absence of a primary stimulus, the lipid specifically enhances secretion of the amine from mouse or rat serosal mast cells activated by IgE-directed or related ligands. The potentiation is specific for these agonists and the compound has no effect or even inhibits the release induced by most chemical histamine liberators (Grosman and Diamant, 1975). Current thinking would suggest that PS may facilitate entry of calcium ions into the mast cell, an integral part of the activation sequence (Pearce, 1982b).

The potentiating action of PS is highly selective for mouse and rat peritoneal and pleural mast cells (Barrett and Pearce, 1982, 1983; Siraganian and Hazard, 1979). In particular, the compound has a limited or negligible effect on isolated peritoneal mast cells of the hamster (Leung and Pearce, 1984), chopped mesentery of the rat (Mongar and Svec, 1972), chopped lung of the rat, guinea pig and man (Lichtenstein and others, 1979; Mongar and Svec, 1972), basophil leucocytes of the rabbit, guinea pig and man (Lichtenstein and others, 1979; Siraganian and Hazard, 1979), and enzymically dispersed mast cells from the mesentery of the rat and guinea pig (Ennis and Pearce, 1980), the intestine (Befus and others, 1982) and skin (Barrett, Ali and Pearce, 1984) of the rat, and the lung of the guinea pig (Barrett, Ennis and Pearce, 1983) and man (Ennis, 1982). The reasons for the striking specificity of PS are not clear but may reflect differences in the membrane lipid composition of diverse mast cells, rendering the peritoneal exudate cells of the mouse and rat peculiarly susceptible to this agent.

INHIBITORS OF HISTAMINE RELEASE

Agents Acting Through Cyclic AMP (cAMP)

Agents which elevate intracellular levels of cAMP have historically been associated with the inhibition of mediator release from the mast cell. Recently this direct, causal relationship has been questioned by some authors but the overall concept seems to be of broad validity (for discussion see Pearce, 1982b).

Concentrations of cAMP may be raised experimentally by a number of methods, namely by application of appropriate analogues of the nucleotide, by activation of adenylate cyclase with cholera toxin, certain prostaglandins or sympathomimetic amines, or by preventing the breakdown of the nucleotide by inhibition of phosphodiesterase with methylxanthines and related compounds. Of these agents, sympathomimetic amines and methylxanthines are used therapeutically in allergic conditions such as asthma. They owe their clinical efficacy largely to their bronchodilator activity but their ability to prevent mediator release from the mast cell may also contribute to their utility. Their selective effects on mast cells are then of some interest.

Phosphodiesterase inhibitors. Methylxanthines, typified by theophylline and its more highly water-soluble derivative aminophylline, inhibit histamine release from a diverse range of mastocytes including those from the lung of man, monkey and the guinea pig (Ishizaka and others, 1971; Orange, Austen and Austen, 1971; Pearce and others, 1978), the skin of the monkey, man and rat (Byars and Ferraresi, 1980; Perper, Sanda and Lichtenstein, 1972; Yamamoto, Greaves and Fairley, 1973) and human basophil leucocytes (Lichtenstein and Margolis, 1968). Strikingly, theophylline has no effect on mediator release from mucosal mast cells from the intestine of the rat (Pearce and others, 1982). Similarly, aminophylline does not inhibit IgE-mediated intestinal anaphylaxis in the rat but blocks the passive cutaneous anaphylactic reaction in this species (Byars and Ferraresi, 1980). Since cAMP analogues inhibit histamine release from isolated rat mucosal mast cells (unpublished work), the cyclic nucleotide phosphodiesterase of this species may possess rather specific properties. Theophylline, unlike sympathomimetic amines (see below), is also inactive against free mastocytes obtained by bronchial lavage of the dog (Tomita, Patterson and Suszko, 1974).

Catecholamines. Mast cells also differ in their sensitivity towards β-adrenoceptor agonists. Sympathomimetic amines are potent inhibitors of mediator release from tissue fragments or enzymically dispersed mast cells of the lung of the dog (Krell and Chakrin, 1976), calf (Burka and Eyre, 1976), guinea pig (Assem and Richter, 1971; Pearce and others, 1978), monkey (Ishizaka and others, 1971) and man (Assem and Richter, 1971; Orange, Austen and Austen, 1971), bronchoalveolar lavage cells of primates and the dog (Butchers and others, 1980; Tomita, Patterson and Suszko, 1974), and human skin (Yamamoto, Greaves and Fairley, 1973), nasal polyps (Kaliner, Wasserman and Austen, 1973), and basophil leucocytes (Lichtenstein and Margolis, 1968). These agents also inhibit cutaneous anaphylactic reactions *in vivo* in man (Assem and Richter, 1971), monkey (Perper, Sanda and Lichtenstein, 1972), and the rat (Assem and Richter, 1971). In total contrast, peritoneal mast cells of the rat, mouse and hamster are resistant to the inhibitory effects of catecholamines (Stechschulte and Austen, 1973; Leung, Barrett and Pearce, 1984). This effect may be attributed to a lack of coupled, functional β-adrenoceptors in these cells or to the generation of cAMP in discrete pools not directly linked to the inhibitory mechanism (see Pearce, 1982b). The situation in the calf leucocyte is even more complex and β-receptor stimulation by catecholamines in this system is associated with a potentiation rather than inhibition of release (Holroyde and Eyre, 1976). No explanation of this effect has yet been offered.

Histamine. Finally, it is of interest to note that histamine may modulate its own release by means of a negative feedback mechanism involving H2-receptors linked to adenylate cyclase on the mast cell membrane. The distribution of these receptors is again highly species specific and they are reportedly present on the basophil leucocyte but not the lung mast cell of man (Schulman and others, 1983), present on the pulmonary or cutaneous mast cell of the dog, monkey and guinea pig (Chakrin and others, 1974; Krell and Chakrin, 1977; Rising and Lewis, 1982) but absent on the lung, skin and peritoneal mast cell of the rat (Chakrin and others, 1974; Rising and Lewis, 1982; Wescott and Kaliner, 1981). The situation in the cow is again complex and stimulatory rather than inhibitory H2-receptors have been reported for both the bovine leucocyte and pulmonary mast cell (Holroyde and Eyre, 1978).

Disodium Cromoglycate

The discovery of the drug disodium cromoglycate in 1965 undoubtedly provided a major advance in the treatment and prophylaxis of asthma and other allergic conditions. Initial studies suggested that the compound had an entirely novel mode of action. Unlike antihistamines and bronchodilators, which were designed to provide essentially symptomatic relief from the inflammatory effects of mast cell mediators, cromoglycate was believed to act directly on the tissue mast cells to prevent the primary release of these substances. However, more recent investigations have suggested that the mechanism of action of the drug may be more complex than initially considered (Stokes and Morley, 1981). In particular, the compound shows a very high degree of tissue and species specificity in its action. Since the clinical success of cromoglycate has stimulated intense efforts to develop new compounds with similar properties (Church, 1978; Garland, Green and Hodson, 1978), these effects are worthy of discussion in some detail.

Sodium cromoglycate is highly active in a number of experimental models in the rat. The compound effectively inhibits cutaneous, peritoneal and pulmonary anaphylactic reactions *in vivo* (Butchers and others, 1979; Church, Collier and James, 1972; Cox, 1967) and blocks histamine release from free peritoneal mast cells and fragments of chopped lung and skin *in vitro* (Greaves, Fairley and Yamamoto, 1971; Leung, Barrett and Pearce, 1984; Sheard and Blair, 1970). In total contrast, the drug has absolutely no effect on isolated mucosal mast cells from rat intestine (Pearce and others, 1982). The data from other species is much less impressive. Cromoglycate produces some inhibition of histamine release from mast cells in primate lung (Assem and Mongar, 1970; Cox, 1967; Sheard and Blair, 1970) but is surprisingly weakly active in this system (Butchers and others, 1979; Church, Holgate and Pao, 1983). The drug is, however, more potent against mastocytes obtained by human bronchoalveolar lavage (Flint and others, 1984). This factor may be of considerable significance in the clinical utility of the drug. These preparations show many of the characteristics of mucosal mast cells and, given their superficial location within the airways and their resulting direct contact with inhaled antigens, may be of primary importance in immediate hypersensitivity reactions in the lung. Cromoglycate does not inhibit cutaneous anaphylactic reactions in the monkey (Patterson, Talbot and Brandfonbrener, 1971), nor Prausnitz-Küstner reactions in man (Assem and Mongar, 1970) and does not prevent mediator release from fragments of human skin (Pearce and others, 1974) or human basophil leucocytes (Assem and Mongar, 1970). The drug is similarly inactive against basophil leucocytes and cutaneous mast cells of the rabbit (Assem and Mongar, 1970; Zvaifler, Bauer and Robinson, 1971) and cow (Holroyde and Eyre, 1978; Wells and Eyre, 1972), cutaneous and peritoneal mast cells of the mouse (Church, 1978; Leung, Barrett and Pearce, 1984), and pulmonary mast cells of the cow (Burka and Eyre, 1975) and dog (Krell and Chakrin, 1976). Hamster peritoneal cells show moderate responsivity (Leung, Barrett and Pearce, 1984). The situation in the guinea pig is the subject of conflicting reports (for discussion see Garland, Green and Hodson, 1978) but most authors would agree that the compound does not inhibit cutaneous or respiratory anaphylaxis *in vivo* (Cox, 1967) and that it is ineffective or very weakly active *in vitro* against guinea pig leucocytes (Greaves, 1969) and mast cells from the lung and skin (Assem and Mongar, 1970; Tay, Yeoh and Greaves, 1972). Representative examples of the effects of cromoglycate on isolated mast cells from a number of different sources are shown in Fig. 2.

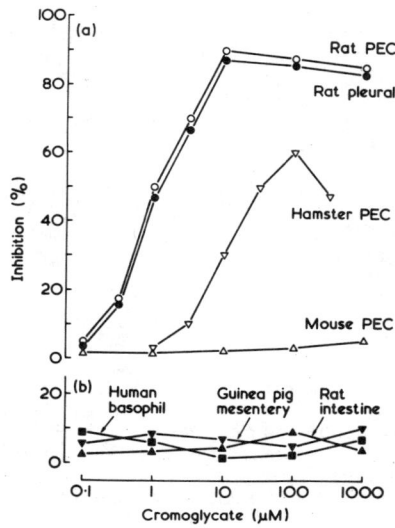

Fig. 2. Inhibition by disodium cromoglycate of IgE-mediated histamine release from mast cells from various sources. PEC denotes peritoneal exudate cells.

In total, the above data clearly emphasize the heterogeneous responsivity of various mast cells to given anti-allergic agents. These observations are of fundamental importance since it cannot be assumed that a drug active against mast cells in one site will necessarily be effective against mast cells in another. If a similar selectivity is observed with other cromoglycate-like drugs, then no single compound can act as a panacea for all allergic conditions. The availability of isolated mast cells from defined locations will then provide a series of ideal test systems for the screening of drugs directed against specific inflammatory problems.

REFERENCES

Ali, H., and F. L. Pearce (1985). Isolation and properties of cardiac and other mast cells from the rat and guinea pig. *Agents and Actions*, in press.
Assem, E. S. K., and G. Atkinson (1973). Histamine release by MCDP (401), a peptide from the venom of the honey bee. *Brit. J. Pharmacol., 48*, 337-338P.
Assem, E. S. K., and J. L. Mongar (1970). Inhibition of allergic reactions in man and other species by cromoglycate. *Int. Arch. Allergy appl. Immunol., 38*, 68-77.
Assem, E. S. K., and A. W. Richter (1971). Comparison of *in vivo* and *in vitro* inhibition of the anaphylactic mechanism by β-adrenergic stimulants and disodium cromoglycate. *Immunology, 21*, 729-739.
Barrett, K. E., H. Ali, and F. L. Pearce (1984). Studies on histamine secretion from enzymically dispersed cutaneous mast cells of the rat. *J. inv. Dermatol.*, in press.
Barrett, K. E., M. Ennis, and F. L. Pearce (1983). Mast cells isolated from guinea pig lung: characterization and studies on histamine secretion. *Agents and Actions, 13*, 122-126.
Barrett, K. E., and F. L. Pearce (1982). A comparative study of histamine secretion from rat peritoneal and pleural mast cells. *Agents and Actions, 12*, 186-188.
Barrett, K. E., and F. L. Pearce (1983). A comparison of histamine secretion from isolated peritoneal mast cells of the mouse and rat. *Int. Arch. Allergy appl. Immunol., 72*, 234-238.
Befus, A. D., F. L. Pearce, J. Gauldie, P. Horsewood, and J. Bienenstock (1982). Mucosal mast cells. I. Isolation and functional characteristics of rat intestinal mast cells. *J. Immunol., 128*, 2475-2480.
Breithaupt, H., and E. Habermann (1968). Mastzelldegranulierendes Peptid (MCD-Peptid) aus Bienengift-Isolierung, biochemische und pharmakologische Eigenschaften. *Naunyn-Schmiedeberg's Arch. Pharmakol., 261*, 252-270.
Burka, J. F., and P. Eyre (1975). Modulation of the formation and release of bovine SRS-A *in vitro* by several anti-anaphylactic drugs. *Int. Arch. Allergy appl. Immunol., 49*, 774-781.
Burka, J. F., and P. Eyre (1976). Modulation of the release of SRS-A from bovine lung *in vitro* by several autonomic and autacoid agents. *Int. Arch. Allergy appl. Immunol., 50*, 664-673.
Bushby, S. R. M., and A. F. Green (1955). The release of histamine by polymyxin B and polymyxin E. *Brit. J. Pharmacol., 10*, 215-219.
Butchers, P. R., J. R. Fullarton, I. F. Skidmore, L. E. Thompson, C. J. Vardey, and A. Wheeldon (1979). A comparison of the anti-anaphylactic activities of salbutamol and disodium cromoglycate in the rat, the rat mast cell and in human lung tissue. *Brit. J. Pharmacol., 67*, 23-32.
Butchers, P. R., C. J. Vardey, I. F. Skidmore, A. Wheeldon, and L. E. Boutal (1980). Histamine-containing cells from bronchial lavage of macaque monkeys. Time course and inhibition of anaphylactic histamine release. *Int. Arch. Allergy appl. Immunol., 62*, 205-212.
Byars, N. E., and R. W. Ferraresi (1980). Inhibition of rat intestinal anaphylaxis by various anti-inflammatory agents. *Agents and Actions, 10*, 252-257.
Chakrin, L. W., R. D. Krell, J. Mengel, D. Young, C. Zaher, and J. R. Wardell

(1974). Effect of a histamine H2-receptor antagonist on immunologically induced mediator release *in vitro*. *Agents and Actions*, *4*, 297-303.

Church, M. K. (1978). Cromoglycate-like anti-allergic drugs: a review. *Drugs of Today*, *14*, 281-341.

Church, M. K., H. O. J. Collier, and G. W. L. James (1972). The inhibition by dexamethasone and disodium cromoglycate of anaphylactic bronchoconstriction in the rat. *Int. Arch. Allergy appl. Immunol.*, *46*, 56-65.

Church, M. K., S. T. Holgate, and G. J.-K. Pao (1983). Histamine release from mechanically and enzymatically dispersed human lung mast cells: inhibition by salbutamol and cromoglycate. *Brit. J. Pharmacol.*, *79*, 374P.

Cox, J. S. G. (1967). Disodium cromoglycate (FPL 670) ("Intal"*): a specific inhibitor of reaginic antibody-antigen mechanisms. *Nature*, *216*, 1328-1329.

Enerbäck, L. (1981). The gut mucosal mast cell. *Monog. Allergy*, *17*, 222-232.

Ennis, M. (1982). Histamine release from human pulmonary mast cells. *Agents and Actions*, *12*, 60-63.

Ennis, M., and F. L. Pearce (1980). Differential reactivity of isolated mast cells from the rat and guinea pig. *Eur. J. Pharmacol.*, *66*, 339-345.

Ennis, M., F. L. Pearce, and P. M. Weston (1980). Some studies on the release of histamine from mast cells stimulated with polylysine. *Brit. J. Pharmacol.*, *70*, 329-334.

Flint, K. C., K. B. P. Leung, F. L. Pearce, B. Hudspith, J. Brostoff, and N. McI. Johnson (1984). Human mast cells recovered by bronchoalveolar lavage: their morphology, histamine release and the effects of sodium cromoglycate. Submitted.

Foreman, J. C., and L. M. Lichtenstein (1980). Induction of histamine release by polycations. *Biochim. biophys. Acta*, *629*, 587-603.

Garland, L. G., A. F. Green, and H. F. Hodson (1978). Inhibitors of the release of anaphylactic mediators. In G. V. R. Born, A. Farah, H. Herken, and A. D. Welch (Eds.), *Handbook of Experimental Pharmacology*, Vol. 50/II. Springer-Verlag, Berlin and Heidelberg. pp. 467-530.

Greaves, M. W. (1969). The effect of disodium cromoglycate and other inhibitors on *in vitro* anaphylactic histamine release from guinea pig basophil leucocytes. *Int. Arch. Allergy appl. Immunol.*, *36*, 497-505.

Greaves, M. W., V. M. Fairley, and S. Yamamoto (1971). Release of histamine from skin during *in vitro* anaphylaxis. Cutaneous anaphylaxis *in vitro*. *Int. Arch. Allergy appl. Immunol.*, *41*, 932-939.

Grosman, N., and B. Diamant (1975). The influence of phosphatidyl serine on the release of histamine from isolated mast cells induced by different agents. *Agents and Actions*, *5*, 296-301.

Harris, J. M., H. Kalmus, and G. B. West (1963). Genetic control of the anaphylactoid reaction in rats. *Genet. Res.*, *4*, 346-355.

Holroyde, M. C., and P. Eyre (1976). Immunological release of histamine from bovine leucocytes: unusual adrenergic modulation. *Immunology*, *31*, 167-170.

Holroyde, M. C. and P. Eyre (1978). Histamine enhances anaphylactic histamine release from bovine lung and leukocytes via histamine H2-receptor. *J. Pharmacol. exp. Thera.*, *204*, 183-188.

Ishizaka, T., K. Ishizaka, R. P. Orange, and K. F. Austen (1971). Pharmacologic inhibition of the antigen-induced release of histamine and slow reacting substance of anaphylaxis (SRS-A) from monkey lung tissues mediated by human IgE. *J. Immunol.*, *106*, 1267-1273.

Kaliner, M. A., S. I. Wasserman, and K. F. Austen (1973). Immunologic release of chemical mediators from human nasal polyps. *New Eng. J. Med.*, *289*, 277-281.

Krell, R. D., and L. W. Chakrin (1976). An *in vitro* model of canine immediate-type hypersensitivity reactions. *Int. Arch. Allergy appl. Immunol.*, *51*, 641-655.

Krell, R. D., and Chakrin, L. W. (1977). The effect of metiamide in *in vitro* and *in vivo* canine models of type I hypersensitivity reactions. *Eur. J. Pharmacol.*, *44*, 35-44.

Leung, K. B. P., K. E. Barrett, and F. L. Pearce (1984). Differential effects of anti-allergic compounds on peritoneal mast cells of the rat, mouse and hamster. *Agents and Actions*, *14*, 461-467.

Leung, K. B. P., and F. L. Pearce (1984). A comparison of histamine secretion

from peritoneal mast cells of the rat and hamster. *Brit. J. Pharmacol., 81,* 693-701.
Lichtenstein, L. M., J. C. Foreman, M. C. Conroy, G. Marone, and H. H. Newball (1979). Differences between histamine release from rat mast cells and human basophils and mast cells. In J. Pepys and A. M. Edwards (Eds.), *The Mast Cell: Its Role in Health and Disease.* Pitman Medical, Tunbridge Wells. pp. 83-96.
Lichtenstein, L. M., and S. Margolis (1968). Histamine release *in vitro*: inhibition by catecholamines and methylxanthines. *Science, 161,* 902-903.
Ludowyke, R. I., G. B. West, J. R. Harris, and T. H. P. Hanahoe (1982). A possible link between the ability of rat isolated peritoneal mast cells to release histamine when challenged with dextran and the proteins in their plasma membranes. *Int. Arch. Allergy appl. Immunol., 68,* 188-191.
Mongar, J. L., and P. Svec (1972). The effect of phospholipids on anaphylactic histamine release. *Brit. J. Pharmacol., 46,* 741-752.
Moodley, I., J. L. Mongar, and J. C. Foreman (1982). Histamine release induced by dextran: the nature of the dextran receptor. *Eur. J. Pharmacol., 83,* 69-81.
Orange, R. P., W. G. Austen, and K. F. Austen (1971). Immunological release of histamine and slow-reacting substance of anaphylaxis from human lung. I. Modulation by agents influencing cellular levels of cyclic 3',5'-adenosine monophosphate. *J. exp. Med., 134,* 136-148s.
Parratt, J. R., and G. B. West (1957). 5-Hydroxytryptamine and the anaphylactoid reaction in the rat. *J. Physiol., 139,* 27-41.
Patterson, R., C. H. Talbot, and M. Brandfonbrener (1971). The use of IgE mediated responses as a pharmacologic test system. The effect of disodium cromoglycate in respiratory and cutaneous reactions and on the electrocardiograms of rhesus monkeys. *Int. Arch. Allergy appl. Immunol., 41,* 592-603.
Peachell, P. T., and F. L. Pearce (1984). Some studies on the release of histamine from mast cells treated with polymyxin. *Agents and Actions, 14,* 379-385.
Pearce, C. A., M. W. Greaves, V. M. Plummer, and S. Yamamoto (1974). Effect of disodium cromoglycate on antigen-evoked histamine release from human skin. *Clin. exp. Immunol., 17,* 437-440.
Pearce, F. L. (1982a). Functional heterogeneity of mast cells from different species and tissues. *Klin. Wochenschr., 60,* 954-957.
Pearce, F. L. (1982b). Calcium and histamine secretion from mast cells. *Prog. med. Chem., 19,* 59-109.
Pearce, F. L. (1983). Mast cell heterogeneity. *Trends pharmacol. Sci., 4,* 165-167.
Pearce, F. L., A. D. Befus, J. Gauldie, and J. Bienenstock (1982). Mucosal mast cells. II. Effects of anti-allergic compounds on histamine secretion by isolated intestinal mast cells. *J. Immunol., 128,* 2481-2486.
Pearce, F. L., U. Blum, G. Poblete-Freundt, and W. Schmutzler (1978). Studies on the release of histamine from isolated guinea pig mast cells stimulated by ionophore A23187 or by the anaphylactic reaction. *Naunyn Schmiedeberg's Arch. Pharmacol., 302,* 165-172.
Perper, R. J., M. Sanda, and L. M. Lichtenstein (1972). The relationship of *in vitro* and *in vivo* allergic histamine release: inhibition in primates by cAMP-active agents. *Int. Arch. Allergy appl. Immunol., 43,* 837-844.
Rising, T. J., and S. Lewis (1982). A species comparison of the histamine H2-receptor on mast cells and basophils. *Agents and Actions, 12,* 263-267.
Rothschild, A. M. (1966). Histamine release by basic compounds. In O. Eichler and A. Farah (Eds.), *Handbook of Experimental Pharmacology,* Vol. 18/I. Springer-Verlag, Berlin und Heidelberg. pp. 386-430.
Schulman, E. S., D. W. MacGlashan, R. P. Schleimer, S. P. Peters, A. Kagey-Sobotka, H. H. Newball, and L. M. Lichtenstein (1983). Purified human basophils and mast cells: current concepts of mediator release. *Eur. J. resp. Disease, 64* (Suppl. 128), 53-61.
Sheard, P., and A. M. J. N. Blair (1970). Disodium cromoglycate: activity in three *in vitro* models of the immediate hypersensitivity reaction in lung. *Int. Arch. Allergy appl. Immunol., 38,* 217-224.
Siraganian, R. P., and K. A. Hazard (1979). Mechanisms of mouse mast cell activation and inactivation for IgE-mediated histamine release. *J. Immunol., 122,* 1719-1725.

Stechschulte, D. J., and K. F. Austen (1973). Control mechanisms of antigen-induced histamine release from rat peritoneal mast cells. *Int. Arch. Allergy appl. Immunol.*, *45*, 110-119.
Stokes, T. C., and J. Morley (1981). Prospects for an oral intal. *Brit. J. Dis. Chest*, *75*, 1-14.
Strobel, S., H. R. P. Miller, and A. Ferguson (1981). Human intestinal mucosal mast cells: evaluation of fixation and staining techniques. *J. clin. Pathol.*, *34*, 851-858.
Tay, C. H., T. S. Yeoh, and M. W. Greaves (1972). Spontaneous and evoked histamine release from guinea pig skin *in vitro* in presence of disodium cromoglycate. *Int. Arch. Allergy appl. Immunol.*, *43*, 390-394.
Tomita, Y., R. Patterson, and I. M. Suszko (1974). Respiratory mast cells and basophiloid cells. II. Effect of pharmacologic agents on 3'5'-adenosine monophosphate content and on antigen-induced histamine release. *Int. Arch. Allergy appl. Immunol.*, *47*, 261-272.
Wells, P. W., and P. Eyre (1972). The pharmacology of passive cutaneous anaphylaxis in the calf. *Can. J. Physiol. Pharmacol.*, *50*, 255-262.
Wescott, S., and M. Kaliner (1981). The effects of histamine and prostaglandin D2 on rat mast cell cyclic AMP and mediator release. *J. Allergy clin. Immunol.*, *68*, 383-391.
Yamamoto, S., M. W. Greaves, and V. M. Fairley (1973). Cyclic AMP-induced inhibition of IgE-mediated hypersensitivity in human skin. *Immunology*, *24*, 77-83.
Zvaifler, N. J., H. Bauer, and J. O. Robinson (1971). IgE immunoglobulin in the rabbit. In K. F. Austen and E. L. Becker (Eds.), *Biochemistry of the Acute Allergic Reactions*. Blackwell, Oxford. pp. 33-44.

ACKNOWLEDGEMENTS

Work from the authors' laboratories was supported by Fisons Pharmaceuticals Limited, The Jules Thorn Trust, The Medical Research Councils of Canada and the United Kingdom, The North Atlantic Treaty Organization, The Science and Engineering Research Council, and The Wellcome Trust.

STUDIES OF THE CALCIUM SIGNAL (QUIN 2 FLUORESCENCE), PHOSPHOLIPID TURNOVER AND HISTAMINE RELEASE IN RAT BASOPHIL LEUKEMIC (2H3) CELLS

M. A. Beaven and E. WoldeMussie

NHLBI, NIH Bethesda, MD 20205, USA

ABSTRACT

Studies with the fluorescent Ca^{2+} indicator, quin 2, in cultured 2H3 cells have established that increases in cytosol Ca^{2+} levels were obligatory for histamine release and have allowed us to define the quantitative relationships between the two events. The increase in cytosol Ca^{2+} levels (from 105 to 1200 nM when cells were maximally stimulated) was a dynamic response in which stimulation with antigen or concanavalin A resulted in at least 10-fold increase of Ca^{2+} influx through La^{3+} inhibitable channels and a corresponding increase in Ca^{2+} efflux across the plasma membrane. Maintenance of response required the continuous presence of cellular ATP, a stimulating ligand and external Ca^{2+} ions. Antigen stimulation also initiated a Ca^{2+}-independent process which led to a progressive inability of cells to generate the Ca signal or to release histamine. In all experiments histamine release was correlated with the magnitude of the Ca signal, except in the presence of Zn^{2+} which appeared to uncouple the Ca signal from histamine release. Substantial breakdown (up to 60%) of phosphatidylinositol and related polyphosphoinositides was associated with generation of the Ca signal. Breakdown was not a consequence of Ca^{2+} influx but appeared to be related to or coincident with generation of the Ca signal.

KEYWORDS

Rat leukemia (2H3) basophils; histamine release; cytosol Ca^{2+}; phosphatidylinositol breakdown; Ca^{2+} signal; polyvalent metal ions; mechanism of degranulation.

INTRODUCTION

Interest in the tissue mast cell and blood basophil lies not only in their involvement in IgE-mediated allergic reactions but also in their utility as a model to study stimulus coupled secretory mechanisms. Their attractiveness is the ease with which these cells can be obtained in reasonable number and purity, the availability of reliable fluorometric and radioenzymatic assays for the major secretory product, histamine, and the availabilty of well defined reactants which include rat and mouse monoclonal IgE antibodies as well as [^{125}I]-labeled and cross linked oligomeric preparations of these antibodies. The existence of a rat leukemic basophil (RBL) cell line (Eccleston and co-workers, 1973) from which histamine releasing and nonreleasing clones have been developed (Barsumian and co-workers, 1981; Siraganian and co-workers, 1982) has facilitated the study of early stimulatory events at the molecular level. A plasma membrane receptor for IgE has been isolated from RBL cells and the general features of the subunit structures of this receptor have now been defined (Metzger and co-workers, 1983; Perez-Montfort and Metzger, 1982).

These cell lines possess 100,000 to 500,000 IgE-receptors per cell as do normal mast cells. IgE binds to the receptors through its F_c region to leave free the antigen recognition site. The receptors have the capacity to migrate into patches and caps (Mendoza and Metzger, 1976) and cell stimulation is initiated by cross-linking bound IgE with antigen or, experimentally, with concanavalin-A or antibody to IgE. Studies with antibodies to IgE (or IgE receptors) and oligomeric preparations of IgE have allowed the process to be defined mathematically. Aggregation of several hundred receptors appears to be sufficient to generate a signal to promote appreciable secretion and cross linking of 2 or a small cluster of receptors are believed to generate a unit signal (see for example Fewtrell and Metzger, 1980; Marone and co-workers, 1981b).

The subsequent cascade of biochemical events that lead to release of histamine-containing granules, arachidonic acid and other inflammatory factors from mast cells (Beaven, 1978; Lewis and Austen, 1981; Metcalfe and associates, 1981) is still unclear. Associated biochemical changes include mobilization of Ca^{2+} ions, enhanced phospholipid metabolism, cyclic AMP production and activation of protein kinases (see Crews and co-workers, 1981; Metcalfe and associates, 1981; Metzger and Ishizaka, 1982). The critical event appears to be either influx of Ca^{2+} from the extracellular space or recruitment of Ca^{2+} from the intracellular pool (Foreman and associates, 1976; Pearce, 1982). External calcium ions are required for degranulation to occur in response to IgE cross-linking agents and large increases in $^{45}Ca^{2+}$ influx are observed during stimulation. Agents such as compound 48/80 or the ionophore A23187, which bypass the IgE-receptor aggregation step, can induce degranulation by release of Ca^{2+} from intracellular pools (Pearce, 1982). Depletion of membrane bound Ca^{2+} stores by prolonged exposure of cells to calcium chelators, for example, renders the cells unresponsive to compound 48/80 but re-exposure of cells to free Ca^{2+} ions leads to rapid repletion of Ca^{2+} stores and restoration of responsiveness to compound 48/80 (WoldeMussie and Moran, 1984). It is assumed that translocation of Ca^{2+} ions results in an increase in free cytosol Ca^{2+} levels ($[Ca]_i$) as a Ca signal to trigger degranulation.

Despite progress thus far, critical pieces of information are lacking. The essential structural features of the IgE receptor as currently defined have yet to provide clues as to how the receptor works (Metzger and co-workers, 1983); whether for example aggregation simply provides additional channels for Ca^{2+} ion influx or trigger biochemical changes that are required for mobilization of Ca^{2+} ions. Until the dynamic aspects of the Ca signal are defined, the biochemical mechanisms (if any) by which it is generated or maintained are still a matter of speculation. With this is mind we thought that it might be instructive to utilize the experience gained in studies with the RBL cell lines at NIH and the calcium fluorescent probe, quin 2 (Tsien, 1980; Tsien and co-workers, 1982a), at Cambridge to observe and quantitate the Ca signal directly. This probe has been used successfully in various cell systems to measure changes in $[Ca]_i$.

To further define the processes involved we also decided to compare the Ca signal, as measured by quin 2 fluorescence, with breakdown of phosphatidylinositol (PI) and related phosphoinositides. Hydrolysis of these membrane phospholipids (to diacylglycerol and inositol phosphates) is thought to be involved in the mobilization of Ca^{2+} ions and is an early event during stimulation of a wide variety of calcium-dependent secretory systems (reviewed by Berridge, 1984; Michell and Kirk, 1981) which include the mast cell (see Beaven and co-workers, 1984b). For reasons discussed below we selected the RBL-2H3 cell line (Barsumian and co-workers, 1981; Siraganian and co-workers, 1982) for our initial studies.

DISCUSSION OF EXPERIMENTAL PROCEDURES

2H3 cells can be grown in either spinner culture (a useful asset in studies with quin 2) or monolayer cultures in cluster plates (useful for studies of mediator release or phospholipid metabolism). They can be primed with a mouse ovalbumin-specific monoclonal IgE or left unprimed for control experiments, an option that is not available in studies with normal mast cells. Additional advantages which became apparent during the course of the study were that, unlike normal rat mast cells, they could be loaded with quin 2 without loss of secretory response and their PI pool could be labelled by incubation overnight with myo [2-^{3}H]-inositol.

2H3 cell cultures were supplied by Reuben Siraganian (National Institute of Dental Research, NIH) and, with his advice, optimal conditions were established for induction of histamine release in both suspension and monolayer cultures. An ovalbumin-specific mouse monoclonal IgE obtained commercially (MAS 038c Sera Laboratory, Crawley, U.K.) was used to sensitize 2H3 cells to ovalbumin. As the antibody was monospecific prior aggregation of ovalbumin (with glutaraldehyde) was required for cross linking of IgE molecules.

In Cambridge only minor modifications of previously established protocols were required. With the experience gained in studies with quin 2 in thymocytes (Hesketh and co-workers, 1983a, 1983b) and by adaptation of assay systems for PI breakdown developed by Berridge and co-workers (1983), the experimental procedures for studies of quin 2 fluorescence and PI breakdown in 2H3 cells were established with few hitches. The radioenzymatic assay of histamine added further flexibility to our investigations as small samples (50 µl) could be withdrawn at frequent intervals from quin 2-loaded cell suspensions in cuvettes and assayed for histamine in cells and medium.

Since these procedures have been published recently (Beaven and co-workers, 1984a, 1984b), only a few points will be emphasized here. Conditions for uptake and hydrolysis of quin 2 acetoxymethyl ester (quin 2 AMe) in cells to form free quin 2 were critical. Inhibition of histamine release or incomplete loading of the cells occurred when the concentrations of quin 2 AMe were respectively > 20 µM or < 5 µM. In the presence of 10^6 cells/ml, 0.1% bovine serum albumin (essential for cell stability) and 10 µM quin 2 AMe complete hydrolysis as indicated by a shift in emission maximum from 435 to 492 nm, was achieved by 60 min. Even though intracellular concentrations of quin 2 reached 7 mM, histamine release in response to a variety of stimulants was not impaired. By contrast in thymocytes (Hesketh and co-workers, 1983a), mast cells (Tsien 1981 and unpublished data) and other cells (Tsien and co-workers, 1982b) intracellular concentrations of quin 2 of 1 to 2 mM may perturb ATP homeostasis and cell function. Thus the 2H3 cells are surprisingly robust, which may be due in part to high ATP levels in these cells (Beaven and co-workers, 1984a). Leakage of quin 2 (and histamine) was, however, a problem with 2H3 cells and useful data could be obtained only within 60 min of loading the cells with quin 2.

In studies of PI breakdown, overnight incubation of 2H3 cells with labelled inositol resulted in the incorporation of 1 to 1.5% of the label into intracellular phospholipids and 0.3% into the inositol pool. In a variety of cell systems the inositol label is incorporated into phosphatidylinositol and, to a lesser extent, phosphatidylinositol (4)-monophosphate and (4,5)-bisphosphate. Breakdown of the phosphoinositides following cell stimulation is catalyzed by a phosphatidylinositol specific phospholipase C to produce diacylglycerol and inositol (1,4,5)-trisphosphate, (1,4)-bisphosphate and (1)-monophosphate. Sequential cleavage of the phosphate groups by phosphatase enzyme(s) yields inositol which is recycled back into the PI pool (Berridge, 1984). In the presence of 5 mM Li^+, which inhibits the conversion of inositol (1)-monophosphate to inositol, the various sugar phosphates accumulate in the cell and can be quantified by adsorption onto Dowex-formate and sequential elution with various buffers (Berridge and co-workers, 1983). Since inositol trisphosphate but not inositol mono- or bisphosphates release Ca^{2+} from endoplasmic reticulum from permeabilized cell systems, it has been proposed that inositol trisphosphate acts as the second messenger to release internal Ca^{2+} (see Berridge, 1984, for citations).

RESULTS

Time Course and Characteristics of Histamine Release, Changes in $[Ca]_i$ and PI Breakdown in 2H3 Cells

As reported recently (Beaven and co-workers, 1984a, 1984b), we have shown that the addition of antigen (cross-linked ovalbumin) to quin 2-loaded 2H3 cell suspensions produced an increase in calcium-dependent fluorescence. The calculated $[Ca]_i$ increased from 0.11 to over 1.0 µM and reached a maximum by 2.75 min. Thereafter $[Ca]_i$ slowly declined over the course of 40 min to concentrations observed before addition of stimulants. Histamine release was apparent within 30-60 sec, but for technical reasons (i.e. time required for removal and centrifuging samples) it was uncertain if the increase in $[Ca]_i$ preceded histamine release. However, curve fitting of all data by computer analysis indicated a correlation between increase in $[Ca]_i$ and rates of histamine release after $[Ca]_i$ had reached a maximum (i.e. after 2.75 min). PI breakdown was observed within 10-40 sec of addition of antigen and at all times thereafter rates of inositol phosphate release were correlated with increase in $[Ca]_i$. Although in some experiments the appearance of inositol phosphates was coincident with the first detectable increase in $[Ca]_i$ there was no indication that PI breakdown preceded $[Ca]_i$ increase. Antigen stimulation also initiated a Ca^{2+}-independent process which led to the progressive inability of cells to generate a Ca signal or to release histamine.

A survey of the effects of various multivalent metal ions and drugs indicated that a number of agents that inhibit histamine release in normal mast cells did not do so in 2H3 cells. Marked inhibition of responses was observed, however, with Zn^{2+} and La^{3+} ions and metabolic inhibitors (Table 1). The responses in 2H3 cells were totally dependent on the presence of external Ca^{2+} ions, but did not require phosphatidyl serine, and were not evoked by compound 48/80 in concentrations of 1 to 100 µg/ml. In these respects, the responses in 2H3 cells were different from those in mast cells (Pearce, 1982) and it seems possible that 2H3 cells do not or cannot mobilize internal Ca^{2+} pools.

These early experiments led to further experimental strategies. All three responses($[Ca_i]$ increase, histamine release and PI breakdown) were highly correlated with concentration of antigen and of external calcium ($[Ca]_o$). All three responses could be blocked by low $[Ca]_o$ (i.e. < 50 µM) but could be initiated by increasing $[Ca]_o$ to 1 mM. In addition to the requirement for external Ca^{2+} ions, all responses were dependent on intracellular ATP. When ATP levels had been reduced to less than 200 µM with sodium azide and 2-deoxyglucose, the cells were completely refractory to antigen stimulation (Table 1). After the responses had been initiated by antigen, the addition of excess EGTA (1.1 mM), La^{3+} (10 µM) or metabolic inhibitors caused a rapid decline in $[Ca]_i$ to prestimulated levels within 30 sec and stopped histamine release. In nonstimulated cells the same reagents produced little or no perturbations in $[Ca]_i$. In the case of concanavalin A stimulated cells, the Ca signal was rapidly reversed by displacement of ligand with α methylmannoside (Beaven and co-workers, 1984a).

As indicated by the above, the signal was dependent on continued presence of ligand, $[Ca]_o$ and cellular ATP and operated through the appearance of La^{3+} sensitive channels, which were absent in nonstimulated cells. Further the Ca signal was not due to a single influx of Ca^{2+} ions but was maintained by a dynamic balance between enhanced Ca^{2+} influx and efflux. Interference in Ca^{2+} influx (with La^{3+} or removal of external Ca^{2+}) led to rapid decline in $[Ca]_i$,

TABLE 1 Effect of Various Agents on Increase in Cytosol Cytosol Ca^{2+} PI Breakdown and Release of Histamine and Labelled Arachidonic Acid

Agent	Conc. (μM)	η	$\Delta[Ca_i^{2+}]$	% Inhibition (Stimulation) Inositol Phosphates	Histamine	Arachidonate
Mn^{2+}	100	2	↑	(18)	8	—
Sr^{2+}	100	2	↑	(18)	9	—
Co^{2+}	100	2	↑	0	36	—
	500	2	↑	15	48	—
Zn^{2+}	10	3	↑	2 ± 1	5 ± 2	(12)
	50	3	↑	12 ± 2	70 ± 9	94 ± 2
	100	3	↑	14 ± 4	99 ± 0.5	97 ± 1
La^{3+}	10	4	70–90	<15	50–90	—
	100	4	>90	>90	>95	91 ± 2
8Br.cAMP	1000	4	<15	19 ± 7⁻	(35 ± 9)	—
Cromolyn Na	1000	2	<10	(3)	(8)	—
Isoproterenol + RO7-2956	100 / 10	6	28 ± 8	—	29 ± 13	—
Methoxyverapamil	50	2	51	29	30	—
Na azide + 2 Dog	1000 / 5000	3	>95	84 ± 1	>98	—

Agents were added 5-10 min before addition of antigen to quin 2 loaded cells previously labeled with [^{3}H]inositol or [^{14}C]-arachidonic acid. An arrow indicates where increases in $[Ca]_i$ were still evident but could not be quantitated because of quenching of quin 2 fluorescence. Values indicate per cent inhibition or, in parenthesis, stimulation of response and are the mean or mean ± SEM for the number (n) of experiments indicated. Where effects were variable, the range of values is given.

presumably through the action of an ATP-dependent Ca^{2+} efflux pump which continued to operate at low ATP levels (i.e. > 200 μM).

Uncoupling of Histamine Release from PI Breakdown and the Ca Signal.

It was also apparent from the data in Table 1 that release of histamine and arachidonate, but not the Ca response and PI breakdown, were blocked by Zn^{2+} at concentrations of 50 to 100 μM. The ability to uncouple the PI response from histamine and arachidonate release is also indicated from the data in figure 1. The effects of Zn^{2+} are of interest because this ion is present in plasma (7 μM in man) and may have potential therapeutic application. Studies in human basophils suggest that Zn^{2+} is a competitive antagonist of Ca^{2+}-dependent IgE mediated release and is a noncompetitive inhibitor (against

Ca^{2+}) of A23187-induced histamine release (Marone and co-workers, 1981a). We too find that antigen- and A23187-induced histamine release in 2H3 cells is inhibited by Zn^{2+} in a dose-dependent manner at concentrations of 10 to 100 μM (K. Maeyama, unpublished data). The site of action of Zn^{2+} is uncertain (Marone and coworkers, 1981) but our bias is that it does uncouple the Ca signal from subsequent histamine release (Beaven and coworkers, 1984a). Other potential modes of action include competition for Ca^{2+} at Ca^{2+} channels, displacement of Ca^{2+} from the calcium binding site of the ionophore or binding to microtubules.

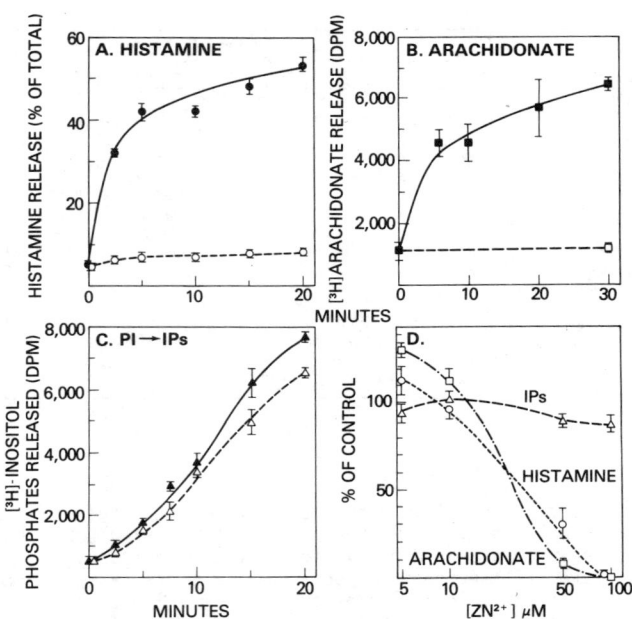

Fig. 1. Ability of Zn^{2+} to block mediator release but not PI breakdown. Monolayer cultures of 2H3 cells were incubated with radiolabelled inositol (4 μCi/ml, 16 hr) or arachidonic acid (0.4 μCi/ml, 3 hr) and primed with IgE. After washing the cultures, Zn^{2+} (100 μM or as indicated in D) was added to medium 10 min before addition of ovalbumin (2.5 μg/ml). In panels A, B and C, release of histamine, labelled inositol phosphates and arachidonate in the presence (open symbols) or absence (filled symbols) of Zn^{2+} was determined at the indicated times. In panel D, the values were obtained at 20 min. Values are the mean ± SEM. Those in panels A and C are taken from a previous publication (Beaven and co-workers, 1984b).

Uncoupling of the Ca signal was also observed when cells were arrested in mitosis by the microtubule-disrupting drug Nocodazole (0.04 µg/ml). Treated cells (92% in mitosis) showed the normal increase in $[Ca]_i$ but did not release histamine. Removal of drug by washing resulted in restoration of histamine-release response within 2 hr. The drug itself had no effect on histamine release in interphase cells. The mechanism by which degranulation was selectively suppressed remains to be determined, but may be related to processes whereby intracellular membrane fusion events are selectively switched-off during cell mitosis (Hesketh and co-workers, 1984).

Detailed Analysis of the PI Breakdown in 2H3 Cells

PI breakdown was always correlated with changes in $[Ca]_i$ when cells were stimulated with IgE cross linking ligands but negligible breakdown was observed upon stimulation with the ionophore A23187 or addition of Ca^{2+} to Ca^{2+} depleted cells. Thus PI breakdown was not a consequence of Ca^{2+} transport into the cell nor was it required for histamine release. Also as discussed above PI breakdown was not a Ca^{2+}-independent event as has been observed in some other cell systems.

Inositol (1,4)-bisphosphate was the predominant breakdown product formed shortly after antigen addition. By 5-10 min inositol (1)-monophosphate was the predominant metabolite. At all times inositol (1,4,5)-trisphosphate remained a minor (< 10% of total inositol phosphates released) product of PI breakdown. The sequence of hydrolysis of the various phosphoinositides and importance of the inositol trisphosphate in the generation of the Ca signal in 2H3 cells is, therefore, unclear at this time (Beaven and co-workers, 1984b).

Effects of Ca^{2+} Channel Blockers and Agents Known to Interact with Intracellular Signal Cascade Mechanisms

Other agents currently under study include the Ca^{2+} channel blockers, calmodulin inhibitors and agents activating protein kinase C. Dramatic and reproducible effects have been observed with some of these agents at low concentrations and further analysis of the signal cascade system in 2H3 cells should be possible in the near future. Studies with Ca^{2+} channel blockers are now well advanced. It appears that these drugs do not have profound effects at therapeutic concentrations and that 'calcium gating' mechanisms in 2H3 cells are probably different to the K^+-activated Ca^{2+} channels in smooth muscle cells. Nifedipine, nitrendipine and verapamil in concentrations up to 100 µM have no effect on the Ca signal, PI breakdown or histamine release in antigen stimulated 2H3 cells. Methoxyverapamil had modest inhibitory actions at 50 and 100 µM and possibly stimulatory actions at lower concentrations. Felodipine had both stimulatory and inhibitory actions but only at concentrations in excess of expected therapeutic levels (Fig. 2).

Studies with Single Cells

A limitation of studies with cell suspensions is that data indicate the average response of a large cell population and not the extent or time course of response within individual cells. Subpopulations of cells may respond differently to other subpopulations. We also do not know whether the response of a single mast cell is 'graded' or an 'all or none'. Refinements in the radioenzymatic assay have reached the point, however, where it is now feasible to measure histamine release in one or two mast cells (Beaven and WoldeMussie, 1984).

Studies with single 2H3 cells have shown that changes in $[Ca]_i$ can be measured by use of quin 2. The fluorescence was uniformly distributed throughout the cytoplasm with no apparent localization in membranes or cell organelles. The increase in fluorescence in single cells in response to antigen, although variable was similar in duration to that observed in cell suspensions (Rogers and co-workers, 1983).

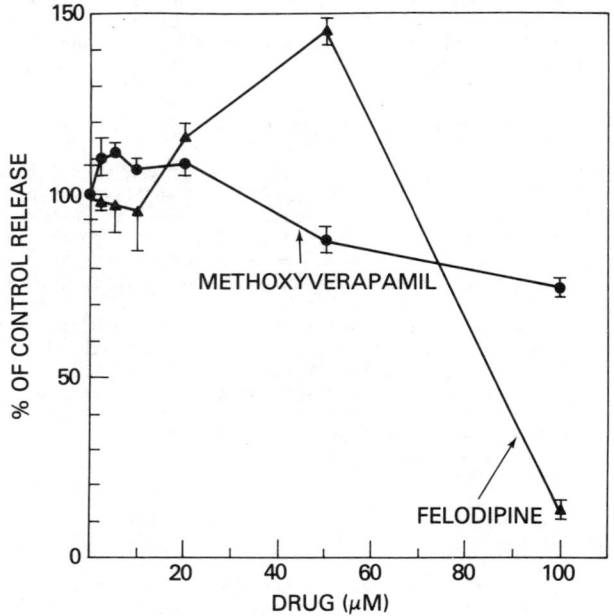

Fig. 2. Effect of two Ca^{2+} channel blockers on PI breakdown in antigen stimulated 2H3 cells. PI breakdown in [^{3}H]inositol labelled 2H3 cells was determined as described previously (Beaven and co-workers, 1984b). Drugs were added to cultures 10 min before addition of antigen (aggregated ovalbumin, 10 µg/ml). In the absence of drugs, 21 ± 2% of the label in the PI pool was released as inositol phosphates over a 30 min period following antigen addition. Values are mean ± SEM of values from 4 cultures. Histamine release (49 ± 1% release in the absence of drugs) was inhibited (23-76%) in the presence of high drug concentrations (50 and 100 µM). Unlike PI breakdown, stimulation of histamine release was not observed (unpublished data).

CONCLUDING COMMENTS

From our studies with 2H3 cells it is not possible to determine whether PI breakdown is obligatory for the Ca signal or is stimulated through receptor aggregation independently of Ca^{2+} influx. These alternatives are presented schematically in Figure 3 (next page). Nevertheless, our studies have established that: 1) IgE receptor aggregation increases membrane permeability to Ca^{2+} ions by an ATP-dependent process; 2) increases in cytosol $[Ca]_i$ are directly correlated with histamine release, but the two events can be uncoupled with Zn^{2+} or mitotic arrest; 3) the calcium signal is a dynamic response maintained by at least a 10-fold enhancement in rates of Ca^{2+} influx which is balanced by enhanced Ca^{2+} efflux; 4) substantial PI breakdown occurs in parallel with changes in Ca^{2+} flux, but further studies are needed to determine whether the two are causal or independent events.

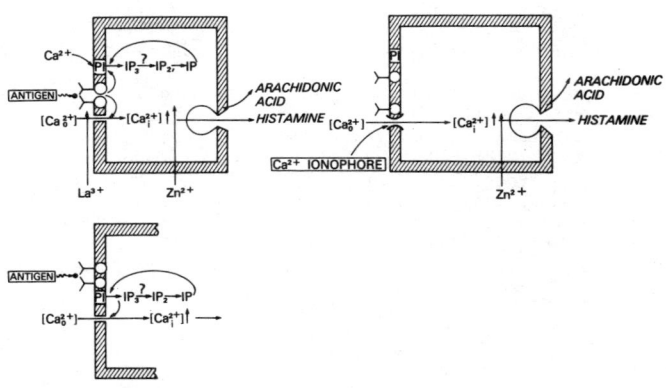

Fig. 3. Proposed sequence of events in antigen and A23187-stimulated 2H3 cells and possible points of intervention for suppression of secretion. The action of Zn^{2+} is uncertain but is believed to uncouple the Ca signal from secretory response. Also, the exact sequence of PI breakdown is unknown, as discussed in text.

REFERENCES

Barsumian, E. L., C. Isersky, M. G. Petrino and R. P. Siraganian (1981). Eur. J. Immunol., 11, 317-323.
Beaven, M. A. (1978). Monogr. Allergy, 13, 1-113.
Beaven, M. A., J. Rogers, J. P. Moore, T. R. Hesketh, G. A. Smith and J. C. Metcalfe (1984a). J. Biol. Chem., 259, 7129-7136.
Beaven, M. A., J. P. Moore, G. A., Smith, T. R. Hesketh and J. C. Metcalfe (1984b). J. Biol. Chem., 259, 7137-7142.
Beaven, M. A. and E. WoldeMussie (1984). New England and Regional Allergy Proceedings, in press.
Berridge, M. J. (1984). Biochem. J., 220, 345-360.
Berridge, M. J., R. M. C. Dawson, C. P. Downes, J. P. Heslop and R. F. Irvine (1983). Biochem. J., 212, 473-482.
Crews, R. T., Y. Morita, A. McGivney, F. Hirata, R. P. Siraganian and J. Axelrod (1981). Arch. Biochem. Biophys., 212, 561-571.
Eccleston, E., B. J. Leonard, J. S. Lowe and H. J. Welford (1973). Nature (New Biol.), 244, 73-76.
Fewtrell, C. and H. Metzger (1980). J. Immunol, 125, 701-710.
Foreman, J. C., M. B. Hallett and J. L. Mongar (1977). J. Physiol., 271, 193-214.
Hesketh, T. R., M. A. Beaven, J. Rogers, B. Burke and G. B. Warren (1984). J. Cell Biol., 98, 2250-2254.

Hesketh, T. R., G. A. Smith, J. P. Moore, M. V. Taylor and J. C. Metcalfe (1983a). J. Biol. Chem., 258, 4876-4882.
Hesketh, T. R., T. Pozzan, G. A. Smith and J. C. Metcalfe (1983b). Biochem. J., 212, 685-690.
Lewis, R. A. and K. F. Austen (1981). Nature (Lond), 293, 103-108.
Marone, G., S. R. Findlay and L . M. Lichtenstein (1981a). J. Pharm. Exptl. Therap., 217, 292-298.
Marone, G., A. Kagey-Sobotka and L. M. Lichtenstein (1981b). Int. Archs. Allergy Appl. Immun., 65, 339-348.
Mendoza, G. and H. Metzger (1976). Nature (Lond.), 264, 548-550.
Metcalfe, D. D., M. Kaliner and M. A. Donlon (1981). CRC Crit. Rev. Immunol., 3, 23-74.
Metzger, H., J-P. Kinet, R. Perez-Montfort, B. Rivnay and S. A. Wank (1983). Progs. Immunol., 5, 493-501.
Metzger, H. and T. Ishizaka (1982). Fed. Proc., 41, 7-34.
Michell, R. H. and C. J. Kirk (1981). Trends Pharmacol. Sci., 2, 86-89.
Pearce, F. L. (1982). Progr. Med. Chem., 19, 59-109.
Perez-Montfort, R. and H. Metzger (1982). Mol. Immunol., 19, 1113-1125.
Rogers, J., T. R. Hesketh, G. A. Smith, M. A. Beaven, J. C. Metcalfe, P. Johnson and P. B. Garland (1983). FEBS Letts., 161, 21-27.
Siraganian, R. P., A. McGivney, E. L. Barsumian, F. T. Crews, F. Hirata and J. Axelrod (1982). Fed. Proc., 41, 30-34.
Tsien, R. Y. (1980). Biochemistry, 19, 2396-2404.
Tsien, R. Y. (1981). Nature (Lond.), 290, 527-528.
Tsien, R. Y., T. Pozzan and T. J. Rink (1982a). Nature (Lond.), 295, 68-71.
Tsien, R. Y., T. Pozzan and T. J. Rink (1982b). J. Cell. Biol., 94, 325-334.
WoldeMussie, E. and N. C. Moran (1984). Agents and Actions, 15, in press.

AUTHOR INDEX

H Ali	University College London, UK	411
J-M Arrang	Centre Paul Broca de l'INSERM, Paris, France	143
J F Bach	Hopital Necker, Paris, France	353
K E Barrett	University College London, UK	411
G Baumann	Technical University of Munich, W. Germany	325
M A Beaven	National Heart, Lung and Blood Inst., Bethesda, USA	423
D J Beer	Boston University School of Medicine, Boston, USA	371
A D Befus	McMaster University, Hamilton, Canada	411
W Beil	Medizinische Hochschule Hannover, W. Germany	275
J S Berman	Boston University School of Medicine, Boston, USA	371
J Bienenstock	McMaster University, Hamilton, Canada	411
R E Birch	Washington University School of Medicine, St. Louis, USA	389
H Blomer	Technical University of Munich, W. Germany	325
R T Borchardt	University of Kansas, Lawrence, USA	163
J Brostoff	Middlesex Hospital Medical School, London, UK	411
U Busch	Technical University of Munich, W. Germany	325
G Buttin	Institute Pasteur, Paris, France	103
S Buyuktimkin	Johannes Gutenberg-Universitat, Mainz, W. Germany	39
R Cacabelos	Osaka University School of Medicine, Japan	225
H Carswell	University of Cambridge, UK	27
D M Center	Boston University School of Medicine, Boston, USA	371
L Chatenoud	Hopital Necker, Paris, France	353
W W Cruikshank	Boston University School of Medicine, Boston, USA	371
D L Cybulsky	University of Toronto, Ontario, Canada	69
P R Daum	University of Cambridge, UK	27
G J Durant	Smith Kline & French Research Ltd., Welwyn, UK	3
M Dy	Hopital Necker, Paris, France	353
S Elz	Johannes Gutenberg-Universitat, Mainz, W. Germany	39
S Emami	Hopital Siant-Antoine, Paris, France	265
M Ennis	University College London, UK	411
L Enerback	University of Goteborg, Sweden	289
J S Fedan	N.I.O.S.H., Morgantown, USA	13
K C Flint	Middlesex Hospital Medical School, London, UK	411

Author Index

C R Ganellin	Smith Kline & French Research Ltd., Welwyn, UK	3,47
M Garbarg	Centre Paul Broca de l'INSER, Paris, France	19,143
G Gerhard	Johannes Gutenberg-Universitat, Mainz, W. Germany	39
C Gespach	Hopital Saint-Antoine, Paris, France	265
S D Glick	Albany Medical College, Albany, USA	131
R C Goldschmidt	Mount Sinai Medical School, New York, USA	131
L M Graver	Cornell University Medical College, New York, USA	305
J P Green	Mount Sinai School of Medicine, New York, USA	185
R Griffiths	Smith Kline & French Research Ltd., Welwyn, UK	3
R W Gristwood	Smith Kline & French Research Ltd., Welwyn, UK	309
P M Gross	State University of New York, Stony Brook, USA	341
S S Gross	Cornell University Medical College, New York, USA	317
H L Haas	Neurochirurgische Universitatsklinik, Zurich, Switzerland	215
C A Harvey	Smith Kline & French Research Ltd., Welwyn, UK	3
B I Hirschowitz	University of Alabama in Birmingham, Birmingham, USA	251
G K Hogaboom	Smith Kline & French Laboratories, Philadelphia, USA	13
D L Horstemeyer	West Virginia University Medical Center, Morgantown, USA	13
L B Hough	Albany Medical College, Albany, USA	131
R Huchet	INSERM, Villejuif, France	365
K S Ice	West Virginia University Medical Center, Morgantown, USA	13
T Ishizaka	Johns Hopkins University School of Medicine, Baltimore, USA	401
N Itoi	Osaka University School of Medicine, Japan	225
A R Jacques	Johns Hopkins University School of Medicine, Baltimore, USA	379
C L Johnson	University of Cincinnati College of Medicine, Cincinnati, USA	79
N McI Johnson	Middlesex Hospital Medical School, London, UK	411
A Kagey-Sobotka	Johns Hopkins University School of Medicine, Baltimore, USA	379
M Kandel	University of Toronto, Ontario, Canada	69
S I Kandel	University of Toronto, Ontario, Canada	69
J K Khandelwal	Mount Sinai School of Medicine, New York, USA	185
S Kiyono	Institute for Developmental Research, Aichi, Japan	225
M Korner	Centre Paul Broca de l'INSERM, Paris, France	19
P Legrain	Institute Pasteur, Paris, France	103
K B P Leung	University College London, UK	411
R Levi	Cornell University Medical College, New York, USA	305,317
K Maeyama	Osaka University School of Medicine, Japan	225
P F Mannaioni	Florence University School of Medicine, Italy	301
B Matuszewska	University of Kansas, Lawrence, USA	163
D Mercader	Technical University of Munich, W. Germany	325
A H Mulder	Free University Medical Faculty, Amsterdam, The Netherlands	119,155
K Nagai	Osaka University, Suita, Japan	225
H Nakagawa	Osaka University, Suita, Japan	225
K Ningel	Technical University of Munich, W. Germany	325
M Nishibori	Okayama University Medical School, Japan	173
D B Norris	Hoechst Pharmaceutical Research Labs., Milton Keynes, UK	61
O Nylander	Biomedical Center, Uppsala, Sweden	281
K J Obrink	Biomedical Center, Uppsala, Sweden	281
J P O'Donnell	West Virginia University Medical Center, Morgantown, USA	13
R Oishi	Okayama University Medical School, Japan	173
D A A Owen	Smith Kline & French Research Ltd., Welwyn, UK	3,309
I Pachot	Centre Paul Broca de l'INSERM, Paris, France	103
J Padawer	Albert Einstein School of Medicine, New York, USA	131

Author Index

P T Peachell	University College London, UK	411
F L Pearce	University College London, UK	411
B Permanetter	Technical University of Munich, W. Germany	325
A Philippu	University of Innsbruck, Austria	335
M Plaut	Johns Hopkins University School of Medicine, Baltimore, USA	379
H Pollard	Centre Paul Broca de l'INSERM, Paris, France	103
S H Polmar	Washington University School of Medicine, St. Louis, USA	389
E Richelson	Mayo Clinic and Foundation, Rochester, USA	237
T J Rising	Hoechst Pharmaceutical Research Labs., Milton Keynes, UK	61
D A Robertson	Cornell University Medical College, New York, USA	305
R E Rocklin	Tufts University Medical School, Boston, USA	357
P Romanec	Smith Kline & French Research Ltd., Welwyn, UK	309
G S Sach	Smith Kline & French Research Ltd., Welwyn, UK	3
K Saeki	Okayama University Medical School, Japan	173
K A Sampford	Smith Kline & French Research Ltd., Welwyn, UK	309
D G Sawutz	University of Cincinnati College of Medicine, Cincinnati, USA	79
W Schunack	Free University of Berlin, W. Germany	39
J-C Schwartz	Centre Paul Broca de l'INSERM, Paris, France	19,103,143
S Schwarz	Johannes Gutenberg-Universitat, Mainz, W. Germany	39
G Sedvall	Karolinska Institutet, Stockholm, Sweden	197
M Seo	Institute for Developmental Research, Aichi, Japan	225
K-Fr Sewing	Medizinische Hochschule Hannover, W. Germany	275
S Shiosaka	Osaka University School of Medicine, Japan	91
R P J M Smits	Free University Medical Faculty, Amsterdam, The Netherlands	155
A H Soll	Wadsworth VA Hospital Center, Los Angeles, USA	253
G H Steinberg	University of Toronto, Ontario, Canada	69
H W M Steinbusch	Free University Medical Faculty, Amsterdam, The Netherlands	119,155
C-G Swahn	Karolinska Institutet, Stockholm, Sweden	197
Y Taguchi	Osaka University School of Medicine, Japan	91
N Takeda	Osaka University School of Medicine, Japan	91
M Tohyama	Osaka University School of Medicine, Japan	91
H Wada	Osaka University School of Medicine, Japan	91,225
T Watanabe	Osaka University School of Medicine, Japan	91,225
D Weinreich	University of Maryland School of Medicine, Baltimore, USA	205
J W Wells	University of Toronto, Ontario, Canada	69
A Wirtzfeld	Technical University of Munich, W. Germany	325
E WoldeMussie	National Heart, Lung and Blood Inst., Bethesda, USA	423
A A Wolff	Cornell University Medical College, New York, USA	305
A Yamatodani	Osaka University School of Medicine, Japan	225
E Yeramian	Centre Paul Broca de l'INSERM, Paris, France	19
J M Young	University of Cambridge, UK	27

SUBJECT INDEX

Acetylcholine 253-64, 283
Acid secretory function in canine fundic mucosa 253-64
Acrivastine 7
ACTH 232
S-Adenosylhomocysteine 163-72
S-Adenosylmethionine 163-72
Adenylate cyclase 326, 331, 343, 402-4
Adrenalectomy 232
β-Adrenergic stimulation mechanism 325, 330
Afterhyperpolarization (AHP) 219
AH 19065 50
AH 22216 53, 268
AH 23844 53
Amino acid analysis of guinea pig brain and rat kidney HMT 165
Amino acid composition of rat kidney and guinea pig brain HMT 170
2-(2-Aminoethyl)thiazole 23, 74, 207, 267, 335-9
Aminopyrine accumulation 253-64
Amino-triazolyl-pyridines 56, 57
Amitriptyline 63, 243, 245
Amoxapine 243, 245
Anti-allergic drugs 411-21
Anti-anaphylactic activity 5
Anticholinergic agents 254, 256
Antidepressants 61, 160, 243, 245
Aplysia californica 205-14
Arachidonic acid metabolism 239, 427
Arachidonic acid release 240, 395, 402
ARL-115 BS 325-33
Arylazide histamine (AAH) 13-17
  effect on histamine concentration-response relationships 14-16
  interactions with histamine receptors 16-17
Astemizole 7

Atopic disease 357-64
Atropine 256
Azatadine 5
Azelastine 5, 6
4(5)-[2-(4-Azido-2-nitroanilino)ethyl] imidazole 13-17

Basophils 295
Basophil, rat leukemic 2H3 423-32
Betahistine 22
Biogenic amines 293
BL 5641 A 49
BL 6341 A 51
Blood-brain barrier 346
Blood histamine 295
Blood pressure, regulation of 335-9
BMY 25260 53
BMY 25271 50
BMY 25368 53
Bradykinin 5
Brain (*see also* Central nervous system)
  histamine levels in brain regions 173-84, 185-96
  monoaminergic neurons in 233
  physiological functions of histamine in 225-35
Brain histamine in regulation of blood pressure 335-9
Brain slices *in vitro* 143-54, 216-17
Bupropion 243
Burimamide 62, 66, 75, 146, 147, 382
d-Butaclamol 242, 244
Butriptyline 243

Ca^{2+} signal 215-24, 423-32
Calcium, effect on ^{3}H-histamine release 150, 155-62, 403

Calcium dependence of response to
  histamine 32-33
Calcium influx 401-10
Calcium paradox 310, 311, 314
Carbachol 33, 257, 258, 283
Carbacyclin 284, 285
Carbamylcholine 269
Cardiac arrhythmias 307
Cardiac contractility 325
Cardiac damage 309-15
Cardiac function 309-16, 317-24
Cardiac histamine 301-8, 309, 317-24
Cardiac histamine release by
  sympathetic nerve stimulation 321-3
Cardiac sympathetic responses 317-24
Cardiovascular dysfunctions 306
Catecholamines 326, 331, 335-9, 416
Central nervous system 119-30
  determination of histamine and tele-
    methylhistamine in 173-84, 185-96
  histamine actions in 215-24
  histamine synthesis and release
    143-53
  histamine turnover see Histamine
    turnover
  neuronal uptake and release of
    histamine in 155-62
  of mollusk *Aplysia californica* 205-14
Cerebral blood flow 342, 345
Cerebral blood vessels 341-9
Cerebral capillary permeability 343,
  346
Cerebral cortical membranes 16-17
Cerebrospinal fluid, histamine
  metabolites in 197-202
Chiral α-substituted histamines 39-46,
  147
Chiral guanidines 39-46, 147
Chiral histamine agonists 39-46, 147
Chlorpheniramine 4, 6, 20, 147, 243
Chlorpromazine 244, 245
Cholinergic agents 255
Cholinergic receptors on nonparietal
  cells 260
Cimetidine 30, 47, 49, 53, 56, 61-67,
  74, 83, 147, 207, 245, 267, 306,
  354-5, 383
Circadian rhythm 225, 230-2
Citalopram 243
Clomipramine 243
Clovoxamine 243
Clozapine 242, 244, 245
Colchicine 84
Compound 48/80 412-13
Congestive cardiomyopathy 325, **326,** 329
Congestive heart failure 325-33
Connective tissue mast cells 289
Creatine kinase 311, 313
Cromoglycate 416-18
Cyclic AMP 80, 82, 87, 257, 267, 275-9,
  283, 328, 386, 393, 402, 415-16

Cyclic AMP assay 81
Cyclic AMP synthesis 237-9
Cyclic GMP synthesis 238, 239
Cytosol Ca^{2+} 423-32
Cytotoxic T lymphocytes (CTL) 379-88

DA 4577 57
Desensitization of H_2 receptors 83,
  270-1
Desipramine 63, 160, 243, 245
Dextran 414
1,2-Diacylglycerol (DAG) 405-8
1,2 Diamino-thiadiazole sulphoxide 51
5,7-Dihydroxytryptamine 155-62
Dimaprit 62, 66, 82-87, 145, 335-9, 383
Dimethylaminomethylfuran 48, 50, 51
Dimethylaminomethyl-furanylphenylene
  derivatives 54
Dimethylaminomethylthiazole 51
Dimethylhistamines 40-46, 144
N^α,N^α-dimethylhistamine 35-37, 74
Dinitrophenol 84
Diphenhydramine 4, 15, 229, 243, 267,
  371
Disodium cromoglycate 416-18
Dobutamine 326
Dopamine 156
Dothiepin 243
Doxepin 5, 63, 243, 245

Enantiomeric histamine agonists see
  Chiral
Enzyme purification 164
Enzyme regional distribution 190
N-Ethylmaleimide (NEM) 19
Etintidine 49, 75
E 1346 65
E 82980 51
E 821308 51

Famotidine 51, 63, 66
α-Fluoromethylhistidine (FMH) 136, 179,
  225-36, 384
  effects on plasma levels of ACTH,
    vasopressin and oxytocin 232
  effects on sleep-wakefulness cycle 229
  effects on spontaneous locomotor
    activity and body temperature 228-9
Fluoxetine 243
Fluphenazine 244
Fluvoxamine 243
Food intake 225, 230-2
Formaldehyde-acetic acid fixative
  (IFAA) 291
Fundic mucosa
  canine 253-64
  histamine cells of 258-60
Furan series of H_2 antagonists 50

Subject Index

Gas chromatography-mass spectrometry 185-95, 197-202
Gastric acid secretion 252, 253, 265
Gastric cell line HGT-1 265-74
Gastric cells 265-74
Gastric glands, histamine action in 281-8
Gastric H_2 receptors
  activity measurement 266-7
  desensitization of 270-1
  interaction of secretagogues or secretory inhibitors on 269
  ontogeny of 271
  pharmacology of 267-8
  tissular, cellular and histological distribution of 268-9
Gastrin 253-64, 269
Gastrointestinal tract 251-2, 289
Glutamine synthetase 210
γ-Glutamyl cysteine synthetase 210
γ-Glutamylhistamine 211
γ-Glutamyltranspeptidase 210
Glycoprotein 19-25
Glycosaminoglycan (GAG) 291, 292
Guanidines 39-46, 74, 147
Guanidinothiazole 48, 51, 52
Guanylylnucleotides on histamine binding 76

H_1-receptors 266
  chiral agonists on 39-46
  cyclic nucleotides 237-250
  inositol phospholipid breakdown 27-38
  NEM action on 19-26
  newer antagonists 3-12
  on lymphocytes 371-8
  photoaffinity labelling of 13-18
  radioligand binding 19-26, 237-50
H_2-receptors 265-74
  chiral agonists on 39-46
  cognitive properties of 69-78
  desensitization 83, 270-1
  display regulation 384-6
  in human leukemia cells 79-88
  radioligand binding studies 61-67, 69-78
  recent antagonists 47-60
  see also Gastric H_2 receptors
H_3-receptors 143-53, 266
  location of 148-9
  pharmacological definition of 144-8
Haloperidol 242, 244, 245
Heart, histamine release from 306-7
  see also Cardiac
High-performance liquid chromatography 173-84
Hippocampal slice 216-17
Histamine
  ^3H 69-78, 143,
  immunopharmacological effects of 353-4
  in brain see Brain
  methyl derivatives see Methylhistamine and dimethylhistamine
  microionophoresis of 215-16
Histamine cells
  isolation of 259-60
  of fundic mucosa 258-60
Histamine-containing neurons (HCNs) 206
Histamine determination
  in CNS 173-84
  neuronal 177, 180-3
Histamine-immunoreactive cell bodies 123-8
Histamine-induced suppressor factor (HSF) 357-64
Histamine liberators
  differential effects of 412-15
  mast cell responses to 411-21
Histamine localization in stomach 270
Histamine metabolism
  in *Aplysia* CNS 209-11
  in stomach 270
  inhibition of 211
Histamine metabolites
  in cerebrospinal fluid 197-202
  in mammalian brain 186
Histamine methylation 163-72, 173-84, 311
Histamine-N-methyltransferase, characterization of guinea pig brain and rat kidney 163-72
Histamine producing cell stimulating factor (HCSF) 355
Histamine receptors see also H_1, H_2, H_3-receptors
  gastric see Gastric H_2 receptors
  in *Aplysia* CNS 208-9
  psychotropic drug interactions with 242-5
  radioligand binding assays for 19-26, 61-67, 69-78, 241-2
  specificity of 381-3
Histamine release
  autoinhibition of 144-8
  cardiac 305-8, 321-3
  central nervous system 144-8, 155-62
  depolarization-induced 161
  effect of calcium and potassium on 150
  from canine heart 307
  from fundic mucosal stores 261
  from human heart 306
  from mast cells 401-9
  histamine modulation of 149-52, 416
  IgE-mediated 401-9, 417
  inhibitors of 415-18
  presynaptic modulation of 149-52
  time course and characteristics of 426-7
  uncoupling from PI breakdown and Ca signal 427-9

Histamine response, cardiac
    sympathetic 318-21
Histamine re-uptake in *Aplysia* ganglia
    212
Histamine suppressor factor (HSF) 359
Histamine synthesis
    autoinhibition mediated by H_3 auto-
        receptors 151-2
    regulation of 383-4
Histamine-synthesising cells 103-17
Histamine transmethylation 163-72, 311
Histamine turnover 173
    regional 178, 180-3, 185-95
Histamine uptake
    central nervous system 155-62
    neuronal 155-62
Histaminergic neurones 91-102, 103-17,
    119-30, 226, 228-32
Histaminergic post-synaptic potentials
    206-8
Histaminergic regulations of myocardial
    functions 301-4
Histaminergic transmission 206
L-Histidine decarboxylase 103-17
    immunohistochemistry 95-99
    partial purification of 104-6
    purification and antibodies against
        91-102, 103-18
HL-60 cells 80-82, 85, 86
6-Hydroxydopamine 155-62
5-Hydroxytryptamine (5-HT) 5, 156,
    293, 294
Hypertension 335-9
Hypothalamus 335-9

IBMX 275-80
ICI 127032 55
IgE-mediated histamine release 305-8,
    401-9, 417
IgE receptors 401-9
Imidazoles 44, 48-50
Imidazolylphenylene 54
Imidazolyl-phenylformamidines 57
Imipramine 63, 243, 245
Immune responses 295
    non IgE-mediated 355-6
    regulation of 353-7, 371
Immunohistochemical methods 95-99,
    119-30
Immunopharmacological effects of
    histamine 353-4
Immunosuppression, Impromidine
    induced 393-4
Impromidine 39-46, 72-74, 145-51,
    218-21, 267-8, 325-33, 344-5
    effect upon T_H-cell function 391-2
    effect upon T-lymphocyte phenotype
        390-1
    induced immunosuppression 393-4
Indomethacin 286, 287

Inflammatory reactions, lymphocyte-
    mediated 372
Inositol 1,2-diacylglycerol 28
Inositol phospholipids 27-38, 423-32
Inositol 1,4, 5-triphosphate 28
Interleukin-1 357-64
Interleukin-2 365-9
Iprindole 63, 243, 245
Ischaemia 305-8, 311, 313, 314
Isobutylmethyl xanthine 287

Kainic acid 113, 148
Ketotifen 5, 6
K^+/H^+-ATPase 275-9

L 643441 53, 85
Lamtidine 53
Lanthanum 258, 423
Leukemia cells 79-88, 423
Leukotrienes 5
Levomepromazine 245
Lithium amplification of response to
    histamine 34-35, 426
Locomotor activity 225, 228-9
Loxapine 242, 244
Loxtidine 53
Lupitidine 50
LY 139037 50
Lymphocyte chemokinetic factor (LCF)
    371-8
Lymphocyte-mediated inflammatory
    responses 377
Lymphocyte migration 371-7
Lymphocytes *see also* T lymphocytes
Lymphokines 357-64
    characterization of 372
    histamine-induced 371-7
    lymphocyte migration inhibitory 372

Magnesium on histamine binding 76
Maprotiline 243, 245
Mast cells
    connective tissue 289
    functional heterogeneity of 411-21
    histamine release from 401-9
    in mammalian CNS 173
    in rat brain 131-40
        biochemical vs. histologic studies
            136-8
        biochemical indices of 135-6
        histology of 132-3
        quantitative studies of 134-5
    mediator release from 407-8
    mucosal 289-98
Mepyramine 4, 8, 9, 16, 20-24, 30-32,
    75, 83, 98, 147, 207, 243, 266, 335-9
Mequitazine 7, 243
Mesoridazine 242, 244

Subject Index

Meta-phenylene see Phenylene
N-Methyldimaprit 72, 83
N^α-Methylhistamine 74, 145
Methylhistamine 197-202
  (see also Prosmethylhistamine and telemethyl histamine)
2-Methylhistamine 22, 35-37, 62, 74, 145
4-Methylhistamine 62, 66, 72-74, 267-8
α-Methylhistamines 40-42, 144
β-Methylhistamine 43
Methylimidazoleacetic acid 197-202
Methyltransferase 45, 163-72, 402-4
Metiamide 66, 219
Mianserin 20, 63, 243, 245
Microionophoresis of histamine 215-16
Mifentidine 57
Molindone 242, 244, 245
Monoaminergic neurons in brain 233
Monoclonal antibody
  against L-histidine decarboxylase 103-17
  immunohistochemical studies 109-13
  production of 106-7
  properties and specificity pattern of 107-9
Mucous cell 278
Muscarinic receptors 253-64
Myocardial contractility 325
Myocardial dysfunction 309-15
Myocardial functions, histaminergic regulations of 301-4
Myocardial ischemia 307
Myocardial metabolism 325

NEM see N-ethylmaleimide
Neoantergan 4
Neuraminidase 375, 376
Neuroblastoma clone 237-50
Neuroendocrine function 225
Neuroleptics and human brain histamine H_1 receptor 242
Neuronal uptake system for histamine 155-62
929F 4
Neutrophils 295
Nisoxetine 243
Nitroglycerin 331, 332
Nitroprusside 331
Nizatidine 50, 52
Nomifensine 243, 245
Noradrenaline 156, 159, 160
Norburimamide 147
Nordimaprit 74, 383
Nortriptyline 243, 245

1517F 4
Ontogeny of gastric H_2 receptors 271
Oxaprotiline 243

Oxatomide 5, 6
Oxmetidine 49, 267-8
Oxytocin 232

Pargyline 179
Parietal cell receptors 255-7
Parietal cells 286
  activation of 255
  function of 255
  histamine action on 283
  isolation of 255
  stimulus-secretion coupling in 275-9
Pentagastrin 284-6
Peptic ulcer 252
Peptide-401 413
Peripheral blood mononuclear cells (PBMC) 372, 381
Perphenazine 244
meta-Phenylene analogues
  of cimetidine 56
  of tiotidine 55
2-Phenylhistamine 22
Phosphatidylinositol 4,5-bisphosphate 28
Phosphatidylinositol breakdown 27-38, 423-32
Phosphatidylserine 415
Phosphodiesterase activity 278
Phosphodiesterase inhibitors 325-33, 415
Phospholipid-diacylglycerol 405-7
Phospholipid methylation 389-400, 405-7
Phospholipid turnover 423-32
Photoaffinity labels 13
Pial circulation 341-5
m-Piperidinomethylphenoxy series of H_2 antagonists 53
Piperoxan 4
Polyacrylamide gel electrophoresis 165
Polylysine 413-14
Polymyxin 413-14
Potassium, effect on ^{3}H-histamine release 150, 158
  see also K
Prazosine 331
Presynaptic modulation of histamine release 149-52
Prochlorperazine 244
Promazine 242, 244
Promethazine 4
Pros-methylimidazoleacetic acid 185-95
Prosmethylhistamine 175, 185
Prostaglandins 80, 283-7, 309, 357-64
Prostanoids 283-6
Protein kinase 81, 82, 275-9
Proteolytic enzymes 404
Protriptyline 243, 245
2-Pyridylethylamine 74, 267, 344, 395-7
Pyrilamine see Mepyramine
Psychotropic drug interactions with histamine receptors 242-5

Quin 2 fluorescence   401-10, 424

Radioligand binding assays for
    histamine receptors   13-18, 19-26,
    61-68, 69-78, 81, 241-2
Ranitidine   50, 54, 62, 75, 147, 245,
    267, 383
Ranitidine analogues   54
Rat leukemia (2H3) basophils   423-32
Receptors see H-receptors
Reperfusion   311, 313
Rheumatoid arthritis   197-202

SCH 29851   7
Schizophrenia   197-202
Secretin   283
Serotonin   160
SKF 91581 see Norburimamide
SKF 91486   74, 147
SK&F 92054 see N-methyldimaprit
SK&F 92334 see Cimetidine
SK&F 92374   75
SK&F 92408   75
SK&F 92456   49
SK&F 92540   75
SK&F 92629   75
SK&F 92994 see Oxmetidine
SK&F 93319   8, 49, 50, 52
SK&F 93479   50, 75, 268
SK&F 93944   8-10
Sleep-wakefulness   225, 229
Somatostatin   260, 269, 283-6
Sopromidine   39-46, 147
Spiperone   242, 244
Spontaneously hypertensive rats (SHR)
    335-9
Stimulus-secretion coupling   275-80,
    281-5
Stomach
  histamine effects on   266
  metabolism and localization of
    histamine in   270
Subarachnoidal hemorrhage   197-202
Suppressor T-cell function   357-64
Synaptic potentials   219
Synaptosomes   148

TAS   53
T-cell-mediated immune reactions   355
Telemethylhistamine   72-74, 185-95,
    197, 311
  determination in CNS   173-84
Telemethylimidazoleacetic acid   185-95
Terfenadine   7
Tetrodotoxin   157, 159
Thalamic histamine   131-42
T-helper cells   389, 391-2

Theophylline   326
Thiazole derivative   52
  see also 2 Aminoethylthiazole
Thiols   19-25
Thioridazine   244
Thiothixene   245
cis-Thiothixene   244
Tiotidine   16, 51, 55, 61-67, 74, 81,
    85, 87, 147, 245, 322, 323, 383
Tiotidine analogues   55
T lymphocytes   353-6, 357-64, 365-70,
    371-7, 379-88
  alterations in phenotype and function
    389-97
  regulation of function of   380
Trazodone   243, 245
Trifluoperazine   244
Trimipramine   243, 245
Triprolidine   4
Trypsin   375, 376
TZU 0460   53

Vasomotor mediators   342-3, 345-6
Vasopressin   232, 283
Viloxazine   243
VIP   269

W/W^v mice   138, 227-8
Wy 45086   53

YM 11170 see Famotidine

Zimelidine   243
Zinc   423